Spinal Cord Injuries: Management and Rehabilitation

Spinal Cord Injuries: Management and Rehabilitation

Editor: Peter Ponce

FOSTER ACADEMICS

www.fosteracademics.com

www.fosteracademics.com

FOSTER ACADEMICS

Cataloging-in-Publication Data

Spinal cord injuries : management and rehabilitation / edited by Peter Ponce.
p. cm.
Includes bibliographical references and index.
ISBN 978-1-63242-568-3
1. Spinal cord--Wounds and injuries. 2. Spinal cord--Wounds and injuries--Treatment.
3. Spinal cord--Wounds and injuries--Patients--Rehabilitation. I. Ponce, Peter.
RA645.S66 S65 2018
617.482 044--dc23

Foster Academics,
118-35 Queens Blvd., Suite 400,
Forest Hills, NY 11375, USA

ISBN 978-1-63242-568-3 (Hardback)

Printed and bound in China.

Contents

Preface

An injury caused to the spinal cord can result in permanent damage. These injuries are either traumatic or nontraumatic. The symptoms of spinal cord injuries vary and depend on the area of the injury. They can cause severe complications like respiratory problems, paralysis and neurogenic shock. This book contains some path-breaking studies in the management of spinal cord injuries. It strives to provide a fair idea about the subject and to help develop a better understanding of the latest advances within this field. The readers would gain knowledge that would broaden their perspective about spinal cord injuries, their management and related rehabilitation techniques.

This book is the end result of constructive efforts and intensive research done by experts in this field. The aim of this book is to enlighten the readers with recent information in this area of research. The information provided in this profound book would serve as a valuable reference to students and researchers in this field.

At the end, I would like to thank all the authors for devoting their precious time and providing their valuable contribution to this book. I would also like to express my gratitude to my fellow colleagues who encouraged me throughout the process.

Editor

1

Human Mesenchymal Cells from Adipose Tissue Deposit Laminin and Promote Regeneration of Injured Spinal Cord in Rats

Karla Menezes[1], Marcos Assis Nascimento[2], Juliana Pena Gonçalves[2], Aline Silva Cruz[1], Daiana Vieira Lopes[1], Bianca Curzio[3], Martin Bonamino[3], João Ricardo Lacerda de Menezes[1], Radovan Borojevic[4], Maria Isabel Doria Rossi[1], Tatiana Coelho-Sampaio[1]*

1 Institute of Biomedical Sciences, Federal University of Rio de Janeiro, Rio de Janeiro, Rio de Janeiro, Brazil, **2** Institute of Biophysics Carlos Chagas Filho, Federal University of Rio de Janeiro, Rio de Janeiro, Rio de Janeiro, Brazil, **3** National Institute of Cancer, Rio de Janeiro, Rio de Janeiro, Brazil, **4** Excellion, Petrópolis, Rio de Janeiro, Brazil

Abstract

Cell therapy is a promising strategy to pursue the unmet need for treatment of spinal cord injury (SCI). Although several studies have shown that adult mesenchymal cells contribute to improve the outcomes of SCI, a descripton of the pro-regenerative events triggered by these cells is still lacking. Here we investigated the regenerative properties of human adipose tissue derived stromal cells (hADSCs) in a rat model of spinal cord compression. Cells were delivered directly into the spinal parenchyma immediately after injury. Human ADSCs promoted functional recovery, tissue preservation, and axonal regeneration. Analysis of the cord tissue showed an abundant deposition of laminin of human origin at the lesion site and spinal midline; the appearance of cell clusters composed of neural precursors in the areas of laminin deposition, and the appearance of blood vessels with separated basement membranes along the spinal axis. These effects were also observed after injection of hADSCs into non-injured spinal cord. Considering that laminin is a well-known inducer of axonal growth, as well a component of the extracellular matrix associated to neural progenitors, we propose that it can be the paracrine factor mediating the pro-regenerative effects of hADSCs in spinal cord injury.

Editor: Eva Mezey, National Institutes of Health, United States of America

Funding: This work was supported by grants from the Conselho Nacional de Desenvolvimento Científico e Tecnológico (CNPq) and Fundação Carlos Chagas Filho de Apoio à Pesquisa do Estado do Rio de Janeiro (FAPERJ). KM and JPG are recipients of fellowships from CNPq, and MAN and DVL received fellowships from Coordenação de Aperfeiçoamento de Pessoal de Ensino Superior (CAPES) and FAPERJ, respectively. ASC received an undergraduate fellowship from CNPq. The funders had no role in study design, data collection and analysis, decision to publish, or preparation of the manuscript.

Competing Interests: Radovan Borojevic is an employee of the company Excellion.

* E-mail: tcsampaio@histo.ufrj.br

Introduction

Traumatic brain and spinal cord injuries affect individuals of all ages, causing various degrees of disability [1,2]. Despite intensive research over the last decade aiming to develop new cell-based therapies to treat trauma in the Central Nervous System (CNS), there is no consensus about the most appropriate cell types to reach this goal [3,4]. Embryonic stem cells previously differentiated into neural precursors, motor neurons, or pre-oligodendrocytes have been used in animal studies [5–8] and more recently, in a clinical study [9]. Adult stem/progenitor cells have also been used in both animal research and clinical studies. The primary source of progenitor cells is the bone marrow, where at least the hematopoietic stem cell and a population of mesenchymal stromal/stem cells co-exist (MSC) [10]. Both cell types have been used to treat experimental spinal cord injury (SCI) in animals, as well as injured human patients [11]. Given the potential of MSC to differentiate into several adult cell types, including neurons [12], these cells have attracted great interest.

In the last years, a growing number of studies have reported the effects of MSCs in promoting functional improvement, tissue sparing, and axonal growth after spine cord injury [13–23]. More recently, a new type of MSC isolated from adipose tissue has been investigated. Adipose tissue constitutes a more readily available deposit of adult progenitors due to its greater abundance of MSC-like cells, if compared to bone marrow, and because liposuction is a minimally invasive procedure. Known as adipose-derived stromal cells (ADSCs), these cells are isolated by selective adhesion and correspond to the perivascular stromal fraction of the adipose tissue [10,24,25]. ADSCs have recently been used to treat SCI in rats and dogs [26–28]. In particular, a recent study compared the effectiveness of hADSCs with that of human bone marrow stromal cells in a model of section injury in immunossupressed rats and reported the superior regenerative effect of hADSCs [29].

In the present study we investigated the regenerative potential of hADSCs in a model of ballon-induced spinal compression using immunocompetent rats. We show that hADSCs promote complete recovery of motor function after 8 weeks, while improving tissue preservation, restricting inflammation and stimulating axonal growth. In addition we propose that the regenerative effects of hADSCs are related to the secretion of the extracellular matrix protein laminin that accumulates in the spinal cord in colocalization with neural precursors.

Results

hADSC Promotes Functional and Morphological Recovery after Compressive SCI

In order to evaluate if human subcutaneous ADSCs (hADSCs) would improve the functional outcome after compressive SCI, we compared the open field locomotion (BBB scores) of animals receiving cells or culture medium (DMEM). Rats were subjected to moderate balloon compression and treated with either hADSCs or DMEM, delivered by intraspinal injection 30 minutes after injury. The BBB score for the DMEM group was 7.2 one week post injury/injection (wpi) and it increased to 15.6 after eight weeks (Fig. 1A). On the other hand, animals treated with hADSCs exhibited superior scores from the first evaluation, whereas such superiority became statistically significant from the fifth week on. From the fourth week on the BBB scores for the treated group were indistinguishable from those found for the sham operated group (Fig. 1A), indicating that hADSCs promoted complete functional recovery after a moderate compressive injury.

Mesenchymal stromal/stem cells are known to have immunosuppressive properties [30,31], enabling the use of human cells in immunocompetent animals as done in this study. We evaluated the distribution of the rat macrophages/microglia marker, ED1 in the spinal cord one week after compression. In the control animals, macrophages/microglia were profusely distributed in both white and gray matter (Fig. 1B). In animals receiving hADSC, macrophages were concentrated in lesion borders (Fig. 1C), suggesting that the injection of hADSC restrained the spread of inflammatory cells in the spinal cord parenchyma.

The compression injury led to the formation of cystic cavities in the spinal cord. Eight weeks after injury, control animals showed a large cavity surrounded by activated astrocytes (Fig. 1D, G). Animals receiving hADSC displayed smaller cavities and a reduction of GFAP expression of approximately 50% (Fig. 1E, H, I). Quantitative analysis of the cavity area was performed in a region encompassing 400 μm of the spinal cord tissue along the dorsal–ventral axis (Fig. 1F). Treatment with hADSCs reduced the cavity area by more than 90% at the lesion epicenter, whereas tissue sparing was seen at all levels analyzed (Fig. 1F). These results demonstrate that hADSC injection results in improved preservation of the nervous tissue after SCI.

hADSC Promotes Regeneration of Axonal Fibers

The presence of descending serotonergic fibers was evaluated in animals one and eight weeks after injury. One week after injury, hADSC-treated rats presented a large number of serotonergic fibers crossing the spared tissue in the lateral funiculus region surrounding the injury site (Fig. 2B). These fibers, which were less abundant in control animals, were apparently thicker than individual axons (Fig. 2A). Their superficial location corresponds to the region of descending serotonergic raphe fibers, indicating that they result from axonal regrowth after injury. In addition, seven days after injury we found several fibers displaying bulging tips, which are indicative of the occurrence of axonal regeneration (Fig. 2B, insert). Rostral to the lesion site the total lengths of serotonergic axons were similar in treated and non-treated rats (Fig. 2C). However, at the level of the epicenter (lateral to it) and caudal to the lesion, the total lengths of serotonergic axons were consistently higher after treatment with hADSC. Eight weeks after injury the fiber lengths decreased in comparison to those found one week after injury (Fig. 2D, E). Nevertheless, the total length of serotonergic fibers in the spinal cord was 8 times higher in the group treated with hADSCs (Fig. 2F). These results indicate that the regeneration of serotonergic axons promoted by hADSCs remains for a considerable time.

Axonal regeneration was further evaluated by using either the Tuj1 antibody, which stains young neurons more intensely [32], or anti-GAP-43, which labels neurons in regeneration [33]. Data are presented in series of three pictures taken from the spare tissue lateral to the lesion area. As shown in Figure 2G–R, the treatment with hADSCs substantially increased axonal regeneration. At both 1 and 8 weeks Tuj1-positive fibers in hADSC-treated animals ran straight and were aligned parallel to each other (Fig. 2J and high magnification in K). On the other hand, in control animals these fibers were tangled and randomly aligned (Fig. 2G and high magnification in H). The thicker bundles and aligned fibers observed in hADSC-treated animals are indicative of axonal fasciculation, which did not occur in control animals (Fig. 2, high magnifications in H and K). Tuj1 labeling presented a very faint and even distribution in normal unlesioned animals as this monoclonal antibody identifies preferentially young neurons [32]. Quantification of Tuj1 labeled fibers after one or eight weeks showed that treatment with hADSC led to an increase in the total length of young fibers of 3 or 3.5 times, respectively. Panels M to Q in Figure 2 show the results obtained by using the anti-GAP-43 antibody. One week after injury the total length of regenerating fibers increased 3-fold in the hADSC group relative to the control (Fig. 2M, P, O). Eight weeks after SCI, a large number of GAP-43 positive fibers was observed in rats treated with hADSCs, while control animals showed little staining (Fig. 2N, Q, R). No labeling was detected when anti-GAP43 was used in sections of normal unlesioned rats.

hADSCs Induce Foci of Increased Cellularity in Spinal Cord

We next sought to investigate the mechanisms by which hADSCs exert regenerative effects in the spinal cord. GFP-transduced hADSCs were injected 30 minutes after compression and animals were euthanized at different times. One day after injection, cells were densely packed and accumulated mainly in the meningeal surface, the central canal, and at the lesion site (Fig. 3A). One week later, the injected cells were detected at the region of the canal and at the injury site (Fig. 3B–D). In the fourth week, only a few isolated clusters of cells were identified near the lesion (Fig. 3E), while cells were not detected at the eighth week after injection.

A remarkable feature of hADSC-treated animals was the increase in tissue cellularity detected in DAPI-stained sections one week after cell injection. One large cluster of cells was found at the lesion site and smaller clusters were distributed along the spinal midline (Fig. 3G). Such clusters were not observed in normal unlesioned rats (Fig. 3F). In transversal sections it was possible to localize the clusters at the midline in the vicinity of the central canal (Fig. 3I–K). GFP-hADSCs were found in the center of these areas of high cellularity (Fig. 3K, L). Analysis of the section containing the central canal revealed that the vimentin-positive ependymal cell layer was enlarged in animals treated with hADSCs (compare Fig. 3M and N). Reconstruction of the central canal in the z axis showed regions with more than 10 stacked cells, indicative of a partial reconfiguration of the canal's architecture (Fig. 3P). We additionally observed an increased number of DAPI-stained nuclei throughout the spinal parenchyma, in the region between the central canal and the individual clusters (Fig. 3N, asterisk) and blood vessels in the vicinity of the reconfigured canal (Fig. S1).

Cell clusters did not correspond to inflammatory infiltrates given that most of them were not positive for the macrophage/microglia marker, CD68 (Fig. 3Q), and neither for the T

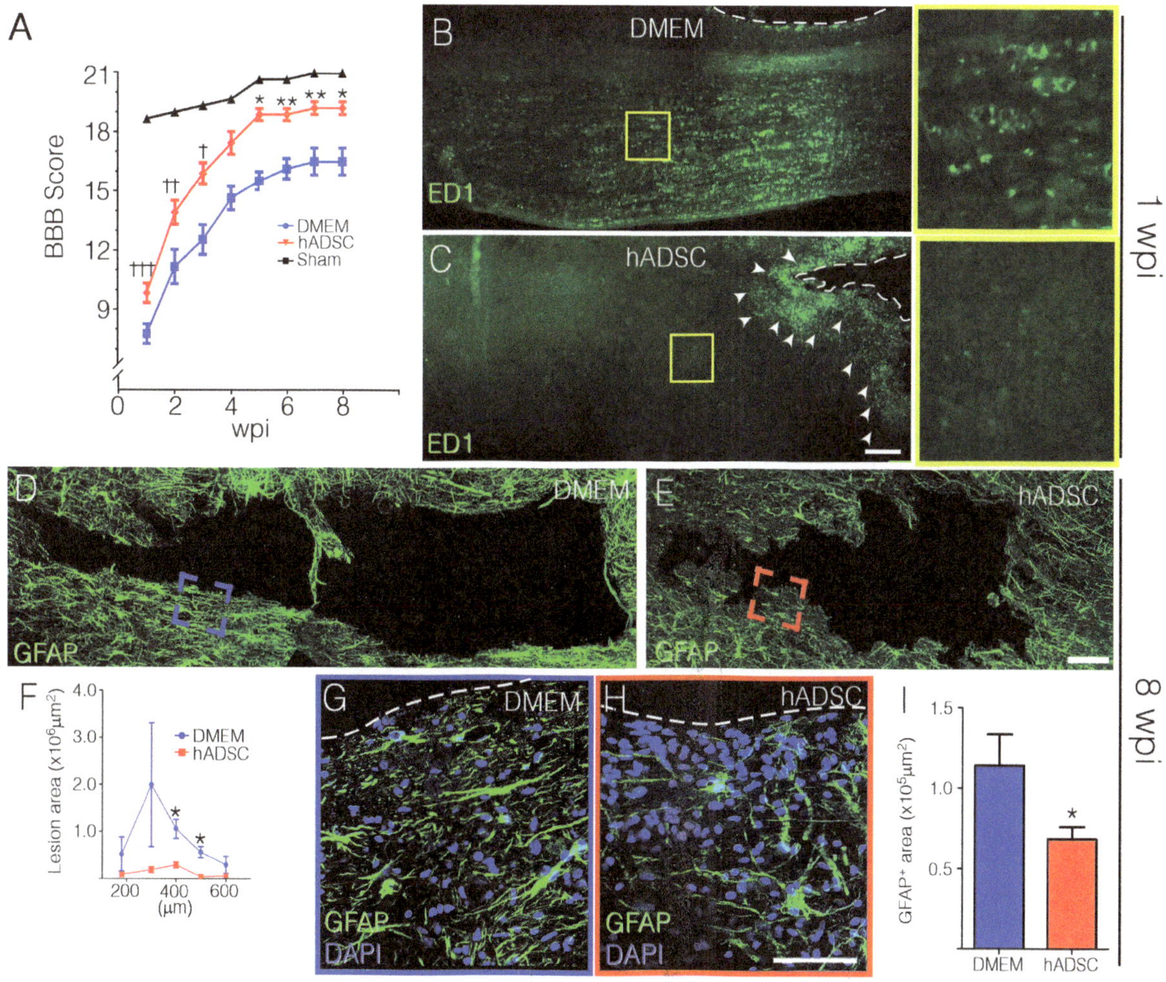

Figure 1. hADSCs induce functional recovery and reduce cavitation and cellular inflammatory response. The locomotor performance was assessed by the BBB score. Animals were evaluated weekly, during eight weeks after spinal compression (A). Asterisks indicate statistic differences between hADSC (n = 9) and DMEM groups (n = 9) and crosses indicate differences between hADSC and sham groups (n = 3). B,C) Low-magnification photomontages showing the marked difference in distribution of macrophages in the spinal cord of rats treated with hADSC (C) and DMEM (B). Note that ED1-positive cells concentrate in the immediate surroundings of the lesion cavity in hADSC-treated animals (arrowheads), in contrast to the dispersed distribution in DMEM-treated animals. D, E) GFAP immunoreactivity delineates the cavity and reveals astrocyte activation following injury, in vehicle (DMEM) (D) and hADSC (E) treated animals. F) Graph representing the area of the lesion cavity of 5 different dorso–ventral sections (represented in the x axis) in DMEM (blue) and hADSC (red) treated animals (n = 3 per condition). Note that cavitation in hADSC-treated animals is smaller. G,H) High magnification images of the boxed areas in *D* (blue) and *E* (red) are shown in G and H, respectively. Note the few GFAP-positive cells at the vicinity of the lesion and that very few cells are seen at the cavity border in hADSC-treated rat (H). I) Graph representing the total area of positive staining for GFAP (see *Materials and Methods*) in the immediate surroundings of the cavity in DMEM (blue) and hADSC (red) treated animals (n = 3 per condition). Dashed line delineates the cavity borders in G and H. *$P<0.05$, **$P<0.01$, ***: $p<0.001$. Bars: B and C = 500 μm, D and E = 100 μm and G and H = 50 μm.

lymphocyte marker, CD3 (Fig. 3R, S). Scattered macrophages were detected in the vicinity of the clusters, as well as T lymphocytes, which tended to form small aggregates surrounding the core of the DAPI-stained clusters. In contrast, DiI-labeled human fibroblasts injected into the intact rat spinal cord attracted large amounts of macrophage/microglial cells (Fig. 3T).

Since the increase in tissue cellularity was not related to injury-induced inflammation, we next investigated whether it would also occur upon injection of the cells into the undamaged spinal cord. We therefore included a third experimental group in which GFP-hADSCs were delivered directly into the spinal cord of normal rats and their distribution was analyzed one week after injection. Cells presented a clear tropism for the spinal midline, where they remained distributed along the central axis of the spinal cord (Fig. 3U'). It was noteworthy that more GFP positive cells were present in uninjured than in the injured spinal cord. Surprisingly we observed a large increase in tissue cellularity, which was more pronounced than that observed when hADSCs were injected after injury (Fig. 3U). Cells within the infiltrate in uninjured spinal cord did not stain for the CD68, which indicate that they were not inflammatory cells (Fig. S2).

hADSCs Led to the Appearance of Perivascular Spaces in between Endothelial and Astrocytic Basement Membranes

Another remarkable feature observed in animals treated with hADSCs was the presence, in the vicinity of the spinal axis, of blood vessels exhibiting two clearly definable separated basal

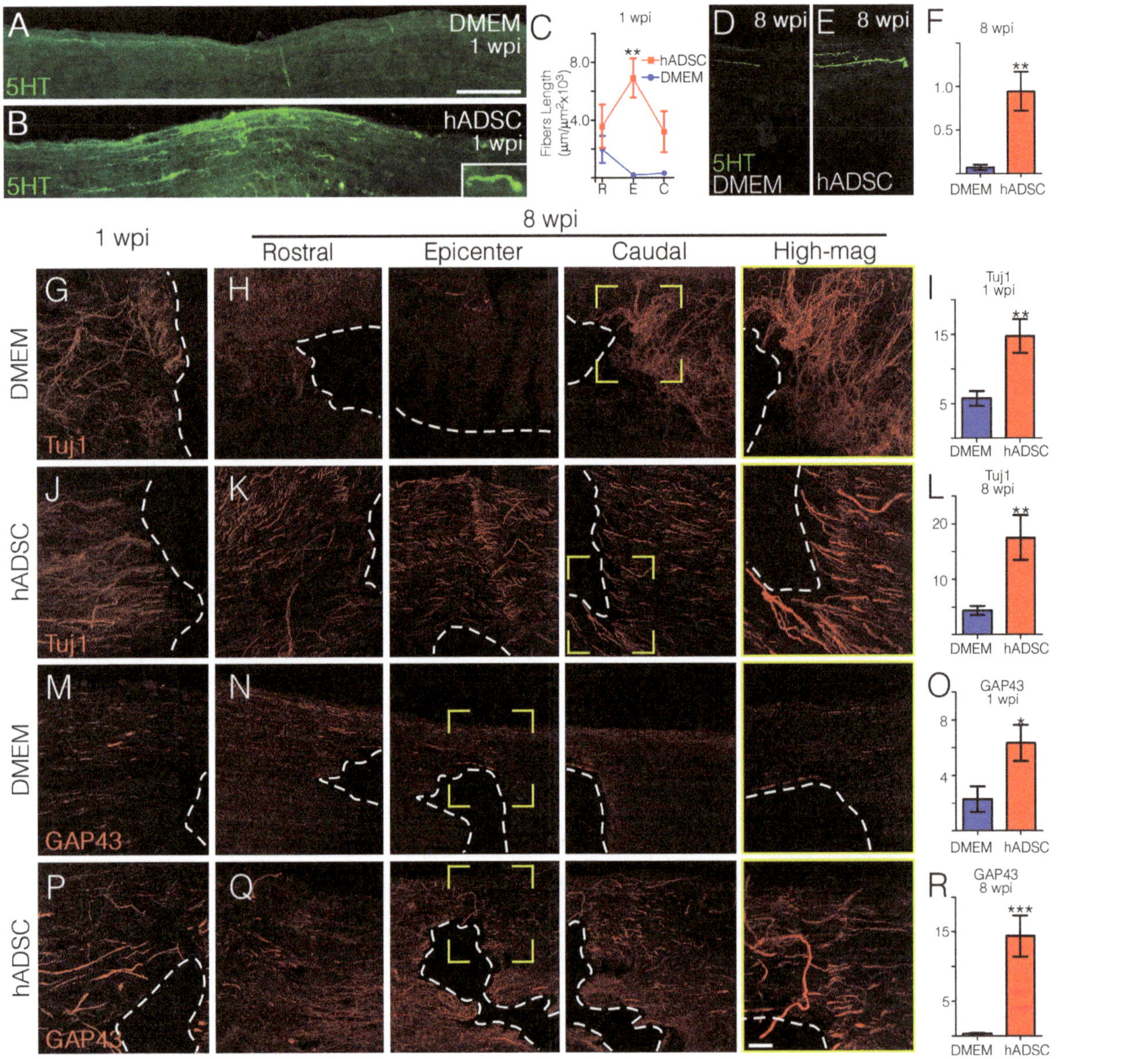

Figure 2. hADSCs promote axonal regeneration. A–D) Photomontages showing the expression pattern of 5HT-positive serotonergic fibers in horizontal sections spanning the pre- and post-lesion regions in DMEM (A) and hADSC (B) treated animals one week after compression. The inset shows an example of a hogback termination in the post-lesion area. Note that the hADSC-treated cord exhibits a larger number of serotoninergic fibers crossing the injury site. C) Graph representing the total length of 5-HT fibers in each experimental group (n = 3 in each group). D–E) 5HT expression was greatly reduced in the chronic phase (8 wks) in DMEM-treated rats (D), while it was slightly reduced in hADSC (E) treated group. F) Quantification of the total length of 5-HT positive axons, eight weeks after SCI (n = 3 in each group). G–R) Progression of axonal regeneration was followed by Tuj1 (G–L) or anti-GAP-43 (M–R) immunoreactivity. Panels on the left show Tuj1 (G, J) or GAP-43 (M, P) positive fibers one week after compression at the epicenter of the lesion. Panels H, K, N, Q and rows on the right show respective rostral (left), epicenter (center), and caudal (right) regions of the same section eight weeks after SCI. Far column on the right (yellow frame) shows boxed areas in higher magnification. The dashed line indicates the border of the lesion cavity. Graphics show the quantification of the total lengths of Tuj1 (I, L) or GAP-43 (O, R) positive fibers one week (I, O) and eight weeks (L, R) after SCI in the peri-cavity region (n = 3 in each group). Tuj1 and GAP-43 positive axons in DMEM (blue) and hADSC (red) treated groups were quantified in an area of approximately 900 μm in extension along the longitudinal axis. Both white and grey matter was analyzed. The y-axes in panels F, I, L, O and R were omitted for aesthetic purpose and they represent fiber length per area ($\mu m/\mu m^2 \times 10^3$). The values in C, F, I, L, O, R represent means ± standard errors. *$P<0.05$, **$P<0.01$, ***$P<0.001$. Bars: A, B = 500 μm, D–Q = 100 μm, high magnification = 50 μm.

lamina, which were identified by immunostaining with an anti-pan-laminin antibody (Fig. 4C, D, Movie S1). The internal lamina corresponds to the basement membrane contributed by the endothelial cells, here identified by immunostaining with the rat endothelial marker, RECA1 (Fig. 4E). The external lamina, which is part of the blood brain barrier in the CNS, is produced by the astrocytes and normally remains connected to the internal one. The separation of these two membranes suggests an increased traffic of cells in the perivascular compartment along blood vessels. A series of confocal images of a blood vessel suggests that cells accumulating in between the two laminas can be released at the spinal parenchyma upon disruption of the outer membrane (Fig. 4F). Separation of two basement membranes around blood

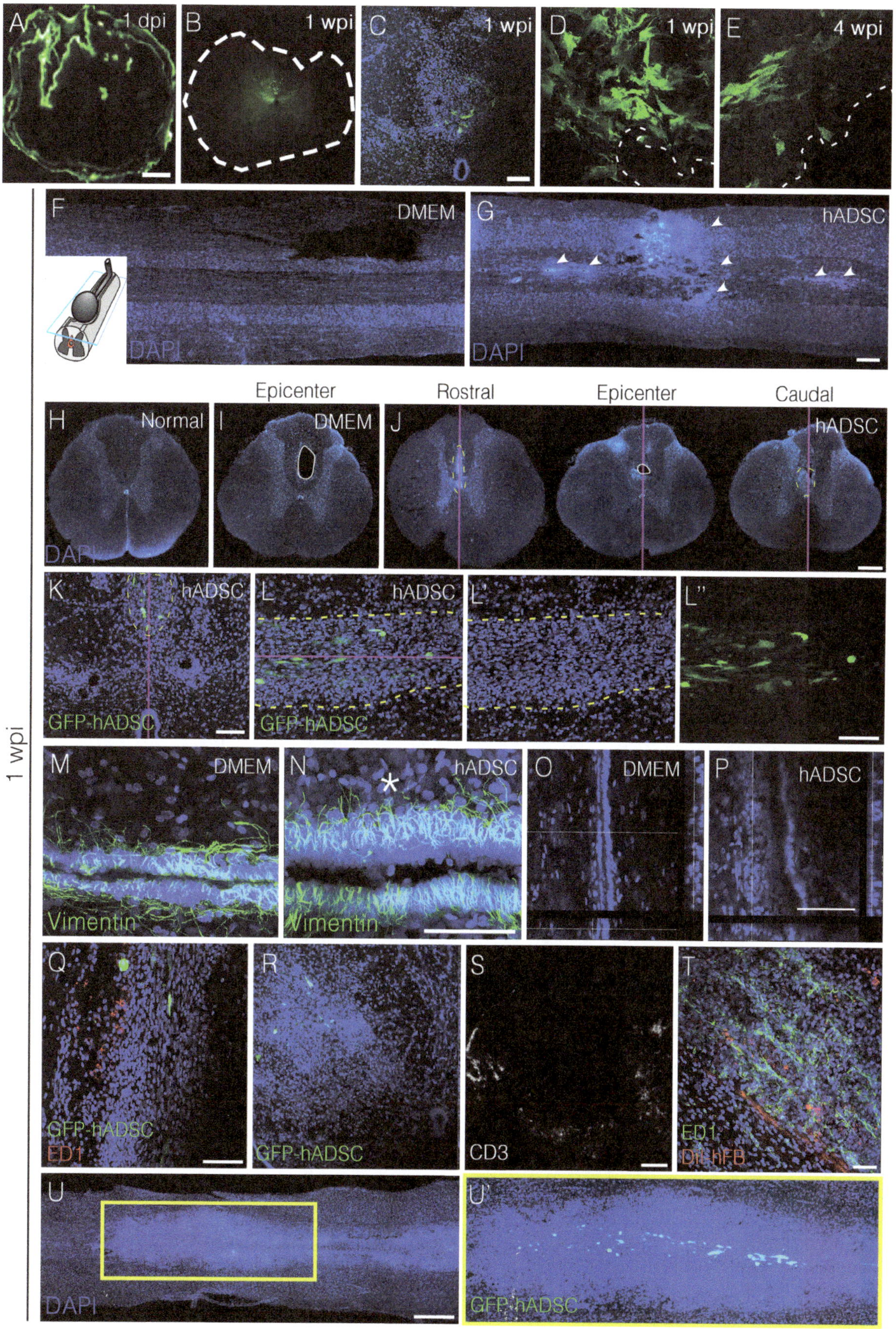
A
1 dpi
B
1 wpi
C
1 wpi
D
1 wpi
E
4 wpi
F
DMEM
DAPI
G
hADSC
DAPI
Epicenter
Rostral
Epicenter
Caudal
H
Normal
DAPI
I
DMEM
J
hADSC
K
hADSC
GFP-hADSC
L
hADSC
GFP-hADSC
L'
L''
M
DMEM
Vimentin
N
hADSC
Vimentin
O
DMEM
P
hADSC
Q
GFP-hADSC
ED1
R
GFP-hADSC
S
CD3
T
ED1
DiI-hFB
U
DAPI
U'
GFP-hADSC
1 wpi

Figure 3. hADSCs increased cellularity in three distinct, but contiguous compartments (the central canal, midline parenchyma, and perivascular region). A–E) Time-course distribution and cell morphology after injection of hADSCs. A) Transverse section of the spinal cord one day after lesion and injection of GFP-transduced hADSCs, showing that these cells accumulate in the pial surface, central canal, and peri-lesional area. After one week (1 wpi), hADSCs were detected predominantly in the canal area and peri-lesionally (B, C). D, E) High magnification images of the GFP-positive cells clusters at one (D) and four wpi (E). F, G) DAPI-stained horizontal sections 200–250 μm above the central canal showing an increase in cellularity (G) mainly along the midline in hADSC-treated cord (arrowheads). H–J) DAPI-stained transversal sections of spinal cord from a normal rat (H), DMEM (I) and hADSCs-treated animals (J), 1 wpi. Sequential analysis of histological sections from treated animals (J) showed that initially there is an increased cellularity along the midline, crossing the region of the central canal of the spinal cord. In the following sections this cell cluster is observed at the margin of the lesion and persisted there until the end of the lesion. K–L") Confocal images of transversal (K) and horizontal (L, L', L") sections of spinal cord of hADSC-treated animal at 1 wpi. Note that the increased cellularity occurs in the region around the GFP-positive cells. M–P) Confocal images of horizontal sections of spinal cord immunostained with anti-vimentin in the central canal at 1 wpi. Note the increased thickness of the ependymal lining of the central canal, and the high cell density in hADSC-treated animal above the canal (asterisk). O, P) Orthogonal views of DAPI-stained section of the central canal. Q–S) Images showing infiltration of macrophages (ED1, panel Q) or T lymphocyte (CD3+ cells, panels R and S). T) Human fibroblasts (stained with CM-Dil, hFB) 1 week post injection into an intact spinal cord. Note the abundance of ED1-positive cells in hFB-treated rat. Confocal images of the cells cluster one week after injection of the hADSC-GFP positive cells into an uninjured spinal cord. The purple line represents the midline of the spinal cord. Bars: A, E, F, H–J = 500 μm; B–D, T = 50 μm; G = 25 μm, K. L, Q, R, S = 100 μm, U = 1 mm.

vessels was also observed when hADSCs were injected into the undamaged spinal cord (Fig. S2).

Cells within the Infiltrates Express Markers of Neural Precursors

In order to indentify the nature of the cells accumulating in the spinal cord of rats treated with hADSC after SCI we used antibodies against pericytes and/or neural cells. Cell within the infiltrates were positive for smooth muscle α-actin (αSMA), a marker for pericytes; Tuj1 and Olig2, markers for neural precursors; and for nestin, vimentin, and NG2, markers for both neural cells and pericytes (Fig. 5,A–F). Cells accumulating in between the two separated vascular basement membranes were negative for Olig2 or Tuj1 and positive for nestin, vimentin, NG2, and αSMA (Fig. 5G–M). Proliferative cells, positive for Ki67 were detected at lesion-associated cell clusters, which correlated with high nestin expression (Fig. 5N–Q). A similar profile of markers expression as well of proliferation was observed after injecting hADSCs into the undamaged spinal cord (Fig. S2), which indicates that the injection of these cells leads to an increased number of neural precursors and/or pericytes in the spinal cord.

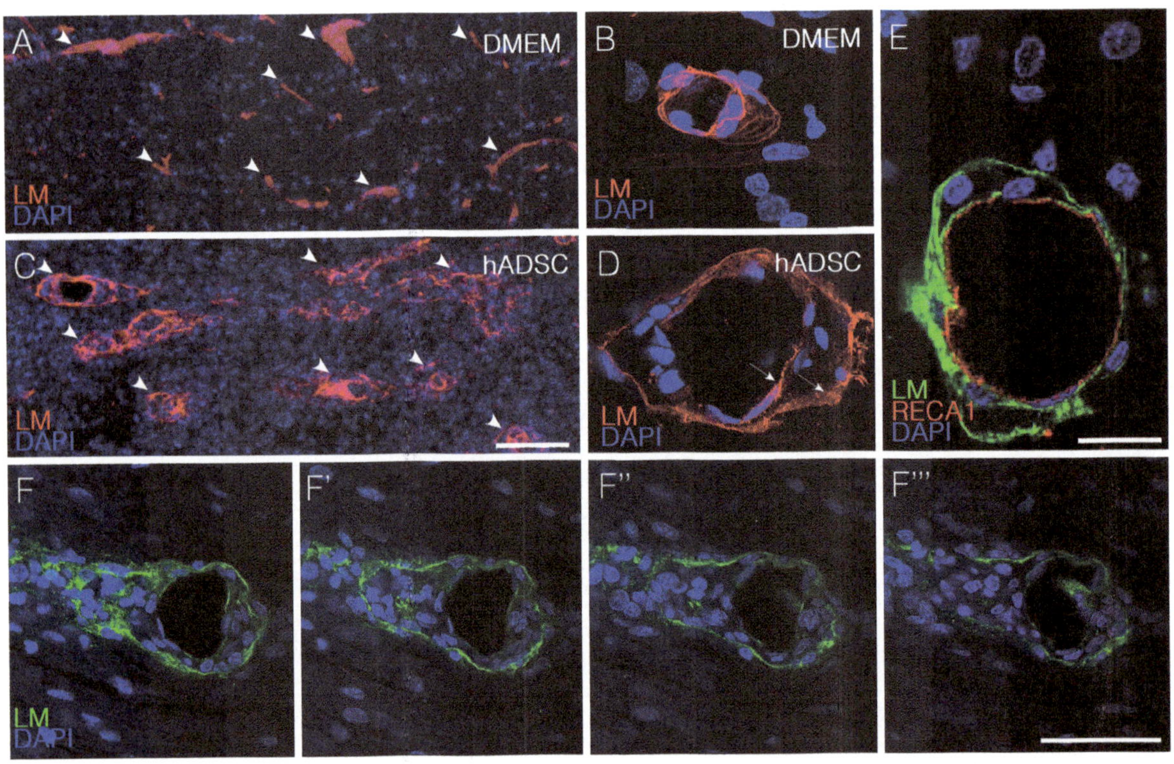

Figure 4. hADSCs led to the appearance of perivascular spaces in between endothelial and astrocytic basement membranes one week after injection. A–D) Confocal images of horizontal sections immunostained with anti-pan-laminin antibody (red) one week after injury. Note that in DMEM animals (A,B) there is no separation between the two membranes whereas in hADSCs-treated animals (C,D) these membranes are separated (arrows in D). E) Confocal images of a horizontal section immunostained with anti-pan-laminin (green) and RECA-1(red). F–F") Confocal imagens of sequential optical sections immunostained with anti-pan-laminin (green) and DAPI (blue) showing the extravasation of cells from the blood vessels. Bars: C, F = 50 μm B, D, E = 25 μm.

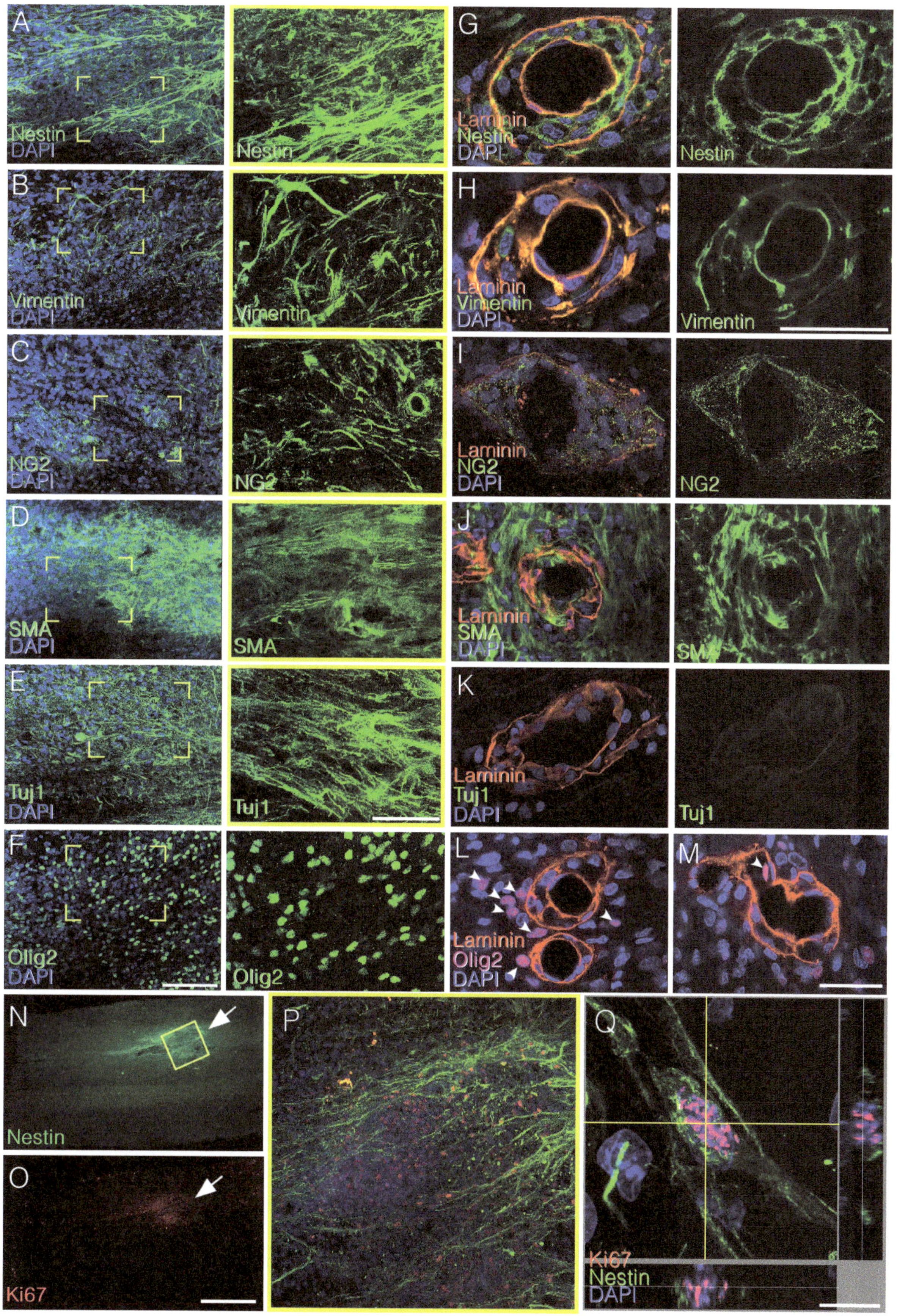
A
Nestin
DAPI
Nestin
G
Laminin
Nestin
DAPI
Nestin
B
Vimentin
DAPI
Vimentin
H
Laminin
Vimentin
DAPI
Vimentin
C
NG2
DAPI
NG2
I
Laminin
NG2
DAPI
NG2
D
SMA
DAPI
SMA
J
Laminin
SMA
DAPI
SMA
E
Tuj1
DAPI
Tuj1
K
Laminin
Tuj1
DAPI
Tuj1
F
Olig2
DAPI
Olig2
L
Laminin
Olig2
DAPI
M
N
Nestin
O
Ki67
P
Q
Ki67
Nestin
DAPI

Figure 5. Areas of increased cellularity induced by hADSC are mainly composed of neural precursors, but cell types differ in the vascular and parenchymal compartments. A–F) Confocal images of horizontal sections of the spinal cord showing immunostaining for nestin (A), vimentin (B), NG2 (C), smooth muscle α-actin (αSMA, D), Tuj1 (E), and Olig2 (F) in clusters of high cell density along the midline, one week after SCI. Note that cells in the clusters are positive for all of these markers, suggesting that clusters are mostly composed of neural progenitors and possibly of invading pericytes. Panels on the right correspond to high-magnification images of the boxed areas, showing the labeling for each phenotypic marker. G–M) Blood vessels immunostained with pan-laminin (red) and nestin (G), vimentin (H), NG2 (I), αSMA (J), Tuj1 (K) (green). Panels L and M show that most Olig2 positive cells (purple) are out of blood vessels (L). Panel M depicts one Olig2-labeled nucleus in close proximity with a region where the basal lamina seems to be disrupted (arrow). (N–Q) Correspondence between immunoreactivities for nestin (N) and Ki67 (O) in photomontages of horizontal sections of an injured spinal cord one week after injury/injection. Confocal images showing proliferative activity (anti-Ki67, red) in the spinal parenchyma (P) and a perivascular region (Q) of nestin positive cells. Bars: A–F = 100 μm; G–M = 50 μm; N, O = 1 mm, Q = 10 μm.

hADSCs Secrete Human Laminin in the Spinal Cord

A distinguished feature of niches of neural stem and neural precursors cells in the central nervous system is the presence of the protein laminin in their extracellular matrix [34–36]. We therefore investigated if hADSCs would produce laminin *in vivo*, which could be related to the accumulation of neural precursors in the tissue. Using monoclonal antibodies specific for laminin of human origin, we searched for a morphological correlation between areas of high cell density and the deposition of the protein. In a photomontage of a whole horizontal section it is possible to appreciate the high degree of co-localization between cell clusters and laminin deposits both in the injured (Fig. 6A–C) and in the uninjured spinal cord (Fig. 6D–E). Immunostainings for human fibronectin and human collagen IV showed that these two proteins were also present in the cell infiltrates but the deposits were less expressive than those of laminin (Fig. S3).

In order to support the interpretation that laminin associated to cell clusters was produced by hADSCs and not by the rat tissue it was important to confirm the specificity of the anti-human laminin antibodies. We used two different anti-human laminin antibodies to detect the protein. The first one was a mouse monoclonal raised against human laminin (clone LAM-89; Fig. 6E), which is commercially available and described as a reagent that does not cross-react with laminin of rat origin. This monoclonal recognizes the α5 chain and has been extensively used in the literature to label basement membranes in human tissue, particularly those associated to blood vessels [37,38]. We found no labeling of blood vessels in the rat spinal cord (Fig. 6, compare E' and E''). The second antibody was an anti-human α2 (clone 5H2; Fig. 6B–D). To assess the specificity of this antibody we performed immunostainings in rat skeletal muscle, a tissue in which laminin α2 is highly expressed. While a polyclonal anti-pan laminin stained the basement membranes around muscle fibers, monoclonal 5H2 did not recognize the rat muscle tissue (Fig. S4). These results indicate that the laminin matrix associated to the infiltrates of neural precursors was not produced by the rat host but, instead, by the injected human cells.

Results up to here indicate that hADSCs produce laminin α2 and α5 *in vivo*. We next used a panel of anti-human laminin antibodies to investigate which laminin chains appeared in the spinal parenchyma injected with hADSCs. Out of the six isoforms tested, we confirmed expression of α2 and α5 and also found positivity for β2 and γ1 laminin chains (Fig. 7A, C, E, F). The matrix associated to cell clusters was negative for α4 and β1 (Fig. 7B, D). In vitro, hADSCs we did not detect expression of α2, α4, α5 or β1 (Fig. 7G–I). We found positivity only for the β2 and the γ1 chains (Fig. 7K, L) and for anti-pan laminin (Fig. 7M).

Based on the recent observation that neurogenic niches in the adult CNS contain a novel type of laminin-rich basal lamina termed fractones [39], we next investigated whether the laminin secreted by hADSCs present the same morphology of fractones. Tissue sections of animals receiving hADSCs into the undamaged spinal cord were immunostained for pan-laminin one week after injection. The polyclonal pan-specific anti-laminin antibody stained all laminin-containing structures present in the tissue. Blood vessels were identified by their overall morphology and diameter above 5 μm (Fig. 8A and E, blue box). Fractones were identified by their organization in puncta with diameter between 1–4 μm and thin lines with 0.1–05 μm width and 5–50 μm length [40] (Fig. 8A and C, red box). In addition, we observed a reticular laminin matrix (Fig. 8A and D, yellow box) similar to the one of human origin secreted by hADSCs (Fig. 6C, E). While a clear increase in cellularity was observed along the whole spinal axis, the location of the most packed cells coincided with the reticular deposit (Fig. 8B, arrowheads). Panels C and D were reconstructed in the z axis to provide views of their 3D organization (Fig. 8F, G). Puncta present in fractones were spherical dense deposits, and the thin lines did not correspond to the side view of sheet-like matrices but instead, resembled essential lines (Fig, 8F). On the other hand, the reticular deposit presented a 3D structure in which each strut was connected to the neighboring one (Fig. 8G). Such reticular mesh is similar to the z-stack obtained using the anti-human α2 laminin antibody (Fig. 8H). DAPI counterstaining showed that cells appearing in the spinal parenchyma seemed trapped into the human laminin mesh secreted by hADSCs (Fig. 8H).

Discussion

In this study, we showed that treatment with cells isolated from human adipose tissue (hADSCs) improve open field locomotion after a compression injury in rats. We also found that hADSCs secreted human laminin, which accumulates in the spinal cord and increases the presence of neural precursors in the tissue.

The lesion area and the expression of the glial scar marker GFAP were both reduced after treatment with hADSCs, characteristics compatible with a resolutive inflammatory reaction. The treatment also resulted in increased numbers of regenerating fibers. A noteworthy finding was the many 5HT-positive descending axons, particularly at the injury epicenter, observed in hADSC rats as early as one week after lesion. Although the number of fibers decreased at the eighth week after lesion, it still remained much higher than that of non-treated animals. To our knowledge, no studies using cell therapy obtained such a marked improvement in axonal growth as the one promoted by hADSCs in our study.

In the present study, we delivered cells immediately after spinal cord injury. The advantage of this experimental design is that the therapy can contribute to reduce the secondary damage, which initiates within hours after trauma. On the other hand, the disadvantage of the early treatment is that the hemorrhagic and ischemic environment of SCI reduces the survival of the injected cells in the host tissue. Accordingly, the number of GFP-labeled cells progressively decreased between 1 and 7 days after injury and virtually disappeared 8 weeks later. In a previous study, Arboleda

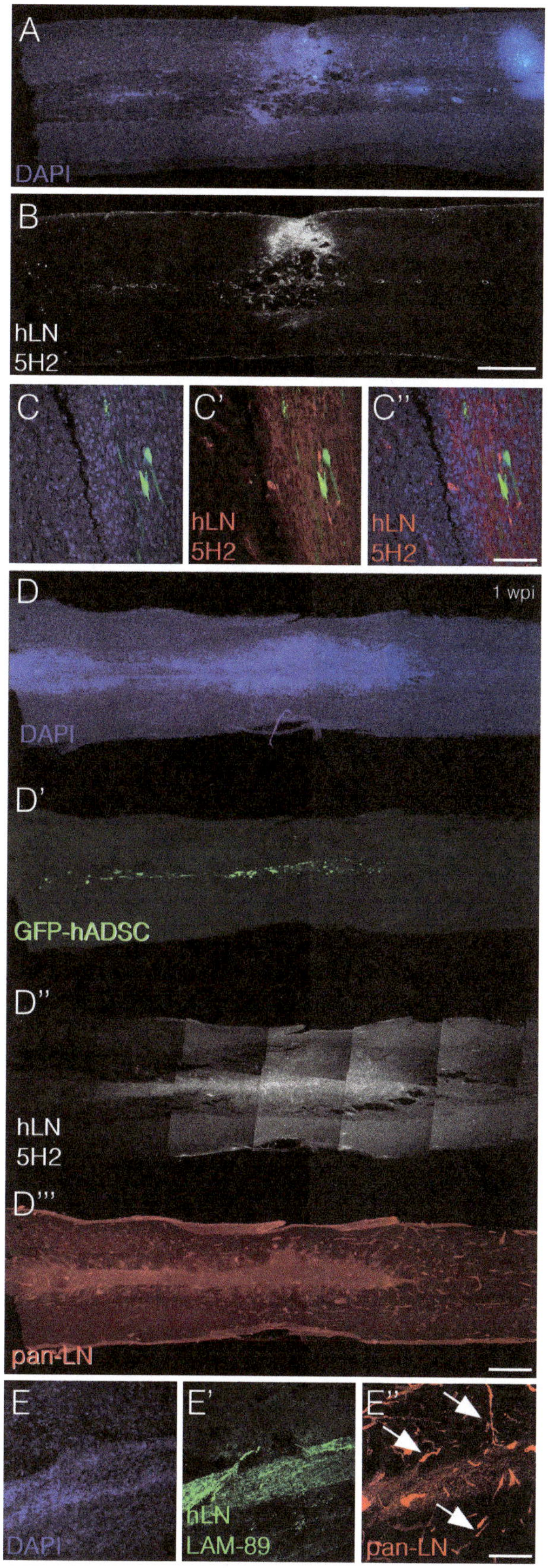

Figure 6. hADSCs secrete laminin in the spinal cord independently of SCI. A–C) Horizontal section of an animal subjected to spinal compression and injected with GFP-hADSCs one week after injury/injection. Panels A and B show photomontages depicting DAPI staining (A) and immunoreactivity for anti-human laminin (B). Note that cell infiltrates and laminin are located in corresponding regions. Panel C shows confocal images demonstrating the coincident localization of GFP-positive hADSCs (green), cell infiltrates (blue) and human laminin (red). D–E) Horizontal section of an uninjured animal one week after transplantation with GFP-hADSCs. Panels D to D''' show photomontages depicting DAPI staining (blue, D), GFP-positive hADSCs (D', green), immunoreactivity for anti-human laminin (D'', white) and immunoreactivity for anti-pan laminin (D''', red). Panel E shows confocal images to demonstrate that while the anti-pan laminin antibody labels rat blood vessels (E'', red), the anti-human laminin does not (E'). Bars: A, B, D = 1 mm, C = 100 μm, E = 200 μm.

and co-workers [26] injected rat ADSCs in immunosuppressed rats one week after injury and reported that living cells remained in the spinal cord during the eight weeks of the experiment. However, these cells did not integrate into the host tissue and their survival did not correlate with the extent of the functional improvements. More recently, Zhou and co-workers [29] reported results compatible with ours, showing that more than 30% of human ADSCs transplanted in immnosuppressed rats survived one week after injection, but that less than 1% remained in the spinal tissue three weeks later. These observations suggest that the regenerative effects of ADSCs were due to the induced secretion of paracrine factors that would stimulate endogenous precursors to regenerate the tissue. It has already been shown that co-culture with BMSCs can prime embryonic stem cells to produce pyramidal neurons able to integrate into the cerebral cortex and to project to the appropriate targets [41,42]. In addition, a recent study has demonstrated that factors produced by BMSCs can indeed prime neural precursors toward an oligodendrocyte fate [43]. Our results in combination with those of the literature suggest that it is not necessary that injected cells remain in the spinal cord during the regeneration process and that their beneficial priming effects are exerted within the first days after injury.

One important effect of hADSCs was the reduction of the spatial diffusion of macrophage/microglia, restraining these cells to the site of injury. To our knowledge, this is the first time that such an effect has been described as a corollary of cell therapy. It is possible that hADSCs accumulating in the lesion secrete cytokines that attract macrophages to the injury site. Indeed, in agreement with a previous study showing that ADSCs secrete 20 times more IL-6 than BMSCs *in vitro* [44], we observed that hADSCs secrete large amounts of IL-6 in the lesion area (MAN, KM, RB, TC-S, unpublished). Secretion of other cytokines such as IL-10, which is largely produced by hADSCs [45], may also play a role in regeneration, due to its ability to favor the differentiation of M2 macrophages. It has already been shown that BMSCs can shift macrophage differentiation towards the M2 pro-regenerative phenotype [46–48].

The present study describes three major novel observations that shed light on the mechanisms of neural tissue regeneration promoted by adult MSC cells. First, hADSCs induced an increase in cellularity at the lesion site and in clusters distributed along the spinal midline above the central canal. Cells in the clusters expressed markers of neural precursors. Likewise, in the non-injured spinal cord progenitor cells accumulated in a single large spindle-like cluster, indicating that the observed increase in cellularity does not depend on the occurrence of a lesion.

In animals receiving hADSCs, the vimentin-positive ependymal cell layer that lines the central canal [49] expanded, indicating that molecules secreted by hADSCs can increase the proliferation of neural precursors in the normal neurogenic area of the spinal cord.

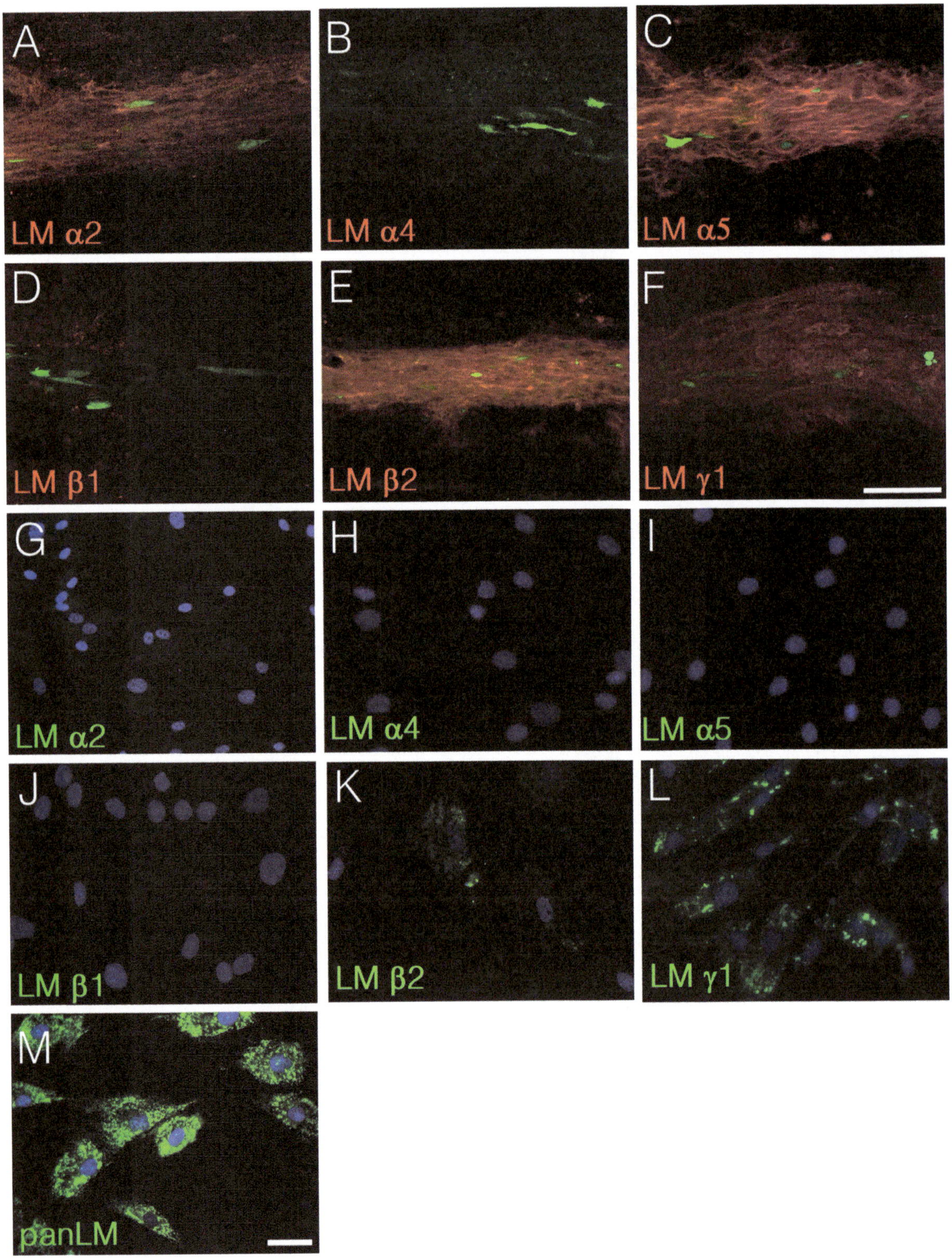

Figure 7. Identification of laminin chains produced by hADSCs *in vivo* and *in vitro*. A–F) Uninjured rats were injected with GFP-hADSCs and the human laminin chains produced in the spinal cord were analyzed one week after transplantation. Confocal images of horizontal sections taken at the spinal midline show that hADSCs are localized in areas rich in human laminin α2 (A), α5 (C), β2 (E) and γ1 (F). Immunoreactivity for human laminin α4 (B) and β1 (D) was not detected in the spinal cord (D). G–M) Analysis of the laminin chains produced by hADSCs cultivated *in vitro*. *In vitro*, the only laminin chains detected were β2 (K) and γ1 (L). Note that hADSCs did not produce α2 (G) nor α5 (I), which suggests that secretion of these two chains is triggered by the contact with the environment of the spinal cord. Panel M shows immunostaining for laminin using an anti-pan laminin antibody. Bars: A–F = 100 μm, G–M = 50 μm.

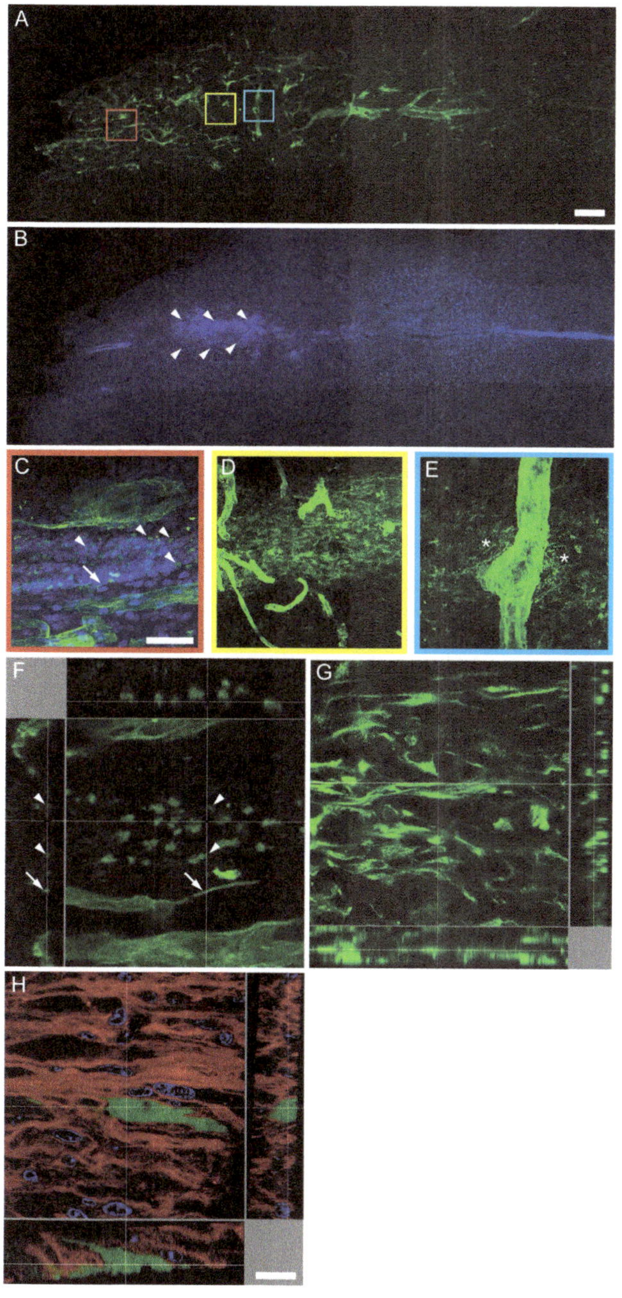

Figure 8. Laminin produced by hADSC forms reticular-like deposits independent of fractones. Photomontage of a horizontal section of the undamaged spinal cord one week after injection of hADSCs (A) immunostained with a pan-specific anti-laminin antibody (green) and (B) counterstained with DAPI (blue). The arrowheads in B delimit the region of the highest increase in cellularity, corresponding to reticular laminin in A. Boxed areas in A were amplified to show the detailed morphology of the types of laminin deposits in the spinal cord. C) The red box shows fractones characterized by the presence of thin lines (arrow) and puncta (arrowhead). D) The yellow box shows an independent reticular-like deposit. E) The blue box shows laminin around a blood vessel. Note that laminin seems to detach from the perivascular basal lamina and to spread in the spinal parenchyma (asterisks). Panels C and D were reconstructed in the z axis to provide a 3D view of the fractones (F) and of the reticular deposits (G). In F, lines (arrow) and puncta (arrowheads) presented similar shapes in 2D or 3D. Panel H shows a 3D view of laminin deposits stained with an antibody specific for the $\alpha 2$ chain of human laminin (red) and counterstained with DAPI (blue). The 3D structure of laminin secreted by hADSCs is similar to the one depicted in G and different from the one depicted in F. Note that DAPI-stained nuclei are nested within reticular laminin (red) and that the protein produced by GFP-transduced hADSCs (green) largely surpasses the borders of the secreting cells.

Cells from the ependymal layer have already been shown to proliferate after spinal cord injury [50]. This phenomenon could account for the scattered cell clusters seen in the white matter above the canal in animals submitted to injury. In these animals, a second focus of increased cellularity was the lesion epicenter. Progenitor cells could migrate from the neurogenic area of the canal toward the lesion using two alternative routes; directly through the parenchyma or along the perivascular space. Although we cannot presently discriminate between these possibilities, the presence of blood vessels near the expanded lining of the central canal reinforces the latter hypothesis. Similar to our results, it has been previously shown that the injection of bone marrow MSCs stimulated subventricular zone neurogenesis in the mouse brain [51].

The second remarkable feature observed in this study was the appearance of perivascular spaces limited by two clearly definable basement membranes in the spinal cord tissue. Separation of the two basal laminas, which are close together in physiological conditions, creates a perivascular compartment suitable for cell trafficking, associated to inflammation [52,53]. Recently, it has been proposed that mesenchymal precursors that differentiate into vascular mural cells use conduits in the extracellular matrix called "vascular guiding tunnels" to approach the newly formed endothelial tubes to which they will associate [54].

Cells located between the two membranes expressed nestin, vimentin, and NG2, which are markers for neural precursors and for perivascular cells. They were also positive for αSMA, which is expressed by pericytes of the nervous system [55], but not considered as a marker for neural precursors. This antigenic profile does not allow us to identify these perivascular cells as neural precursors derived from remote neurogenic areas into the lesion site or to perivascular cells with the potential to divide and differentiate into neural lineages. Corroborating the latter, pericytes have recently been proposed to correspond to a heterogeneous population [56] containing multipotent mesenchymal cells with the potential to differentiate into neural precursors [57]. Nevertheless, at this point we cannot determine if neural progenitors originate from the central canal or from the perivascular compartment. Tuj1 and Olig2 expression were not detected in the perivascular compartment, but were detected in the cellular infiltrate at the lesion site and also in the spindle-like cluster in non-damaged spinal cord. Thus, if progenitor cells do in fact migrate through the perivascular compartment they must differentiate into neuroblasts or glial precursors only upon contact with the neural parenchyma.

The third finding providing new information on the mechanisms involved in hADSC-induced regeneration is the accumulation of human laminin in the same areas of the spinal cord where precursor cells have also accumulated. Grafted cells produced a cloud-like pattern of laminin deposition, which corresponded to the location of neural precursors in both injured and non-injured spinal cord. Given that laminins, particularly those containing the $\alpha 2$ and $\alpha 5$ chains [36], are present in CNS regions where neural stem and progenitor cells reside, both during development and in the adult [34,35,58,59], we hypothesize that laminin can be the molecule produced by hADSCs that mediated the accumulation of neural precursors along the midline and at the injury site. In line with this hypothesis is our previous demonstration that acute injection of the protein laminin alone, as long as it is delivered in its polymeric form, promotes regeneration after spinal cord injury [60]. Although in that study we did not search for the presence of neural precursors in the tissue, we did find that laminin treatment led to regeneration of descending axons, to decreases in astrogliosis and cystic cavity size and to an expressive reduction of macrophage spreading in the spinal parenchyma, all events similar to those described here as elicited by hADSC.

This is the first time that a link between laminin and the pro-regenerative effects of mesenchymal cells in the central nervous system is proposed. Previous studies had proposed a connection between laminin and MSCs in other tissues such as the peripheral nerve and skeletal muscle [61,62]. However, those studies were conducted in laminin deficient animals in which MSCs were injected exactly as an attempt to restore tissue integrity. Furthermore, none of these two studies demonstrated a strong correlation between the localization of endogenous progenitors and laminin deposited by MSC, as shown here.

Bone marrow stromal cells have been shown to express laminin α4, α5, β1, β2 and γ1 [63]. Here we tested whether hADSCs *in vitro* produced these laminin chains, but we found reactivity only for β2 and γ1. In addition, we found no positivity for the α2 chain, which, together with α5, β2 and γ1, was detected *in vivo*. Considering that laminin α2 and α5 of human origin appeared in spinal cord of rats injected with hADSCs (injured or uninjured), we propose that the exposure of the cells to the spinal cord environment was capable of switching the production of laminin chains α2 and α5. These laminin chains secreted only after transplantation of hADSC may stimulate the proliferation and migration of neural precursors from the ependymal layer around the central canal or from other neurogenic niches around blood vessels. The attracted precursor cells accumulate mainly in the lesion site, contributing to regeneration of the nervous tissue and ultimately to functional recovery. In line with this hypothesis, it has previously been shown that laminin isoforms containing the α chains 2, 4 and 5 are essential components of the subependymal neurogenic niche of adult mice [36].

Our results show that hADSCs are efficient in promoting regeneration after SCI and suggest laminin as a mediator of the beneficial effects of these cells. A better understanding of the mechanisms underlying the regenerative effects of stem/progenitor cells in the nervous system is essential for development of future cell-based therapies to treat spinal cord injury in humans.

Experimental Procedures

Ethics Statement

All experimental procedures adhered to the guidelines of the American National Institute of Health and the Brazilian COBEA and were approved by the animal welfare committee of the Federal University of Rio de Janeiro/Center of Health Sciences [DAHEICB 041]. All the procedures involving human samples were approved by the Investigational Review Board at HUCFF (protocol numbers 043/09 and 088/04). Bone marrow samples were collected from discharged bone marrow collection kits after aspirates were transferred to infusion bags. Informed consent exemption was approved by the Investigational Review Board at HUCFF since data were analyzed anonymously and derived from discarded samples. Adipose tissue and lipoaspirates were collected after the patients signed a written informed consent.

Animals

We used adult female Sprague-Dawley rats (200–250 g), bred at the animal facility of the Federal University of Rio de Janeiro. Rats were kept in 12-hour light/dark cycles with free access to food and water in an isolated animal room. Sixty seven rats were used in this study. Forty-eight animals were included in the injured group submitted to spinal cord compression and were further subdivided in cell treated group (n = 27; 3 euthanized at 1 dpi, 12 at 1 wpi, 3 at 4 wpi and 9 at 8 wpi) and vehicle control (n = 21; 3 euthanized at 1 dpi, 6 at 1 wpi, 3 at 4 wpi and 9 at 8 wpi). Non-injured animals that received cells (n = 12; euthanized at 1 wpi) and sham operated animals (n = 6; 3 euthanized at 1 wpi and 3 at 8 wpi) were included. One uninjured animal was injected with human fibroblasts and euthanized one week later.

Samples and Cells

Fragments of subcutaneous adipose tissue and lipoaspirates were obtained from the abdominal region of patients undergoing plastic surgery at the Clementino Fraga Filho University Hospital (HUCFF), Federal University of Rio de Janeiro, Brazil. Human skin fibroblast cell line was obtained from the Cell Bank of Rio de Janeiro (BCRJ, Rio de Janeiro, RJ, Brazil).

Plasmid Construct and Lentivirus Production

The pLL3.7 plasmid, originally described by Dr. van Parijs's group [64], was provided by Dr. Guido Lenz (UFRGS – Porto Alegre, Brazil). Lentiviral vectors were produced as previously described [65,66].

Isolation and Transduction of hADSCs

Human adipose tissue-derived stromal cells were obtained as previously described [24,25,67]. Briefly, subcutaneous adipose tissue fragments and lipoaspirates were submitted to enzymatic digestion with 10 mg/mL collagenase IA (Sigma-Aldrich, St. Louis, MO) for 1 hour at 37°C under agitation. Cells were plated at $1–2 \times 10^4$ cells/cm^2 in Dulbecco's (DMEM Low-glucose, LGC, São Paulo, SP, Brazil) supplemented with 10% fetal bovine serum (FBS, Cultilab, Campinas, SP, Brazil) and antibiotics (100 U/ml of penicillin and 100 μg/ml of streptomycin, both from Sigma-Aldrich) and maintained overnight at 37°C with 5% CO_2. Non-adherent cells were removed and adherent cells were maintained as above and expanded by enzymatic digestion with 0.125% trypsin and 0.78 mM EDTA (Sigma-Aldrich). Lentivirus transduction was performed by addition of 1 mL of lentiviral vector stock with polybrene at the concentration of 8 μg/mL and 7 mL of DMEM. Cells were then incubated at 5% $C0_2$ and 37°C overnight. After incubation, the medium was replaced by fresh DMEM medium with 10% FCS. Cells were kept under these conditions until they were prepared for *in vivo* analysis. The typical multiplicity of infection (MOI) used for ADSC transduction ranged from 10 to 50. Transduced cells were trypsinized, fixed with 4% paraformaldehyde in PBS, and GFP expression was analyzed by flow cytometry (BD FACScalibur Flow Cytometer; Becton Dickinson) using CellQuest software.

Surgical Procedures

Animals were anesthetized with an i.m. injection (300 μl) of a cocktail containing xylazine (3.2 mg/kg; Syntec, Cotia, SP, Brazil), ketamin (62.5 mg/kg; Syntec), and acepromazin (0.625 mg/kg; Syntec) diluted in water, and were subjected to dorsal laminectomy. For the compression injury, T7 vertebra was removed and a 2-French Fogarty catheter (Baxter Healthcare Corporation, Irvine, CA) was inserted into the dorsal epidural space caudally to T8–T9 spinal level (1 cm distance from the incision). The balloon was inflated with 15 μl of water for 5 min. Rats were kept anesthetized for 30 min before application of acute experimental treatment or control buffers. Soft tissue and skin were sutured in anatomical layers and the animals were allowed to recover in warmed cages and kept in pairs during survival. As specific surgical and post-surgical care, all animals had their eyes lubricated during surgery, received subcutaneous 10 ml injections of Ringer solution for hydration immediately after being sutured, and were treated with gentamicin sulfate (40 mg/kg; Neoquímica, Anápolis, GO, Brazil) for 3 days to avoid urinary infection. The bladder was manually expressed until spontaneous function was reestablished 3 days after injury.

Spinal Cord Injections

Cell suspensions or vehicle (10 μl) were stereotaxically injected using a 10 μl Hamilton syringe, immediately after injury or after laminectomy in non-injured animals. The total volume was injected once, 1 cm rostrally to the lesion epicenter. In animals, which were not subjected to SCI, injections were made at T8–9 level.

Histology and Immunofluorescence

Rats were anesthetized and perfused transcardially with 4% paraformaldehyde in 0.1 M phosphate buffer (pH 7.4). Spinal cords were removed and a 1 cm segment between T7–T10 levels was removed. For immunofluorescence analysis, segments were cut in the transversal or horizontal planes in a vibratome (model 3000, Vibratome Co; 40 μm thick), and collected serially onto gelatin-coated glass slides. Tissue samples of gastrocnemius muscle of rats were cut in a cryostat for the anti-human laminin immunolabeling.

Prior to immunolabeling, slides were extensively washed with PBS, permeabilized with 0.3% Triton-X-100 (Sigma), blocked with 10% bovine serum albumin (Sigma) or normal goat serum (Sigma), and finally incubated overnight at 4°C with primary antibodies. The following mouse antibodies were used: anti-GAP-43 (1:4.000; Sigma); anti-GFAP (1:500; Sigma); anti-CD68 (ED1; 1:30; AbD Serotec, Oxford, UK); anti-RECA-1 (1:100; AbD Serotec), anti-CD3 (clone 1F4; 1:100; BioLegend, San Diego, CA); anti-αSMA (1:400; Sigma), anti-class III β-tubulin (Tuj1; 1:500; Covance, Princeton, NJ), anti-vimentin (1:100; Sigma), anti-human fibronectin (1:400; Sigma), anti-human collagen IV (1:500; Sigma), anti-human laminin α5 chain (clone LAM-89; 1:1000; Sigma), anti-human laminin α2 chain (clone 5H2; 1:1000; Millipore), anti-human laminin α2, α4, α5, β1, β2 and γ1, corresponding to clones 5A4, 3D12, 6A11, IIID9, 9F8 and IIID10, were kindly provided by Dr. Lydia Sorokin (University of Muenster, Germany). The following rabbit antibodies were used: anti-serotonin (5HT; 1:1000; Sigma); anti-Ki67 (1:100; Abcam); anti-nestin (1:500; Millipore); anti-Olig2 (1:500; Millipore); anti-NG2 (1:150; Millipore); and pan-laminin (polyclonal antibody raised against EHS laminin; 1:50; Sigma). After rinsing with PBS, sections were incubated for 2 h at room temperature with fluorescent dye-conjugated goat anti-mouse or anti-rabbit IgGs (1:500; Cy3-conjugated from Sigma and Alexa 488-conjugated from Molecular Probes/Invitrogen). After an additional wash with PBS and one with distilled water, slides were mounted with n-propyl galate (Sigma). In negative controls the primary antibodies were omitted (Fig. S5).

Image Analysis

Tissue and cells were analyzed in a TE200 fluorescence inverted microscope (Nikon), with standard DAPI/FITC/TRITC filters coupled to a color CCD camera (Evolution vf, Media Cybernetics) and using the software Image Pro Plus 6.0 for image processing (Media Cybernetics Inc.). Images were alternatively acquired with a TCS-SP5 confocal microscope (Leica).

Lesion epicenters and the largest diameter of cavity size were determined by digitalizing the cavity contours of GFAP-stained horizontal sections of the dorsal–ventral plane of the injured cord. The analyses were confined to the middle 640 μm, ranging from 120 to 760 μm below the first section from the top of the spine. For quantification, the section with the largest cavity size was chosen as the epicenter and 5 sections in 5 successive slides on each side of this putative epicenter had their areas calculated using the software Image Pro Plus 6.0 (Media Cybernetics Inc.) and plotted against a spatial axis. We evaluated three animals of each experimental group.

GAP-43 and 5-HT fibers were evaluated in conventional fluorescence images and plotted as the sum of the total length of positive fibers, at 3 different regions (injury epicenter; 500 μm rostral and caudal to epicenter), in 3 animals (1 section per animal).

Behavioral Assessment

Locomotor activity was evaluated using the open-field walking test, BBB [68]. One animal at a time was allowed to move freely inside a circular plastic tray for 5 min, and two independent examiners who were blinded to the experiment attributed scores. The final score of each animal was the mean value of both examiners.

Statistics

Comparisons between different experimental groups were performed using GraphPad Prism version 5.00 for Windows (GraphPad Software, San Diego, USA) to analyze the variance (ANOVA) with post-hoc Kruskal-Wallis test for multiple comparisons (BBB assays). For comparison between 2 groups we used the Student's t test (cavity size, ED1, GAP-43, and 5-HT labeling). Differences were considered significant when $p<0.05$.

Supporting Information

Figure S1 Neighboring blood vessels interact with the expanded wall of the central canal. (A–F) Consecutive confocal images in the z axis of a horizontal section at the level of the central canal processed for DAPI staining (blue) 1 week after injury. It is possible to see the transition between a single cell (A) and a multiple cell (B) lining of the canal wall (dashed line); the progressive thickening of the canal wall (D–E); a blood vessel approaching the canal area (arrows in B–F); and cells from the canal wall contacting the lumen of this blood vessel (F). (G–I) Higher magnification images of boxed areas in D–F, showing the area of interaction between the blood vessel and the central canal with high cell density. GFAP immunoreactivity (red) reveals the areas of tissue as opposed to hollow structures such as the blood vessel and the canal. Dashed lines delineate the border between the wall of the central canal and the spinal grey matter. Bars: A–F = 50 μm and G–I = 25 μm.

Figure S2 Areas of increased cellularity in the uninjured spinal cord injected with hADSC contain neural precursors and/or pericytes. A–C) Confocal images of a transverse section of the spinal cord immunostained with anti-CD68 (ED1, red), one week after the injection of GFP-hADSC into the undamaged spinal cord. Note that only a few scattered cells correspond to macrophages/microglial cells appearing in cell infiltrates (DAPI, blue). D–S) Confocal images of horizontal sections of the undamaged spinal cord one week after injection of hADSCs, showing the presence of neural precursors and/or pericytes, identified by immunostaining with anti-nestin (D–G, R,

S, green), anti-vimentin (H, I, red; J, K, green), Tuj1 (L,M, red), anti-SMA (N,O, red) and anti-Olig2 (P, Q, green). Note that the phenomenon of separation of the two laminas around blood vessels also occurs in the absence of lesion (F, G, J, K). Nestin-positive cells (green) present Ki67-positive nuclei (red), indicating that neural precursors proliferate in the cell infiltrates (R, S). Bars: A, H, I, P, Q = 100 μm; B, C, F–I, K, S = 25 μm; D, E, L–O, R: = 50 μm.

Figure S3 Extracellular matrix proteins secreted by the hADSCs in the undamaged spinal cord. Confocal images of horizontal sections of the spinal cord, one week after injection of GFP-hADSCs (green). Images show immunoreactivity for anti-human fibronectin (B, C, red), anti-human collagen IV (E, F, red) and anti-human laminin (clone 5H2, H, I, red) counterstained with DAPI (blue) to reveal cell infiltrates (A, D, G). Note that human laminin is more abundant than the other proteins. Bars: A–I = 100 μm.

Figure S4 The anti-human α2 laminin antibody does not cross-react with rat α2 laminin. The specificity of the anti-human laminin α2 antibody (clone 5H2) was investigated by testing its ability to recognize the rat muscle, where α2 is the major component of the basal lamina. Rat gastrocnemius muscle was cut transversally and stained with an anti-pan laminin antibody (A) or with 5H2 (B). Note that basement membranes around muscle fibers were labeled by anti-pan but not by anti-human α2 laminin. A negative control obtained by omitting the primary antibodies is shown in panel C. DAPI counterstaining appears in panels D–F. Scale bar = 100 μm.

Figure S5 Negative controls for immunolabeling analyses. A–F) Confocal images of horizontal sections of the spinal cord incubated with fluorescent dye-conjugated goat Cy3-anti-rabbit (A, red), Alexa 488-anti-mouse (B, green), Cy3-anti-mouse (D, red), Alexa 488-anti-rabbit (E, green). Red and green channels are shown superimposed (C, F) together with DAPI counterstaining (blue). Bars: A–F = 200 μm.

Movie S1 Cells accumulate in between the two laminin-rich basement membranes around blood vessels in the spinal cord of hADSC-treated animals. The animation was generated from a series of confocal optical slices of a horizontal section (50 μm thick) of the rat spinal cord 1 week after injury and injection of hADSC. The slice was immunostained for PAN-laminin (red) and nestin (green) and counterstained with DAPI (blue). Cells tend to accumulate in nestin-rich areas both between the two basement membranes and in the spinal parenchyma. Note that in the inferior part of the image cells seem to escape from the vessel in a region where the laminin membrane appears disrupted. Confocal micrographs were analyzed using a free trial version of Imaris software (version 7.2, Bitplane Scientific Software).

Acknowledgments

We would like to thank Laina Martins Cunha and Rosana Maria Assis Silva for excellent technical assistance. The authors are indebted to Dr. César Cláudio da Silva and Dr. Marcelo C. Acineto Souza, both from the Faculty of Medicine (UFRJ), who provided the adipose tissue fragments and lipoaspirates for isolation of hADSCs and to Dr. Lydia Sorokin from the University of Muenster for the kind gift of anti-laminin antibodies.

This manuscript was reviewed by a professional science editor and by a native English-speaking copy editor to improve readability.

Author Contributions

Conceived and designed the experiments: KM MB JRLM RB MIDR TCS. Performed the experiments: KM MAN JPG ASC DVL BC JRLM. Analyzed the data: KM MAN JRLM RB MIDR TCS. Contributed reagents/materials/analysis tools: MB JRLM RB MIDR TCS. Wrote the paper: KM JRLM MIDR TCS.

References

1. Burns AS, O'Connell C (2012) The challenge of spinal cord injury care in the developing world. J Spinal Cord Med 35: 3–8.
2. Devivo MJ (2012) Epidemiology of traumatic spinal cord injury: trends and future implications. Spinal Cord 50: 365–372.
3. Bradbury EJ (2002) Re-wiring the spinal cord: introduction to the special issue on plasticity after spinal cord injury. Exp Neurol 235: 1–4.
4. Ruff CA, Wilcox JT, Fehlings MG (2012) Cell-based transplantation strategies to promote plasticity following spinal cord injury. Exp Neurol 235: 78–90.
5. Hatami M, Mehrjardi NZ, Kiani S, Hemmesi K, Azizi H, et al. (2009) Human embryonic stem cell-derived neural precursor transplants in collagen scaffolds promote recovery in injured rat spinal cord. Cytotherapy 11: 618–630.
6. Keirstead HS, Nistor G, Bernal G, Totoiu M, Cloutier F, et al. (2005) Human embryonic stem cell-derived oligodendrocyte progenitor cell transplants remyelinate and restore locomotion after spinal cord injury. J Neurosci 25: 4694–4705.
7. McDonald JW, Howard MJ (2002) Repairing the damaged spinal cord: a summary of our early success with embryonic stem cell transplantation and remyelination. Prog Brain Res 137: 299–309.
8. Wyatt TJ, Rossi SL, Siegenthaler MM, Frame J, Robles R, et al. (2011) Human motor neuron progenitor transplantation leads to endogenous neuronal sparing in 3 models of motor neuron loss. Stem Cells Int 2011: 207230.
9. Lebkowski J (2011) GRNOPC1: the world's first embryonic stem cell-derived therapy. Interview with Jane Lebkowski. Regen Med 6: 11–13.
10. da Silva Meirelles L, Caplan AI, Nardi NB (2008) In search of the in vivo identity of mesenchymal stem cells. Stem Cells 26: 2287–2299.
11. Wright KT, El Masri W, Osman A, Chowdhury J, Johnson WEB (2011) Concise review: Bone marrow for the treatment of spinal cord injury: mechanisms and clinical applications. Stem Cells 29: 169–178.
12. Scuteri A, Miloso M, Foudah D, Orciani M, Cavaletti G, et al. (2011) Mesenchymal stem cells neuronal differentiation ability: a real perspective for nervous system repair? Curr Stem Cell Res Ther 6: 82–92.
13. Ankeny DP, McTigue DM, Jakeman LB (2004) Bone marrow transplants provide tissue protection and directional guidance for axons after contusive spinal cord injury in rats. Exp Neurol 190: 17–31.
14. Chopp M, Zhang XH, Li Y, Wang L, Chen J, et al. (2000) Spinal cord injury in rat: treatment with bone marrow stromal cell transplantation. Neuroreport 11: 3001–3005.
15. Cízková D, Rosocha J, Vanický I, Jergová S, Cízek M (2006) Transplants of human mesenchymal stem cells improve functional recovery after spinal cord injury in the rat. Cell Mol Neurobiol 26: 1167–1180.
16. Führmann T, Montzka K, Hillen LM, Hodde D, Dreier A, et al. (2010) Axon growth-promoting properties of human bone marrow mesenchymal stromal cells. Neurosci Lett 474: 37–41.
17. Hofstetter CP, Schwarz EJ, Hess D, Widenfalk J, El Manira A, et al. (2002) Marrow stromal cells form guiding strands in the injured spinal cord and promote recovery. Proc Natl Acad Sci USA 99: 2199–2204.
18. Osaka M, Honmou O, Murakami T, Nonaka T, Houkin K, et al. (2010) Intravenous administration of mesenchymal stem cells derived from bone marrow after contusive spinal cord injury improves functional outcome. Brain Res 1343: 226–235.
19. Pal R, Gopinath C, Rao NM, Banerjee P, Krishnamoorthy V, et al. (2010) Functional recovery after transplantation of bone marrow-derived human mesenchymal stromal cells in a rat model of spinal cord injury. Cytotherapy 12: 792–806.
20. Park H-W, Lim M-J, Jung H, Lee S-P, Paik K-S, et al. (2010) Human mesenchymal stem cell-derived Schwann cell-like cells exhibit neurotrophic effects, via distinct growth factor production, in a model of spinal cord injury. Glia 58: 1118–1132.
21. Pedram MS, Dehghan MM, Soleimani M, Sharifi D, Marjanmehr SH, et al. (2010) Transplantation of a combination of autologous neural differentiated and undifferentiated mesenchymal stem cells into injured spinal cord of rats. Spinal Cord 48: 457–463.
22. Zhang W, Yan Q, Zeng Y-S, Zhang X-B, Xiong Y, et al. (2010) Implantation of adult bone marrow-derived mesenchymal stem cells transfected with the

neurotrophin-3 gene and pretreated with retinoic acid in completely transected spinal cord. Brain Res 1359: 256–271.
23. Zurita M, Vaquero J, Bonilla C, Santos M, De Haro J, et al. (2008) Functional recovery of chronic paraplegic pigs after autologous transplantation of bone marrow stromal cells. Transplantation 86: 845–853.
24. Baptista LS, da Silva KR, da Pedrosa CSG, Claudio-da-Silva C, Carneiro JRI, et al. (2009) Adipose tissue of control and ex-obese patients exhibit differences in blood vessel content and resident mesenchymal stem cell population. Obes Surg 19: 1304–1312.
25. Zuk PA, Zhu M, Mizuno H, Huang J, Futrell JW, et al. (2001) Multilineage cells from human adipose tissue: implications for cell-based therapies. Tissue Eng 7: 211–228.
26. Arboleda D, Forostyak S, Jendelova P, Marekova D, Amemori T, et al. (2011) Transplantation of predifferentiated adipose-derived stromal cells for the treatment of spinal cord injury. Cell Mol Neurobiol 31: 1113–1122.
27. Oh JS, Kim KN, An SS, Pennant WA, Kim HJ, et al. (2011) Cotransplantation of mouse neural stem cells (mNSCs) with adipose tissue-derived mesenchymal stem cells improves mNSC survival in a rat spinal cord injury model. Cell Transplant 20: 837–849.
28. Park S-S, Lee YJ, Lee SH, Lee D, Choi K, et al. (2012) Functional recovery after spinal cord injury in dogs treated with a combination of Matrigel and neural-induced adipose-derived mesenchymal Stem cells. Cytotherapy 14: 584–597.
29. Zhou Z, Chen Y, Zhang H, Min S, Yu B, et al. (2013) Comparison of mesenchymal stem cells from human bone marrow and adipose tissue for the treatment of spinal cord injury. Cytotherapy, 15: 434–448.
30. Aggarwal S, Pittenger MF (2005) Human mesenchymal stem cells modulate allogeneic immune cell responses. Blood 105: 1815–1822.
31. Le Blanc K, Mougiakakos D (2012) Multipotent mesenchymal stromal cells and the innate immune system. Nat Rev Immunol 12: 383–396.
32. Menezes JR, Luskin MB (1994) Expression of neuron-specific tubulin defines a novel population in the proliferative layers of the developing telencephalon. J Neurosci 14: 5399–5416.
33. Benowitz LI, Routtenberg A (1997) GAP-43: an intrinsic determinant of neuronal development and plasticity. Trends Neurosci 20: 84–91.
34. Lathia JD, Patton B, Eckley DM, Magnus T, Mughal MR, et al. (2007) Patterns of laminins and integrins in the embryonic ventricular zone of the CNS. J Comp Neurol 505: 630–643.
35. Shen Q, Wang Y, Kokovay E, Lin G, Chuang S-M, et al. (2008) Adult SVZ stem cells lie in a vascular niche: a quantitative analysis of niche cell-cell interactions. Cell Stem Cell 3: 289–300.
36. Kazanis I, Lathia JD, Vadakkan TJ, Raborn E, Wan R, et al. (2010) Quiescence and activation of stem and precursor cell populations in the subependymal zone of the mammalian brain are associated with distinct cellular and extracellular matrix signals. J Neurosci 30: 9771–9781.
37. Hamann GF, Okada Y, Fitridge R, del Zoppo GJ (1995) Microvascular basal lamina antigens disappear during cerebral ischemia and reperfusion. Stroke 26: 2120–2126.
38. Chen X, Ai Z, Rasmussen M, Bajcsy P, Auvil L, et al. (2003) Three-dimensional reconstruction of extravascular matrix patterns and blood vessels in human uveal melanoma tissue: techniques and preliminary findings. Invest Ophthalmol Vis Sci 44: 2834–2840.
39. Mercier F, Kitasako JT, Hatton GI (2002) Anatomy of the brain neurogenic zones revisited: fractones and the fibroblast/macrophage network. J Comp Neurol 451: 170–188.
40. Mercier F, Schnack J, Chaumet MSG (2011) Fractones: Home and conductors of the neural stem cell niche. In Neurogenesis in the adult brain I: Neurobiology, eds Seki T et al. (Springer, Heidelberg), 109–133.
41. Barberi T, Klivenyi P, Calingasan NY, Lee H, Kawamata H, et al. (2003) Neural subtype specification of fertilization and nuclear transfer embryonic stem cells and application in parkinsonian mice. Nat Biotechnol 21: 1200–1207.
42. Ideguchi M, Palmer TD, Recht LD, Weimann JM (2010) Murine embryonic stem cell-derived pyramidal neurons integrate into the cerebral cortex and appropriately project axons to subcortical targets. J Neurosci 30: 894–904.
43. Steffenhagen C, Dechant F-X, Oberbauer E, Furtner T, Weidner N, et al. (2012) Mesenchymal stem cells prime proliferating adult neural progenitors toward an oligodendrocyte fate. Stem Cells Dev 21: 1838–1851.
44. Nakanishi C, Nagaya N, Ohnishi S, Yamahara K, Takabatake S, et al. (2011) Gene and protein expression analysis of mesenchymal stem cells derived from rat adipose tissue and bone marrow. Circ J 75: 2260–2268.
45. Castelo-Branco MTL, Soares IDP, Lopes DV, Buongusto F, Martinusso CA, et al. (2012) Intraperitoneal but not intravenous cryopreserved mesenchymal stromal cells home to the inflamed colon and ameliorate experimental colitis. PloS One 7: e33360.
46. Busch SA, Hamilton JA, Horn KP, Cuascut FX, Cutrone R, et al. (2011) Multipotent adult progenitor cells prevent macrophage-mediated axonal dieback and promote regrowth after spinal cord injury. J Neurosci 31: 944–953.
47. Kim J, Hematti P (2009) Mesenchymal stem cell-educated macrophages: a novel type of alternatively activated macrophages. Exp Hematol 37: 1445–1453.
48. Nakajima H, Uchida K, Guerrero AR, Watanabe S, Sugita D, et al. (2012) Transplantation of mesenchymal stem cells promotes an alternative pathway of macrophage activation and functional recovery after spinal cord injury. J Neurotrauma 29: 1614–1625.
49. Alfaro-Cervello C, Soriano-Navarro M, Mirzadeh Z, Alvarez-Buylla A, Garcia-Verdugo JM (2012) Biciliated ependymal cell proliferation contributes to spinal cord growth. J Comp Neurol 520: 3528–3552.
50. Meletis K, Barnabe?-Heider F, Carlén M, Evergren E, Tomilin N, et al. (2008) Spinal cord injury reveals multilineage differentiation of ependymal cells. PLoS Biol 6: e182.
51. Kan I, Barhum Y, Melamed E, Offen D (2011) Mesenchymal stem cells stimulate endogenous neurogenesis in the subventricular zone of adult mice. Stem Cell Rev 7: 404–412.
52. Sixt M, Engelhardt B, Pausch F, Hallmann R, Wendler O, et al. (2001) Endothelial cell laminin isoforms, laminins 8 and 10, play decisive roles in T cell recruitment across the blood-brain barrier in experimental autoimmune encephalomyelitis. J Cell Biol 153: 933–946.
53. Takigawa T, Yonezawa T, Yoshitaka T, Minaguchi J, Kurosaki M, et al. (2010) Separation of the perivascular basement membrane provides a conduit for inflammatory cells in a mouse spinal cord injury model. J Neurotrauma 27: 739–751.
54. Stratman AN, Davis GE (2012) Endothelial cell-pericyte interactions stimulate basement membrane matrix assembly: influence on vascular tube remodeling, maturation, and stabilization. Microscopy Microanal 18: 68–80.
55. Krueger M, Bechmann I (2010) CNS pericytes: concepts, misconceptions, and a way out. Glia 58: 1–10.
56. Göritz C, Dias DO, Tomilin N, Barbacid M, Shupliakov O, et al. (2011) A pericyte origin of spinal cord scar tissue. Science 333: 238–242.
57. Paul G, Özen I, Christophersen NS, Reinbothe T, Bengzon J, et al. (2012) The adult human brain harbors multipotent perivascular mesenchymal stem cells. PloS One 7: e35577.
58. Belvindrah R, Hankel S, Walker J, Patton BL, Müller U (2007) Beta1 integrins control the formation of cell chains in the adult rostral migratory stream. J Neurosci 27: 2704–2717.
59. Loulier K, Lathia JD, Marthiens V, Relucio J, Mughal MR, et al. (2009) Beta1 integrin maintains integrity of the embryonic neocortical stem cell niche. PLoS Biol 7: e1000176.
60. Menezes K, de Menezes JR, Nascimento MA, Santos RS, Coelho-Sampaio T (2010) Polylaminin, a polymeric form of laminin, promotes regeneration after spinal cord injury. FASEB J 24: 4513–4522.
61. Carlson KB, Singh P, Feaster MM, Ramnarain A, Pavlides C, et al. (2011) Mesenchymal stem cells facilitate axon sorting, myelination, and functional recovery in paralyzed mice deficient in Schwann cell-derived laminin. Glia 59: 267–277.
62. Fukada S-I, Yamamoto Y, Segada M, Sakamoto K, Nakajima M, et al. (2008) CD90-positive cells, an additional cell population, produce laminin α2 upon transplantation to dy^{3k}/dy^{3k} mice. Exp Cell Res 314: 193–203.
63. Siler U, Seiffert M, Puch S, Richards A, Torok-Storb B, et al. (2000) Characterization and functional analysis of laminin isoforms in human bone marrow. Blood 96: 4194–4203.
64. Rubinson DA, Dillon CP, Kwiatkowski AV, Sievers C, Yang L, et al. (2003) A lentivirus-based system to functionally silence genes in primary mammalian cells, stem cells and transgenic mice by RNA interference. Nat Genet 33: 401–406.
65. Lima LG, Oliveira AS, Campos LC, Bonamino M, Chammas R, et al. (2011) Malignant transformation in melanocytes is associated with increased production of procoagulant microvesicles. Thromb Haemost 106: 712–723.
66. Bonamino M, Serafini M, D'Amico G, Gaipa G, Todisco E, et al. (2004) Functional transfer of CD40L gene in human B-cell precursor ALL blasts by second-generation SIN lentivectors Gene therapy 11: 85–93.
67. Baptista LS, Pedrosa CSG, Silva KR, Otazú IB, Takiya CM, et al. (2007) Bone marrow and adipose tissue-derived mesenchymal stem cells: How close are they? J Stem Cells, 2: 73–90.
68. Basso DM, Beattie MS, Bresnahan JC (1995) A sensitive and reliable locomotor rating scale for open field testing in rats. J Neurotrauma 12: 1–21.

2

Abundant Expression of Guidance and Synaptogenic Molecules in the Injured Spinal Cord

Anne Jacobi[1], Anja Schmalz[1], Florence M. Bareyre[1,2]*

1 Institute of Clinical Neuroimmunology, Ludwig-Maximilians University Munich, Munich, Germany, **2** Munich Cluster for Systems Neurology (SyNergy), Munich, Germany

Abstract

Background: Spinal interneurons have emerged as crucial targets of supraspinal input during post-injury axonal remodelling. For example, lesioned corticospinal projections use propriospinal neurons as relay stations to form intraspinal detour circuits that circumvent the lesion site and contribute to functional recovery. While a number of the molecules that determine the formation of neuronal circuits in the developing nervous system have been identified, it is much less understood which of these cues are also expressed in the injured spinal cord and can thus guide growing collaterals and initiate synaptogenesis during circuit remodelling.

Methodology/Principal Findings: To address this question we characterized the expression profile of a number of guidance and synaptogenic molecules in the cervical spinal cord of healthy and spinal cord-injured mice by *in situ* hybridization. To assign the expression of these molecules to distinct populations of interneurons we labeled short and long propriospinal neurons by retrograde tracing and glycinergic neurons using a transgenically expressed fluorescent protein. Interestingly, we found that most of the molecules studied including members of slit-, semaphorin-, synCAM-, neuroligin- and ephrin-families as well as their receptors are also present in the adult CNS. While many of these molecules were abundantly expressed in all interneurons examined, some molecules including slits, semaphorin 7a, synCAM4 and neuroligin 1 showed preferential expression in propriospinal interneurons. Overall the expression pattern of guidance and synaptogenic molecules in the cervical spinal cord appeared to be stable over time and was not substantially altered following a midthoracic spinal cord injury.

Conclusions: Taken together, our study indicates that many of the guidance and synaptogenic cues that regulate neuronal circuit formation in development are also present in the adult CNS and therefore likely contribute to the remodelling of axonal connections in the injured spinal cord.

Editor: Norbert Weidner, Heidelberg University Hospital, Germany

Funding: Work in F.M.B.'s lab is supported by grants from the Deutsche Forschungsgemeinschaft (DFG, SFB 870) and the German Federal Ministry of Education and Research (BMBF). The funders had no role in study design, data collection and analysis, decision to publish, or preparation of the manuscript.

Competing Interests: The authors have declared that no competing interests exist.

* E-mail: Florence.Bareyre@med.uni-muenchen.de

Introduction

For successful wiring of the nervous system axons need to navigate and establish synaptic contacts with their proper target cells. Work in the developing nervous system has established that this process is regulated by target derived guidance and synaptogenic cues (for review see [1], [2]). A number of the molecules that can guide growing axons in the developing nervous system have been identified and include among others netrins [3], semaphorins [4], slits [5] and ephrins [6]. Similarly, molecules that can facilitate pre- and postsynaptic differentiation following axon-target contact have been studied in neuronal development. Among these, synCAMs [7] and neuroligins [8], for example, can act as pre-synaptic organizers while neurexins [9], and ephrinBs [10] are postsynaptic organizers. To what extend these molecules also regulate pathfinding and synapse formation of re-growing axons in the damaged adult nervous system is so far only incompletely understood.

During the recent years, it has become increasingly clear that new axonal connections are not only formed during development but also following nervous system injury. For example, we and others have shown that the corticospinal tract (CST) undergoes extensive remodelling following spinal cord injury [11–14]. A key element of this remodelling process is the formation of intraspinal detour circuits [11,13]. For detour circuits to form, the hindlimb CST sprouts new collaterals in response to a midthoracic dorsal hemisection. These collaterals then enter the gray matter of the cervical spinal cord and contact different populations of spinal interneurons including C3–C4 short propriospinal neurons (SPSN) - which are important for visually-guided target reaching with the forelimb [15] - and C3–C5 long propriospinal neurons (LPSN) - which contribute to locomotion and in particular mediate the coupling of forelimbs and hindlimbs during walking [16]. Initially CST collaterals equally contact long and short propriospinal neurons, however over time contacts onto SPSN are partially removed while contacts onto LPSN are refined and maintained [11,13]. LPSN in turn increase their projections onto lumbar motoneurons and thereby complete an intraspinal detour circuit that can relay information from hindlimb motor cortex to the lumbar spinal cord. The importance of intraspinal detour circuits has been further emphasized by a number of subsequent studies that demonstrate that similar detour circuits (i) mediate the recovery of the supraspinal control of stepping after spinal cord injury [12], (ii) also form in response to inflammatory insults to the spinal cord [17,18], and (iii) are the target of therapeutic strategies that can promote remarkable recovery of locomotor function in rodents [19,20]. While the importance of intraspinal detour circuits for functional recovery is thus well-established, it is unclear how the initiation and stabilization of the synaptic contacts that form the new circuits is regulated. To identify candidate cues that can guide the formation of intraspinal detour circuits we investigated the expression pattern of a number of membrane-bound guidance and synaptogenic molecules in the cervical spinal cord of healthy mice and spinal-cord injured mice by *in situ* hybridization. In particular we assessed the expression in the following populations of spinal interneurons: (i) C3–C4 SPSN, (ii) C3–C5 LPSN and (iii) glycinergic neurons which are located in similar spinal laminae as propriospinal neurons and served as control population. Our results show that members of the slit-, semaphorin-, synCAM-, neuroligin- and ephrinB- families are abundantly expressed in spinal interneurons both before and after spinal cord injury. While most of these molecules are equally expressed in the different interneuronal populations, some molecules like slits, semaphorin 7a and neuroligin 1 are present in many propriospinal neurons but in only few glycinergic interneurons. These results suggest that similar molecular mechanisms might regulate the initial formation of circuits in development and their re-formation after injury.

Materials and Methods

Ethics Statement

All animal experiments conformed to the institutional guidelines and were approved by the Animal Study Committee of the Regierung von Oberbayern. Approval ID: 55.2-1-54-2531-127-05.

Mice

Adult mice between 6 and 12wks of age were used in this study. C57/Bl6 mice (Janvier SAS) were used to study stereotactically labeled long and short propriospinal neurons. *GlyT2*- EGFP mice that express enhanced green fluorescent protein (EGFP; [21]) under the control of the GlyT2 promoter were used to label inhibitory glycinergic neurons.

Surgery procedure

For hemisection procedures mice were anesthetized by i.p. injections of ketamine/xylazine (ketamine 87 mg/kg, xylazine 13 mg/kg). The dorsal spinal cord was exposed by a laminectomy at thoracic level 8 (Th8) and a dorsal hemisection which completely interrupts the main dorsal and minor dorsolateral CST was made with fine iridectomy scissors as previously described [13]. After surgery the mice were kept on a heating pad (38°C) until fully awake and treated with Metacam (0.05 mg/kg, Boehringer Ingelheim) for two more days. Spinal cord and cortex that were used for further analysis were derived from the same mice.

Retrograde labelling of propriospinal neurons and cortical projection neurons

To co-localize the *in situ* hybridization (ISH) signal with propriospinal neurons, these neurons were retrogradely-labeled two weeks before sacrifice for all time points investigated. One µl of Fluoro-Emerald (10% in 1 x PBS, Life Technologies) was stereotactically injected with a glass capillary filled into the lower thoracic cord (Th12) to label LPSN and into the lower cervical cord (C8-Th1) to label SPSN on both sides of the spinal cord (±1.0 mm lateral from spinal midline, depth 1.0 mm). The micropipette remained in place for 2min after completing the injection. To co-localize the ISH signal with the cortical projection neurons of the transected CST, these neurons were retrogradely-labeled 7 days before sacrifice. Briefly, after laminectomy at thoracic level 8 of the spinal cord, 0,5 µl of TexasRed® (5% in 0.1 M PB, Life Technologies) was stereotactically injected rostrally to the lesion with a glass capillary into each side of the spinal cord (±0,2 mm lateral from spinal midline, depth 0.3 mm). The micropipette remained in place for two minutes after completing the injection to avoid backflow. After retrograde labelling mice were kept on a heating pad (38°C) until fully awake and treated with Metacam for 2 more days.

Tissue preparation

Animals were deeply anesthetized with isoflurane and perfused transcardialy with saline solution followed by 4% paraformaldehyde (PFA) in 0.1 M phosphate buffer (PBS). After post-fixation in 4% PFA at 4°C overnight the spinal cord and brains were dissected, incubated in 30% sucrose for 2–3 d, frozen and stored at −20° until use.

Immunohistochemistry (IHC). To assess the presence of the ISH signal in NeuN positive neurons, the cervical spinal cord was sectioned in coronal orientation (30 µm) with a cryostat (Leica CM1850) and sections were then washed three times for 10min in 1x PBS. All solutions used for the IHC contained DEPC to prevent degradation of target RNAs for later ISH. After washing the sections were blocked for 45min in 1x PBS containing 10% horse serum and 0.1% Triton. The primary antibody anti-NeuN (1:500; Millipore MAB377) was incubated in 1x PBS solution containing 0.1% Triton and 2.5% goat serum overnight at 4°. On day 2 the tissue was washed three times for 10min in 1x PBS before the application of the secondary antibody (1:500, Alexa-Fluor 488 goat anti-mouse; Life Technologies). After 3hrs of incubation the tissue was washed three times for 10min in 1x PBS and mounted in VectaShield.

In situ Hybridization (ISH)

Spinal cord tissue (cervical region C2–C5) and brain tissue (Bregma −1.06 till −1.70) were sectioned in coronal orientation (50 µm thick) with a cryostat (Leica CM1850) and washed two times for 10min in 2X SSC (from 20X stock solution containing 3M NaCl and 0,3M Na Citrate). All steps were carried out with DEPC treated solutions to prevent degradation of target RNAs. Before the prehybridization step, the sections were incubated in a 1:1 mixture of 2X SSC and hybridization buffer (50% Formamide, 5X SSC, 5X Denhardt's solution (Sigma-Aldrich D2532), 250 µg/ml yeast tRNA, 500 µg/ml salmon sperm DNA) for 15min at RT. Afterwards the sections were incubated for 1hr in hybridization buffer at the appropriate (pre-) hybridization temperatures for each probe (see Table 1). For hybridization, the probe (200–400 ng/ml in hybridization buffer) was heated for 10min at 80°C, applied to the tissue and incubated overnight in an oven (for temperatures see Table 1). Sections were then rinsed at RT in 2X SSC and washed in decreasing concentration of SSC (2X to 0.1X SSC at hybridization temperature) before applying an alkaline-phosphatase-conjugated sheep anti-digoxigenin antibody, Fab fragments (1:2000; Roche Diagnostics) in blocking buffer overnight at 4°C. Alkaline phosphatase activity was detected using nitroblue tetrazolium chloride (337.5 mg/ml) and 5-Bromo-4-chloro-3-indolyl phosphate (175 mg/ml) (Carl Roth). The sections

Table 1. Hybridization and pre-hybridization temperatures for the different probes used in the study.

	Origin of the probe	Prehybridization Temperature	Hybridization Temperature	Washing Temperature
Slit-1	rat	45°C	48°C	55°C
Slit-2	rat	45°C	48°C	55°C
Slit-3	rat	45°C	48°C	55°C
Robo-1	rat	50°C	54°C	60°C
Robo-2	rat	50°C	54°C	60°C
Robo-3	rat	50°C	58°C	65°C
Sema6A	mouse	50°C	50°C	60°C
Sema7A	rat	50°C	55°C	65°C
PlexinA2	mouse	48°C	48°C	55°C
PlexinC1	mouse	50°C	55°C	65°C
SynCAM1	mouse	55°C	60°C	65°C
SynCAM3	mouse	55°C	65°C	65°C
SynCAM4	mouse	55°C	60°C	65°C
NL1	mouse	55°C	55°C	55°C
NL4	mouse	55°C	55°C	55°C
EphB2	mouse	50°C	52°C	55°C
EphrinB1	mouse	50°C	55°C	55°C

Table 2. Distribution and intensity of the ligands in the unlesioned cervical spinal cord of adult mice.

Area	Slit-1	Slit-2	Slit-3	Sema6a	Sema7a	SynCam1	SynCam3	SynCam4	NL1	NL4	EphB2	EphrinB1
Gray Matter												
Laminae I – IV	++	+++	+	+	++	++	+	++	+	++	+++	+
Laminae V	++	++++	++	+++	+++	++++	+++	+++	++	++	+++	++
Laminae VI – IX	+++	++++	++	++++	+++	+++	++++	+++	+++	++	+++	++
White Matter												
Dorsal Column	+	+	– .	–	+	–	–	+	–	–	+	+
Ventral Funiculus	+	+	–	–	+	–	–	+	–	–	–	+

Relative intensities were estimated by visual comparison with sense probe in situ hybridization slides: +: weak; ++: moderate; +++: strong; ++++: very strong; –: not detected.

were washed in ddH_2O after the staining procedure. When applied, the fluorescent Nissl stain Neurotrace 435 was applied for 2h at RT, the sections were washed and mounted with Gel Mount (Sigma Aldrich).

Imaging and image processing

As the ISH procedure interferes with the fluorescent labels we analyzed fluorescence and ISH signals using a two-step approach. For visualizing the co-localization of ISH signals and NeuN

Table 3. Distribution and intensity of the receptors in the unlesioned adult mouse cortex.

Area	Robo1	Robo2	Robo3	PlexinA2	PlexinC1	SynCam1	SynCam3	SynCam4	EphB2	EphrinB1
LayerI	+	–	–	–	–	+	–	–	–	–
Layer II	+	+	+	+	+	++	++	++	++	++
Layer III	++	++	–	++	++	++	++	+	++	++
Layer IV	++	++	–	–	–	++	+	+++	–	–
Layer V	++++	+++	++	++	+++	++	++	++++	+++	+++
Layer VI	++	+	+	+	–	++	+	++	–	–

Relative intensities were estimated by visual comparison with sense probe in situ hybridization slides: +: weak; ++: moderate; +++: strong; ++++: very strong; –: not detected.

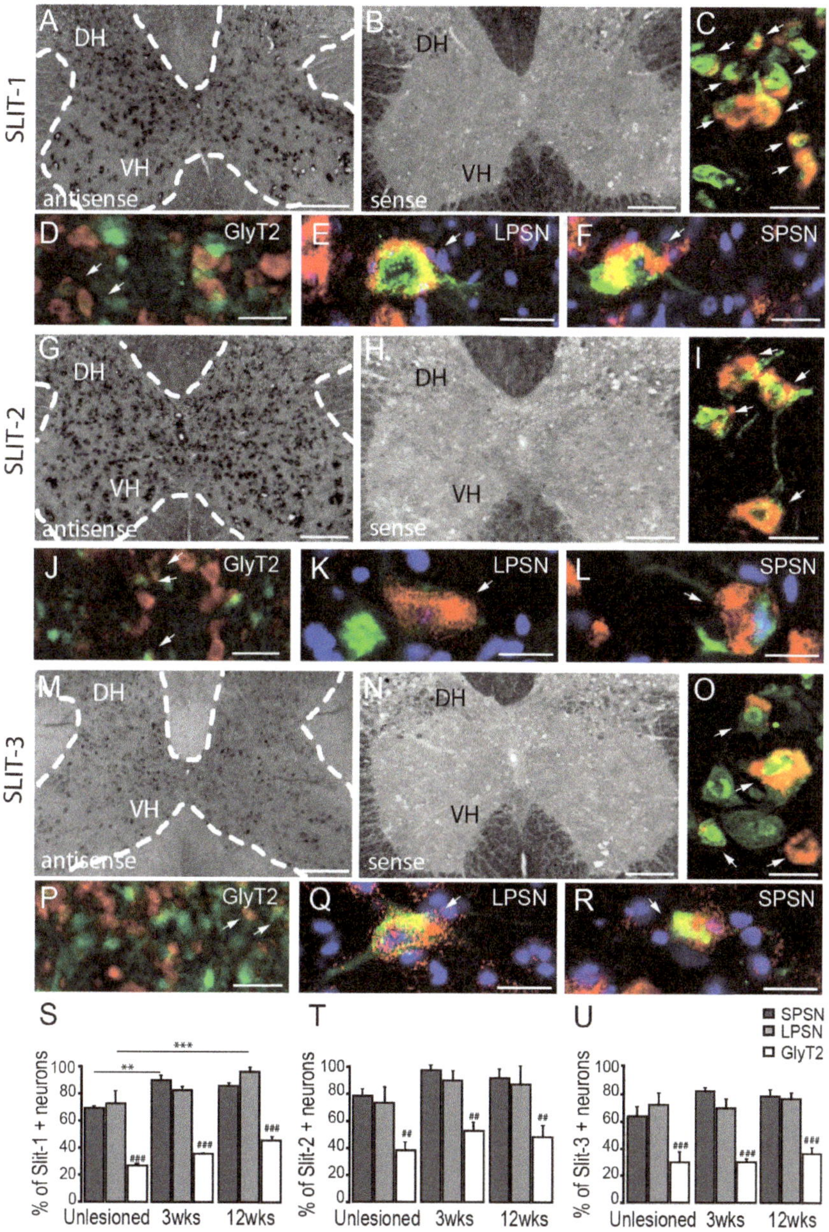

Figure 1. *In Situ* hybridization pattern of Slit-1,-2,-3 in the cervical spinal cord. *In situ* hybridization of slit-1 (A-F), slit-2 (G-L), slit-3 (M-R) mRNA in the unlesioned cervical spinal cord. Strong signals for slit-1 (A) and slit-2 (G) are detected with the anti-sense probe in cervical interneurons and motoneurons while slit-3 (M) shows a weaker signal. No signals are detected with the sense probes for slit-1 (B), slit-2 (H) or slit-3 (N). (C, I, O) Epifluorescence images of double-labeled neurons in the ventral horn (NeuN: green; *In situ* signal: red). (D-F) Co-localization of slit-1 mRNA in glycinergic neurons (D; GlyT2: green; slit-1: red), LPSN (E; LPSN: green; slit-1: red; NT435: blue) and SPSN (F; SPSN: green; slit-1: red; NT435: blue) in the cervical spinal cord. (J-L) Co-localization of slit-2 mRNA in glycinergic neurons (J; GlyT2: green; slit-2: red), LPSN (K; LPSN: green; slit-2: red; NT435: blue) and SPSN (L; SPSN: green; slit-2: red; NT435: blue) in the cervical spinal cord. (P-R) Co-localization of slit-3 mRNA in glycinergic neurons (P; GlyT2: green; slit-3: red), LPSN (Q; LPSN: green; slit-3: red; NT435: blue) and SPSN (R; SPSN: green; slit-3: red; NT435: blue) in the cervical spinal cord. (S-U) Quantification of the proportion of glycinergic neurons, LPSN and SPSN expressing slit-1 (S), slit-2 (T) and slit-3 (U) in the unlesioned and lesioned cervical spinal cord. Scale bars in A,B,G,H,M,N, 250 μm; Scale bars in C,I,O, 25 μm; Scale bars in D-F,J-K,P-R, 25 μm.

immunolabelling, we first imaged sections immunostained for NeuN using a confocal microscope (FV1000, Olympus). The sections were then unmounted, ISH was performed as described above before the same sections were then re-imaged with a confocal microscope using bright field illumination. Both images (that were acquired with the same magnification) were overlaid in Photoshop (Adobe) and a number of anatomical landmarks including the central canal and the ventral and dorsal border between the gray and white matter were used as fiduciary marks to co-register the images and adjust for tissue shrinkage due to the ISH process. For imaging retrogradely-labeled CST neurons, we first imaged the fluorescence signals using a confocal microscope (FV1000, Olympus) using standard filter settings before we unmounted the sections, performed ISH and image alignment as described above. To assess the presence of ISH signals in transgenically-labeled glycinergic interneurons, we first imaged

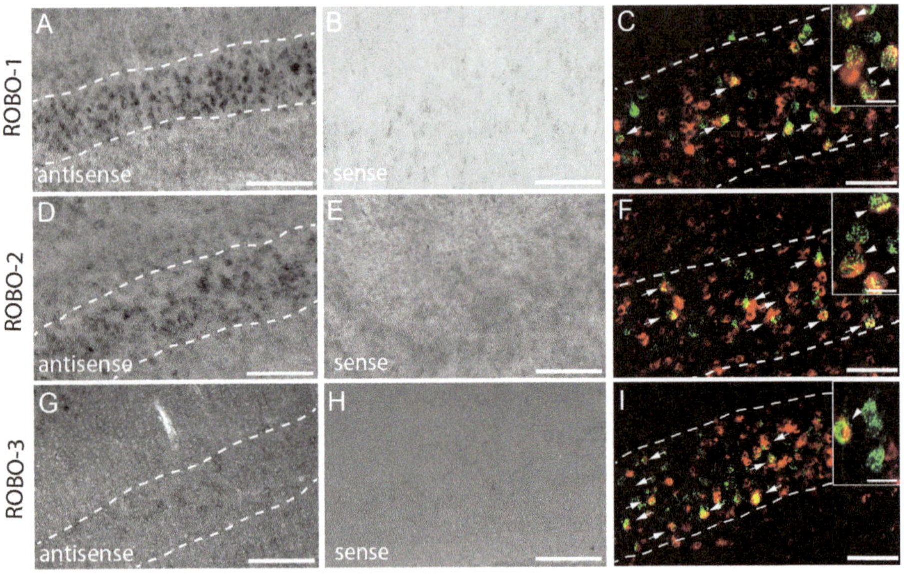

Figure 2. ***In Situ*** **hybridization pattern of Robo-1,-2,-3 in the cortex.** *In situ* hybridization of Robo-1 (A), Robo-2 (D) and Robo-3 (G) mRNA in the cortex. No signals are detected with the sense probes (B: Robo-1; E: Robo-2; H: Robo-3). Dotted lines in A, D, and G represent layer V. (C,F, I) Epifluorescence images of double-labeled neurons of layer V (Retrogradely-labeled CST neurons: green; *In situ* signal: red).Scale bars in A,B,D,E,G,H: 100 μm; Scale bars in C,F,I: 50 μm (25 μm in insets).

the fluorescence signals using an epifluorescence Olympus IX71 microscope using standard filter settings before we unmounted the sections, performed ISH and image alignment as described above. Retrogradely-labeled propriospinal neurons were imaged using an epifluorescence Olympus IX71 concomitantly for fluoro-emerald and ISH signals as the ISH did not interfere with this fluorescent label.

Image analysis and cell counts

Retrogradely-labeled cortical projection neurons and propriospinal neurons were assessed under the fluorescent microscope by alternating between the fluorescence and the bright field. Glycinergic neurons were assessed on the acquired images.

To determine the proportion of cortical projection neurons that express a given molecule, we counted all retrogradely-labeled neurons on every third sections of the cortex (n = 3 mice). Sections were assessed from anterior to posterior and the analysis began with the first section in which retrogradely-labeled CST neurons appeared. To determine the proportion of glycinergic neurons that express a given molecule, three sections at C3/C4 and three sections at C5 were randomly selected. Then, all glycinergic neurons in lamina VI to IX (which are the laminae in which long and short propriospinal neurons are located) were assessed (n = 3 mice). To determine the proportion of long and short propriospinal neurons that express a given molecule, all retrogradely-labeled neurons located from C3 to C5 were counted until the number of cells reached 30 per animal (about 10 sections per animal, n = 3 mice) taking the first section as the section in which propriospinal neurons were first detected. Results were expressed as a ratio of the number of double-labeled neurons compared to the total number of assessed neurons. All counts were performed by an independent blinded-observer. To assess co-localization we used the following evaluation criteria: A cell was considered countable when the contour of its soma could be clearly identified either based in the retrograde label or based on the fluorescent transgenic label. ISH signals were considered to be overlaying when they followed the contour of the soma and did not extend beyond it.

For generating the rating in Table 2 and 3, we first defined the area for the analysis e.g. laminae VI to IX for the spinal cord or in the cortex at −1.3 from bregma starting at +/− 1 mm from the midline. To assess the expression in different cortical layers we used a box of 35 μm^2 that was overlaid on layer 1, or 2 or 3 or 4 or 5 or 6 of the cortex. We then set the threshold for detection and measured the grayscale intensity of the selected area with the ImageJ Measurement Tool. Values below 500 were defined as not detected; Values between 500 and 1500 were defined as +; Values between 1500 and 2500 were defined as ++; Values between 2500 and 3500 were defined as +++; Values above 3500 were defined as ++++.

Statistical analysis

Results are given as mean ± SEM unless indicated otherwise. Data were analyzed in GraphPad Prism5.01 software using a two-way ANOVA (factors: time and interneuron-type) followed by Bonferroni post hoc tests. Significance levels was taken with $p < 0.01$.

Results

Expression of the repulsive axon guidance cues slit-1, -2 and -3 and their receptors in the adult CNS

The process of axon pathfinding is mediated by a number of guidance molecules, among them slits (slit-1,-2,-3) and their receptors (robo-1,-2,-3), which have been shown to have a repulsive effect on axons during development [22–23] and have been proposed to restrict axonal growth at the lesion site following spinal cord injury [24]. To assess whether slits can also regulate axon growth during axonal remodelling distant from the lesion site we first investigated the expression of slit family members in the unlesioned mouse spinal cord by *in situ* hybridization. Hybridization with the anti-sense probe shows that slit-1, slit-2 and slit-3 mRNAs are detected in all laminae of the cervical gray matter (Fig. 1A,G,M) while hybridization with the sense probe showed no signal (Fig. 1B,H,N). In particular, slit-1 and slit-2 show high

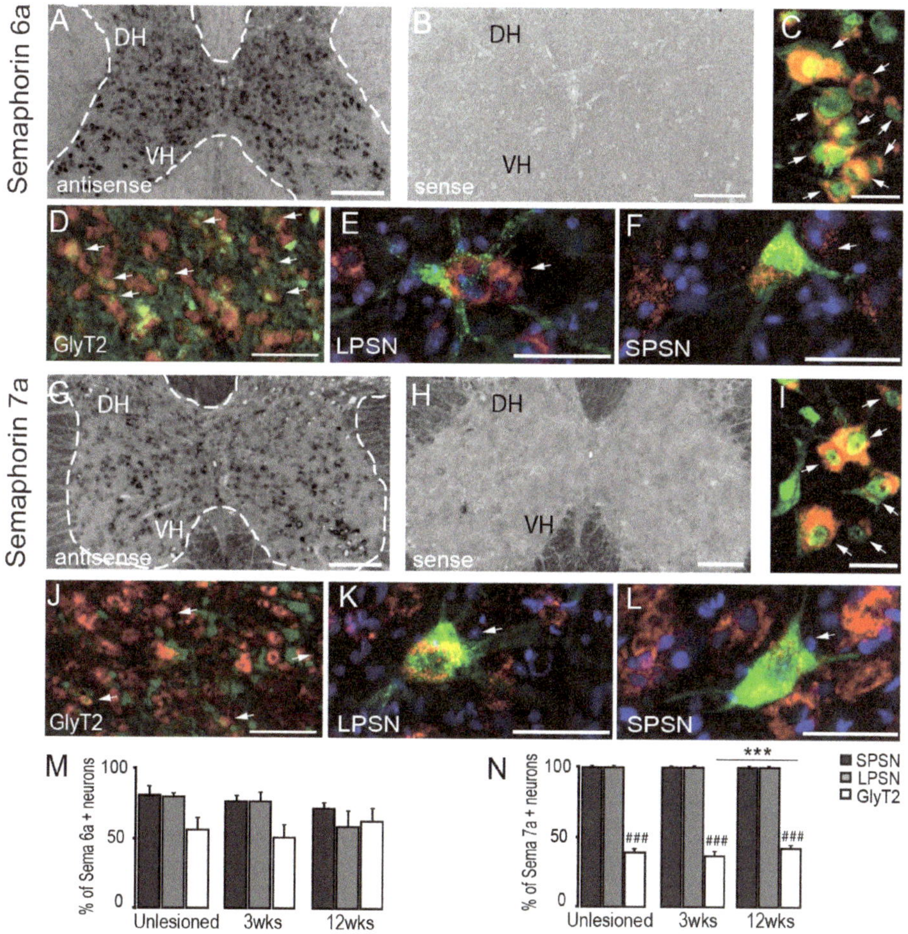

Figure 3. *In Situ* hybridization pattern of Semaphorin 6a and Semaphorin 7a in the cervical spinal cord. *In situ* hybridization of Semaphorin 6a (A) mRNA in the unlesioned cervical spinal cord. Strong signal for Semaphorin 6a (A) is detected with the anti-sense probe. No signal is detected with the sense probe (B). (C) Confocal picture of double-labeled neurons in the ventral horn (NeuN: green; Semaphorin 6a: red). (D-F) Co-localization of Semaphorin 6a mRNA in glycinergic neurons (D; GlyT2: green, Semaphorin6a: red), LPSN (E; LPSN: green, Semaphorin 6a: red, NT435: blue), and SPSN (F; SPSN: green, Semaphorin 6a: red, NT435: blue) in the cervical spinal cord. *In situ* hybridization of Semaphorin 7a (G) mRNA in the unlesioned cervical spinal cord. Moderate signals for semaphorin 7a in inter- and motoneurons for Semaphorin 7a (G) is detected with the anti-sense probe. No signal is detected with the sense probes (H). (I) Confocal image of double-labeled neurons in the ventral horn (NeuN : green; Semaphorin 7a: red). (J-L) Co-localization of Semaphorin 7a mRNA in glycinergic neurons (D; GlyT2: green, Semaphorin 7a: red), LPSN (E; LPSN: green, Semaphorin 7a: red, NT435: blue), and SPSN (F, SPSN: green, Semaphorin 7a: red, NT435: blue) in the cervical spinal cord. (M, N) Quantification of the number of GlyT2, LPSN and SPSN expressing Semaphorin 6a (M) and semaphorin 7a (N) in unlesioned and lesioned cervical spinal cord. DH: dorsal horn; VH: ventral horn. Arrows in D and J show double-labeled glycinergic neurons. Scale bars in A, B, G, H: 250 µm; Scale bars in C, I: 25 µm; Scale bars in E, F, K, L: 25 µm; Scale bars in D, J: 50 µm.

expression levels throughout the spinal gray matter and in particular in the ventral horn (Table 2) while slit-3 mRNA seems to be expressed at a lower level. Analysis after counterstaining with NeuN suggests that slits are expressed by neurons including by interneurons and motoneurons (Fig. 1C,I,O). To better understand which populations of spinal interneurons express slit mRNA, we visualized glycinergic interneurons using a transgenic label (Fig. 1D,J,P) and LPSN (Fig. 1E,K,Q) and SPSN (Fig. 1F,L,R) using retrograde labelling . Our results show that, 60 to 80% of all propriospinal neurons but only about 30% of glycinergic interneurons express slit-1, -2 and -3 (Fig. 1S-U). While overall this expression pattern is rather unchanged in the cervical spinal cord of mice at 3 and 12 weeks after injury, there is a moderate but significant increase in the proportion of propriospinal neurons that expressed slit-1 or slit-3 after injury (Fig. 1 S-U).

To determine whether the corticospinal collaterals that enter the spinal gray matter can respond to slits expressed by spinal interneurons we examined the expression of the corresponding slit-receptors (robo-1, -2, -3) in the mouse cortex by *in situ* hybridization . In the cortex, robo-1 can be detected in layer I to VI, with its strongest expression in the cells of layer V (Table 3 and Fig. 2A). Robo-2 is expressed from layer II to VI in the cortex, with a slightly more intense labelling in layer V (Fig. 2D). Additionally, robo-3 mRNA is detectable in layer II, V and VI although the expression level is very low (Fig. 2G). Specificity of the staining was validated by hybridization of the tissue with the sense probe which showed no signals (Fig. 2 B,E,H). Retrograde labelling with Texas Red® revealed that 90,2±3,4% of CST projection neurons in layer V express robo-1, 55,2±5,2% of CST projection neurons express robo-2 and that 26,4±1,9% of CST projection neurons express robo-3 (Fig. 2 C,F,I).

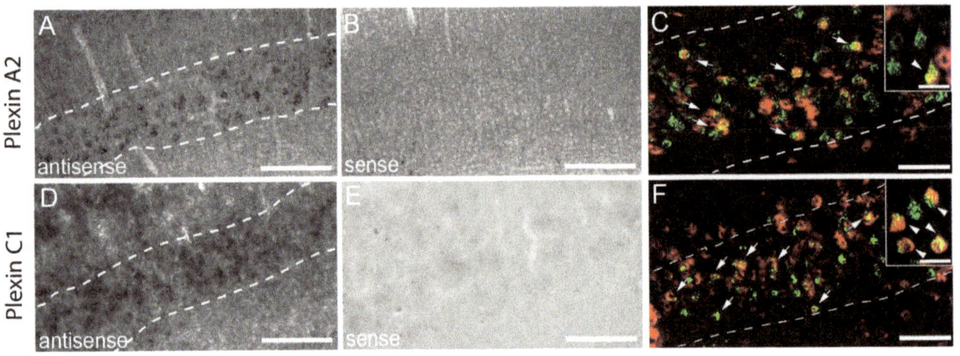

Figure 4. ***In Situ*** **hybridization pattern of plexin A2 and plexin C1 in the cortex.** *In situ* hybridization of PlexinA2 in the cortex (A). No signal is detected with the Sema6a sense probe (B). Dotted lines in A represent layer V of the cortex. (C) Confocal image of double-labeled neurons of layer V (retrogradely-labeled CST projection neurons, green; plexin A2, red). *In situ* hybridization of PlexinC1 in the cortex (D). No signal is detected with the Sema7a sense probes (E). Dotted lines in D represent layer V of the cortex. (F) Confocal picture of double-labeled CST projection neurons identified by retrograde tracing (retrogradely-labeled CST projection neurons, green; plexin C1, red). Scale bars in A,B,D,E: 100 μm; Scale bars in C, F: 50 μm (25 μm in insets).

Expression of the guidance cues semaphorin 6a (Sema6a) and semaphorin 7a (Sema7a) and their receptors plexin A2 and plexin C1 in the adult CNS

The repulsive membrane associated Sema6a has been shown to control axon guidance in different parts of the nervous system [25-27] and specifically to affect the growth of the developing CST at multiple choice points [28]. We now investigated the expression pattern of Sema6a in the cervical spinal cord of healthy mice by *in situ* hybridization. While Sema6a mRNA is specifically present throughout the spinal gray matter (Fig. 3A,B) the hybridization signals are more intense in the middle and ventral laminae (IV – IX) of the spinal cord than in the dorsal horn (Fig. 3A and Table 2). Morphology analysis after counterstaining with NeuN suggests that in the gray matter Sema6a is primarily expressed by neurons and in particular by interneurons (Fig. 3C). Sema6a mRNA is also present in cells in the dorsal and ventral white matter (Table 2), consistent with the reported expression of Sema6a in oligodendrocytes, [25].

Analysis of different interneuronal populations revealed that the majority of glycinergic interneurons as well as LPSN and SPSN contain Sema6a mRNA (Fig. 3D-F) both before and at 3 and 12 weeks after a thoracic spinal cord injury (Fig. 3M).

In contrast to Sema6a, semaphorin7a (Sema7a) is an attractive guidance cue that supports axonal growth [29]. In order to determine the expression pattern of Sema7a, we hybridized a Sema7a anti-sense probe to sections from the cervical spinal cord of healthy mice. We can show that Sema7a is specifically expressed in all laminae of the spinal cord (I – IX; Table 2 and Fig. 3G,H) with the strongest expression in ventral and intermediate laminae (Table 2). Cells that expressed Sema7a morphologically resembled interneurons (Fig. 3I) and further anaylsis revealed that all long and short propriospinal neurons but only about 40% of glycinergic interneurons expressed Sema7a both in the healthy spinal cord as well as 3 and 12 weeks after spinal cord injury (Fig. 3J-L, N).

To determine whether corticospinal axons can integrate attractive or repulsive signals from Sema6a or 7a, we detected the mRNA coding for the main receptor of Sema6a, plexinA2, and the receptor for Sema7a, plexinC1 in the mouse cortex by *in situ* hybridization. Our results show specific expression of plexinA2 in layers II-III and V-VI of the cortex (Fig. 4.A,B and Table 3) and specific expression of plexinC1 in in layers II-III and V (Fig. 4D,E and Table 3) Notably, both plexinA2 and plexinC1 are expressed in retrogradely-labeled CST projection neurons in layer V(plexinA2: 54,0±3,65%; plexinC1: 70,0±2,00%) (Fig. 4C,F).

Expression of the bidirectional synaptogenic cues SynCAM1, SynCAM3 and SynCAM4 in the adult CNS

Once the newly growing collaterals have been guided to their target cells, they need to make appropriate synaptic connections. During development this process is regulated by molecules like the synaptic cell adhesion molecules (SynCAM) that promote synapse formation and maturation [7]. In order to determine the expression pattern of these bidirectional synaptic cues we analysed the mRNA expression of SynCAM1, 3 and 4 in the cervical spinal cord. In adult healthy mice SynCAM1, 3, 4 expression appears to be limited to the gray matter with particular strong signals seen in the ventral horn (Fig. 5A,B,G,H,M, N and Table 2). Morphology analysis after counterstaining with NeuN indicates that SynCAMs are primarily expressed by neurons including by interneurons and motoneurons (Fig. 5C,I,O). Expression in motoneurons was confirmed by ChAT immunostaining (data not shown).

In line with these findings, mRNAs for SynCAM1, 3 and 4 can be detected in the majority of LPSN, SPSN and glycinergic interneurons (Fig. 5D-F,J-L,P-R,S-U). Mostly similar expression patterns were observed in the cervical spinal cord of healthy mice and the cervical cord of mice perfused at 3 or 12 weeks following a thoracic spinal cord injury (Fig. 5 S-U).

Further analysis showed that SynCAM1 and SynCAM4 and to a lesser extent SynCAM3 are also expressed in the cortex (Table 3 and Fig. 6A,B,D,E,G,H). In all cases expression seems to be strongest in layer V neurons. In particular, we show that 69,8±6,5% of retrogradely-labeled layer V CST projection neurons express SynCAM1; 73,1±7,3% SynCAM3 and 94,7±0,3% SynCAM4 (Fig. 6C,F,I).

Expression of pre-synaptic organizers neuroligin-1 (NL1) and neuroligin-4 (NL4) in the adult spinal cord

Neuroligins are postsynaptic adhesion proteins, which have been shown to promote synapse maturation and synaptic function [30]. Their receptors, the neurexins, have been shown to be widely expressed not only in development but also in the adult cortex and in particular in layer V where pyramidal cells reside [31]. We analyzed NL1 and NL4 expression in the cervical spinal cord of adult mice by *in situ* hybridization. Both NLs are strongly

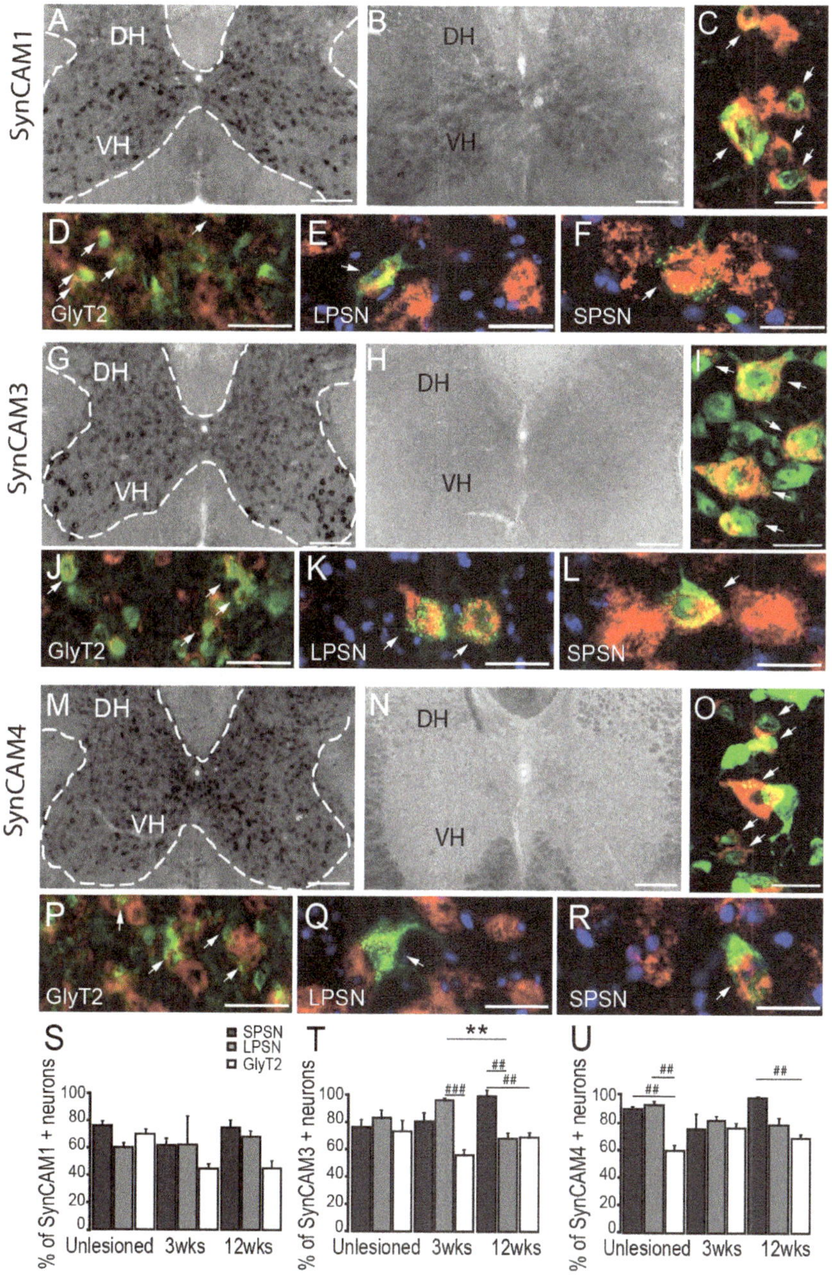

Figure 5. *In Situ* hybridization pattern of SynCAM1, SynCAM 3, SynCAM 4 in the cervical spinal cord. *In situ* hybridization of SynCAM1 (A) mRNA in the unlesioned spinal cord. Strong signal for SynCAM1 (A) is detected with the anti-sense probe. No signal is detected with the sense probe (B). (C) Epifluorescence picture of double-labeled neurons in the ventral horn (NeuN: green; SynCAM1: red). (D-F) Co-localization of SynCAM1mRNA in glycinergic neurons (D; GlyT2: green; SynCAM1: red), LPSN (E; LPSN: green; SynCAM1: red; NT435: blue) and SPSN (F; SPSN: green; SynCAM1: red; NT435: blue) in the cervical spinal cord. *In situ* hybridization of SynCAM3 (G) in the unlesioned spinal cord. Moderate signal for SynCAM3 (G) mRNA is detected with the anti-sense probe. No signal is detected with the sense probe (H). (I) Epifluorescence picture of double-labeled neurons in the ventral horn (NeuN: green; SynCAM3: red). (J-L) Co-localization of SynCAM3 in glycinergic neurons (J; GlyT2: green; SynCAM3: red), in LPSN (K; LPSN: green; SynCAM3: red; NT435: blue) and SPSN (L, SPSN, green; SynCAM3, red; NT435: blue) in the cervical spinal cord. *In situ* hybridization of SynCAM4 (M) in the unlesioned spinal cord. Strong signal for SynCAM4 (M) is detected with the anti-sense probe. No signal is detected with the sense probe (N). (O) Epifluorescence image of double-labeled neurons in the ventral horn (NeuN: green; SynCAM4: red). (P-R) Co-localization of SynCAM4 in glycinergic neurons (P; GlyT2: green; SynCAM4: red), in LPSN (Q; LPSN, green; SynCAM4, red; NT435: blue) and SPSN (R; SPSN, green; SynCAM4, red; NT435: blue) in the cervical spinal cord. (S-U) Quantification of the number of GlyT2 neurons, LPSN and SPSN expressing SynCAM1 (S), SynCAM3 (T) and SynCAM4 (U) in unlesioned and lesioned cervical spinal cord. DH: dorsal horn; VH: ventral horn. Arrows in D, J and P show double-labeled glycinergic neurons. Scale bar in A,B,G,H,M,N: 250 μm; Scale bar in C,I,O: 25 μm; Scale bars in D,J,P: 40 μm; Scale bars in E,F,K,L,Q,R: 25 μm.

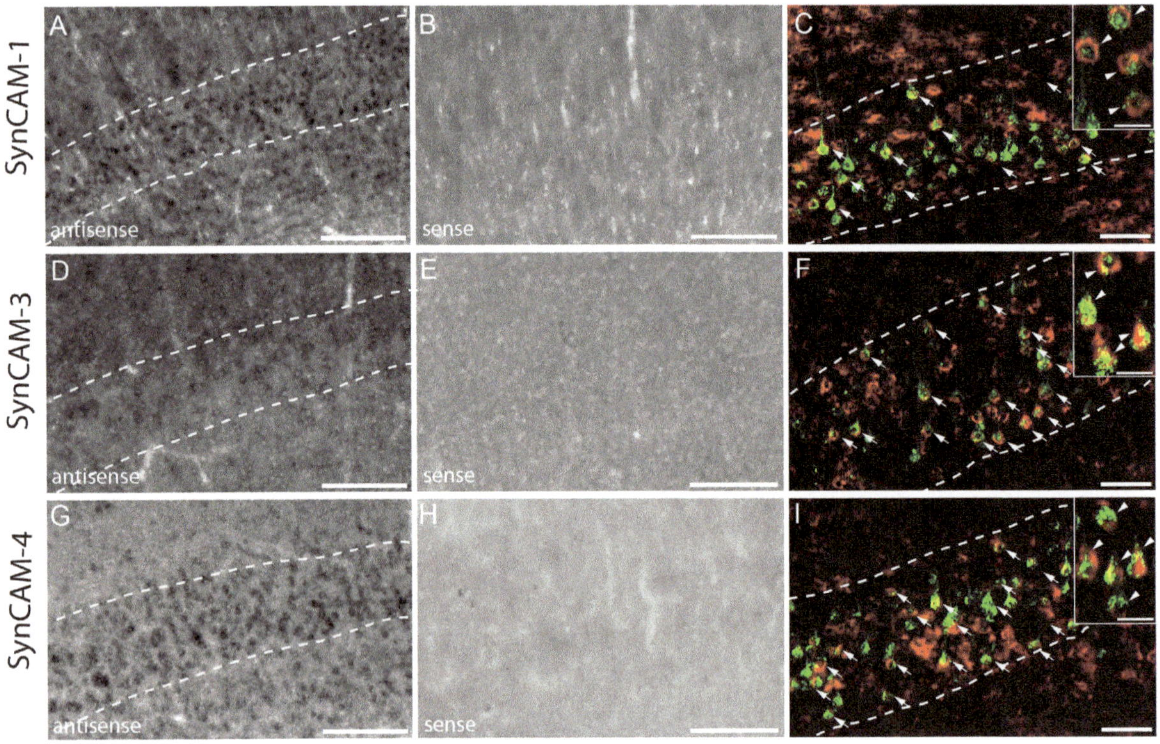

Figure 6. ***In Situ*** **hybridization profile of SynCAM1, SynCAM 3, SynCAM 4 in the cortex.** Profile of expression of SynCAM1 (A) mRNA in the cortex. No signal is detected with the SynCAM1 sense probe (B). Dotted lines in A represent layer V of the cortex. (C) Confocal image of double-labeled neurons of layer V (retrogradely-labeled CST neurons: green; SynCAM1: red). Profile of expression of SynCAM3 (D) mRNA in the cortex. No signal is detected with the sense SynCAM3 probe (E). Dotted lines in D represent layer V of the cortex. (F) Confocal image of CST projection neurons (retrogradely-labeled CST neurons: green, SynCAM3: red).). Profile of expression of SynCAM4 (G) mRNA in the cortex. No signal is detected with the sense SynCAM4 probe (H). Dotted lines in G represent layer V of the cortex. (I) Confocal image of double-labeled CST projection neurons (retrogradely-labeled CST projection neurons: green; SynCAM4: red). Scale bar in A, B, D, E, G, H: 100 μm; Scale bar in C,F,I: 50 μm (25 μm in insets).

expressed throughout all laminae of the spinal gray matter (Table 2 and Fig. 7A,F). The analysis of different groups of spinal interneurons reveals that significantly higher percentage of long and short propriospinal neurons express NL1 compared to glycinergic neurons (Fig. 7B-E). In contrast no prominent differences in NL4 expression were observed between the different interneuronal populations studied (Fig. 7G-J). Further, the presence of a thoracic spinal cord injury did not change the expression pattern of either NL1 or NL4 in the cervical spinal cord (Fig. 7 I,J).

Expression of bidirectional guidance and synaptogenic cues ephrinB1 and ephB2 in the adult CNS

Ephrins and their receptors (Eph) are pleiotropic molecules involved in cell migration, axon guidance [32] and synapse formation [33] during nervous system development. Interestingly, eph-ephrin interactions can mediate both repulsive and attractive forces between cells [34]. EphB-ephrinB interaction has been shown to be important for proper ipsilateral targeting of CST and retinal axons [35–37]. *In situ* hybridization revealed that both ephB2 and ephrinB1mRNA are expressed throughout all laminae of the gray matter of the cervical spinal cord (Fig. 8A,B,G,H) with EphrinB1 having a dimmer expression in laminae I-IV (Table 2). Morphology analysis after counterstaining with NeuN suggests that both molecules are primarily expressed by neurons including by interneurons and at least in the case of EphB2 also motoneurons (Fig. 8C,I). Further characterization indeed showed that both EphB2 and Ephrin B1 are expressed in different interneuronal population located in the cervical spinal cord including LPSN, SPSN and glycinergic interneurons (Fig. 8D-F, J-L). While EphB2 mRNA is expressed by a similar proportion of these interneurons, Ephrin B1 was particularly prominently expressed in short propriospinal neurons in the healthy cervical spinal cord. Mostly, these expression patterns in the cervical spinal cord were not affected by the presence of a thoracic spinal cord injury (Fig. 8 M,N). The only exception is that the percentage of glycinergic interneurons expressing EphB2 was increased in the cervical spinal cord at 3 weeks post injury and decreased at 12 weeks after injury. Further expression analysis of cortical sections showed that both, Ephrin B1 and EphB2, were also expressed in layer II-III and layer V of the cortex (Fig. 9 A,B,D,E and Table 3). Retrograde labelling of layer V CST projection neurons revealed that 84, 6±3,5% of CST projection neurons express EphrinB1 and 74,1±2,2% EphB2 (Fig. 9 C,F).

Discussion

While a number of the cues that determine the formation of neuronal circuits during the development of the nervous system have been identified, it is currently unclear which molecular signals can attract growing axon collaterals and initiate the formation of synapses during the remodelling of circuits in the injured adult CNS. The aim of this work was to study the expression of chemotropic and synaptogenic factors in the cervical spinal cord of adult mice to determine which of these cues are presented by spinal interneurons in the mature CNS. We focused

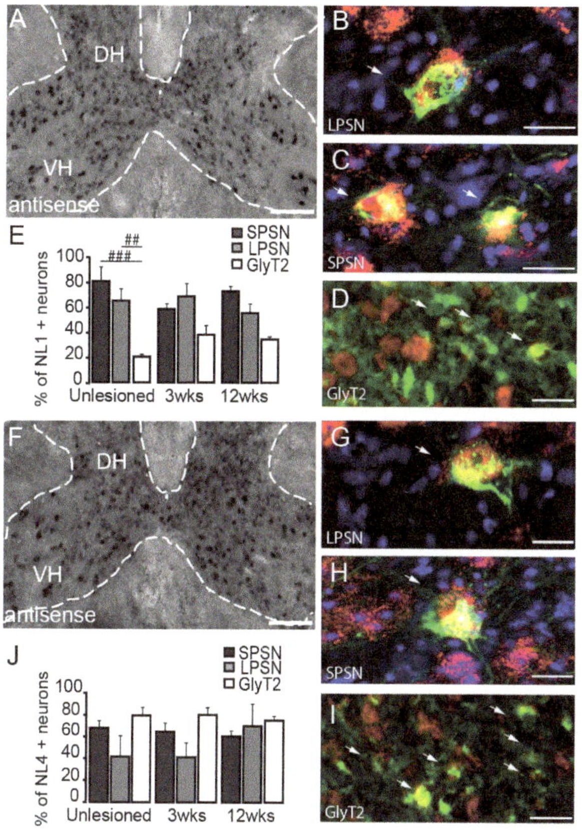

Figure 7. *In Situ* hybridization pattern of NL-1 and NL-4 in the cervical spinal cord. *In situ* hybridization of NL1 (A) and NL4 (F) mRNA in the unlesioned cervical spinal cord. Intense signals for NL1 (interneurons, A) and NL4 (inter- and motoneurons, F) are detected with the anti-sense probe. (B-D) Co-localization of NL1 in LPSN (B; LPSN: green; NL1: red; NT435: blue), SPSN (C; SPSN: green; NL1: red; NT435: blue) glycinergic neurons (D; GlyT2, green; NL1, red) in the cervical spinal cord. (E) Quantification of the number of GlyT2, LPSN and SPSN expressing NL1 in unlesioned and lesioned cervical spinal cord. (G-I) Co-localization of NL4 in LPSN (G; LPSN: green; NL4: red; NT435: blue), SPSN (H; SPSN: green; NL4: red; NT435: blue) glycinergic neurons (I; GlyT2: green; NL4: red) in the cervical spinal cord. (J) Quantification of the number of GlyT2, LPSN and SPSN expressing NL4 in normal and lesioned cervical spinal cord. DH: dorsal horn; VH: ventral horn. Arrows in D and I show double-labeled glycinergic neurons.Scale bar in A and F: 250 µm; Scale bar in B,C,G,H: 25 µm; Scale bar in D,I: 40 µm.

our analysis on the cervical spinal cord – an area remote from the lesion site – as we and others have previously shown that new CST contacts with local cervical interneurons such as long propriospinal neurons play a key role during axonal remodelling following spinal cord injury [11–13]. While gene expression changes are certainly magnified at the lesion site [38–41], first reports indicate that a spinal lesion might also affect, although more moderately, gene expression changes more remote from the lesion site [38;41;42]. We mostly concentrated our efforts on membrane-bound molecules [7,26,43–47] as these are best suited to explain the attraction or repulsion of growing CST collaterals towards or from distinct spinal interneurons. To elucidate if and how the expression of these molecules in the cervical spinal cord changes following injury we analyzed the expression pattern at two time points following a midthoracic spinal cord injury. At 3 weeks after lesion when newly formed CST collaterals first initiate contact with spinal interneurons and 9 weeks later when these contacts have been refined [11,13]. Our study now shows that (i) all the guidance and synaptogenic cues studied were not only expressed in the developing CNS but also expressed in the adult nervous system. (ii) While we did not detect cues that were exclusively expressed in a subpopulation of spinal interneurons, some molecules studied e.g. slits, Sema7a, SynCAM4 and NL1 were preferentially expressed in propriospinal neurons compared to glycinergic neurons. (iii) The expression pattern of guidance and synaptogenic molecules appeared to be stable over time and was by large not affected by a thoracic hemisection. It is interesting to note that the individual cues appear to be quite uniformly expressed throughout the different laminae of the adult spinal cord. This expression pattern is distinct from the region-specific pattern observed during neuronal development. For example, Semaphorin 3 mRNA is expressed between E13 and E 17 in the entire ventral half of the spinal cord but not in the floor plate [48]. Conversely, Slits are essentially expressed in the floor plate during development [49,50]. Similarly it has been shown that expression of EphrinB ligands is confined to discrete regions of the spinal cord during development with for example EphrinB3 expression being localized to the floor plate around the ventral midline while EphrinB2 and B1 are primarily present in the dorsal spinal cord [51,52]. The different regional expression pattern observed in the developing and adult spinal cord also indicates that the role of guidance and synaptogenic molecules might evolve in adulthood - classical repulsive cues in development might indeed become attractive in adulthood or conversely. While the exact role of these molecules in adulthood thus still needs to be better defined, their abundant expression suggests that they also can influence the formation and stabilization of circuits in the adult spinal cord. This view is supported by our finding that all receptors for guidance and synaptogenic molecules that we probed for were expressed in the cell bodies of CST projection neurons that reside in lamina V of the cortex. While we can formally only show that mRNAs are expressed in the neuronal cell body we believe that it is highly likely that functional receptors are present on growing CST axons as numerous studies in development show that the guidance and synaptogenic molecules that bind to these receptors factors can influence the behavior of CST axons [28,35,53]. In the following paragraphs, we summarize the expression pattern of the different families of chemotropic and synaptogenic cues and discuss their potential relevance in the context of the post-injury remodelling of axonal connections.

Slit and Robo family

The attractive or repulsive action of axonal guidance cues in the developing nervous system has been documented extensively (for reviews see [54,55]). One family of these guidance cues are the slit molecules (slit-1, slit-2 or slit-3) and their binding partners the Robo-receptors [56]. These molecules have, for example, been shown to prevent commissural neurons from re-crossing the midline in *Drosophila* [23]. More recently it has been suggested that slits are also expressed after spinal cord injury and can contribute to the failure of axon regeneration at the lesion site in the adult CNS [24]. We can show that slits are not only expressed at the lesion site [24,56] but also in the cervical spinal cord of unlesioned animals. Their receptors in particular robo-1 and robo-2 are expressed throughout the forebrain while robo-3 is more sparsely expressed. This wide-spread expression of slits and robos in the adult CNS has previously been reported and suggests that these molecules also play an important role in the adult nervous system [57]. It is interesting to note that the slits were preferentially expressed by propriospinal neurons compared to glycinergic neurons. As propriospinal neurons are efficiently contacted by

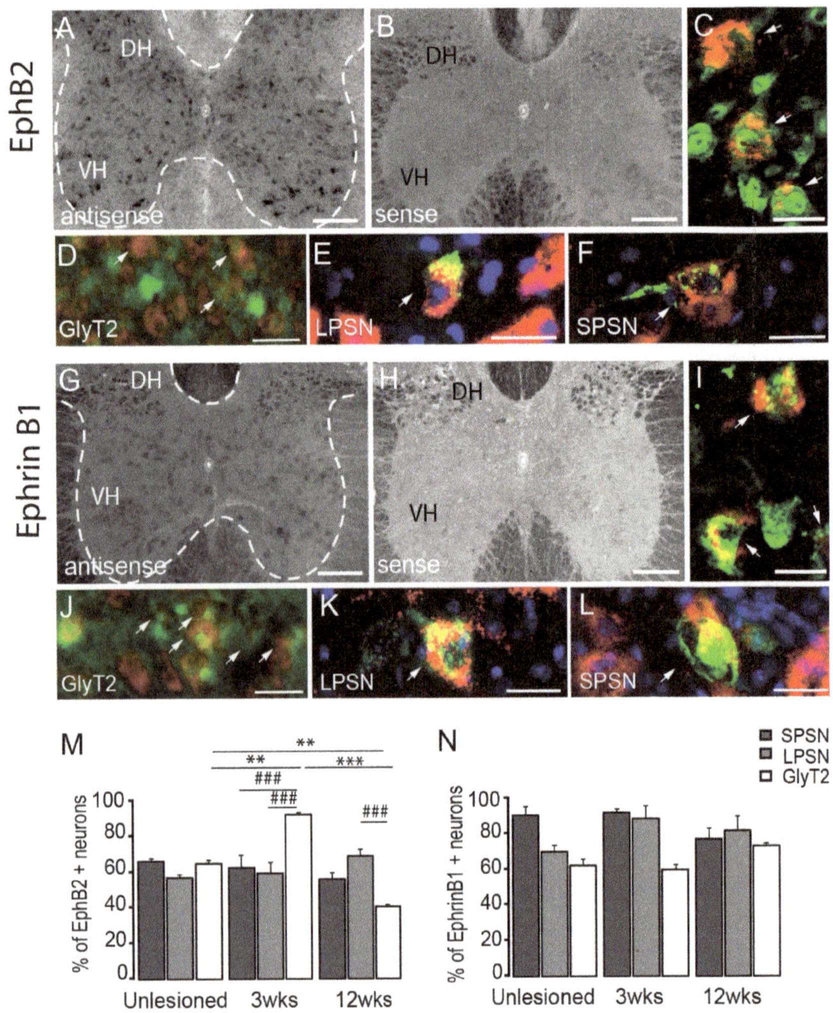

Figure 8. ***In Situ*** **hybridization pattern of EphB2 and EphrinB1 in the cervical spinal cord.** *In situ* hybridization of EphB2 (A), mRNA in the unlesioned cervical spinal cord. Intense signals for EphB2 is detected in inter- and motoneurons with the anti-sense (A). No signal is detected with the sense probe (B). (C) Confocal picture of double-labeled neurons in the ventral horn (NeuN, green; EphB2, red). (D-F) Co-localization of EphB2 in glycinergic neurons (D; GlyT2, green; EphB2, red), in LPSN (E; LPSN: green; EphB2: red; NT435: blue) and SPSN (F; SPSN, green; EphB2, red; NT435: blue) in the cervical spinal cord. *In situ* hybridization of EphrinB1 (G), mRNA in the unlesioned cervical spinal cord. Moderate signal for EphrinB1 is detected in inter- and motoneurons with the anti-sense probe (G). No signal is detected with the sense probe (H). (I) Confocal picture of double-labeled neurons in the ventral horn (NeuN: green; EphrinB1: red). (J-L) Co-localization of EphrinB1 in glycinergic neurons (J; GlyT2: green; EphrinB1: red), in LPSN (K; LPSN, green; EphrinB1, red; Neurotrace, blue) and SPSN (L; SPSN: green; EphrinB1: red; NT435: blue) in the cervical spinal cord. DH: dorsal horn; VH: ventral horn. Arrows in D and J show double-labeled glycinergic neurons.Scale bars in A, B,G,H: 250 μm; Scale bar in C,I: 25 μm; Scale bars in D,J: 40 μm; Scale bars in E,F,K,L: 25 μm.

growing CST collaterals this might indicate that, in adulthood after injury, slit expression preferentially triggers neurite growth and arborisation rather than neurite repulsion as it has been shown for cortical interneurons during corticogenesis [58,59].

Semaphorin 6a and 7a and PlexinA2 and C1

Similarly to slits and robos, semaphorins and their receptors, the plexins [4,28,29,60] have been implicated in the control of multiple aspects of neural development, including cell migration and axon guidance [61,62]. In particular the transmembrane class 6 and 7 semaphorins, have been shown to be crucial regulators of axon growth, guidance and cell migration in many different parts of the brain [26–29,62]. In this study we observed that Sema6a and Sema7a are expressed throughout the cervical gray matter. As previously reported, we found that plexinA2 and plexinC1, the respective receptors of Sema6a and Sema7a are expressed in the cortex in particular layer V where the cell bodies of the corticospinal tract resides [63,64]. Interestingly, Sema7a is expressed by all propriospinal neurons but only some glycinergic neurons. As Sema7a is an attractive cue [63] that has been shown to promote axon growth [29] its expression might help to direct growing corticospinal collaterals towards propriospinal neurons during post-injury remodelling. A thoracic hemisection did not change the expression of semaphorin 6a and 7a in the cervical cord. This is in contrast to changes at the site of injury where Sema7a expression is increased in neurons, endothelial cells and components of the glial scar [65].

SynCAMs

For circuits to remodel successfully growing collaterals not only need to reach their appropriate target cells but also form new synaptic connection. The formation of synapses requires the

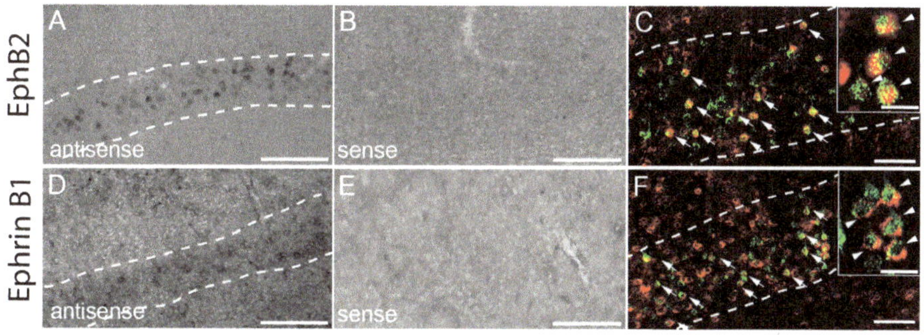

Figure 9. *In Situ* hybridization profile of EphB2 and EphrinB1 in cervical interneurons. *In situ* hybridization of EphB2 (A), EphrinB1 (B) mRNA in the cortex. No signal is detected with the sense probes for EphB2 (B) and EphrinB1 (E). Dotted lines in A and B represent layer V of the cortex. (C, F) Confocal images of double-labeled CST projection neurons (C; retrogradely-labeled CST projection neurons: green; EphB2: red and F; retrogradely-labeled CST projection neurons: green; EphrinB1: red). Scale bars in A, B, D, E: 100 μm; Scale bars C,F: 50 μm (25 μm in insets).

involvement of trans-synaptic adhesion molecules which span the synaptic cleft [66]. How the tight and precise alignment of the pre- and postsynaptic sites is achieved is currently under close investigation. In vertebrates this process is thought to be mediated via synaptic adhesion molecules. Synaptic Cell Adhesion Molecules (SynCAMs) comprise a group of four immunoglobulin (Ig) superfamily members that are crucial for the establishment of new synapses during development [66]. Interestingly these molecules are also prominently expressed in the adult brain [7,66] and spinal cord [67,68]. In line with these findings we detected the expression of SynCAM1, 3 and 4 throughout the cortex with a prominent expression in layer V of the cortex. SynCAMs are also present in interneurons and motoneurons in the spinal gray matter. In addition we detected SynCAM expression in the white matter which is consistent with expression in oligodendrocytes that has been reported by Thomas and colleagues [67]. While SynCAM1 and SynCAM3 were similarly expressed in all interneurons studied, SynCAM4 is preferentially expressed in propriospinal neurons. The latter is reminiscent of the differential presence of SynCAMs in excitatory and inhibitory neurons has been reported previously in the hippocampus [67]. Overall however the abundant expression of SynCAMs in the spinal cord suggests that while they might contribute to formation of synaptic contacts between CST collaterals and spinal interneurons [68] they are unlikely to explain the differential targeting and stabilization of contacts observed during intra-spinal remodelling.

Neuroligins

Neuroligins [46,47] and their presynaptic partners, the neurexins [69,70], are another family of molecules that have been shown to regulate the maturation of functional synapses [30,71,72]. The expression of neurexins in the adult murine cortex has been previously documented [31]. In this study we now show that NL1 and NL4 are expressed throughout the cervical gray matter in both interneurons and in particular in the case of NL1 also in motoneurons. This is consistent with studies showing expression of NL2 and NL3 in spinal motoneurons [73]. Interestingly, NL1 was prominently expressed by propriospinal interneurons. As NL1 is known to be important for excitatory synapse formation [74] it might contribute to the establishment of mature synapses between CST collaterals and propriospinal neurons. Overall neuroligin expression in the neurons located distant from the lesion site in the cervical spinal cord did not changes substantially in response to a thoracic spinal cord injury while a downregulation of neuroligin mRNA expression has been previously reported to occur in transected neurons [73].

Ephrin B1 and EphB2

Ephrins and their receptors (Eph) regulate synaptic function and eph-ephrin interactions can activate both repulsive and attractive forces between cells [32]. As a result these interactions can influence crucial aspects of nervous system development including cell migration, axon guidance, and topographic mapping [32]. Interestingly ephB-ephrinB interaction has been shown to control proper ipsilateral targeting in the visual system and in the developmental CST [35–37]. We now find that ephrinB1 and ephB2 are expressed in neurons throughout the spinal gray matter as well as in parts of the white matter. While expression of ephrinB1 and ephB2 in spinal interneurons has not been reported so far, expression in the white matter has already been shown to occur following SCI and expression of ephB2 has been reported in meningeal cells and of ephrinB1 and ephBs in astrocytes [75]. We also show that both ligands are expressed in layer II-III and V of the cortex consistent with previous reports of ephB2 expression in the brain [76,77]. EphrinB1 and ephB2 were expressed in a large proportion of all interneurons studied both before and after spinal cord injury indicating that, similar to SynCAMs, ephrinB1-ephB2 interactions might contribute to the establishment of functional synapses but are unlikely to explain the differential stabilization of synaptic contacts during post-injury remodelling.

In summary, our systematic characterization of the expression pattern of guidance and synaptogenic molecules in the adult cervical spinal cord demonstrates that a large proportion of the cues that regulate developmental circuit formation are also present during the remodelling of circuits after injury. This suggests that many of the mechanistic insights gained by studying the developing nervous system might also help to better understand how the adult nervous system reacts to injury. Clearly, further studies are warranted to define the roles that each of these molecules play during the formation and maturation of new circuits after injury and ultimately to provide new avenues for the therapeutic support of axonal remodelling.

Acknowledgments

We would like to thank Dana Matzek for excellent animal husbandry, Martin Adrian for excellent technical help and Martin Kerschensteiner for critical reading of the manuscript. Additionally we would like to thank J. Pasterkamp, University of Utrecht; R. Klein, Max-Plank-Institute Munich; J. Burré, Stanford University, Palo Alto; F. Suto, Tohoku University,

Sendai; T. Biederer, Yale University, New Haven and I. Dusart, Paris University, Paris for the generous gift of plasmids.

Author Contributions

Conceived and designed the experiments: AJ FMB. Performed the experiments: AJ AS. Analyzed the data: AJ AS. Wrote the paper: AJ FMB.

References

1. Kolodkin AL, Tessier-Lavigne M (2011) Mechanisms and molecules of neuronal wiring: a primer. Cold Spring Harb Perspect Biol 3(6).
2. Fox MA, Umemori H (2006) Seeking long-term relationship: axon and target communicate to organize synaptic differentiation. J Neurochem 97(5): 1215–1231.
3. Kennedy TE, Wang H, Marshall W, Tessier-Lavigne M (2006) Axon guidance by diffusible chemoattractants: a gradient of netrin protein in the developing spinal cord. J Neurosci 26(34): 8866–8874.
4. Behar O, Golden JA, Mashimo H, Schoen FJ, Fishman MC (1996) Semaphorin III is needed for normal patterning and growth of nerves, bones and heart. Nature 383(6600): 525–528.
5. López-Bendito G, Flames N, Ma L, Fouquet C, Di Meglio T, et al. (2007) Robo1 and Robo2 cooperate to control the guidance of major axonal tracts in the mammalian forebrain. J Neurosci 27(13): 3395–3407.
6. Eberhart J, Swartz M, Koblar SA, Pasquale EB, Tanaka H, et al. (2000) Expression of EphA4, ephrin-A2 and ephrin-A5 during axon outgrowth to the hindlimb indicates potential roles in pathfinding. Dev Neurosci 22(3): 237–250.
7. Biederer T, Sara Y, Mozhayeva M, Atasoy D, Liu X, et al. (2002) SynCAM, a synaptic adhesion molecule that drives synapse assembly. Science 297(5586): 1525–1531.
8. Scheiffele P, Fan J, Choih J, Fetter R, Serafini T (2000) Neuroligin expressed in nonneuronal cells triggers presynaptic development in contacting axons. Cell 9; 101(6): 657–669.
9. Graf ER, Zhang X, Jin SX, Linhoff MW, Craig AM (2004) Neurexins induce differentiation of GABA and glutamate postsynaptic specializations via neuroligins. Cell 119(7): 1013–1026.
10. Henkemeyer M, Itkis OS, Ngo M, Hickmott PW, Ethell IM (2003) Multiple EphB receptor tyrosine kinases shape dendritic spines in the hippocampus. J Cell Biol 163(6): 1313–1326.
11. Bareyre FM, Kerschensteiner M, Raineteau O, Mettenleiter TC, Weinmann O, et al. (2004) The injured spinal cord spontaneously forms a new intraspinal circuit in adult rats. Nat Neurosci 7(3): 269–277.
12. Courtine G, Song B, Roy RR, Zhong H, Herrmann JE, et al. (2008) Recovery of supraspinal control of stepping via indirect propriospinal relay connections after spinal cord injury. Nat Med 14(1): 69–74.
13. Lang C, Guo X, Kerschensteiner M, Bareyre FM (2012) Single collateral reconstructions reveal distinct phases of corticospinal remodelling following spinal cord injury. PLoS ONE 7(1): e30461.
14. Weidner N, Ner A, Salimi N, Tuszynski MH (2001) Spontaneous corticospinal axonal plasticity and functional recovery after adult central nervous system injury. Proc Natl Acad Sci U S A 98(6):3513–3518.
15. Alstermark B, Gorska T, Lundberg A, Pettersson LG (1990) Integration in descending motor pathways controlling the forelimb in the cat. 16. Visually guided switching of target-reaching. Exp Brain Res 80(1): 1–11.
16. Alstermark B, Lundberg A, Pinter M, Sasaki S (1987) Subpopulations and functions of long C3-C5 propriospinal neurones. Brain Res 404(1–2): 395–400.
17. Kerschensteiner M, Bareyre FM, Buddeberg BS, Merkler D, Stadelmann C, et al. (2004) Remodelling of axonal connections contributes to recovery in an animal model of multiple sclerosis. J Exp Med 200(8): 1027–1038.
18. Muramatsu R, Takahashi C, Miyake S, Fujimura H, Mochizuki H, et al. (2012) Angiogenesis induced by CNS inflammation promotes neuronal remodelling through vessel-derived prostacyclin. Nat Med 18(11):1658–1664.
19. Dominici N, Keller U, Vallery H, Friedli L, van den Brand R, et al. (2012) Versatile robotic interface to evaluate, enable and train locomotion and balance after neuromotor disorders. Nat Med 18(7): 1142–1147.
20. van den Brand R, Heutschi J, Barraud Q, DiGiovanna J, Bartholdi K, et al. (2012) Restoring voluntary control of locomotion after paralyzing spinal cord injury. Science 336(6085): 1182–1185.
21. Zeilhofer HU, Studler B, Arabadzisz D, Schweizer C, Ahmadi S, et al. (2005) Glycinergic neurons expressing enhanced green fluorescent protein in bacterial artificial chromosome transgenic mice. J Comp Neurol 482(2): 123–141.
22. Brose K, Bland KS, Wang KH, Arnott D, Henzel W, et al. (1999) Slit proteins bind Robo receptors and have an evolutionarily conserved role in repulsive axon guidance. Cell 96(6): 795–806.
23. Kidd T, Brose K, Mitchell KJ, Fetter RD, Tessier-Lavigne M, et al. (1998) Roundabout controls axon-crossing of the CNS midline and defines a novel subfamily of evolutionarily conserved guidance receptors. Cell 92, 205–215.
24. Wehrle R, Camand E, Chedotal A, Sotelo C, Dusart I (2005) Expression of netrin-1, slit-1 and slit-3 but not of slit-2 after cerebellar and spinal cord lesions. Eur J Neurosci 22(9): 2134–2144.
25. Mauti O, Domanitskaya E, Andermatt I, Sadhu R, Stoeckli ET (2007) Semaphorin6A acts as a gate keeper between the central and peripheral nervous system. Neural Dev 2: 28.
26. Kerjan G, Dolan J, Haumaitre C, Schneider-Maunoury S, Fujisawa H, et al. (2005) The transmembrane semaphorin Sema6A controls cerebellar granule cell migration. Nat Neurosci 8: 1516–1524.
27. Suto F, Tsubio M, Kamiya H, Mizuno H, Kiyama Y, et al. (2007) Interactions between Plexin-A2, Plexin-A4, and Semaphorin6A controls lamina-restricted projection of hippocampal mossy fibers. Neuron 53: 535–547.
28. Rünker AE, Little GE, Suto F, Fujisawa H, Mitchell KJ (2008) Semaphorin-6A controls guidance of corticospinal tract axons at multiple choice points. Neural Dev 3: 34.
29. Pasterkamp RJ, Peschon JJ, Spriggs MK, Kolodkin AL (2003) Semaphorin 7A promotes axon outgrowth through integrins and MAPKs. Nature 424(6947): 398–405.
30. Varoqueaux F, Aramuni G, Rawson RL, Mohrmann R, Missler M, et al. (2006) Neuroligins determine synapse maturation and function. Neuron 51: 741–754.
31. Ullrich B, Ushkaryov YA, Südhof TC (1995) Cartography of neurexins: more than 1000 isoforms generated by alternative splicing and expressed in distinct subsets of neurons. Neuron 14(3): 497–507.
32. Klein R (2004) Eph/ephrin signaling in morphogenesis, neural development and plasticity. Curr Opin Cell Biol 16(5): 580–9.
33. Aoto J, Ting P, Maghsoodi B, Xu N, Henkemeyer M, et al. (2007) Postsynaptic ephrinB3 promotes shaft glutamatergic synapse formation. J Neurosci 27(28): 7508–7519.
34. Klein R (2001) Excitatory Eph receptors and adhesive ephrin ligands. Curr Opin Cell Biol 13(2): 196–203.
35. Yokoyama N, Romero MI, Cowan CA, Galvan P, Helmbacher F, et al. (2001) Forward signaling mediated by ephrin-B3 prevents contralateral corticospinal axons from recrossing the spinal cord midline. Neuron 29: 85–97.
36. Nakagawa S, Brennan C, Johnson KG, Shewan D, Harris WA, et al. (2000) Ephrin-B regulates the ipsilateral routing of retinal axons at the optic chiasm. Neuron 25: 599–610.
37. Williams SE, Mann F, Erskine L, Sakurai T, Wei S, et al. (2003) Ephrin-B2 and EphB1 mediate retinal axon divergence at the optic chiasm. Neuron 39, 919–935.
38. Aimone JB, Leasure JL, Perreau VM, Thallmair M, Christopher Reeve Paralysis Foundation Research Consortium (2004) Spatial and temporal gene expression profiling of the contused rat spinal cord. Exp Neurol 189(2):204–221.
39. Chamankhah M, Eftekharpour E, Karimi-Abdolrezaee S, Boutros PC, San-Marina S, et al. (2013) Genome-wide gene expression profiling of stress response in a spinal cord clip compression injury model. BMC Genomics 28; 14(1):583.
40. Di-Giovanni S, Knoblach SM, Brandoli C, Aden SA, Hoffman EP, et al. (2003) Gene profiling in spinal cord injury shows role of cell cycle in neuronal death. Ann Neurol 53(4):454–468.
41. De-Biase A, Knoblach SM, Di-Giovanni S, Fan C, Molon A, et al. (2005) Gene expression profiling of experimental traumatic spinal cord injury as a function of distance from impact site and injury severity. Physiol Genomics 22(3):368–381.
42. Bareyre FM, Haudenschild B, Schwab ME (2002) Long-lasting sprouting and gene expression changes induced by the monoclonal antibody IN-1 in the adult spinal cord. J Neurosci 22(16):7097–7110.
43. Xu X, Ng S, Wu ZL, Nguyen D, Homburger S, et al. (1998) Human semaphorin K1 is glycosylphosphatidylinositol-linked and defines a new subfamily of viral-related semaphorins. J Biol Chem 273: 22428–22434.
44. Pasquale EB (1997) The Eph family of receptors. Curr Opin Cell Biol 9(5): 608–15.
45. Flanagan JG, Vanderhaeghen P (1998) The ephrins and Eph receptors in neural development. Annu Rev Neurosci 21: 309–345.
46. Ichtchenko K, Hata Y, Nguyen T, Ullrich B, Missler M, et al. (1995) Neuroligin 1: a splice site-specific ligand for beta-neurexins. Cell 81: 435– 443.
47. Boucard AA, Chubykin AA, Comoletti D, Taylor P, Sudhof TC (2005) A splice code for trans-synaptic cell adhesion mediated by binding of neuroligin 1 to alpha- and beta-neurexins. Neuron 48: 229 –236.
48. Wright DE, White FA, Gerfen RW, Silos-Santiago I, Snider WD (1995) The guidance molecule semaphorin 3 is expressed in regions of spinal cord and periphery avoided by growing sensory axons. J Comp Neurol 361(2): 321–333.
49. Hammond R, Vivancos V, NaeemA, Chilton J, Mambetisaeva E, et al. (2005) Slit-mediated repulsion is a key regulator of motor axon pathfinding in the hindbrain. Dev 132(20): 4483–4495.
50. Philipp M, Niederkopfler V, Debrunner M, Alther T, Kunz B, et al. (2012) RabGDI controls axonal midline crossing by regulating Robo1 surface expression. Neural Dev 7:36
51. Jevince AR, Kadison SR, Pittman AJ, Chien CB, Kaprielian Z (2006) Distribution of EphB receptors and ephrin-B1 in the developing vertebrate spinal cord. J Comp Neurol 497(5):734–750.
52. Kadison SR, Murakami F, Matise MP, Kaprielian Z (2006) The role of floor plate contact in the elaboration of contralateral commissural projections within the embryonic mouse spinal cord. Dev Biol 296(2): 499–513.
53. Bagri A, Marín O, Plump AS, Mak J, Pleasure SJ, et al. (2002) Slit proteins prevent midline crossing and determine the dorsoventral position of major axonal pathways in the mammalian forebrain. Neuron 33(2):233–248.

54. Tessier-Lavigne M, Goodman CS (1996) The molecular biology of axon guidance. Science 274: 1123–1133.
55. Mueller BK (1999) Growth cone guidance: first steps towards a deeper understanding. Annu Rev Neurosci 22: 351–358.
56. Lu YJ, Xu NW, Yang WQ (2008) Immunofluorescence laser confocal expression and localization study of rat nerve growth guidance cues Netrin-1 and Slit2 after spinal cord injury. Chin J Traumatol 11(2): 98–103.
57. Marillat V, Cases O, Nguyen-Ba-Charvet KT, Tessier-Lavigne M, Sotelo C, et al. (2002) Spatiotemporal expression patterns of slit and robo genes in the rat brain. J Comp Neurol 442(2): 130–155.
58. Sang Q, Wu JY, Rao Y, Hsueh Y-P, Tan S-S (2002) Slit promotes branching and elongation of neurites of interneurons but not projection neurons from the developing telencephalon. Mol Cell Neurosci 21: 250–265.
59. Whitford KL, Marillat V, Stein E, Goodman CS, Tessier-Lavigne M, et al. (2002) Regulation of cortical dendrite development by slit–robo interactions. Neuron 33: 47–61.
60. Kolodkin AL, Matthes D, Goodman CS (1993) The *semaphorin* genes encode a family of transmembrane and secreted growth cone guidance molecules. Cell 75(7): 1389–1399.
61. Muller B K, Bonhoeffer F, Drescher U (1996) Novel gene families involved in neural pathfinding. Curr Opin Genet Dev 6: 469–474.
62. Mann F, Chauvet S, Rougon G (2007) Semaphorins in development and adult brain: Implication for neurological diseases. Prog Neurobiol 82: 57–79.
63. Pasterkamp RJ, Kolk SM, Hellemons AJ, Kolodkin AL (2007) Expression patterns of semaphorin7A and plexinC1 during rat neural development suggest roles in axon guidance and neuronal migration. BMC Dev Biol 7: 98.
64. Shim SO, Cafferty WB, Schmidt EC, Kim BG, Fujisawa H, et al. (2012) PlexinA2 limits recovery from corticospinal axotomy by mediating oligodendrocyte-derived Sema6A growth inhibition. Mol Cell Neurosci 50(2): 193–200.
65. Kopp MA, Brommer B, Gatzemeier N, Schwab JM, Prüss H (2010) Spinal cord injury induces differential expression of the profibrotic semaphorin 7A in the developing and mature glial scar. Glia 58(14): 1748–1756.
66. Biederer T (2006) Hooking up new synapses. Nat Neurosci 9(10): 1203–1204.
67. Thomas LA, Akins MR, Biederer T (2008) Expression and adhesion profiles of SynCAM molecules indicate distinct neuronal functions. J Comp Neurol 510(1): 47–67.
68. Zelano J, Berg A, Thams S, Hailer NP, Cullheim S (2009) SynCAM1 expression correlates with restoration of central synapses on spinal motoneurons after two different models of peripheral nerve injury. J Comp Neurol 517(5): 670–682.
69. Ushkaryov YA, Petrenko AG, Geppert M, Südhof TC (1992) Neurexins: synaptic cell surface proteins related to the alpha- latrotoxin receptor and laminin. Science 257: 50–56.
70. Ushkaryov YA, Südhof TC (1993) Neurexin III alpha: extensive alternative splicing generates membrane-bound and soluble forms. Proc Natl Acad Sci USA 90: 6410–6414.
71. Scheiffele P, Fan J, Choih J, Fetter R, Serafini T (2000) Neuroligin expressed in nonneuronal cells triggers presynaptic development in contacting axons. Cell 101: 657–669.
72. Dean C, Scholl FG, Choih J, DeMaria S, Berger J, et al. (2003) Neurexin mediates the assembly of presynaptic terminals. Nat Neurosci 6: 708–716.
73. Zelano J, Wallquist W, Hailer NP, Cullheim S (2007) Down-regulation of mRNAs for synaptic adhesion molecules Neuroligin-2 and -3 and SynCAM1 in spinal motoneurons after axotomy. J Comp Neurol 503: 308–318.
74. Song JY, Ichtchenko K, Suedhof TC, Brose N (1999) Neuroligin 1 is a postsynaptic call-adhesion molecule of excitatory synapses. Proc Natl Acad Sci USA 96: 1100–1105.
75. Bundesen LQ, Scheel TA, Bregman BS, Kromer LF (2003) Ephrin-B2 and EphB2 regulation of astrocyte-meningeal fibroblast interactions in response to spinal cord lesions in adult rats. J Neurosci 23(21): 7789–800.
76. Moreno-Flores MT, Wandosell F (1999) Up-regulation of Eph tyrosine kinase receptors after excitotoxic injury in adult hippocampus. Neurosci 91(1): 193–201.
77. Wang Y, Ying GX, Liu X, Wang WY, Dong JH, et al. (2005) Induction of ephrin-B1 and EphB receptors during denervation-induced plasticity in the adult mouse hippocampus. Eur J Neurosci 21(9): 2336–46.

3

The Multifaceted Effects of Agmatine on Functional Recovery after Spinal Cord Injury through Modulations of BMP-2/4/7 Expressions in Neurons and Glial Cells

Yu Mi Park[1,2], Won Taek Lee[1], Kiran Kumar Bokara[1], Su Kyoung Seo[1,2], Seung Hwa Park[3], Jae Hwan Kim[1], Midori A. Yenari[4], Kyung Ah Park[1], Jong Eun Lee[1,2]*

1 Department of Anatomy, Yonsei University College of Medicine, Seoul, Republic of Korea, **2** BK 21 Project for Medical Science, Yonsei University College of Medicine, Seoul, Republic of Korea, **3** Department of Anatomy, Konkuk University College of Medicine, Seoul, Republic of Korea, **4** Department of Neurology, University of California San Francisco and Veterans Affairs Medical Center, San Francisco, California, United States of America

Abstract

Presently, few treatments for spinal cord injury (SCI) are available and none have facilitated neural regeneration and/or significant functional improvement. Agmatine (Agm), a guanidinium compound formed from decarboxylation of L-arginine by arginine decarboxylase, is a neurotransmitter/neuromodulator and been reported to exert neuroprotective effects in central nervous system injury models including SCI. The purpose of this study was to demonstrate the multifaceted effects of Agm on functional recovery and remyelinating events following SCI. Compression SCI in mice was produced by placing a 15 g/mm^2 weight for 1 min at thoracic vertebra (Th) 9 segment. Mice that received an intraperitoneal (i.p.) injection of Agm (100 mg/kg/day) within 1 hour after SCI until 35 days showed improvement in locomotor recovery and bladder function. Emphasis was made on the analysis of remyelination events, neuronal cell preservation and ablation of glial scar area following SCI. Agm treatment significantly inhibited the demyelination events, neuronal loss and glial scar around the lesion site. In light of recent findings that expressions of bone morphogenetic proteins (BMPs) are modulated in the neuronal and glial cell population after SCI, we hypothesized whether Agm could modulate BMP- 2/4/7 expressions in neurons, astrocytes, oligodendrocytes and play key role in promoting the neuronal and glial cell survival in the injured spinal cord. The results from computer assisted stereological toolbox analysis (CAST) demonstrate that Agm treatment dramatically increased BMP- 2/7 expressions in neurons and oligodendrocytes. On the other hand, BMP- 4 expressions were significantly decreased in astrocytes and oligodendrocytes around the lesion site. Together, our results reveal that Agm treatment improved neurological and histological outcomes, induced oligodendrogenesis, protected neurons, and decreased glial scar formation through modulating the BMP- 2/4/7 expressions following SCI.

Editor: Ulrike Schmidt, Max Planck Institute of Psychiatry, Germany

Funding: This research was supported by Basic Science Research Program through the National Research Foundation of Korea (NRF) funded by the Ministry of Education, Science and Technology (MEST) (2012-0002340) and National Institutes of Health (NS40516, to MY), the Veteran's Merit Award (to MY). Grants to MY were administered by the Northern California Institute for Research and Education, and supported by resources of the Veterans Affairs Medical Center, San Francisco, California. This work was also supported by the Brain Korea 21 Project for Medical Science, Yonsei University. The funders had no role in study design, data collection and analysis, decision to publish, or preparation of the manuscript.

Competing Interests: The authors have declared that no competing interests exist.

* E-mail: jelee@yuhs.ac

Introduction

Spinal cord injury (SCI) often results in permanent disability or loss of movement (paralysis) and sensation below the site of injury leading either to paraplegia (thoracic level injury) or tetraplegia (cervical level injury) [1]. SCI rostral to the lumbosacral level disrupts voluntary and supraspinal control of voiding and induces a considerable reorganization of the micturition reflex pathway. The urinary bladder is initially are flexic, but then becomes hyperreflexic because of the emergence of spinal micturition reflex pathway following SCI [2]. SCI leads to neuronal and glial cell death, induces glial scar formation [3] and inhibits axonal regeneration and remyelination [4]. Oligodendrocytes produce myelin that wraps around the axons of neurons to enable them to conduct electrical impulses [5,6] and neurotrophic factors to support the maintenance of nerve cells. Oligodendrocytes are lost during SCI, resulting in the loss of myelin and motor function that cause paralysis in animals.

Agmatine (Agm) (4-aminobutyl guanidine), NH_2-CH_2-CH_2-CH_2-CH_2-NH-C (-NH_2) (=NH), is an endogenous amine and four carbon guanidine compound formed by decarboxylation of arginine [7]. Agm was implicated in modulation of neurotransmission functions. It interacts with various neurotransmitter receptors, including nicotine, N-methyl-d-aspartate (NMDA) α_2-adrenoceptors and imidazoline receptors [7,8]. In addition, this molecule can interfere with second messenger pathways by acting as an adenosine diphosphate (ADP)-ribose acceptor thereby inhibiting ADP-ribosylation of proteins [9]. Exogenous administration of Agm significantly reduces pain induced by inflammation following SCI [10]. The above characteristics of Agm led us to hypothesize that it might serve as a neuroprotective agent following neurotrauma.

Bone morphogenetic proteins (BMPs) are multifunctional growth factors that belong to the transforming growth factor-β (TGF-β) super family. BMPs signal through serine/threonine kinase receptors, composed of type I and II BMP receptors [11]. BMPs play important roles as trophic factors that may act in cell death regulation/differentiation [12], proliferation of neural progenitor cells and are also involved in restoration of injured neurons following various central nervous system (CNS) injuries [12,13]. Among the various types of BMPs, BMP- 2/7 in particular promotes differentiation and boosts dendrite growth in cultured striatal neurons [14] and modulates the balance between glial cells and neurons [15]. Earlier reports suggested that the BMP levels are altered following SCI [16]. BMP- 7 given intravenously showed neuroprotective effects following SCI [17,18]. Furthermore, BMP- 4 signaling was reported to be essential for astrocytes lineage proliferation following SCI [19]. Conversely, disruption of BMP signaling in vivo negatively affects astrogliogenesis [20]. Several groups have studied the effects of BMP signaling after SCI with mixed results. It was also demonstrated that BMP signaling enhances axonal outgrowth and locomotor recovery after SCI. These observations suggest that BMP signaling may be involved in both the beneficial and the detrimental effects following SCI [21,22]. Agm treatment following SCI was shown to improve locomotor functions and reduce collagen scar formation accompanied with TGF-β and BMP- 7 expressions suggesting that BMPs may regulate neural cell lineage commitment in vivo [23]. Based on the previous evidences reporting the beneficial effects of Agm, we hypothesized that Agm treatment, a well-known neuroprotector, may have effects on (1) recovery of locomotory and physiological functions, (2) facilitate axonal remyelination, (3) promote protection of neurons, (4) attenuate glial scar formation, and (5) modulate the BMP- 2/4/7 expressions in neuronal and glial cells following SCI. In this study, the mice subjected to SCI were divided into agmatine treatment group (Agm treated group) and saline treatment group (EC group) along with parallel controls. All the experimental groups were examined for functional recovery and urinary bladder functions which included open field test and urine residual volume measurement respectively following SCI. Histological sections were examined to measure glial scar using an imaging program and the axonal remyelination was confirmed with myelin basic proteins (MBPs) staining. The surviving neurons, oligodendrocytes, and astrocytes were confirmed by counting the total cell numbers of microtubule-associated protein-2 (MAP-2), oligodendrocyte transcription factor-2 (Olig-2), and glial fibrillary acidic protein (GFAP) immunopositive cells in the total spinal cord (Th 8–Th 10 segments) and also in the rostral (Th 8), lesion (Th 9) and caudal regions (Th 10) separately using computer assisted sterological toolbox analysis (CAST) following SCI.

This first study provides robust evidence of the beneficial effects of Agm treatment leading to lasting improvements of structure and function through modulating the BMP- 2/4/7 expressions in neurons, oligodendrocytes, and astrocytes, which could be vital for directing the axonal remyelination and protect damaged neurons following SCI.

Materials and Methods

Animals

Studies were conducted on male Imprinting Control Region (ICR) mice, 8 weeks old, weighing 28±5 g (Sam tako, South Korea). All animal experiments were performed in accordance with the Korean Food and Drug Administration (KFDA) guidelines. Protocols were reviewed and approved by the Institutional Animal Care and Use Committee (IACUC) of the Yonsei Laboratory Animal Research Center (YLARC) (Permit #: 10-114). All mice were maintained in the specific pathogen-free facility of the YLARC.

Compression Spinal Cord Injury (SCI) and Agmatine (Agm) Treatment

The mice ($n = 280$) were anesthetized with a combination of ketamine (100 mg/kg) and xylazine (rompun) (10 mg/kg) by intraperitoneal (i.p.) injection. Body temperatures of the animals were monitored with rectal probes maintained between 36.5°C and 37.5°C with heating pads and lamps. A laminectomy of thoracic vertebra (Th) segment 8– Th 10 (potentially Th 9 as a result of surgical variability) was performed using a fine pair of rongers without damaging the durameter. The spinal cord at Th 9 was injured with a bilateral micro clamp clip (Fine Science Tools Inc in Foster City, CA, USA). A compression of 15 g/mm^2 was applied to the exposed spinal cord for 1 minute. The clip was then removed and the skin sutured. Bladders were manually pressed twice daily until spontaneous voiding occurred, and any hematuria or urinary tract infection was treated with ampicillin (1 mg/kg) daily for one week. Food and water were freely accessible at a lowered height in their cages. Agmatine (Agm treated group, $n = 101$) was administered at a dose 100 mg/kg/day (Sigma) by intraperitoneal injection within 1 hour after SCI until 35 days post injury (DPI). Experimental control mice (EC group, $n = 101$) received intraperitoneal (i.p.) injections of saline instead of Agm. Normal control mice without spinal cord injury (NC group, $n = 78$) were maintained all through the experiment (see Table S1).

Behavior Test

Mice were tested for locomotor deficits at 1 day, 3 days, 7 days, 10 days, 14 days ($n = 30$, per group), 21 days, 28 days and 35 days ($n = 15$, per group) after SCI in an open field using the Basso Mouse Scale (BMS) as previously described [24,25] (see Table S1). The BMS test scores were rated on a scale of 0 to 9 with 0 being no function (complete paralysis of the hind limbs) and 9 being normal (normal movement of the hind limbs). The performance of both left and right limbs of the mice were assessed depending on the average BMS test scale scores obtained until 35 DPI.

Bladder Function Analysis

Assessment of bladder function was carried in all the experimental groups until 14 DPI. The bladders were manually stimulated twice a day until 14 days ($n = 10$, per group) till they regained to normal autonomic bladder function (approximately 11–15 DPI) (see Table S1). Retained urine from each mouse was collected and measured from all the experimental groups both in the morning and evening sessions (12 hours interval) until 14 DPI [26].

Ultra Structural Studies of Spinal Cord using Transmission Electron Microscope

Transmission electron microscopic studies were done to assess micro structural changes of myelin sheath after SCI. Briefly, mice were perfused with normal saline followed by a solution containing 2% glutaraldehyde - 4% paraformaldehyde. After thermal stresses for 12 hours, each sample was fixed with 2% glutaraldehyde - paraformaldehyde in 0.1 M phosphate buffer (PB), pH 7.4 for 2 hour and washed three times for 30 min in 0.1 M PB. They were post fixed with 1% OsO_4 dissolved in 0.1 M PB for 2 hour and dehydrated in ascending gradual series (50–100%) of ethanol and infiltrated with propylene oxide. Specimens were embedded by

Poly/Bed 812 kit (Polysciences). After embedding in pure fresh resin they were polymerized at 60°C in electron microscope oven (TD-700, DOSAKA, Japan) for 24 hours. After incubation, 350 nm thick sections were initially cut and stained with toluidine blue for light microscope to confirm the quality of embedding. Later, 70 nm thin sections were cut by LEICA Ultracut UCT Ultra-microtome (Leica Microsystems, Austria) and were double stained with 7% uranyl acetate for 20 min and lead citrate for contrast staining. All of the thin sections were observed under transmission electron microscopy (JEM-1011, JEOL, Japan) at the acceleration voltage of 80 kv.

Luxol Fast Blue Staining

To confirm the myelination at the injury site before and after Agm treatment, the luxol fast blue staining was performed. The spinal cord tissue section (20 µm) from NC, EC and Agm treated groups were placed directly into 1:1 alcohol/chloroform for a few hours/overnight and then were hydrated back with 95% ethyl alcohol. Later the tissue slides were incubated with luxol fast blue stain for 16 hrs at 56°C in oven and then excess stain was rinsed with 95% alcohol. The tissue sections were counterstained with cresyl violet solution for 30–40 seconds and mounted onto slides.

Tissue Processing for Immunohistochemistry

At 1, 7, 14 and 35 DPI, mice were deeply anaesthetized with a combination of ketamine (100 mg/kg) and xylazine (rompun) (10 mg/kg) and were perfused transcardially with 0.9% saline containing 0.1% heparin, followed by 4% paraformaldehyde (PFA). The spinal cords were removed and incubated in the same fixative for 2 h at room temperature and then cryoprotected in 30% sucrose PBS solution overnight. A segment of each cord, extending from 3 mm rostral to 3 mm caudal to the lesion site representing Th 8 - Th 10 segments of the spinal cord was embedded in medium (Tissue - Tek O.C.T. compound, Sakura Finetek USA, Inc., Torrance, CA, USA). Serial transverse sections were cut at 20 µm for immmunohistochemistry ($n = 18$, per group) and 40 µm ($n = 60$, per group) for CAST analysis on a cryostat and mounted onto slides (ColorFrost/Plus; Fisher, Pittsburgh, PA, USA) (see Table S1).

GFAP Positive Area Measurement

To quantify the glial scar area in the EC group ($n = 4$) and the Agm treated group ($n = 4$) (see Table S1), 20 µm thick spinal cord sections were sequentially immunoreacted with GFAP antibody (1:500, mouse, monoclonal; Thermo) at 4°C overnight. Later on the tissue slides were incubated with appropriate biotinylated secondary antibody. Immunostaining of GFAP was visualized using the ABC kit (Vector, Burlingame, CA, USA), then reacted with 3, 3′– diaminobenzidine tetra hydrochloride (DAB, sigma, St.Lousi, MO, USA). Negative controls were prepared without adding primary antibody. The entire GFAP positive area around the lesion site of the spinal cord both in EC and Agm treated group was measured by computer-associated scanning image analysis system (Optimas ver 6.1, Optimas, Bothwell, WA, USA) for considering the glial scar area.

3, 3′- diaminobenzidine Tetra Hydrochloride (DAB) Immunostaining for CAST Analysis

The 40 µm thick spinal cord sections ($n = 60$, per group) (see Table S1) were treated with 10% blocking serum at 37°C for 1 hour. Primary antibodies: anti-mouse GFAP (1:500, monoclonal antibody; Thermo), anti-mouse MAP-2 (1:500, monoclonal antibody; Sigma), anti-goat Olig-2 (1:500, polyclonal antibody; Santa-cruz), anti-mouse BMP-2 (1:500, monoclonal antibody; Abcam), anti-mouse BMP-4 (1:250, polyclonal antibody; Santa-cruz), and anti-rabbit BMP-7 (1:500, monoclonal antibody; Abcam) diluted in antibody diluents solution (Invitrogen, Carlsbd, CA) were added to the tissue section samples and incubated at 4°C overnight. Primary antibody was removed and tissue slides were washed 3 times for 3 min each with PBS. Later samples were incubated with appropriate secondary antibody prepared in dilution buffer conjugated to peroxidase (1:500; Abcam) for 2 h at room temperature. Tissue sections were washed again 3 times for 3 min each with PBS and stained with 3, 3′ - diamino-benzidine tetra hydrochloride (DAB, sigma, St. Louis, MO, USA) and SG substrate kit (Vector, Burlingame, CA, USA) for 5 min at room temperature. Staining with DAB results in the deposition of a brown insoluble precipitate and staining with SG substrate results in blue-gray precipitate at the antigenic sites containing the specific epitopes recognized by the primary antibody and were visualized using light microscope. Immunostaining negative controls were prepared without the primary antibody.

Computer Assisted Stereological Toolbox (CAST) Analysis

The spinal cord segments (Th 8–Th 10) were obtained from control mice without SCI (NC group), SCI mice treated with saline (EC group) and SCI mice treated with agmatine (Agm treated group). Briefly, 40–50 longitudinal cryotissue sections (40 µm thick) of the spinal cord were obtained from each animal and were collected sequentially on histology slides. Every 5th slide was chosen from the total of 40–50 tissue sections for the CAST analysis. The tissue slides were incubated with respective primary antibodies and washed in PBS three times followed by appropriate biotinylated secondary antibody incubation. The DAB and SG stained antigens in the spinal cord (Th 8–Th 10 segments) were quantified using computer assisted stereological toolbox (CAST stereological analysis of cells) (software Ver. 2.3.1.5, applied to an Olympus BX-51, Melville, NY, USA). CAST is a data collection program for obtaining efficient and unbiased estimates of cell number, cell density, cell size, and other stereological quantities. CAST evaluation was performed using a morphometric system consisting of an Olympus BX-51 microscope equipped with a motorized stage, which was controlled by a computer for manual interactive counting on the computer screen. The software CAST-grid version 2.3.1.5 (Olympus, Albertslund, Denmark) was used to generate counting areas. A counting frame was placed randomly and it was systematically moved throughout the encircled counting area until 20% of the entire area was sampled using a 1,000×objective. The cells showing the plasma membrane, a visible nucleus, located within the counting frame were considered positive. The mean number of immunopositive cells per square millimeter of tissue was assessed from each mouse spinal cord tissue [27].

$$N\,\text{total} = Q\,\text{total} \times \frac{100}{\text{areal sampling fraction (\%)}} \times \frac{1}{\text{section sampling fraction (\%)}} \times \frac{\text{section number}}{\text{analzed section number}}$$

The formula to count the total number of cells using the CAST analysis software program as described by the manufacturer was as follows; N total, represents the total number of immunopositive cells stained per one subject; Q total, a raw count of immunopositive cells per one set per animal group; areal sampling fraction (%), the percentage of the selected area in the total spinal cord (Th 8–Th 10 segments); section sampling fraction (%), the total immunostained area of the selected tissue; section number, the total number of tissue sections prepared from the total spinal cord (Th 8–Th 10 segments); analyzed section number, the number of tissue sections selected for the CAST analysis.

The spinal cord (Th 8–Th 10 segments) was divided into three regions and each segment was identified as: 1) Th 8 is considered as rostral site of the spinal cord from the lesion site, 2) Th 9 is considered as lesion site of the spinal cord and 3) Th 10 is considered as caudal site of the spinal cord from the lesion site.

Note: All experimenters involved with CAST analysis were blinded to treatment group identity.

Immunofluorescence Studies Using Confocal Microscopy

The frozen sections ($n = 18$, per group) (see Table S1) were air dried at room temperature for 20 min and were blocked for 1 hour using blocking solution at 37°C for 1 hour. The following primary antibodies were used overnight at 4°C: anti-mouse GFAP (1:500, monoclonal antibody; Thermo), anti-mouse BMP-2 (1:500, monoclonal antibody; Abcam), anti-mouse BMP-4 (1:250, polyclonal antibody; Santa-cruz), anti-rabbit BMP-7 (1:500, monoclonal antibody; Abcam), anti-mouse MAP-2 (1:500, monoclonal antibody; Sigma), anti-goat Olig-2 (1:250, polyclonal antibody; Santa-cruz), anti-rat MBP (1:500, Abcam), anti-mouse Neuronal Nuclei (NeuN) (1:500, monoclonal antibody; Millipore), and anti-rabbit neurofilament (NF) (1:500, monoclonal antibody; Millipore), anti-rabbit 5-HT (1:10000, monoclonal antibody; Abcam), anti-rabbit p53 (1:500, monoclonal antibody; santa-cruz) and anti-rabbit NG2 (1:500, monoclonal antibody; Millipore). Then the slides were washed in PBS three times and were incubated with appropriate secondary antibodies conjugated either with fluorescein isothiocyanate (*FITC*) (1:500, Chemicon) or rhodamine (1:500, Chemicon) at 37°C for 2 hours. The slides were stained with 4′-6-diamidino-2-phenylindole (DAPI) (Vector, Burlingame, USA) to counterstain the nuclei and were coverslipped with mounting medium. Images were taken using a confocal microscopy (LSM700; Zeiss, Thornwood, NY, USA).

Western Blot Analysis

For immunoblotting, spinal cords from each experimental group ($n = 20$–25, per group) (see Table S1) were dissected, placed in ice-cold artificial CSF (124 mM NaCl, 3 mM KCl, 1 mM NaHPO4, 26 mM NaHCO3, 1.5 mM MgSO4, 1.5 mM CaCl2, and 10 mM glucose), and cleaned from meninges and nerve roots. Spinal cord tissue samples were homogenized on ice using a homogenizer in 500 μL radio immunoprecipitation assay buffer (RIPA) containing 150 mM sodium chloride, 1% nonidet-p40 (NP-40), 0.5% sodium deoxycholate, and 0.1% sodium dodecyl sulphate (SDS), 50 mM Tris (pH 8.0) and phosphatase inhibitor solution, 20 mM/L Tris -HCl (pH 7.5), 2 μg/ml aprotinin, 5 μg/ml leupeptin, 1 μg/ml pepstatin A, 1 mM phenylmethylsulphonyl fluoride (PMSF), 5 mM ethylenediaminetetraacetic acid (EDTA), 1 mM EGTA, 5 mM sodium fluoride (NaF), and 1 mM Sodium Orthovanadate (Na_3VO_4). The homogenates were centrifuged at 15,000 g for 15 minutes and protein concentrations were determined by BCA protein assay. Equal amounts of protein (50 μg) were loaded onto 8–10% polyacrylamide gel and were transferred onto PVDF membranes by electrophoresis. The membranes were then blocked with Tris buffered saline with tween -20 (TBST) buffer containing 20 mM Tris-HCI, 5% skim milk, 150 mM NaCI, and 0.05% Tween 20 at pH 7.6, for 1hour at 37°C. The following primary antibodies were used overnight at 4°C: anti-mouse GFAP (1:1000, monoclonal antibody; Thermo), anti-rabbit S100β (1:1000, monoclonal antibody; Abcam), anti-mouse BMP-2 (1:1000, monoclonal antibody; Abcam), anti-mouse BMP-4 (1:1000, polyclonal antibody; Santa-cruz), anti-rabbit BMP-7 (1:1000, monoclonal antibody; Abcam), anti-mouse MAP-2 (1:1000, monoclonal antibody; Sigma), and anti-goat Olig-2 (1:1000, polyclonal antibody; Santa-cruz). The membranes were washed with TBST and incubated with horseradish peroxidase-conjugated with anti-mouse, anti-rabbit and anti-goat, secondary antibody (1:2000; Chemicon) at 37°C for 2 hours. Following the incubation, membranes were incubated in super-signal west pico chemiluminescent substrate according to the manufacturer's specifications. Immunoreactive bands were digitally scanned and analyzed with Image J software (National Institutes of Health). To control for equal protein loading, membranes were also probed for β-actin and the protein values were normalized to β-actin (1:3000, monoclonal antibody; Abcam).

Statistical Analysis

All statistical analyses were performed using SPSS 18.0. The data were presented as means and standard errors (S.E.M.).One-way or two-way repeated measures ANOVA was used to compare the experimental groups, with post-hoc Tukey's test for multiple comparisons. Differences were considered statistically significant at $P<0.05$.

Results

Agmatine Treatment Enhanced Functional Outcome and Prevented Cell Death Following SCI

The functional recovery of the mice subjected to SCI was assessed using the Basso Mouse Scale (BMS) scores. After SCI, the EC group ($n = 30$) and Agm treated group ($n = 30$) showed no ankle movement at 1 DPI (BMS score 0). Subsequently, the Agm treated group showed extensive ankle movements (BMS score 2) at 7 DPI and reached frequent or consistent plantar stepping, paws parallel at initial contact and lift off, and severe trunk instability (BMS score 6.8) at 21 DPI. At 35 DPI, the Agm treated group demonstrated frequent or consistent plantar stepping, some or mostly coordinated, paws parallel at initial contact and lift off, and normal trunk stability with up and down tail movement (BMS score 8). Even though the EC group showed occasional plantar stepping but the mice failed to frequent or consistent plantar stepping and their BMS scores were reached only up to a maximum of 4 points at 35 DPI. Our behavioral test results suggested that Agm treated mice showed improvement in the functional recovery compared with that of the saline treated mice (Fig. 1). SCI results in the blockage of the reflex signals between the brain and the bladder and consequently, the self urination fails [2,28,29]. Regaining bladder, bowel, and sexual function are some of the highest priorities following SCI and urinary function should be monitored as an outcome measure in SCI models [30,31]. In this study we assessed whether Agm treatment could improve the bladder function following SCI ($n = 10$, per group). Residual urine was collected and the volumes were measured until 14 DPI. Assessment of bladder function revealed that Agm treatment significantly reduced peak residual urine volumes from 4 day until 10 days compared to saline treated group. This effect of low residual volumes of urine was observed both in the EC and Agm treatment group after 10 DPI and the EC group showed improvement in self voiding and at the end of 14 DPI, both the

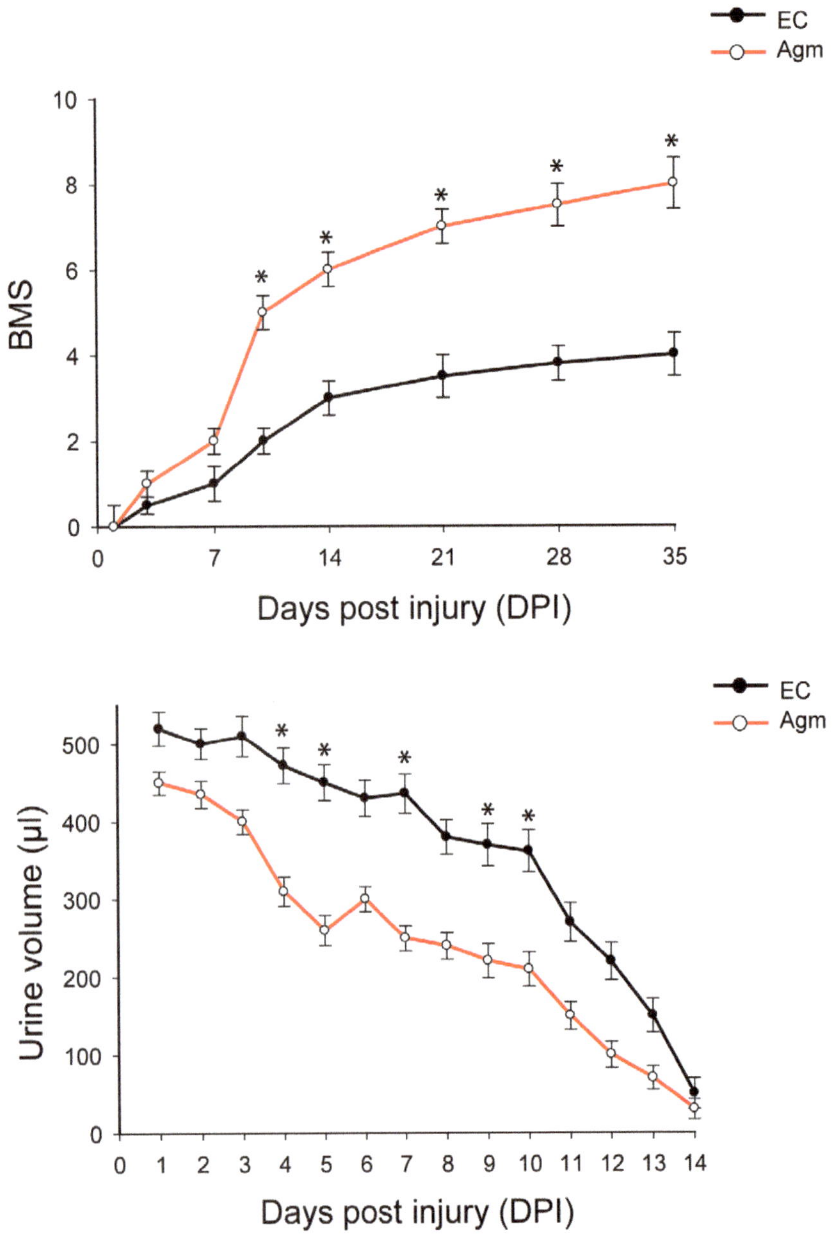

Figure 1. Agmatine treatment enhanced functional outcome following compression SCI. The BMS score was used to evaluate hindlimb locomotor function. The BMS scores in the Agm treated mice (Agm treated group, $n=30$) were significantly higher than the saline treated mice (EC group, $n=30$) at 1, 3, 7, 10, 14, 21, 28 and 35 DPI. The Bladder residual urine volumes were measured in Agm treated group ($n=10$) and in the EC group ($n=10$). The graph showed that the amount of residual urine was significantly decreased in the Agm treated group compared with the EC group until 14 DPI. *, $p<0.05$ EC group vs Agm treated group. Results represent mean ± S.E.M.

Agm treated and EC group totally regained the normal voiding function with no urine residual volumes while manual pressing of the bladders. These results depict that Agm treatment could retain the balance between the brain and spinal cord and helps in maintaining the reflex signals for self-urination. This effect was not due to altered fluid intake because fluid consumption did not differ between Agm and saline treated groups (Data not shown). SCI induces a series of endogenous biochemical changes that lead to secondary degeneration, including apoptosis. The p53-mediated apoptosis is likely to be an important mechanism of cell death in SCI [32,33]. Our immunohistochemical staining results revealed that SCI induced the activation of p53 expression following SCI in the EC group. But fewer number of $p53^+$ cells were seen in the lesion site in the Agm treated group compared with EC group both at 14 and 35 days DPI (Fig. S1).

Agmatine Treatment Promoted Remyelination Following SCI

SCI induces local inflammation and demyelination of the white matter around the lesion site, resulting in disrupted axonal conduction. Enhancement of oligodendrocytes or progenitors proliferation to enhance remyelination and functional recovery may lead to repair and restoration of locomotory function after SCI [34]. To ascertain whether Agm could enhance the remyelination process following SCI, transmission electron microscopic studies (TEM) were performed to assess the micro-structural changes of the myelin sheath after SCI. TEM results suggested that Agm treated group ($n = 3$) showed better pattern of myelination in the white matter of lesioned spinal cords compared to EC group ($n = 3$) at 14 days following SCI. In the EC group, a number of large swollen axons with broken myelin sheaths were found across the degenerative white matter in the lesioned area. Thick myelin sheaths broke down and compact layers split apart irregularly and demyelinated axons were amongst the degenerative axons with enlarged spaces between the axolemma and deteriorating sheaths were also prominent in the EC group. Contrast to EC group, Agm treated group showed less broken myelin sheaths and more compact myelination around the lesion site. Moreover, demyelinated axons were found less across the degenerating area in the Agm treated group (Fig. 2A). The myelination was also checked by luxol fast blue staining in NC group, EC group and Agm treated group ($n = 3$, per group) at 14 and 35 DPI. The staining results showed a remarkable increase of myelin (blue) and neurons (violet) stained cells indicating the reconstruction of lost myelin and neurons in the Agm treated group compared with the EC group (Fig. 2B).

Following SCI, the fibers (serotonergic) originated from brain stem which extend the projections to the spinal cord get completely damaged at the lesion site which results in sensorimotor dysfunctions. To determine the effect of Agm ($n = 3$) on regeneration of serotonergic fibers, which are important for the motor functional recovery of hind limbs [35,36], 5-HT immunostaining was performed in the distal segment of the spinal cord at 14 and 35 DPI. The staining results showed bead like structures with broken morphology of the serotogenic nerve fibers both at 14 and 35 DPI in the EC group ($n = 3$). Conversely Agm treated group showed dense network of serotogenic fibers both at 14 and 35 DPI (Fig. S2) representing the restoration of sensorimotor dysfunctions.

These remyelination effects were further confirmed by checking the Olig-2 (oligodendrocyte marker) expression by western blotting. Western blot analysis showed that the Olig-2 protein expression in Agm treated group ($n = 5$) was increased at all the time periods (from 1 DPI to 35 DPI) after compression SCI compared with that of the EC group ($n = 5$) and the values reached significance at 35 DPI (Fig. 3A). Furthermore the number of Olig-2^{+} cells were counted in the EC group ($n = 5$) and Agm treated group ($n = 5$) using CAST analysis program. The CAST counting results showed that the numbers of Olig-2^{+} cells were higher in the total spinal cord (Th 8 - Th 10 segments) at 1, 7, 14 and 35 DPI and significant increase was recorded at 14 and 35 DPI (Fig. 3B). There was an increase in the intensification of Olig-2^{+} cells in the rostral (Th 8), the lesion (Th 9), and the caudal segments (Th 10) of the injured spinal cord in the Agm treated group at 1, 7, 14, and

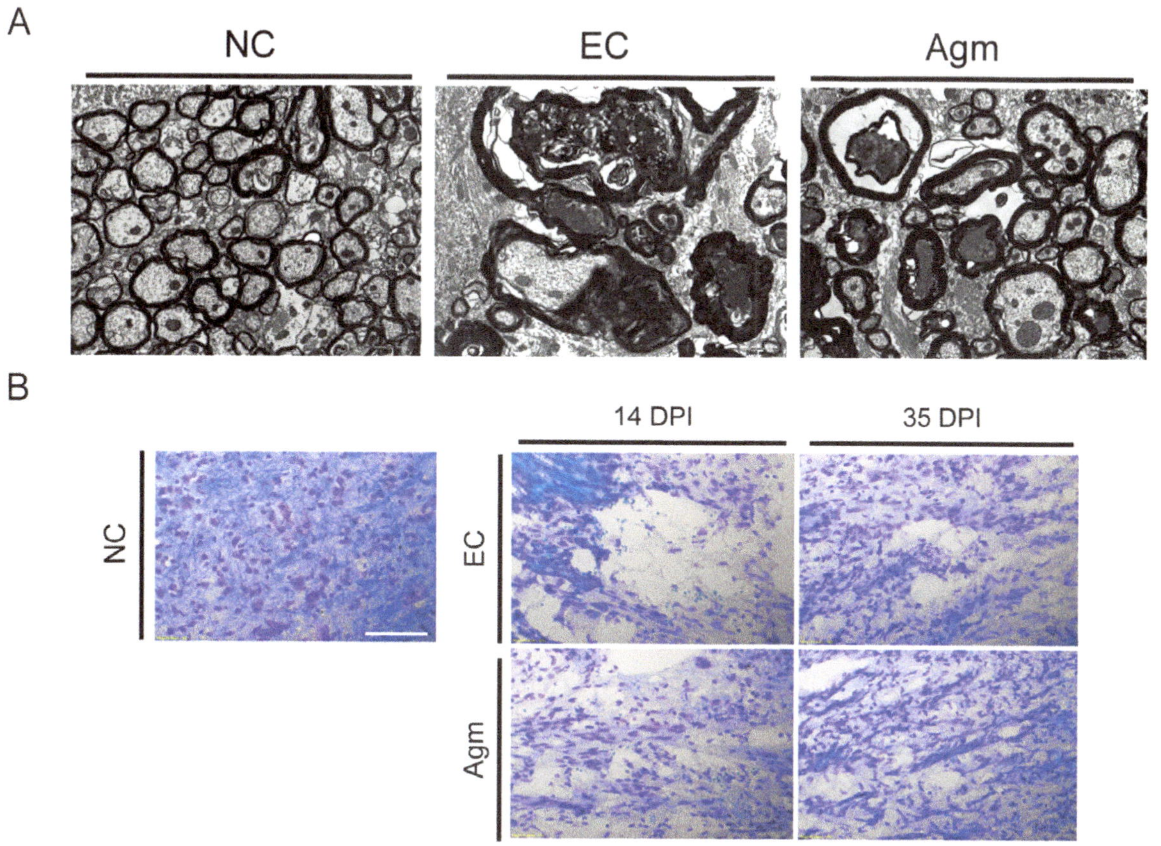

Figure 2. Agmatine treatment promoted remyelination following SCI. (A) Myelin sheath formation in white matter of normal and injured spinal cord was observed by transmission electron microscope (TEM) (1,0000x). The myelination of white matter was ultrastructurally improved with less degenerated myelin in the Agm treated group while swollen axons with broken myelin sheaths were found across the degenerative white matter in the lesioned area in the EC group at 14 DPI. (B) Luxol fast blue staining results showed a remarkable increase of myelin (blue) and neuron (violet) stained cells indicating the reconstruction of lost myelin and neurons in the Agm treated group compared with the EC group at 14 and 35 DPI. Scale bars: 20 μm.

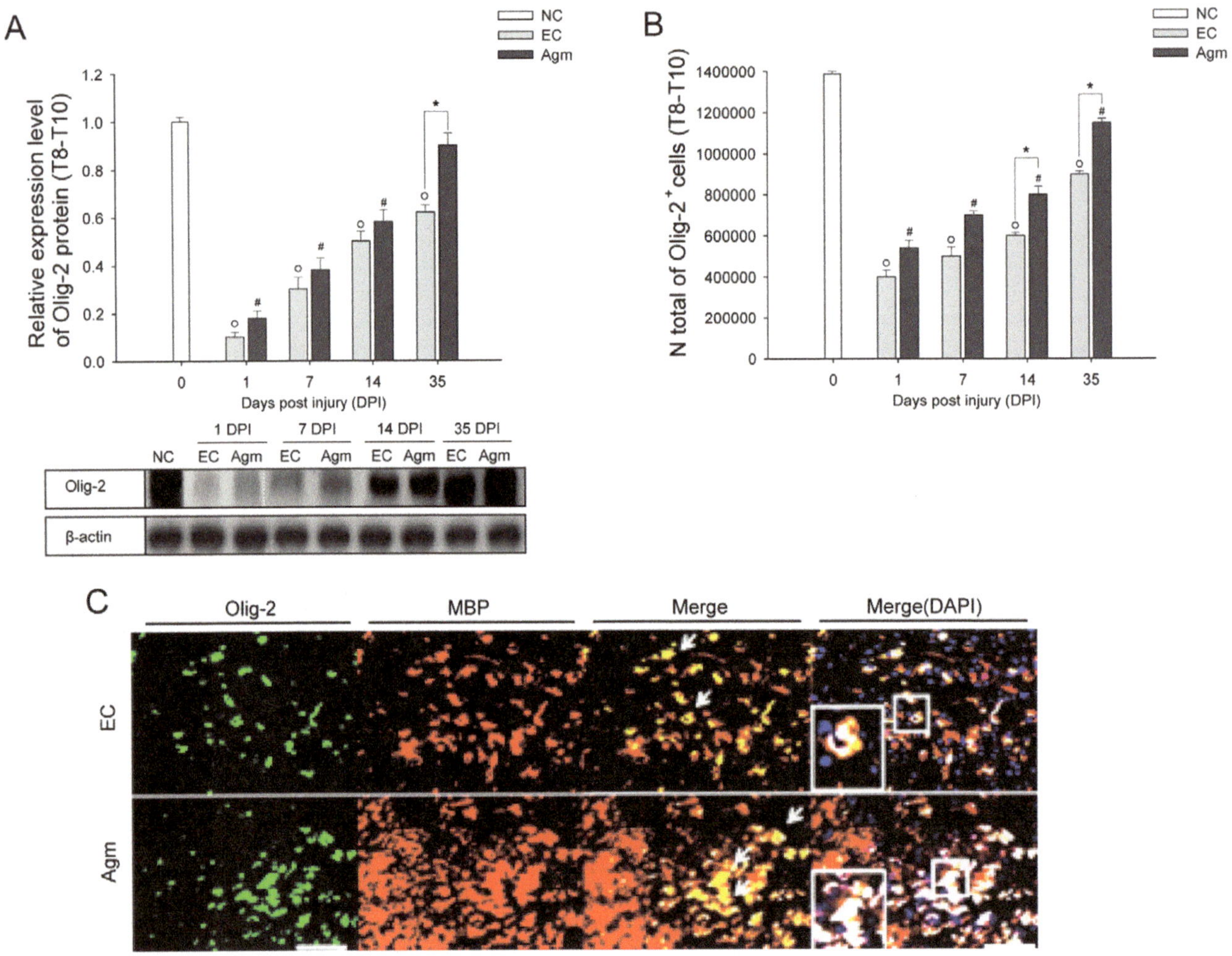

Figure 3. Agmatine treatment increased the expansion of oligodendrocytes following SCI. (A) Quantification of Olig-2 expression was determined by western blot analysis. The bar graph represents densitometry of the mean Olig-2 expression. Olig-2 expression was significantly higher in the Agm treated group ($n = 5$) compared with the EC group ($n = 5$) at 35 DPI. (B) Olig-2^+ cell number were acquired using CAST analysis in the Th 8 - Th 10 segments of the injured spinal cord. The number of Olig-2^+ cells in the Agm treated group ($n = 5$) were significantly increased compared to EC group ($n = 5$) at 14 and 35 DPI. (C) The spinal cords were immunostained with Olig-2 (green) and MBP (red) antibodies at 35 DPI. The number of Olig-2^+/MBP$^+$ cells were higher in the Agm treated group ($n = 5$) than in the EC group ($n = 5$) around the lesion site at 35 DPI. Higher magnification images revealed intact myelin rings surrounding the axons in Agm treated group, whereas disrupted myelin was found in EC group (see figure in the box). Scale bars: 50 µm. †, $p<0.05$ NC group vs EC group; #, $p<0.05$ NC group vs Agm treated group; *, $p<0.05$ EC group vs Agm treated group. Results represent mean ± S.E.M.

35 DPI and the significant difference between the groups (Agm treated group vs EC group) were recorded at 35 DPI (Fig. S4). Furthermore, remyelination (within the perimeter of the lesion site) in the injured spinal cord was confirmed by double immunostaining with Olig-2 (green) and MBP (red) at 35 DPI (Fig. 3C). Confocal microscopy results showed higher intensity of Olig-2^+/MBP$^+$ cells (rings formation indicated by a white arrow in Fig. 3C) in the Agm treated group ($n = 5$) compared with the EC group ($n = 5$). Considering that endogenous oligodendrocyte progenitor cells (NG2^+) local to the lesion site are to be the source of new myelinating cells, experiments were done to check the expression of NG2^+ cells in Olig-$2^+$and GFAP$^+$ cell population at 7 and 35 DPI. Our immunohistochemical staining results showed that the expansion of NG2^+/Olig-2^+ cells outnumbered in the Agm treatment group both at 7 days and 35 DPI compared to EC group. But the NG2^+/GFAP$^+$ cells were less in Agm treated group both at 7 and 35 days DPI compared to EC group (Fig. S3).

These results depict that Agm treatment could promote the formation of myelin sheath and might facilitate the remyelination process following SCI.

Agmatine Treatment Protects the Damaged Neurons Following SCI

Approaches to treat SCI include prevention of damaged neurons and regeneration of tissue loss. Strategies aimed to prevent neuronal damage will arise from secondary injury processes providing some hope for tissue sparing and improved functional outcome [37]. To ascertain this, quantitative measurement of MAP-2 protein expression was done using western blot analysis after SCI. The densitometry results showed that the MAP-2 expression in the Agm treated group ($n = 5$) was increased at 1, 7, 14 and 35 DPI ($n = 5$) and the values reached significance at 14 and 35 DPI compared with the EC group (Fig. 4A). CAST analysis showed that the expansion of total number of surviving

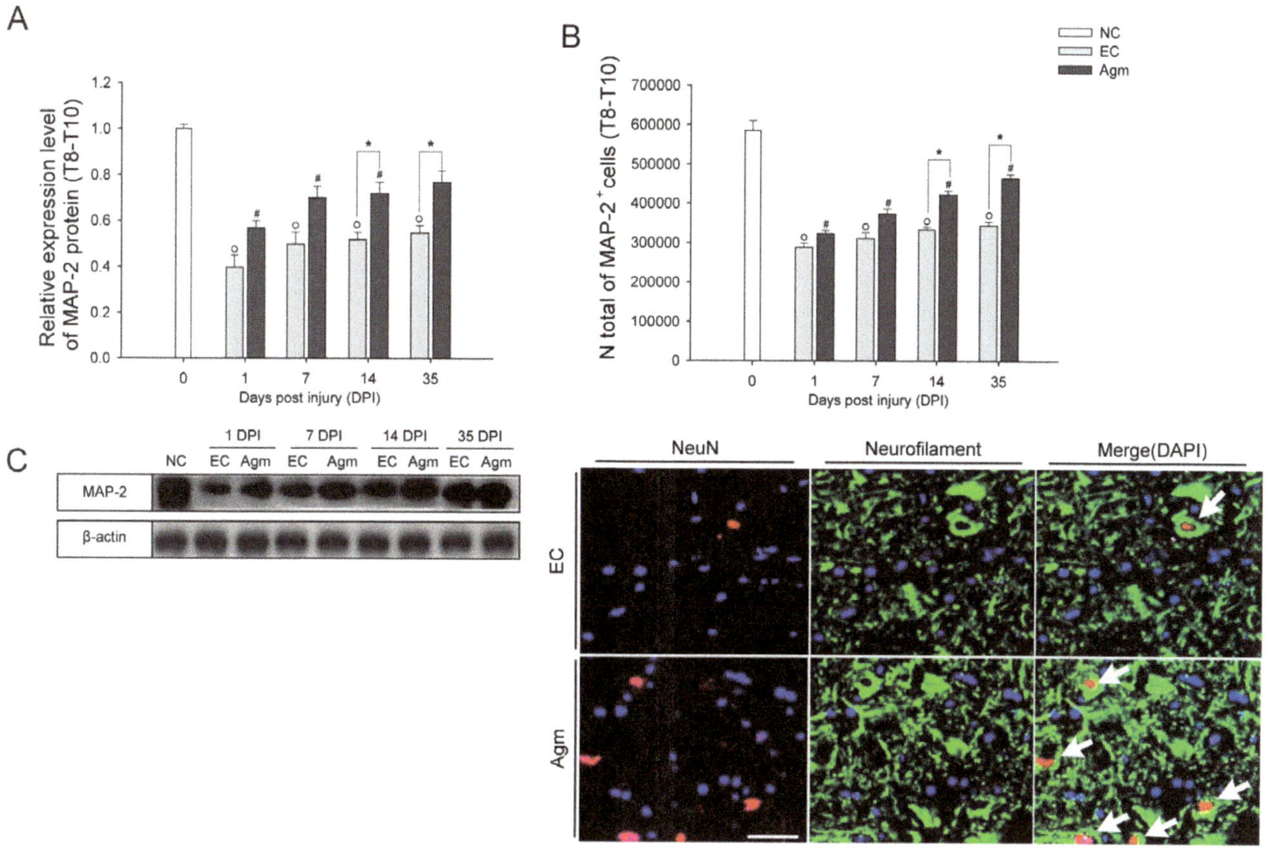

Figure 4. Agmatine treatment prevented neuronal cell loss following SCI. (A) Western blots of MAP-2 protein expression at 1, 7, 14, and 35 DPI. The representative graphs showed that the MAP-2 expression in Agm treated group ($n = 5$) was increased from 1 to 35 DPI and the increase was significant at 14 and 35 DPI compared to EC group ($n = 5$). (B) Stereological count of MAP-2$^+$ cells. The number of MAP-2$^+$ cells were increased in the Agm treated group ($n = 5$) at 1, 7, 14 and 35 DPI compared with the EC group ($n = 5$) in Th 8 - Th 10 segments of the spinal cord. (C) The injured spinal cord tissues were immunostained with NeuN (red) and Neurofilament (green). Results showed higher number of NeuN$^+$/Neurofilament$^+$ cells in the Agm treated group ($n = 5$) compared with the EC group ($n = 5$) at 35 DPI. Scale bars: 50 µm. †, $p<0.05$ NC group vs EC group; #, $p<0.05$ NC group vs Agm treated group; *, $p<0.05$ EC group vs Agm treated group. Results represent mean ± S.E.M.

neurons (immunostained with MAP-2 antibody) in the total spinal cord (Th 8–Th 10 segments) (Fig. 4B) and in the rostral (Th 8), the lesion (Th 9) and the caudal (Th 10) segments of the spinal cord were increased in Agm treated group at all the time intervals compared with EC group ($n = 15$, per group) (Fig. S5) and the increase was significant at 14 and 35 DPI compared with the EC group in the total spinal cord and in the rostral and caudal segments ($n = 15$, per group). These results suggest that Agm treatment rescue the damaged neurons and accelerate the regeneration of damaged neurons after SCI. The neuronal nucleus (NeuN) and neurofilament (NF) expressions were found almost exclusively in neuronal cells and support the cytoskeleton following SCI. In our study immunofluorescence staining was done to detect the expressions of NeuN$^+$/NF$^+$ cells in EC and Agm treated groups. Immunofluorescence results showed higher number of NeuN$^+$/NF$^+$ cells in Agm treated group ($n = 5$) compared with the EC group ($n = 5$) and it seems that Agm treatment preserved the formation of dendrites and cell bodies of neurons around the lesion site in the injured spinal cord at 35 DPI (Fig. 4C).

These findings suggest that Agm treatment attenuate the neuronal damage and aid for the neuronal survival following SCI.

Agmatine Treatment Attenuated Glial Scar Formation and Reactive Gliosis at the Injury Site Following SCI

SCI often results in permanent neurological impairment and axonal regeneration is made difficult due to astrocytes activation, oxidative stress, inflammation, cell death, and axon disruption [38]. Recently it was reported that Agm treatment could support neuroregeneration by reducing the collagen scar area by decreasing the expression of TGFß-2 and increasing the expression of BMP-7 following SCI [17,23].

In our study, the western blot results demonstrated significant decrease in the GFAP protein expression in the Agm treated group ($n = 5$) at all the time periods (1, 7, 14, and 35 DPI) and the decrease was statistically significant at 14 DPI (Fig. 5A) compared with EC group ($n = 5$). The number of GFAP$^+$ cells were counted using CAST analysis from total spinal cord (Th 8–Th 10 segments) and at the rostral (Th 8), the lesion (Th 9), and the caudal (Th 10) segments of the spinal cord in EC and Agm treated groups ($n = 5$, per group). The CAST analysis revealed significant decrease in the total number of GFAP$^+$ cells in the total spinal cord and also in the rostral, lesion and caudal segments of the spinal cord in Agm treated group compared with the EC group at 7, 14, and 35 DPI. (Fig. 5B, S6). And also, the glial scar formation after SCI was determined by GFAP immunoreactivity at the injured site. The GFAP immunoreactivity was measured using the image analysis

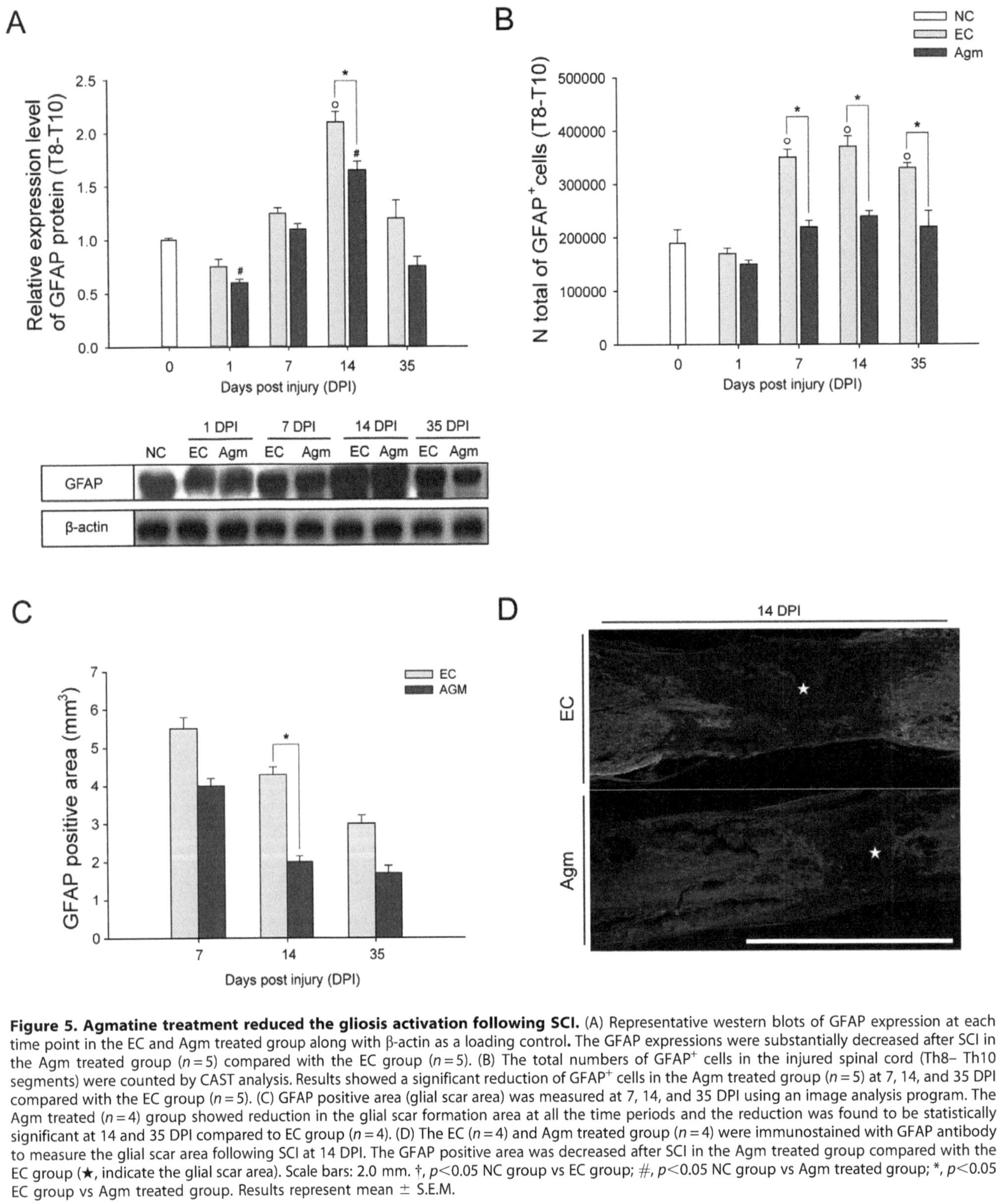

Figure 5. Agmatine treatment reduced the gliosis activation following SCI. (A) Representative western blots of GFAP expression at each time point in the EC and Agm treated group along with β-actin as a loading control. The GFAP expressions were substantially decreased after SCI in the Agm treated group ($n=5$) compared with the EC group ($n=5$). (B) The total numbers of $GFAP^+$ cells in the injured spinal cord (Th8– Th10 segments) were counted by CAST analysis. Results showed a significant reduction of $GFAP^+$ cells in the Agm treated group ($n=5$) at 7, 14, and 35 DPI compared with the EC group ($n=5$). (C) GFAP positive area (glial scar area) was measured at 7, 14, and 35 DPI using an image analysis program. The Agm treated ($n=4$) group showed reduction in the glial scar formation area at all the time periods and the reduction was found to be statistically significant at 14 and 35 DPI compared to EC group ($n=4$). (D) The EC ($n=4$) and Agm treated group ($n=4$) were immunostained with GFAP antibody to measure the glial scar area following SCI at 14 DPI. The GFAP positive area was decreased after SCI in the Agm treated group compared with the EC group (★, indicate the glial scar area). Scale bars: 2.0 mm. †, $p<0.05$ NC group vs EC group; #, $p<0.05$ NC group vs Agm treated group; *, $p<0.05$ EC group vs Agm treated group. Results represent mean ± S.E.M.

program. The results showed that Agm treatment significantly decreased the GFAP immunopositive area ($n=5$) compared with the EC group ($n=5$) at 7, 14 and 35 DPI and the decrease was found to be statistically significant at 14 and 35 DPI (Fig. 5C) suggesting that Agm treatment significantly attenuated the glial scar formation at 14 days following SCI (★, indicate glial scar area Fig. 5D).

Agmatine Treatment Prevented the Neuronal & Oligodendrocytes Cell Loss and Attenuated the Astrocytes Formation Around the Lesion Site Following SCI

Earlier it was reported that in the intact adult spinal cord the glial progenitor cells occupy 80% of the total cells. However, there is a substantial net increase in the progeny of damaged ependymal and astrocytes lineage cells following SCI [39,40]. Our present study first aimed to count the total cell numbers of surviving neurons, astrocytes and oligodendrocytes in the NC, EC and Agm treated groups ($n = 5$, per group) in Th 8–Th 10 segments of the spinal cord using CAST analysis program (cells were read as actual number; $\times 10^6$ cells/mm^3) at 1, 7, 14 and 35 DPI using MAP-2, GFAP and Olig-2 antibodies. The CAST results showed that in the control mice (NC group) the average cell number representing neurons were 5.742±0.274 ($\times 10^6$ cells/mm^3). After SCI the total neuronal cell numbers were decreased in the EC group. However, Agm treatment dramatically attenuated the total neuronal cell loss following SCI and the average cell count number were significantly higher at all the time points compared with the EC group and the average numbers compared with EC group (EC vs Agm) were: 2.875±0.043 vs 3.268±0.065 at 1 day, 3.127±0.065 vs 3.745±0.056 at 7 days, 3.359±0.095 vs 4.251±0.109 at 14 days and 3.517±0.144 vs 4.622±0.273 ($\times 10^6$ cells/mm^3) at 35 DPI. Specifically, the average numbers of surviving neurons in the Agm treated group were recorded to be almost similar to that NC group at 35 DPI.

The total number of oligodendrocytes were also counted using CAST analysis. The CAST counting results revealed that the average Olig-2$^+$ cell numbers in the NC group were 14.078±2.037 ($\times 10^6$ cells/mm^3). SCI resulted in the significant loss of oligodendrocytes. But, and the average cell count number from the CAST results showed 4.018±0.030, 4.997±0.205, 5.993±0.082 and 9.018±0.206 ($\times 10^6$ cells/mm^3) at 1, 7, 14 and 35 DPI respectively in EC group. But, Agm treatment prevented the oligodendrocytes cell loss and the average Olig-2$^+$ cells were 5.404±0.008, 6.964±0.04, 8.030±0.112 & 12.004±0.431 ($\times 10^6$ cells/mm^3) at 1, 7, 14 and 35 DPI and the average cell numbers were found to be significant at 7 and 14 days compared to the EC group.

The total numbers of GFAP$^+$ cells were counted in the NC, EC and Agm treated groups. CAST analysis showed that in the NC group the average total cell numbers of GFAP$^+$ cells were 2.092±0.281 ($\times 10^6$ cells/mm^3). Following SCI the total number of GFAP$^+$ cells were decreased in the Agm treated group compared to the EC group and the decrease between EC vs Agm were: 1.702±0.007 vs 1.502±0.005 at 1 day, 3.502±0.171 vs 2.205±0.108 at 7 days, 3.701±0.148 vs 2.395±0.086 at 14 days and 3.752±0.086 vs 2.503±0.055 ($\times 10^6$ cells/mm^3) at 35 DPI.

The overall CAST results suggest that Agm treatment significantly prevented the neurons and oligodendrocytes cell loss and inhibited the formation of astrocytes. Moreover, the average cell numbers of all the cell types (neurons, oligodendrocytes and astrocytes) in Agm treated group at 35 DPI were almost reached to the normal control group (Table 1).

Table 1. The average numbers of neurons and glial cells in injured spinal cord in Th 8–Th 10 segments following SCI.

		EC	Agm	NC
Neurons	**1 DPI**	2.875±0.043†	3.268±0.065$^\#$	5.742±0.274
	7 DPI	3.127±0.065†	3.745±0.056$^\#$	5.742±0.274
	14 DPI	3.359±0.095†	4.251±0.109$^{\#,*}$	5.742±0.274
	35 DPI	3.517±0.144†	4.622±0.273$^\#$ *	5.742±0.274
Oilgo dendrocytes	**1 DPI**	4.018±0.030†	5.404±0.008$^\#$	14.078±2.037
	7 DPI	4.997±0.205†	6.964±0.043$^\#$	14.078±2.037
	14 DPI	5.993±0.082†	8.030±0.112$^{\#,*}$	14.078±2.037
	35 DPI	9.018±0.206†	12.004±0.431$^{\#,*}$	14.078±2.037
Astrocytes	**1 DPI**	1.702±0.007	1.502±0.005	2.092±0.281
	7 DPI	3.502±0.171†	2.205±0.108*	2.092±0.281
	14 DPI	3.701±0.148†	2.395±0.086*	2.092±0.281
	35 DPI	3.752±0.086†	2.503±0.055*	2.092±0.281

For the computer assisted stereological toolbox (CAST) analysis the spinal cord containing Th 8–Th 10 segments were chosen for the study. The table showing the distribution of neurons, oligodendrocytes and astrocytes in NC group ($n = 5$), EC group ($n = 5$) and Agm treated group ($n = 5$) at 1, 7, 14, and 35 DPI. The cells were measured per mm^3 (Units: $\times 10^6$ cells/mm^3). The Agm treated group showed an overall increase of the total number of cells with high proportions of MAP-2$^+$ and Olig-2$^+$ cells and less GFAP$^+$ cells compared with the EC group at all the time periods following SCI. †, $p < 0.05$ NC group vs EC group; #, $p < 0.05$ NC group vs Agm treated group;*, $p < 0.05$ EC group vs Agm treated group. Results represent mean ± S.E.M.
Data are means ± S.E.M.
†, $P < 0.05$ for NC group vs EC group; #, $P < 0.05$ for NC group vs Agm group; *, $P < 0.05$ for EC vs Agm group.
NC: normal control group; EC: experimental control group; Agm: agmatine treated group; DPI: days post injury.
Cell number: $\times 10^6$ cells/mm^3; $n = 5$ per group.

Agmatine Treatment Modulated the BMP-2/4/7 Expressions Following SCI

Bone morphogenetic proteins (BMPs) play a critical role in regulating cell fate determination during central nervous system (CNS) development and BMP- 2/4/7 expressions in particular modulates cell differentiation at the injury site following SCI [16]. Taking into consideration the important roles of BMP- 2/4/7 expressions following SCI, here, we intended to investigate whether Agm treatment could modulate the BMP- 2/4/7 protein expressions and contribute for neurological recovery following SCI.

The quantitative western blot results showed that the BMP- 2/7 protein expressions were increased at 1, 7, 14, and 35 DPI and the values reached significant at 1 & 7 DPI and 7 & 14 DPI respectively in Agm treated group ($n = 5$) compared with the EC group ($n = 5$) (Fig. 6A, 6B). Conversely, the quantitative results of the BMP- 4 protein expression was decreased at 1, 7, 14, and 35 DPI and the values were significant at 7, 14 and 35 DPI in the Agm treated group ($n = 5$) compared with those of the EC group ($n = 5$) (Fig. 6C).

Agmatine Treatment Modulates the Expansion of Oligodendrocytes Progenitor Cells (NG2$^+$) via BMP- 2/4/7 Expressions Following SCI

Endogenous oligodendrocyte progenitor cells (NG2) local to the lesion site differentiate into oligodendrocytes and are responsible for myelin repair [41,42]. The expression pattern of NG2$^+$ in BMP- 2/4/7$^+$ cell populations was determined by immunofluorescence staining. The results suggested that the NG2$^+$/BMP- 2$^+$ cells were higher in the Agm treated group compared with EC group at 7 and 35 DPI. However, the NG2$^+$/BMP- 4$^+$ cell population were decreased at 7 DPI and the NG2$^+$/BMP- 4$^+$ cells were almost disappeared in the Agm group at 35 DPI. Conversely the expansion of NG2$^+$/BMP- 7$^+$ cells was increased around the lesion site in Agm treated group at 35 DPI compared to EC group ($n = 5$) (Fig. S8).

Agmatine Treatment Increased the BMP- 2/7 Expressions in Neurons and Oligodendrocytes and Decreased the BMP- 4 Expressions in Astrocytes and Oligodendrocytes Following SCI

BMPs are known to regulate proliferation or differentiation of neurons, oligodendrocytes, and astrocytes during CNS develop-

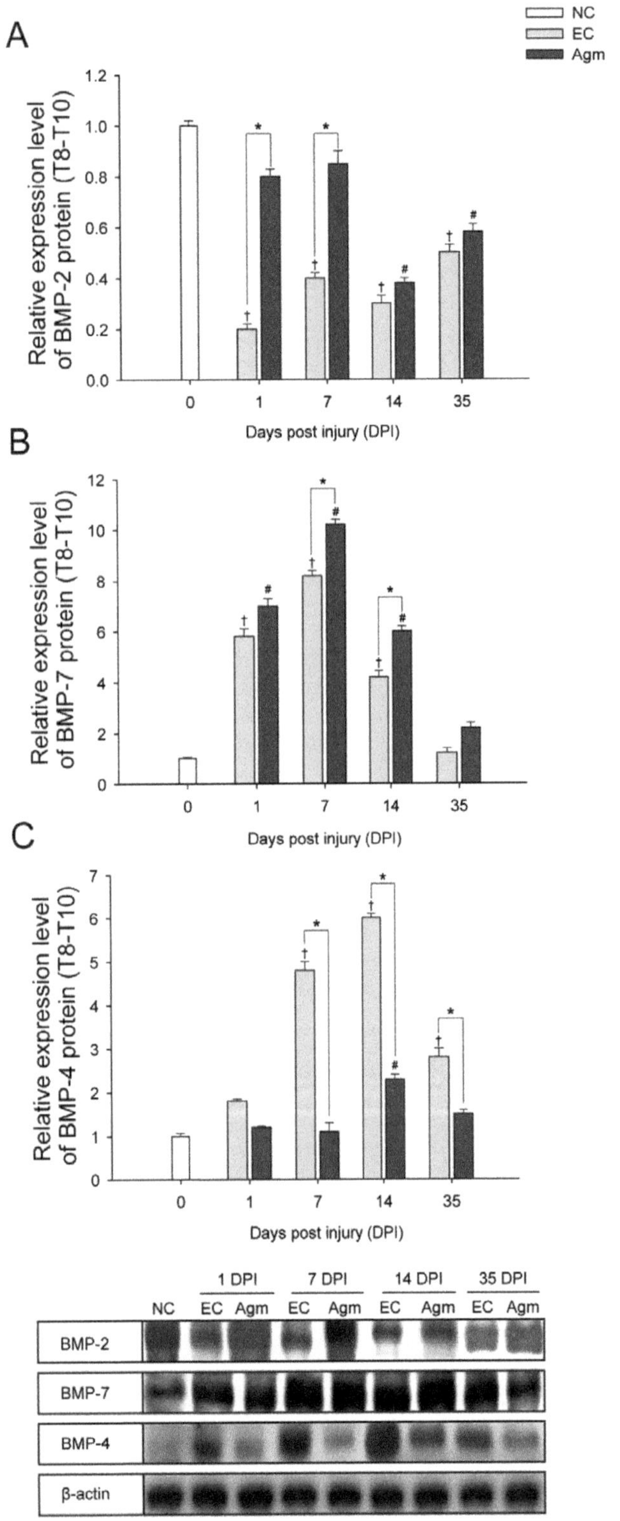

Figure 6. Agmatine treatment modulated the BMP- 2/4/7 expressions after SCI. Quantification of BMP- 2/4/7 protein expressions was determined by western blot analysis. The bar graph represents densitometry measurement of BMP- 2/4/7 protein expressions. (A) BMP- 2 protein expression was significantly higher in the Agm treated group ($n = 5$) compared with the EC group ($n = 5$) at 1 and 7 DPI. (B) BMP- 7 protein expression was higher in the Agm treated group ($n = 5$) compared with the EC group ($n = 5$) at 1, 7, 14, and 35 DPI and the increase was significant at 7 & 14 DPI. (C) BMP- 4 expression was significantly lower in the Agm treated group ($n = 5$) compared with the EC group ($n = 5$) at 7, 14 & 35 DPI following SCI. †, $p<0.05$ NC group vs EC group; #, $p<0.05$ NC group vs Agm treated group; *, $p<0.05$ EC group vs Agm treated group. Results represent mean ± S.E.M.

ment [43]. We hypothesized whether Agm treatment could modulate BMPs expression in neurons, astrocytes and oligodendrocytes after SCI. Recent findings demonstrated that BMPs show potential relationship with neurons and glial cells in the normal/ injured spinal cord [16]. In this study immunofluorescence and DAB staining (CAST analysis) were performed to co-localize and count the BMP- $2/4/7^+$ cells in neurons, oligodendrocytes and astrocytes at 1, 7, 14 and 35 DPI.

The immunofluorescence staining results showed higher number of BMP- 2^+/MAP-2^+ & BMP- 2^+/Olig-2^+ cells in Agm treated group compared to the EC group at 7 and 14 days respectively following SCI (Fig. 7A). Similarly, CAST results showed the total number of BMP- 2^+/MAP-2^+ and BMP- 2^+/Olig-2^+ cells were higher in the Agm treated group ($n = 5$) compared with the EC group ($n = 5$) at 1, 7, 14 and 35 DPI and the increase in numbers were significant at 7 & 35 DPI and 7 & 14 DPI respectively in the Agm treated group ($n = 5$) compared with EC group ($n = 5$) (Fig. 8A, 8B). The average cell numbers representing the BMP- 2 co-localized cells with MAP-2 and Olig-2 expressions were provided in the Table S2.

It was reported that BMP- 7 has been shown to exert neuroprotective effect after traumatic SCI and promote the functional recovery after contusion SCI [17]. Here, we investigated whether Agm could modulate the BMP- 7 expressions in neurons and oligodendrocytes after SCI. Dual immunofluorescence staining was performed to localize the BMP- 7^+/MAP-2^+ and BMP- 7^+/Olig-2^+ cells following SCI. The immunofluorescence staining results showed increased number of BMP- 7^+/ MAP-2^+ and BMP- 7^+/Olig-2^+ cells at 7 and 14 DPI in the Agm treated group ($n = 4$) compared with the respective EC group ($n = 4$) (Fig. 7B). DAB immunostaining was also performed to localize the BMP- 7 expression in neurons and oligodendrocytes and the total number of BMP- 7^+/MAP-2^+ and BMP- 7^+/Olig-2^+ cells were counted using the CAST analysis program. The CAST data showed that the number of BMP- 7^+/MAP-2^+ and BMP- 7^+/ Olig-2^+ cells were increased in the Agm treated group ($n = 5$) compared with the EC group ($n = 5$) at 1, 7, 14, and 35 DPI and the values were significant at 7 & 14 DPI and 7 DPI respectively compared with that of the EC group (Fig. 8C, 8D). The average cell numbers representing the BMP-7 co-localized cells with MAP-2 and Olig-2 expressions was provided in the Table S2.

BMP- 4 can take part in inhibiting oligodendrocytes specification and differentiation to promote astrocytes proliferation after injury [16]. Previous findings suggest that BMP- 4 increases reactive gliosis and glial scar formation at the lesion site following SCI [44,45]. To ascertain the involvement of BMP- 4 expression in modulating gliosis, immmunofluorescence staining was performed to localize the BMP- 4^+ cells in astrocytes and oligodendrocytes. Results showed that Agm treatment decreased the BMP- 4^+/GFAP$^+$ cell population at 7 DPI and increased the BMP- 4^+/Olig-2^+ cells expansion at 35 DPI (Fig. 7C). However, BMP- 4 expression was not found to be co-localized with MAP-2 both in the EC and the Agm treated group (Fig. S7).

Simultaneously, CAST analysis was performed to count the total number of BMP- 4^+ cells in astrocytes and oligodendrocytes in the EC ($n = 5$) and Agm treated group ($n = 5$) at 1, 7, 14, and 35 DPI. The CAST results showed that the total numbers of BMP- 4^+/GFAP$^+$ and BMP- 4^+/Olig-2^+ cells in the Agm treated group were decreased at all the time periods compared with the EC

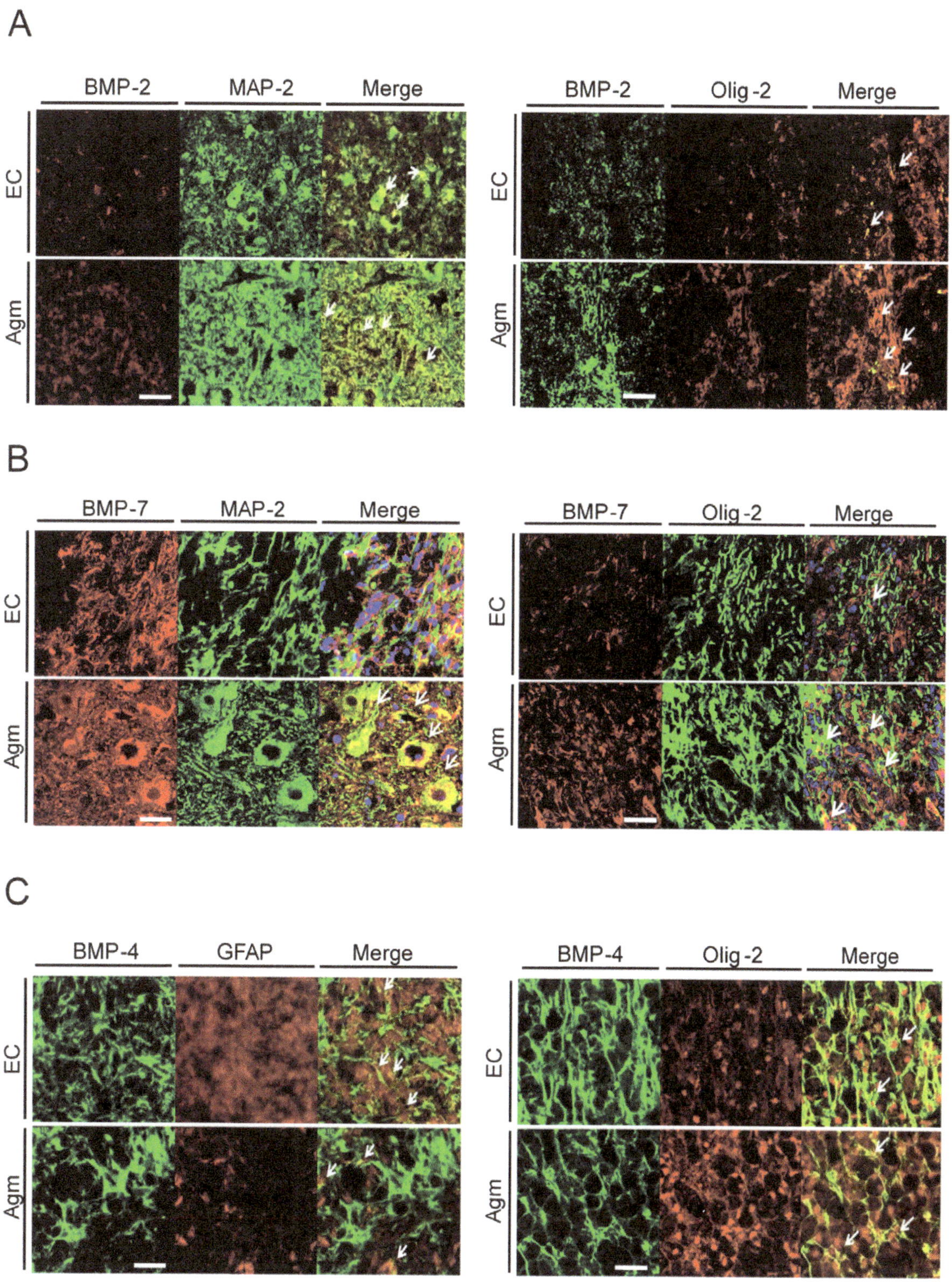

Figure 7. Confocal microscopic images of BMP- 2/4/7 expressions in neurons, oligodendrocytes and astrocytes after agmatine treatment following SCI. (A) Dual immunofluorescence was done to localize the BMP- 2 expression in neurons (MAP-2) and oligodendrocytes (Olig-2) after SCI. The BMP- 2^+/MAP- 2^+& BMP- 2^+/Olig-2^+ cells around the lesion site were higher in the Agm treated group ($n = 4$) compared with the EC group ($n = 4$) at7 DPI. Scale bars: 50 μm. (B) The immunostaining of BMP- 7 (red) with MAP-2 (green) showed increased number of BMP- 7^+/MAP-2^+ cells in the Agm treated group ($n = 5$) when compared with the EC group ($n = 5$) at 7 days after SCI. The immunostaining of BMP- 7 with Olig-2 showed an increased number of BMP- 7^+/Olig-2^+ cells in the Agm treated group ($n = 5$) compared to EC group ($n = 5$) at 14 DPI. Scale bars: 10 μm. (C) The immuno co-localization of BMP- 4^+ cells in astrocytes (GFAP) showed reduced number of BMP- 4^+/GFAP$^+$ cellsaround the lesion site in the Agm treated group ($n = 4$) compared with the EC group ($n = 4$) at7 DPI. Whereas, BMP- 4^+/Olig-2^+ cells were higher in the Agm treated group compared with EC at 35 DPI. The scale bars: 10 μm.

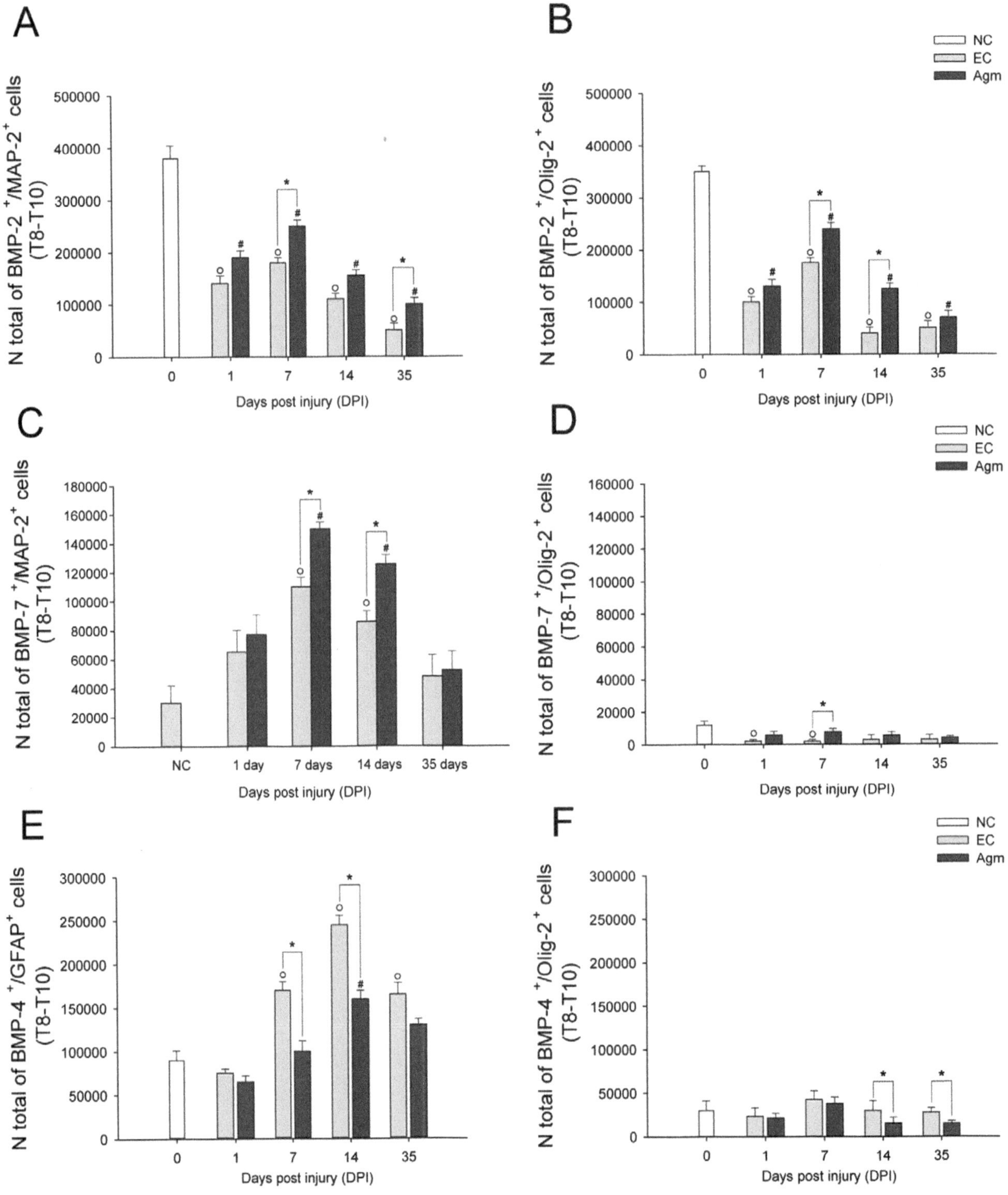

Figure 8. CAST analysis showed that agmatine treatment modulated BMP- 2/7 expressions in neurons & oligodendrocytes and BMP- 4 expressions in astrocytes & oligodendrocytes following SCI. (A) Stereological counting of BMP- 2^+/MAP-$2^+$and (B) BMP- 2^+/Olig-2^+ cells in the injured spinal cord (Th 8–Th 10 segments). The number of BMP- 2^+/MAP-2^+ and BMP- 2^+/Olig-2^+ cells were significantly increased in the Agm treated group ($n = 5$) compared with the EC group ($n = 5$) at 7 & 35 DPI and 7 & 14 DPI (C) BMP- 7^+/MAP-2^+ and (D) BMP- 7^+/Olig-2^+ cells in the Th 8–Th 10 segments of the injured spinal cord. The number of BMP-7^+/MAP-2^+ and BMP-7^+/Olig-2^+ cells were significantly increased in the Agm treated group ($n = 5$) compared with the EC group ($n = 5$) at 7 & 14 days and 7 days respectively following SCI. (E) BMP- 4^+/GFAP$^+$ and (F) BMP- 4^+/Olig-2^+ cells in Th 8–Th 10 segments of the injured spinal cord. The number of BMP- 4^+/GFAP$^+$ and BMP- 4^+/Olig-2^+ cells were decreased at all the time periods in the Agm treated group ($n = 5$) compared with the EC group ($n = 5$) and the decrease was significant at 7 & 14 days and 14 & 35 days respectively following SCI. †, $p<0.05$ NC group vs EC group; #, $p<0.05$ NC group vs Agm treated group; *, $p<0.05$ EC group vs Agm treated group. Results represent mean ± S.E.M.

group and the decrease was found to be statistically significant at 7 & 14 DPI in astrocytes and at 14 & 35 DPI in oligodendrocytes (Fig. 8E, 8F) compared with EC group. The average cell numbers representing the BMP- 4 co-localized cells with GFAP and Olig-2 expressions was provided in Table S2.

Discussion

Agmatine (Agm), an N-methyl-D-aspartate receptor (NMDAR) antagonist and nitric oxide synthase (NOS) inhibitor prevent adaptive changes in neuronal function and selectively relieves allodynic, hyperalgesic, and autotomy-like states accompanying spinal cord injury (SCI) [10]. In neurons of the brain and spinal cord, Agm is packaged in synaptic vesicles and released upon neuronal depolarization. The evidence of neuromodulatory role for Agm is shown to antagonize NMDAR [46–48].

In the present study, Agm treatment (1) improved locomotory and physiological functions, (2) facilitated axonal remyelination, (3) promoted protection of neurons, (4) attenuated glial scar formation, and (5) modulated the BMP- 2/4/7 expressions in neuronal and glial cells which might be critical factor for the improvements of the impairments following SCI. Previous studies suggested that mice and rat recovered from locomotor dysfunctions after Agm treatment in contusion and transaction SCI models [23,49]. Corroborating with the earlier studies our funtional recovery test results also demonstrated that Agm treated mice significantly regained the ability to make weight-supported steps with their hind limbs, which was in stark contrast to EC group (saline treated mice) that only regained the ability to make rhythmic sweeping motions with their hind limbs after SCI. SCI leads to bladder and renal dysfunctions resulting in failure of self urination and ultimately delay the overall recovery process [50]. In our study, injury induced bladder dysfunction was restored with Agm treatment is of particular clinical relevance for quality of life, since restoration of bladder function is consistently ranked as a higher priority than walking [30]. SCI is a devastating disease and the resultant pathology arises from both primary and secondary injury mechanisms resulting in inflammation and oxidative stress leading to low survival rate of the oligodendrocytes [51]. In general oligodendrocytes provide myelin sheath formation for enhanced axonal transmission [52,53]. But, SCI results in the loss of myelin forming cells which leads to exposure of surviving axons, impairs their conductive capacity and limits the recovery of neural function [54]. Oligodendrocytes that survive the demyelinating insult are not thought to be able to contribute to remyelination [55,56]. Instead endogenous oligodendrocyte progenitor cells, $NG2^+$ cells, local to the lesion are believed to be the source of new myelinating cells and there are evidences that these cells are responsible for myelin repair [57–59]. Our transmission electron microscopic (TEM) studies suggested that Agm treatment showed better pattern of myelination in the lesioned cords compared to EC group and luxol fast blue staining indicated the reconstruction of lost myelin and neurons. Immunostaining results suggested that Agm treatment increased the intensification of oligodendrocyte progenitor cells ($NG2^+$) associated with mature oligodendrocytes ($Olig\text{-}2^+$) with less expansion of $NG2^+/GFAP^+$ cells in Agm treated group compared to EC group following SCI. These events of remyelination were further confirmed by quantification of Olig-2 expression by western blotting and CAST analysis. The $Olig\text{-}2^+/MBP^+$ cells were increased in the Agm treated group compared to those in the EC group after SCI, suggesting that Agm treatment might boost the regeneration of damaged oligodendrocytes, prevent myelin loss, and assist in enhancing axonal remyelination following SCI.

In the spinal cord, neurons coordinate rhythmic locomotor movements [60,61] and these spinal neurons require neuromodulators like serotonin (5-hydroxytryptamine or 5-HT) to function, setting them into a state of readiness for sensiromotor integration [62,63]. The neuromodulator, 5-HT is one of the important endogenous monoamine synthesized by specialized neurons in the brainstem (ie, raphe nucleus and parapyramidal region) with extended projections throughout the brain as well as in the spinal cord as far as into the lumbar and sacral segments [1]. During the chronic phase of SCI, drugs that activate 5-HT may contribute for regaining the sensiromotor integration showing the strong correlation between locomotor recovery and lumbosacral spinal 5-HT status after SCI [64,65]. Our immunostaining results with 5-HT antibody (represents serotogenic fiber staining) showed increase in the caudal 5-HT fiber density in the Agm treated group and the morphology of the serotogenic fibers were almost similar compared to normal control mice. However the serotogenic fibers showed broken morphology in the EC group and were appeared like beads both at 14 and 35 DPI. These results depicts that local sprouting of the serotogenic fibers could accout for the improvement of functional recovery in the Agm treated mice.

SCI causes neuronal and glial cells loss resulting in motor neuron dysfunctions. SCI repair focuses on finding ways to improve the axonal re-growth, the axonal re-connection and replace or protect damaged neurons and glial cells [66,67]. Given that Agm has been reported to possess neuroprotective effects, our western blot and immunostaining data demonstrated that Agm treatment increased the MAP-2, NeuN, and NF expressions following SCI. Parallel to our western blot and immunostaining results, CAST analysis also revealed an increased expansion of $MAP\text{-}2^+$ cell population in the Agm treated group. The p53 associated apoptosis is considered to be one of the common mechanisms of cell death in neurodegenerative diseases. Our immunohistochemical staining results revealed fewer number of p53 positive cells in the Agm treated group compared with EC group both at 14 and 35 DPI. The above findings suggest that Agm treatment rescued the neuronal cell loss and exerted neuroprotection in the damaged cords.

Following SCI one of the physical barriers for regenerating axons is glial scar formation, which consists predominately of reactive astrocytes. Axons cannot regenerate beyond the glial scar, and they take a dystrophic appearance of stalled growth [51] and GFAP is one of the major intermediates reported to be localized in the cytoplasm responsible for the surrounding astrocytes population [68]. Finding means of inhibiting the glial scar formation offers a potential strategy for facilitating axonal regeneration. Recently, it was demonstrated that Agm treatment reduced collagen scar formation in a transected SCI mice [23]. In agreement with the above findings our current study results also demonstrated that the expansion of glial scar formation area was significantly attenuated in Agm treatment compared with the EC group. The beneficial effects of Agm on functional outcome may in part be due to increased tissue preservation within the injury site (glial scar attenuation), since the amount of preserved tissue has previously been positively correlated with functional outcome [69]. Interestingly, our western blot and CAST results also showed that the expansion of $GFAP^+$ cells were significantly decreased in the Agm treated group which might facilitate the reduction in the glial scar formation following SCI.

The bone morphogenic proteins (BMPs) signalling enhances axonal outgrowth and locomotory recovery following SCI [70]. Previous studies demonstrated that BMPs play key roles as neurotrophic and growth factors during CNS development [4,71]. In addition BMPs also play important role in regulating the development of many tissues, protecting nerve cells, promoting their re-growth, and promoting a substantial improvement in locomotor function following CNS injuries [72]. Moreover, the BMPs signaling are implicated in multiple developments such as proliferation, differentiation and dendrite formation of neuronal cells [73,74]. In light of above evidences we intended to investigate whether Agm treatment could modulate the BMPs (BMP- 2/4/7 in particular) expressions in neurons and glial cells which might promote the glial and neuronal cell survival following SCI. Among the BMPs family, BMP- 2 promotes the differentiation of neurons and dendrite growth in cultured striatum neurons [75] and the percentage of MAP-2^+ cells were greatly increased with BMP- 2 stimulation in a mouse embryonic telencephalon culture, however, the percentage of $GFAP^+$ cells were decreased [76]. Our study results showed that the BMP- 2 expression in neurons and oligodendendrocytes were increased in Agm treated group following SCI showing the role of BMP- 2 in controlling neurogenesis and oligodendrogenesis. The expression of BMP- 7 was known to increase after CNS injury in motor neurons and might regulate differentiation of glial cells from neural progenitors which induced functional recovery after CNS injury [77,78]. In addition, the expression of BMP- 7 was reported to exert both neuroprotective and neuroregenerative effects in animals with stroke and SCI [18,79]. In agreement to the previous findings, our results show that Agm treatment increased the BMP- 7 expression in neurons and oligodendrocytes following SCI which might be one of the critical factor for restoration of damaged neurons and oligodendrocytes. It was reported that the expression of BMP- 4 enhanced the astrocytic lineage during CNS development and contributed to the formation of glial scar in injured spinal cord [45,80]. BMP- 4 can induce oligodendroglial lineage cells and promote functional recovery in paraplegic mice [13,16]. Recently, it was demonstrated that transected axons can be regenerated with the adeno-associated virus (AAV) vector encoding BMP- 4 treatment following SCI [81]. In parallel with the available literature reporting the BMP- 4 function in regulating the astrocytes formation, our CAST results showed that the number of BMP- 4^+ cells were lessened in astrocytes and oligodendrocytes after SCI in the Agm treated group compared with the EC group, suggesting that Agm treatment could be beneficial in controlling glial scar formation through modulating BMPs expression following SCI. Inhibitory role of BMP- 4 in neural differentiation of murine embryonic stem cells further confirmed our immunostaining results of the non-colocalization of BMP- 4^+ and MAP-2^+ co-localized cells [82,83]. While contemplating the BMP- 2/4/7 expression in oligodendrocyte precursor cell population (NG2), our immunofluroscence staining showed no co-localized cells at the injury site (data not shown). However, co-localized cells were identified little away from the injury site and staining pictures suggested that Agm treatment activated $NG2^+$/Olig-2^+ cells and this increase is thought to be associated with $NG2^+$/BMP- 2^+/7^+cells. The attenuation of $NG2^+/GFAP^+$ cells seems to be related with the decreased population of $NG2^+$/BMP- 4^+ cells.

Immunohistochemical techniques that enable the detection of specific molecular markers at the single-cell level are essential tools for identifying and characterizing cells in healthy and pathological tissue. Previous report demonstrated the random quantification of oligodendrocytes, ependymal and astrocytes in SCI mice [39]. We for the first time provided the un-biased distribution data of MAP-2 (neurons), Olig-2 (oligodendrocytes), GFAP (astrocytes) immunopositive cells and BMP- 2/4/7 expressions in neurons, astrocytes and oligodendrocytes in Th 8–Th 10 segments of the spinal cord by CAST analysis program. Our results suggested that the total number of surviving neurons and oligodendrocytes were increased and the astrocytes poulation was decreased and the total cell number of the surviving cells almost reached almost to that of normal control group in the Agm treated mice at 35DPI. And also, Agm treatment increased the BMP- 2/7 expressions in neurons and oligodendrocytes and decreased in the astrocytes following SCI. Moreover, the reduction of gliosis and glial scar formation following SCI is thought to be controlled with the decreased expression of BMP- 4 in astrocytes in the Agm treated group following SCI.

Conclusions

Taken together our results suggest that Agm treatment apparently improved the neurological & functional outcomes, improved the remyelination, rescued the damaged neurons and attenuated the glial scar formation after SCI. These beneficial effects are thought to be related with differential expression of BMP- 2/4/7 in neurons, oligodendrocytes and astrocytes with Agm treatment. However, further studies are necessary to elucidate the pharmacokinetics of Agm in the CNS, which may in turn open a new window into the clinical treatment of human SCI.

Supporting Information

Figure S1 Agmatine treatment attenuated apoptosis following SCI. The EC ($n=4$) and Agm treated group ($n=4$) were immunostained with p53 antibody at (A) 14 and (B) 35 DPI. The p53 expression was substantially decreased after SCI in the Agm treated group compared with the EC group at 14 and 35 DPI. Scale bars: 50 μm.

Figure S2 Agmatine treatment increased serotogenic fiber following SCI. Images were taken from the mice which received either Agm or saline ($n=3$, per group) following SCI. Agm treated mice showed dense network of 5-HT^+ serotonergic fibers in the caudal region of the spinal cord almost showing the same morphology to that of the normal control group ($n=3$). EC group showed the beaded and broken morphology of serotogenic fibers both at 14 and 35 DPI. Scale bars: 50 μm.

Figure S3 Agmatine treatment increased the expansion of oligodendrocyte progenitor cells ($NG2^+$) following SCI. Immunolocalization of $NG2^+$ cells in astrocytes ($GFAP^+$) and oligodendrocytes (Olig-2^+) at (A) 7 and (B) 35 DPI. The number of $NG2^+/GFAP^+$ cells were reduced in the Agm treated group ($n=5$) compared with the EC group ($n=5$) at (C) 7 & (D) 35 DPI. The $NG2^+$/Olig-2^+ cells expansion were outnumbered in the Agm treated group both at 7 & 35 DPI compared with EC group.

Figure S4 Agmatine treatment increased the number of oligodendroyctes following SCI. The quantitative measurements of the total Olig-2^+ cells by CAST analysis in (A) the rostral (Th 8), (B) lesion (Th 9) and (C) caudal (Th 10) regions after SCI. The results showed a significant increase of the Olig-2^+ cells in Th 8, Th 9 and Th 10 segments of the injured spinal cord in the Agm treated group compared with the EC group and the values reached significance at 35 DPI ($n=5$). †, $p<0.05$ NC group vs EC group; #, $p<0.05$ NC group vs Agm treated group; *, $p<0.05$ EC group vs Agm treated group. Results represent mean ± S.E.M.

Figure S5 Agmatine treatment prevented neuronal cells death following SCI. The quantitative measurement of the total

MAP-2$^+$ cells using CAST analysis in (A) the rostral (Th 8), (B) the lesion (Th 9) and (C) the caudal (Th 10) regions of the injured spinal cord ($n = 5$, per group).The results showed an increase of MAP-2$^+$ cells in Th 8, Th 9, and Th 10 segments of the spinal cord in the Agm treated group ($n = 5$) compared with the EC group ($n = 5$) and significant increase was recorded at 14 and 35 DPI in rostral and caudal segments. †, $p<0.05$ NC group vs EC group; #, $p<0.05$ NC group vs Agm treated group; *, $p<0.05$ EC group vs Agm treated group. Results represent mean ± S.E.M.

Figure S6 Agmatine treatment reduced the number of astrocytes following SCI. The quantitative measurement of the GFAP$^+$ cells using CAST analysis in the (A) rostral (Th 8), (B) lesion (Th 9) and (C) caudal (Th 10) regions of injured spinal cord. The results showed a significant decrease of the GFAP$^+$ cells in Th 8, Th 9, and Th 10 segments of the injured spinal cord in the Agm treated group ($n = 5$) compared with the EC group ($n = 5$) at 7, 14, and 35 DPI. †, $p<0.05$ NC group vs EC group; #, $p<0.05$ NC group vs Agm treated group; *, $p<0.05$ EC group vs Agm treated group. Results represent mean ± S.E.M.

Figure S7 Non co-localization of neurons and BMP- 4 following SCI. There were no BMP- 4 & MAP-2 co-localized cells both in the EC group ($n = 4$) and Agm treated group ($n = 4$) at (A) 7 days and (B) 35 days around the lesion site following SCI. Scale bars: in A, 100 μm & in B, 10 μm.

Figure S8 Agmatine treatment increased oligodendrocyte progenitor cells (NG2$^+$) following SCI. The expression of NG2$^+$ in BMP- 2/4/7$^+$ cell population was determined by immunofluorescence staining. The NG2$^+$/BMP- 2$^+$ cells were higher in the Agm treated group compared with EC group at (A) 7 and (B) 35 DPI. (C) Conversely the expansion of NG2$^+$/BMP- 7$^+$ cells were increased around the lesion site in Agm treated group at 35 DPI compared to EC group. (D) NG2$^+$/BMP- 4$^+$ cell population was decreased at 7 days and the (E) NG2$^+$/BMP- 4$^+$ cells were almost disappeared in the Agm treated group at 35 DPI.

Table S1 The table showing the allocation of animals in normal control (NC), saline treated mice (EC group) and Agm treated mice (Agm treated group) following SCI.

Table S2 The average numbers of BMP- 2/4/7$^+$ cells in neurons and glial cells in Th 8–Th 10 segments following SCI. The table showing the total number of BMP- 2/4/7$^+$ cells co-localized with MAP-2$^+$,Olig-2$^+$ and GFAP$^+$ cell population in Th 8–Th 10 segments at 1, 7, 14, and 35 DPI in NC group ($n = 5$), EC group ($n = 5$) and Agm treated group ($n = 5$) using computer assisted stereological toolbox (CAST) analysis. The immunopositive cells were measured per mm^3 (Units: $\times 10^6$cells/mm^3). †, $p<0.05$ NC group vs EC group; #, $p<0.05$ NC group vs Agm treated group; *, $p<0.05$ EC group vs Agm treated group. Results represent mean ± S.E.M.

Author Contributions

Conceived and designed the experiments: JEL YMP WTL KAP JHK. Performed the experiments: JEL YMP SKS. Analyzed the data: JEL YMP. Contributed reagents/materials/analysis tools: JEL YMP SKS KKB. Wrote the paper: JEL YMP KKB SHP MAY.

References

1. Guertin PA (2008) Anxiolytics may promote locomotor function recovery in spinal cord injury patients. Neuropsychiatr Dis Treat 4: 759–763.
2. Yoshimura N (1999) Bladder afferent pathway and spinal cord injury: possible mechanisms inducing hyperreflexia of the urinary bladder. Prog Neurobiol 57: 583–606.
3. Rasouli A, Bhatia N, Dinh P, Cahill K, Suryadevara S, et al. (2009) Resection of glial scar following spinal cord injury. J Orthop Res 27: 931–936.
4. McDonald JW, Belegu V (2006) Demyelination and remyelination after spinal cord injury. J Neurotrauma 23: 345–359.
5. Kotter MR, Stadelmann C, Hartung HP (2011) Enhancing remyelination in disease–can we wrap it up? Brain 134: 1882–1900.
6. Kulbatski I, Mothe AJ, Keating A, Hakamata Y, Kobayashi E, et al. (2007) Oligodendrocytes and radial glia derived from adult rat spinal cord progenitors: morphological and immunocytochemical characterization. J Histochem Cytochem 55: 209–222.
7. Li G, Regunathan S, Barrow CJ, Eshraghi J, Cooper R, et al. (1994) Agmatine: an endogenous clonidine-displacing substance in the brain. Science 263: 966–969.
8. Piletz JE, Chikkala DN, Ernsberger P (1995) Comparison of the properties of agmatine and endogenous clonidine-displacing substance at imidazoline and alpha-2 adrenergic receptors. J Pharmacol Exp Ther 272: 581–587.
9. Murayama T, Tsai SC, Adamik R, Moss J, Vaughan M (1993) Effects of temperature on ADP-ribosylation factor stimulation of cholera toxin activity. Biochemistry 32: 561–566.
10. Fairbanks CA, Schreiber KL, Brewer KL, Yu CG, Stone LS, et al. (2000) Agmatine reverses pain induced by inflammation, neuropathy, and spinal cord injury. Proc Natl Acad Sci U S A 97: 10584–10589.
11. Chen D, Zhao M, Mundy GR (2004) Bone morphogenetic proteins. Growth Factors 22: 233–241.
12. Karimi-Abdolrezaee S, Schut D, Wang J, Fehlings MG (2012) Chondroitinase and growth factors enhance activation and oligodendrocyte differentiation of endogenous neural precursor cells after spinal cord injury. PLoS One 7: e37589.
13. Obermair FJ, Schroter A, Thallmair M (2008) Endogenous neural progenitor cells as therapeutic target after spinal cord injury. Physiology (Bethesda) 23: 296–304.
14. Reiriz J, Espejo M, Ventura F, Ambrosio S, Alberch J (1999) Bone morphogenetic protein-2 promotes dissociated effects on the number and differentiation of cultured ventral mesencephalic dopaminergic neurons. J Neurobiol 38: 161–170.
15. Lein PJ, Beck HN, Chandrasekaran V, Gallagher PJ, Chen HL, et al. (2002) Glia induce dendritic growth in cultured sympathetic neurons by modulating the balance between bone morphogenetic proteins (BMPs) and BMP antagonists. J Neurosci 22: 10377–10387.
16. Xiao Q, Du Y, Wu W, Yip HK (2010) Bone morphogenetic proteins mediate cellular response and, together with Noggin, regulate astrocyte differentiation after spinal cord injury. Exp Neurol 221: 353–366.
17. de Rivero Vaccari JP, Marcillo A, Nonner D, Dietrich WD, Keane RW (2009) Neuroprotective effects of bone morphogenetic protein 7 (BMP7) treatment after spinal cord injury. Neurosci Lett 465: 226–229.
18. Setoguchi T, Yone K, Matsuoka E, Takenouchi H, Nakashima K, et al. (2001) Traumatic injury-induced BMP7 expression in the adult rat spinal cord. Brain Res 921: 219–225.
19. Chalazonitis A, D'Autreaux F, Pham TD, Kessler JA, Gershon MD (2011) Bone morphogenetic proteins regulate enteric gliogenesis by modulating ErbB3 signaling. Dev Biol 350: 64–79.
20. See J, Mamontov P, Ahn K, Wine-Lee L, Crenshaw EB III, et al. (2007) BMP signaling mutant mice exhibit glial cell maturation defects. Mol Cell Neurosci 35: 171–182.
21. Matsuura I, Taniguchi J, Hata K, Saeki N, Yamashita T (2008) BMP inhibition enhances axonal growth and functional recovery after spinal cord injury. J Neurochem 105: 1471–1479.
22. Setoguchi T, Nakashima K, Takizawa T, Yanagisawa M, Ochiai W, et al. (2004) Treatment of spinal cord injury by transplantation of fetal neural precursor cells engineered to express BMP inhibitor. Exp Neurol 189: 33–44.
23. Kim JH, Lee YW, Park YM, Park KA, Park SH, et al. (2011) Agmatine-reduced collagen scar area accompanied with surface righting reflex recovery after complete transection spinal cord injury. Spine (Phila Pa 1976) 36: 2130–2138.
24. Basso DM, Fisher LC, Anderson AJ, Jakeman LB, McTigue DM, et al. (2006) Basso Mouse Scale for locomotion detects differences in recovery after spinal cord injury in five common mouse strains. J Neurotrauma 23: 635–659.
25. Pajoohesh-Ganji A, Byrnes KR, Fatemi G, Faden AI (2010) A combined scoring method to assess behavioral recovery after mouse spinal cord injury. Neurosci Res 67: 117–125.
26. Sharp KG, Dickson AR, Marchenko SA, Yee KM, Emery PN, et al. (2012) Salmon fibrin treatment of spinal cord injury promotes functional recovery and density of serotonergic innervation. Exp Neurol 235: 345–356.
27. Hvid M, Jensen HK, Deleuran B, Kemp K, Andersson C, et al. (2009) Evaluation of FITC-induced atopic dermatitis-like disease in NC/Nga mice and

BALB/c mice using computer-assisted stereological toolbox, a computer-aided morphometric system. Int Arch Allergy Immunol 149: 188–194.
28. de Groat WC, Yoshimura N (2006) Mechanisms underlying the recovery of lower urinary tract function following spinal cord injury. Prog Brain Res 152: 59–84.
29. Widerstrom-Noga E, Cruz-Almeida Y, Krassioukov A (2004) Is there a relationship between chronic pain and autonomic dysreflexia in persons with cervical spinal cord injury? J Neurotrauma 21: 195–204.
30. Estores IM (2003) The consumer's perspective and the professional literature: what do persons with spinal cord injury want? J Rehabil Res Dev 40: 93–98.
31. Anderson KD (2004) Targeting recovery: priorities of the spinal cord-injured population. J Neurotrauma 21: 1371–1383.
32. Amar AP, Levy ML (1999) Pathogenesis and pharmacological strategies for mitigating secondary damage in acute spinal cord injury. Neurosurgery 44: 1027–1039.
33. Crowe MJ, Bresnahan JC, Shuman SL, Masters JN, Beattie MS (1997) Apoptosis and delayed degeneration after spinal cord injury in rats and monkeys. Nat Med 3: 73–76.
34. Thuret S, Moon LD, Gage FH (2006) Therapeutic interventions after spinal cord injury. Nat Rev Neurosci 7: 628–643.
35. Bregman BS, Kunkel-Bagden E, Reier PJ, Dai HN, McAtee M, et al. (1993) Recovery of function after spinal cord injury: mechanisms underlying transplant-mediated recovery of function differ after spinal cord injury in newborn and adult rats. Exp Neurol 123: 3–16.
36. Nygren LG, Fuxe K, Jonsson G, Olson L (1974) Functional regeneration of 5-hydroxytryptamine nerve terminals in the rat spinal cord following 5, 6-dihydroxytryptamine induced degeneration. Brain Res 78: 377–394.
37. Shoichet MS (2008) Strategies for Regeneration and Repair in the Injured Central Neurous System. Taylor & Francis Group, LLC.CRC press. 221 p.
38. Boido M, Garbossa D, Vercelli A (2011) Early graft of neural precursors in spinal cord compression reduces glial cyst and improves function. J Neurosurg Spine 15: 97–106.
39. Barnabe-Heider F, Goritz C, Sabelstrom H, Takebayashi H, Pfrieger FW, et al. (2010) Origin of new glial cells in intact and injured adult spinal cord. Cell Stem Cell 7: 470–482.
40. Choi BH (1986) Myelin-forming oligodendrocytes of developing mouse spinal cord: immunocytochemical and ultrastructural studies. J Neuropathol Exp Neurol 45: 513–524.
41. Wu J, Yoo S, Wilcock D, Lytle JM, Leung PY, et al. (2010) Interaction of NG2(+) glial progenitors and microglia/macrophages from the injured spinal cord. Glia 58: 410–422.
42. Lytle JM, Wrathall JR (2007) Glial cell loss, proliferation and replacement in the contused murine spinal cord. Eur J Neurosci 25: 1711–1724.
43. Ille F, Atanasoski S, Falk S, Ittner LM, Marki D, et al. (2007) Wnt/BMP signal integration regulates the balance between proliferation and differentiation of neuroepithelial cells in the dorsal spinal cord. Dev Biol 304: 394–408.
44. Fuller ML, DeChant AK, Rothstein B, Caprariello A, Wang R, et al. (2007) Bone morphogenetic proteins promote gliosis in demyelinating spinal cord lesions. Ann Neurol 62: 288–300.
45. Gomes WA, Mehler MF, Kessler JA (2003) Transgenic overexpression of BMP4 increases astroglial and decreases oligodendroglial lineage commitment. Dev Biol 255: 164–177.
46. Auguet M, Viossat I, Marin JG, Chabrier PE (1995) Selective inhibition of inducible nitric oxide synthase by agmatine. Jpn J Pharmacol 69: 285–287.
47. Galea E, Regunathan S, Eliopoulos V, Feinstein DL, Reis DJ (1996) Inhibition of mammalian nitric oxide synthases by agmatine, an endogenous polyamine formed by decarboxylation of arginine. Biochem J 316 (Pt 1): 247–249.
48. Halaris A, Plietz J (2007) Agmatine : metabolic pathway and spectrum of activity in brain. CNS Drugs 21: 885–900.
49. Yu CG, Marcillo AE, Fairbanks CA, Wilcox GL, Yezierski RP (2000) Agmatine improves locomotor function and reduces tissue damage following spinal cord injury. Neuroreport 11: 3203–3207.
50. Shunmugavel A (2010) Simvastatin protects bladder and renal functions following spinal cord injury in rats. J Inflamm (Lond).
51. Silver J, Miller JH (2004) Regeneration beyond the glial scar. Nat Rev Neurosci 5: 146–156.
52. Franklin RJ, Ffrench-Constant C (2008) Remyelination in the CNS: from biology to therapy. Nat Rev Neurosci 9: 839–855.
53. Jarjour AA, Zhang H, Bauer N, Ffrench-Constant C, Williams A (2012) In vitro modeling of central nervous system myelination and remyelination. Glia 60: 1–12.
54. Wu B, Ren X (2009) Promoting axonal myelination for improving neurological recovery in spinal cord injury. J Neurotrauma 26: 1847–1856.
55. Keirstead HS, Blakemore WF (1997) Identification of post-mitotic oligodendrocytes incapable of remyelination within the demyelinated adult spinal cord. J Neuropathol Exp Neurol 56: 1191–1201.
56. Redwine JM, Armstrong RC (1998) In vivo proliferation of oligodendrocyte progenitors expressing PDGFalphaR during early remyelination. J Neurobiol 37: 413–428.
57. Chang A, Nishiyama A, Peterson J, Prineas J, Trapp BD (2000) NG2-positive oligodendrocyte progenitor cells in adult human brain and multiple sclerosis lesions. J Neurosci 20: 6404–6412.
58. Nishiyama A (2007) Polydendrocytes: NG2 cells with many roles in development and repair of the CNS. Neuroscientist 13: 62–76.
59. Cigognini D, Satta A, Colleoni B, Silva D, Donega M, et al. (2011) Evaluation of early and late effects into the acute spinal cord injury of an injectable functionalized self-assembling scaffold. PLoS One 6: e19782.
60. Butt SJ, Harris-Warrick RM, Kiehn O (2002) Firing properties of identified interneuron populations in the mammalian hindlimb central pattern generator. J Neurosci 22: 9961–9971.
61. Grillner S, Zangger P (1979) On the central generation of locomotion in the low spinal cat. Exp Brain Res 34: 241–261.
62. Jacobs BL, Martin-Cora FJ, Fornal CA (2002) Activity of medullary serotonergic neurons in freely moving animals. Brain Res Brain Res Rev 40: 45–52.
63. Jordan LM, Liu J, Hedlund PB, Akay T, Pearson KG (2008) Descending command systems for the initiation of locomotion in mammals. Brain Res Rev 57: 183–191.
64. Fouad K, Rank MM, Vavrek R, Murray KC, Sanelli L, et al. (2010) Locomotion after spinal cord injury depends on constitutive activity in serotonin receptors. J Neurophysiol 104: 2975–2984.
65. Saruhashi Y, Matsusue Y, Fujimiya M (2009) The recovery of 5-HT transporter and 5-HT immunoreactivity in injured rat spinal cord. Arch Orthop Trauma Surg 129: 1279–1285.
66. Boulenguez P, Vinay L (2009) Strategies to restore motor functions after spinal cord injury. Curr Opin Neurobiol 19: 587–600.
67. Hawryluk GW, Rowland J, Kwon BK, Fehlings MG (2008) Protection and repair of the injured spinal cord: a review of completed, ongoing, and planned clinical trials for acute spinal cord injury. Neurosurg Focus 25: E14.
68. do Carmo Cunha J, de Freitas Azevedo Levy B, de Luca BA, de Andrade MS, Gomide VC, et al. (2007) Responses of reactive astrocytes containing S100beta protein and fibroblast growth factor-2 in the border and in the adjacent preserved tissue after a contusion injury of the spinal cord in rats: implications for wound repair and neuroregeneration. Wound Repair Regen 15: 134–146.
69. Basso DM, Beattie MS, Bresnahan JC (1996) Graded histological and locomotor outcomes after spinal cord contusion using the NYU weight-drop device versus transection. Exp Neurol 139: 244–256.
70. Hampton DW, Asher RA, Kondo T, Steeves JD, Ramer MS, et al. (2007) A potential role for bone morphogenetic protein signalling in glial cell fate determination following adult central nervous system injury in vivo. Eur J Neurosci 26: 3024–3035.
71. Tsujii M, Akeda K, Iino T, Uchida A (2009) Are BMPs involved in normal nerve and following transection?: a pilot study. Clin Orthop Relat Res 467: 3183–3189.
72. Davies JE, Proschel C, Zhang N, Noble M, Mayer-Proschel M, et al. (2008) Transplanted astrocytes derived from BMP- or CNTF-treated glial-restricted precursors have opposite effects on recovery and allodynia after spinal cord injury. J Biol 7: 24.
73. Liu A, Niswander LA (2005) Bone morphogenetic protein signalling and vertebrate nervous system development. Nat Rev Neurosci 6: 945–954.
74. Henriquez JP, Krull CE, Osses N (2011) The Wnt and BMP Families of Signaling Morphogens at the Vertebrate Neuromuscular Junction. Int J Mol Sci 12: 8924–8946.
75. Pisano JM, Colon-Hastings F, Birren SJ (2000) Postmigratory enteric and sympathetic neural precursors share common, developmentally regulated, responses to BMP2. Dev Biol 227: 1–11.
76. Nakashima K, Takizawa T, Ochiai W, Yanagisawa M, Hisatsune T, et al. (2001) BMP2-mediated alteration in the developmental pathway of fetal mouse brain cells from neurogenesis to astrocytogenesis. Proc Natl Acad Sci U S A 98: 5868–5873.
77. Chang CF, Lin SZ, Chiang YH, Morales M, Chou J, et al. (2003) Intravenous administration of bone morphogenetic protein-7 after ischemia improves motor function in stroke rats. Stroke 34: 558–564.
78. Harvey BK, Hoffer BJ, Wang Y (2005) Stroke and TGF-beta proteins: glial cell line-derived neurotrophic factor and bone morphogenetic protein. Pharmacol Ther 105: 113–125.
79. Reissmann E, Ernsberger U, Francis-West PH, Rueger D, Brickell PM, et al. (1996) Involvement of bone morphogenetic protein-4 and bone morphogenetic protein-7 in the differentiation of the adrenergic phenotype in developing sympathetic neurons. Development 122: 2079–2088.
80. White RE, Jakeman LB (2008) Don't fence me in: harnessing the beneficial roles of astrocytes for spinal cord repair. Restor Neurol Neurosci 26: 197–214.
81. Parikh P, Hao Y, Hosseinkhani M, Patil SB, Huntley GW, et al. (2011) Regeneration of axons in injured spinal cord by activation of bone morphogenetic protein/Smad1 signaling pathway in adult neurons. Proc Natl Acad Sci U S A 108: E99–107.
82. Finley MF, Devata S, Huettner JE (1999) BMP-4 inhibits neural differentiation of murine embryonic stem cells. J Neurobiol 40: 271–287.
83. Gambaro K, Aberdam E, Virolle T, Aberdam D, Rouleau M (2006) BMP-4 induces a Smad-dependent apoptotic cell death of mouse embryonic stem cell-derived neural precursors. Cell Death Differ 13: 1075–1087.

4

Transplantation of Oligodendrocyte Precursor Cells Improves Locomotion Deficits in Rats with Spinal Cord Irradiation Injury

Yan Sun[1]‡, Chong-Chong Xu[1]‡, Jin Li[2], Xi-Yin Guan[3], Lu Gao[1], Li-Xiang Ma[1], Rui-Xi Li[1], Yu-Wen Peng[1]*, Guo-Pei Zhu[3]*

1 Department of Anatomy, Histology and Embryology, Shanghai Medical College, Fudan University, Shanghai, China, **2** Institutes of Biomedical Sciences, Fudan University, Shanghai, China, **3** Department of Radiation Oncology, Shanghai Cancer Hospital, Fudan University, Shanghai, China

Abstract

Demyelination contributes to the functional impairment of irradiation injured spinal cord. One potential therapeutic strategy involves replacing the myelin-forming cells. Here, we asked whether transplantation of Olig2$^+$-GFP$^+$-oligodendrocyte precursor cells (OPCs), which are derived from Olig2-GFP-mouse embryonic stem cells (mESCs), could enhance remyelination and functional recovery after spinal cord irradiation injury. We differentiated Olig2-GFP-mESCs into purified Olig2$^+$-GFP$^+$-OPCs and transplanted them into the rats' cervical 4–5 dorsal spinal cord level at 4 months after irradiation injury. Eight weeks after transplantation, the Olig2$^+$-GFP$^+$-OPCs survived and integrated into the injured spinal cord. Immunofluorescence analysis showed that the grafted Olig2$^+$-GFP$^+$-OPCs primarily differentiated into adenomatous polyposis coli (APC$^+$) oligodendrocytes (54.6±10.5%). The staining with luxol fast blue, hematoxylin & eosin (LFB/H&E) and electron microscopy demonstrated that the engrafted Olig2$^+$-GFP$^+$-OPCs attenuated the demyelination resulted from the irradiation. More importantly, the recovery of forelimb locomotor function was enhanced in animals receiving grafts of Olig2$^+$-GFP$^+$-OPCs. We concluded that OPC transplantation is a feasible therapy to repair the irradiated lesions in the central nervous system (CNS).

Editor: Brahim Nait-Oumesmar, Université Pierre et Marie Curie-Paris6, INSERM, CNRS, France

Funding: This study was supported the by the National Natural Science Foundation of China (No. 30770637, 30901615 and 81201029). The funders had no role in study design, data collection and analysis, decision to publish, or preparation of the manuscript.

Competing Interests: The authors have declared that no competing interests exist.

* E-mail: antica@gmail.com (GPZ); ywpeng@fudan.edu.cn (YWP)

‡ These authors contributed equally to this work.

Introduction

The spinal cord is one of the important dose-limiting normal tissues in clinical radiotherapy. Excessive doses of radiation to the spinal cord result in radiation injury, which is a rare but serious complication of radiotherapy for cancer [1,2]. The pathophysiology involved in irradiation-induced spinal cord injury is demyelination caused by death of oligodendrocytes [3,4]. Reduction in the number of oligodendrocytes was observed as early as 24 hours after X-ray irradiation [5,6]. There is a persistent decline in the number of OPCs from two weeks to three months after X-ray irradiation [7,8]. Remyelination often fails because of primary deficiency in the precursor cells, failure of precursor cells' recruitment, or incompetence of differentiation and maturation of precursor cells [9]. Persistent demyelination may result in further axonal loss. Such changes could be associated with permanent motor and sensory deficits [10], which become fatal if the damage occurs at the upper cervical level [11]. There are currently no therapeutic approaches that promote remyelination available in a clinical setting.

Cell therapy offers an attractive option as grafted cells may replace the lost ones as well as provide neurotrophic benefits to surrounding tissue [9,12]. To date, primary cultured adult neural stem cells, Schwann cells and olfactory ensheathing cells have been transplanted into the radiation-injured spinal cord [13,14,15,16,17]. However, these cells have limited capacity in producing oligodendrocytes, the primary cell type that is damaged in radiation injury. Oligodendrocyte precursor cells (OPCs), which can be isolated from brain tissues [18,19], offer an alternative source. Nevertheless, they need to be derived from brain tissues. Embryonic stem cells (ESCs) may become a suitable candidate because they are genetically normal, pluripotent, and capable of indefinite replication, and they can be differentiated to all the cell types in the body, including OPCs [20,21,22]. Although the induced differentiation of ESCs is a well-developed approach, there are still problems, especially the purity of target cells [23]. Therefore, it is important to develop strategies for the directed differentiation of ESCs into specialized functional cell types and/or purification of the target cells *in vitro* before transplantation.

In the present study, we employed a mESCs line that carries a GFP reporter in the locus of Olig2, a transcription factor that is critical for OPCs development [24]. Following transplantation of Olig2$^+$-GFP$^+$-OPCs into the spinal cord of rat that underwent irradiation injury, the grafted OPCs survived, differentiated to myelinating oligodendrocytes and improved locomotor function of the injured rats.

Materials and Methods

Ethics Statement

This study was carried out in strict accordance with the recommendations in the Guide for the Care and Use of Laboratory Animals of the National Institutes of Health. The protocol was approved by the Committee on the Ethics of Animal Experiments of Fudan University (Permit Number: SCXK 2009-0019). All efforts were made to minimize suffering.

Irradiation Injury of the Spinal Cord

Female Wistar adult rats (180–200 g, Slrc Laboratory Animal, China) were anesthetized by an intraperitoneal injection of 7.5 mg/kg ketamine, 60 mg/kg xylazine and immobilized during irradiation. The rats' cervical spinal cords were irradiated using a 6 Mev Electron Beam Linear Accelerator (Elekta AB, Stockholm, Sweden). A 22 Gy radiation dose was delivered to a 2 cm×2 cm radiation field, maintaining cervical 4–5 as the center of the electron-irradiated zone. Radiographs were taken before and after X-irradiation to confirm that all the animals were in the same position. After irradiation, the animals were given subcutaneous saline (5 ml) and housed in a 25°C warm room.

Derivation of Olig2$^+$-GFP$^+$-OPCs from Olig2-GFP-mESCs

Olig2-GFP-mESCs were the gift of Dr. Su-Chun Zhang (University of Wisconsin, USA) and have been previously described [25]. Olig2-GFP-mESCs were differentiated according to a modified protocol [25]. Briefly, mESCs were trypsinized and placed onto low attachment flasks (Greiner, Germany) in a neural differentiation medium containing DMEM/F12, N2 supplement, leukemia inhibitory factor (LIF), nonessential amino acids, L-glutamine, 2-mercaptoethanol and 10% knockout serum replacement (all from Invitrogen, Carlsbad, CA, USA). Under this condition for 2 days, mESCs formed small aggregates. Retinoic acid (RA, 0.5 μM, Sigma, St Louis, MO, USA) and Purmorphamine (Pur, 0.5 μM, Calbiochem, San Diego, CA, USA) were added at days 2–6 to induce neural progenitors. The aggregates were cultured in suspension in the neural differentiation medium with bFGF (20 ng/ml, R&D systems) and heparin (2 μg/ml, Sigma) for another 6 days. On day 12, the differentiated aggregates were dissociated with trypsin-EDTA (0.05%, Gibco) and plated onto flasks coated with Matrigel in modified Bottenstein-Sato medium. The modified Bottenstein-Sato medium contained insulin (10 μg/ml), BSA (100 μg/ml), human transferrin (100 μg/ml), progesterone (60 μg/ml), sodium selenite (40 μg/ml), N-acetyl-cysteine (60 μg/ml), putrescine (16 μg/ml), biotin (10 ng/ml) and cAMP (5 μM) (all reagents from Sigma). T3 (40 ng/ml, Sigma), PDGF-AA (10 ng/ml) and NT3 (5 ng/ml) (all from R&D systems) were added to promote the proliferation of the OPCs.

For immunofluorescence, dissociated spheres (2×10^4 cells/μl) were plated on coverslips coated with poly-L-lysine and human laminin (Sigma).

For fluorescence activated cell sorting (FACS), cells were harvested at day 12, gently dissociated to single cells and washed with a FACS buffer (PBS, 1%N2, 200 mM L-glutamine, 55 mM β-ME, 50 ng/ml NAC). Cells were analyzed by a Becton Dickinson FACSCaliber with CellQuest Pro (BD Biosciences, San Diego, CA, USA).

For transplantation, FACS-sorted Olig2$^+$-GFP$^+$-OPCs were resuspended in a fresh culture medium and cultured for 2 days. At day 14, cells were dissociated with accutase (Invitrogen) and prepared at approximately 100,000 cells/μl in artificial cerebrospinal fluid (aCSF). Trypan blue exclusion testing indicated that this preparation consisted of 95% viable cells at time of transplantation.

Cell Transplantation

Transplantation was performed as described [26]. The animals were immunosuppressed using cyclosporine A (10 mg/kg/d, s.c; Novartis Pharma Schweiz AG, Switzerland) 1 day prior to transplantation and then every day for the duration of the study. Cell transplantation occurred 4 months after irradiation surgery. The animals were anesthetized as above, and the spinal cord was exposed by laminectomy at the cervical 4–5 vertebral level. After immobilization of the spinal cord, a 10 μl Hamilton syringe (Hamilton, Reno, NV) was lowered into the spinal cord using a stereotactic manipulator arm. Cell suspension (2 μl) was injected into two sites along the midline at a depth of 1.2 mm, 4 mm cranial and 4 mm caudal to the lesion epicenter, at a rate of 1.0 μl/min. The needle was removed after 5 min. The animals in which the injected solution was observed to exit from the needle track during injection or after withdrawal of the needle were omitted from the experiment. Animals receiving the same surgery and injection of 2 μl aCSF solution (without cells) were served as controls.

Histology

For the histological analysis, the animals were deeply anesthetized with an overdose of 3% pentobarbitone and perfused with 0.9% saline following by 4% ice-cold paraformaldehyde prepared with phosphate buffer (0.1 M, pH7.4). The spinal cord was divided into eight 1 mm blocks that extended 4 mm cranial to and 4 mm caudal to the injury epicenter. Alternate blocks were processed to produce cryostat sections. Some of the cryostat sections were stained with LFB/H&E to examine general morphology and the extent of demyelination. Some of the cryostat sections were used for immunofluorescent analysis of grafted cells.

To quantify the demyelination of injured spinal cord, we used Image J (http://rsbweb.nih.gov/ij/index.html) to measure the relative optical density of the dorsal funiculus from all groups. A pre-defined region of interest was selected to encompass the dorsal funiculus. Color images were acquired at the same exposure level, coverted to 8-bit gray scale, and the mean density calculated from the threshold pixels excluding the background. Density was analyzed in four regions of the dorsal funiculus per section. Eight sections per spinal cord were analyzed. There were six animals in each group.

Immunofluorescence

Immunostaining was performed on cultured cells or cryosectioned spinal cord using standard protocols [27]. Primary antibodies used in present study included mouse anti-Oct4 (1:2000, Santa Cruz Biotechnology, Santa Cruz, CA), goat anti-Sox2 (1:1000, R&D Systems), rabbit anti-NG2 (1:500, Chemicon International Inc, Temecula, CA, USA), rabbit anti-O4 (1:50, Santa Cruz), rabbit anti-PDGFRα (1:500, Santa Cruz), rabbit anti-MBP (1:500, Abcam, Cambridge, MA), goat anti-GFP (1:200; Abcam), mouse anti-APC (1:1000; Abcam), mouse anti-p75 (1:1000; Chemicon), rabbit anti-GFAP (1:500; Chemicon), and mouse anti-NF (1:2000; Chemicon). Coverslip cultures or spinal cord sections were incubated in a blocking buffer (10% donkey serum and 0.2% Triton X-100 in phosphate buffer saline) for 60 min at room temperature before being incubated in the primary antibodies overnight at 4°C. Fluorescently conjugated secondary antibodies were used to reveal the binding of primary antibodies (1:2000, Invitrogen) and nuclei were stained with 4,6-dianidina-2-phenylindole (DAPI) (0.1 μg/ml, Sigma). The immu-

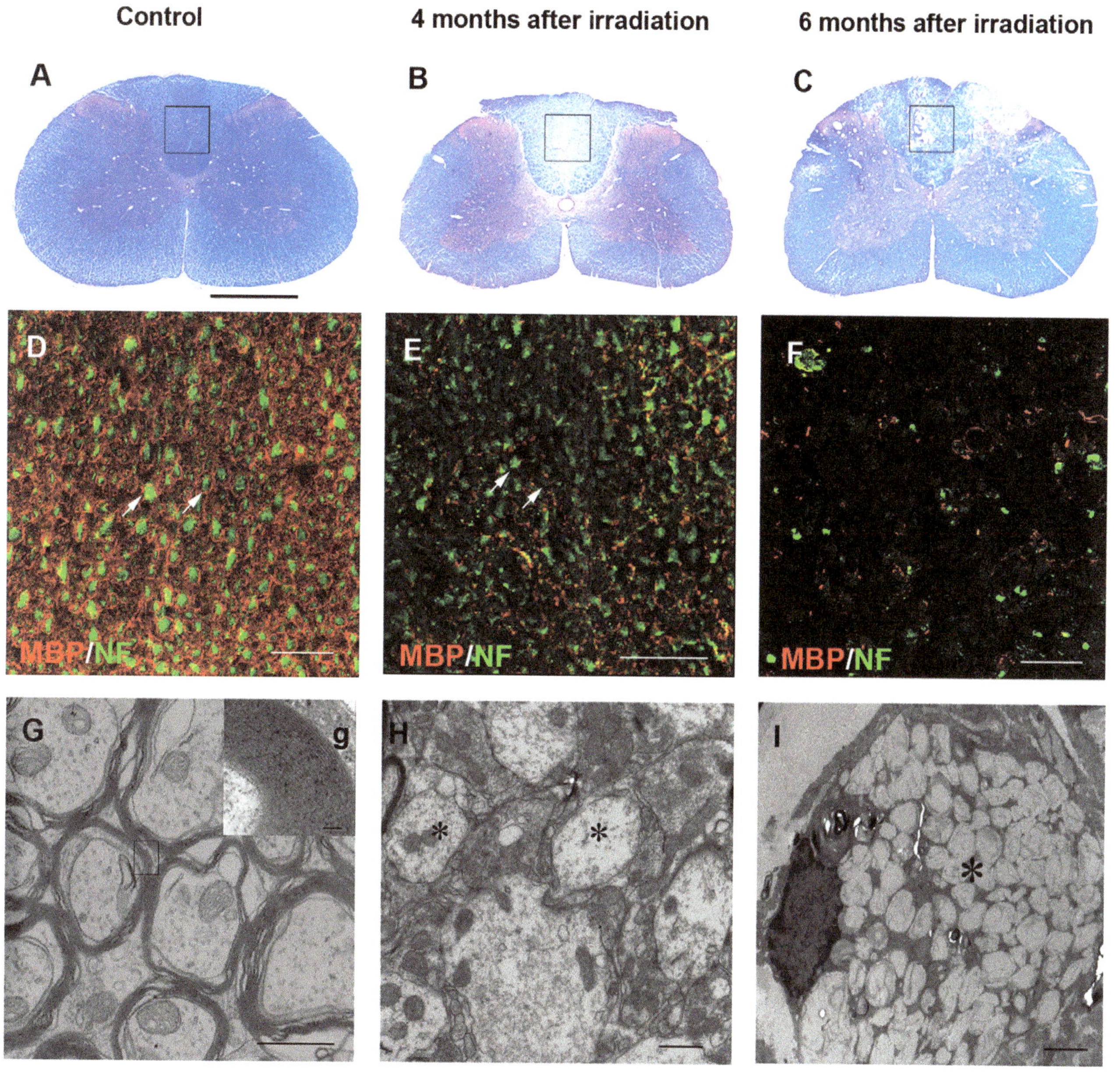

Figure 1. Radiation-induced demyelination in the dorsal funiculus of cervical spinal cord. (A) LFB/H&E staining showed normal spinal cord without irradiation. (B) Four months after irradiation, there was a focal demyelinated zone in the dorsal funiculus. (C) Six months following injury, focal necrosis was seen in the dorsal funiculus. (D) Immunostaining for MBP and NF, enlargement of framed area in A, depicted that non-irradiated myelin surrounding the axons (arrows). (E) Four months after irradiation, most of the axons lost myelin (arrows). (F) At six months, axons began to show necrosis. (G) Electron microscopy confirmed the normal structure of myelin. *g*, Higher magnification of the tissue in the box in G, indicated the compact myelin sheath. (H) Four months after irradiation, most of axons remained demyelinated (asterisk). (I) Six months following damage, axons necrosis was found (asterisk). Bar, 200 μm (A–C); bar, 50 μm (D–F); bar, 1 μm (G, H); bar, 100 nm (g); bar, 2 μm (I).

nofluorescent samples were visualized using a Nikon-Eclipse TE 2000-S fluorescence microscope (Nikon Instruments, Sterling Heights, MI, USA) or a Leica TCS-SP5 laser-scanning confocal microscope (Leica, Germany).

To quantify the differentiation pattern *in vitro*, the percentage of immunopositive cells was determined by dividing the total number of immunopositive cells by the total number of GFP/DAPI positive cells in each imaging field and then averaging the result from three fields per marker. These fixed fields were randomly selected from biological replicates using "Image J".

To assess the differentiation of grafted Olig2^{+}-GFP^{+}-OPCs in the injured spinal cord, four coronal sections, 200 μm apart, were taken spanning the lesion epicenter. The percentage of engrafted OPCs that co-expressed NG2, APC, MBP, p75 and GFAP was quantified for the grafted animals.

Electron Microscopy

For electron microscopic processing, the animals were sacrificed by aortic perfusion with isotonic, heparinized saline followed with 4% paraformaldehyde and 1% glutaraldehyde in 0.1 M phosphate buffer. The fixed spinal cords were washed in 0.1 M phosphate

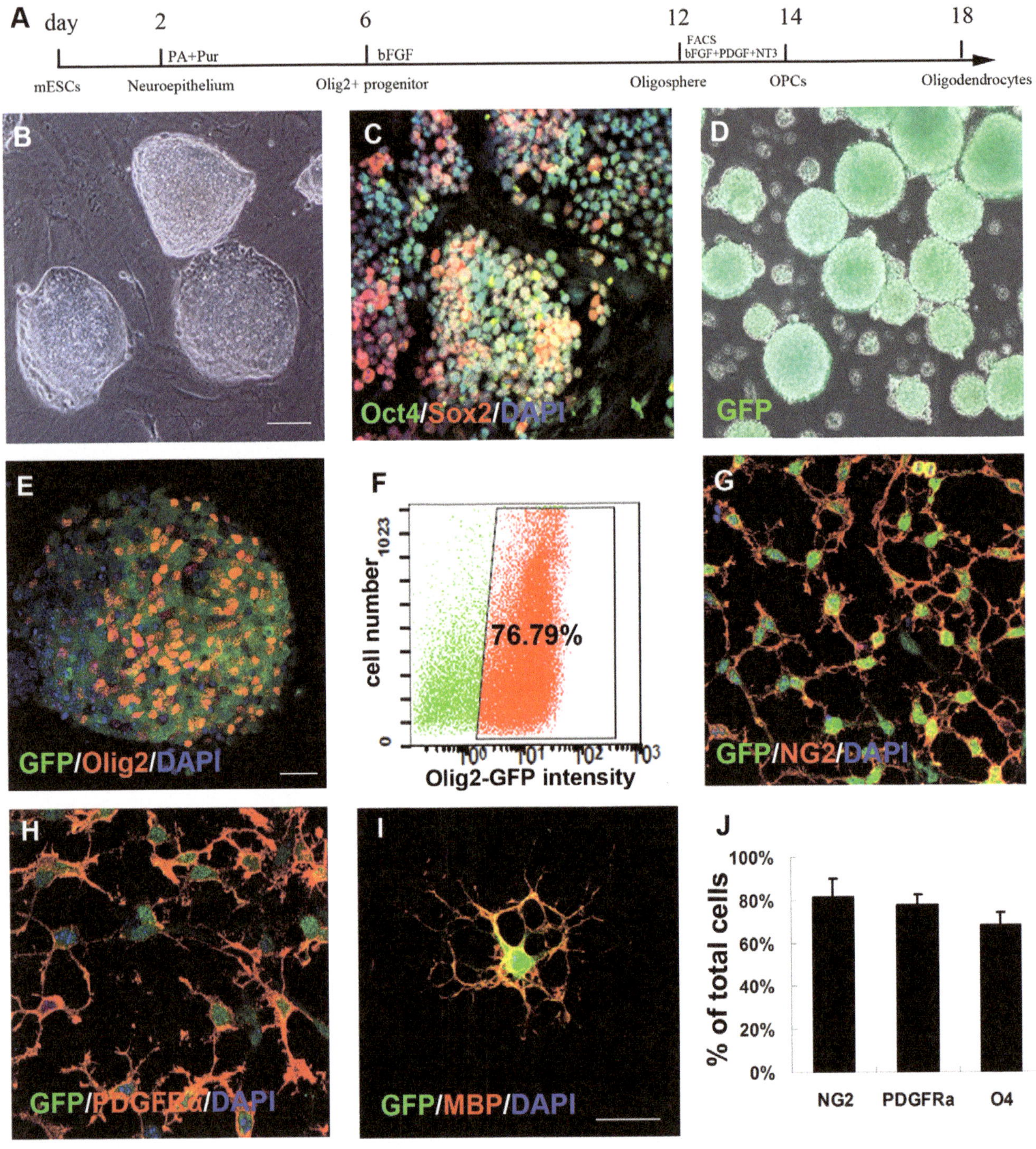

Figure 2. ***In vitro*** **differentiation of Olig2-GFP-mouse mESCs into Olig2$^+$-GFP$^+$- OPCs.** (A) Schematic procedure for differentiation of Olig2-GFP-mESCs into Olig2$^+$-GFP$^+$-OPCs. (B) Phase contrast photograph of mESCs colonies on mouse embryonic fibroblast. (C) mESCs remained undifferentiated and stained positive for Oct4/Sox2. (D) Phase contrast photograph of Olig2$^+$-GFP$^+$ spheres at day 12. (E) GFP$^+$ spheres expressed Olig2. (F) At day 12, the percentage of GFP$^+$ cells was 76.79%±1.35%, sorted by FACS method. At day 14, all purified OPCs expressed GFP as well as the OPC markers NG2 (G) and PDGFRα (H). At day 18, plated cells adopted a typical oligodendrocyte morphology characterized by multiple branches and expressed GFP and MBP (I). (J) Quantification of immunostaining: 81.69±8.16% of cells expressed NG2, 78±4.31% of cells expressed PDGFRα, and 68.47±5.59% of cells expressed O4. Data in J are expressed as the mean±SEM, n = 3 independent experiments, 6 total replicates. Bar, 200 μm (B–D); bar, 50 μm (E–H); bar, 30 μm (I).

buffer and embedded in 3% agar. Transverse sections (40 μm thick) were obtained on a vibrotome (Leica, VT1000S, Nussloch, Germany) and mounted onto slides. The sections were washed in PB and subjected to an additional fixation in 2% OsO_4 in phosphate buffer for 2 h at room temperature. After sequential dehydration in increasing concentrations of ethanol (50–100%) and pure acetone, the sections were embedded in Epon 812. Ultrathin sections (80 nm) obtained using an ultramicrotome (UI-

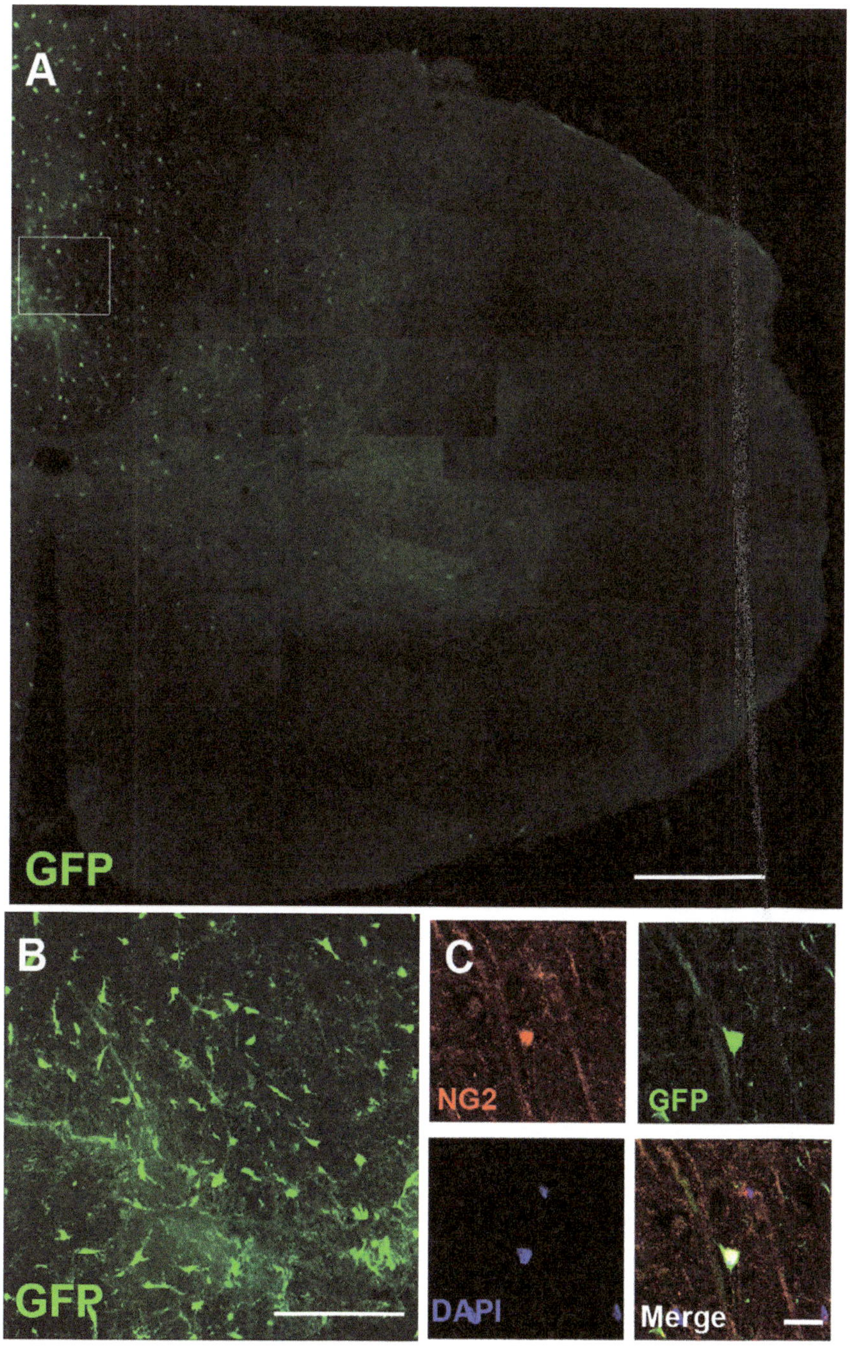

Figure 3. Distribution and morphology of Olig2$^+$-GFP$^+$-OPCs in irradiated spinal cord at four weeks after transplantation. (A) GFP$^+$ cells were observed and distributed in the damaged spinal cord. (B) At higher magnification of the boxed area from (A), the GFP$^+$ cells exhibited typical bipolar OPC morphology. (C) Many grafted Olig2$^+$-GFP$^+$-OPCs co-expressed the OPCs marker NG2. Bar, 250 μm (A); bar, 100 μm (B); bar, 20 μm (C).

tracut E, Reicher-Jung, NY, USA) were stained with uranyl acetate and lead citrate, examined and photographed under a transmission electron microscope (Philips CM120, Amsterdam Netherlands).

Behavioral Assessments

The clinical degree of weakness was graded according to a scale developed by Ushio et al. [28,29]: grade 0 = normal; grade 1 = forelimb instability seen only when the animal jumps or runs; grade 2 = mild weakness, but able to run; grade 3 = moderate weakness, able to walk but not run; grade 4 = marked weakness, attempts to walk; grade 5 = severe weakness, purposeless movements of legs or complete paraplegia. All rats were allowed to live for 8 weeks after transplantation.

Statistical Analysis

All data are reported as Mean±SEM. Repeated measures ANOVA followed by the Tukey-Kramer test was used for

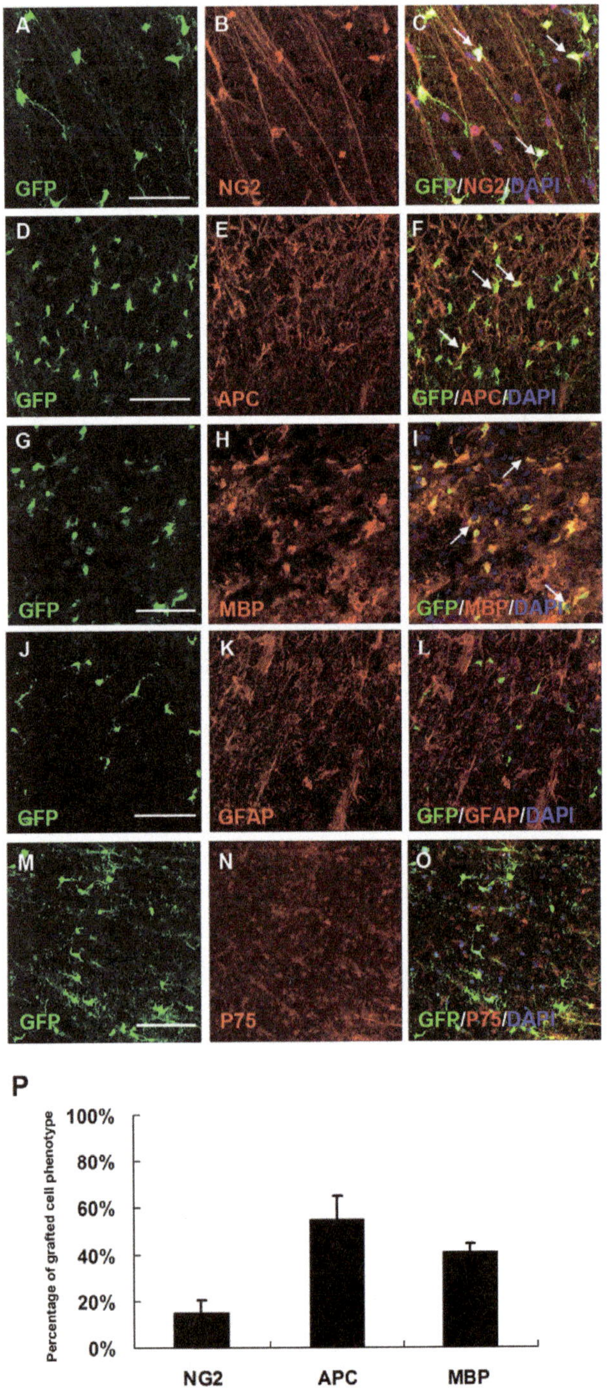

Figure 4. Olig2$^+$-GFP$^+$-OPCs primarily differentiate along the oligodendrocyte lineage. At eight weeks after transplantation, a certain number of grafted GFP$^+$ cells still expressed NG2 (A–C, arrows) and most of the grafted GFP$^+$ cells became APC-positive mature oligodendrocytes (D–F, arrows). Double staining for GFP and MBP in cross-sections further confirmed that GFP-immunoreactive rings were composed of MBP$^+$ myelin (G–I, arrows). The grafted GFP$^+$ cells did not co-expressed GFAP (J–L) or P75 (M–O). (P) Quantification of GFP$^+$ cell populations in the spinal cord. Data are expressed as the mean number of cells/spinal cord±SEM (n = 6). GFP$^+$ cells expressed NG2 (15.1±5.53%), APC (54.6±10.5%) and MBP (40.5±3.8%). Bar, 50 μm (A–C); bar, 35 μm (D–O).

comparison of clinical grade scores at each time point. The difference between the two was compared using Student's tests. Statistical analysis was performed using SPSS 16.0. Differences were considered to be statistically significant at $p<0.05$.

Results

Demyelination Induced by Irradiation

Non-irradiated animals (n = 6) did not show any evidence of demyelination (Fig. 1A, D and G). Even though there was no histological evidence of demyelination observed from 1 to 3-month after irradiation, 80% of the animals (n = 60) developed a focally demyelinated zone in the dorsal funiculus from the fourth month, as shown by LFB/H&E staining (Fig. 1B). This was confirmed by immunostaining for myelin basic protein (MBP) and neurofilment (NF), showing the presence of many axons but sharply reduced MBP staining (Fig. 1E). Electron microscopy showed many viable demyelinated axons in the dorsal funiculus (Fig. 1H). Six months after irradiation, focal areas of necrosis were apparent in the white matter (Fig. 1C), with MBP loss and axonal degeneration (Fig. 1F). Axon necrosis was also found by electron microscopy (Fig. 1I).

The clinical degree of weakness was consistent with the histological changes. The mean interval between irradiation and manifestation of the first neurological symptoms (grade 1 = forelimb instability seen only when the animal jumps or runs) was 112±14 days. Four months after irradiation, the animals (n = 12) that did not manifest neurological symptoms (grade 0 = normal) were omitted from the experiment.

Generation and Purification of Olig2$^+$-GFP$^+$-OPCs from mESCs

We used an established mESCs line (Olig2-GFP-mESCs) in which GFP was knocked into the locus of Olig2, a transcription factor expressed by ventral spinal cord progenitors [24]. In order to identify and purify OPCs, we used a modified protocol established in the Zhang Lab to differentiate mESCs into OPCs [25] (Fig. 2A). The Olig2-GFP-mESCs, expanding as discrete colonies on mouse embryonic fibroblast (Fig. 2B) and expressing Oct4/Sox2 (Fig. 2C), were detached from mouse embryonic fibroblasts to initiate differentiation and grown as free floating embryoid bodies (EB) for 2 days in the medium before being treated with RA (0.5 μM) and Pur (0.5 μM). At day 6, GFP$^+$ spheres began to appear and by day 12 almost all the spheres were green (Fig. 2D). FACS analysis, confirmed by confocal microscopy, indicated that 76.79± 1.35% of the total differentiated cells expressed Olig2 and GFP (Fig. 2E, F). To further purify the OPCs, we used FACS based on GFP expression. FACS isolated cells were plated in the presence of FGF2, PDGF-AA and NT3. The majority of GFP cells expressed NG2 (81.69±8.16%) (Fig. 2G, J), PDGFRα (78±4.31%) (Fig. 2H, J) and O4 (68.47±5.59%) (Fig. 2J). Further differentiation of the OPCs for 6 days resulted in generation of highly branched oligodendrocytes, as indicated by positive staining for MBP (Fig. 2I).

Survival and Migration of Transplanted OPCs within the Spinal Cord

A total of 24 injured animals received transplantation of Olig2$^+$-GFP$^+$-OPCs 4 months after irradiation. Four weeks after transplantation, grafted cells revealed by GFP, were found in the spinal cord of all transplanted animals. The animals (n = 24) without cell transplantation did not exhibit such labeling. The GFP-expressing cells were mainly distributed in the dorsal funiculus with a small number of cells migrating into the gray matter (Fig. 3A). At a higher magnification, the GFP$^+$ cells

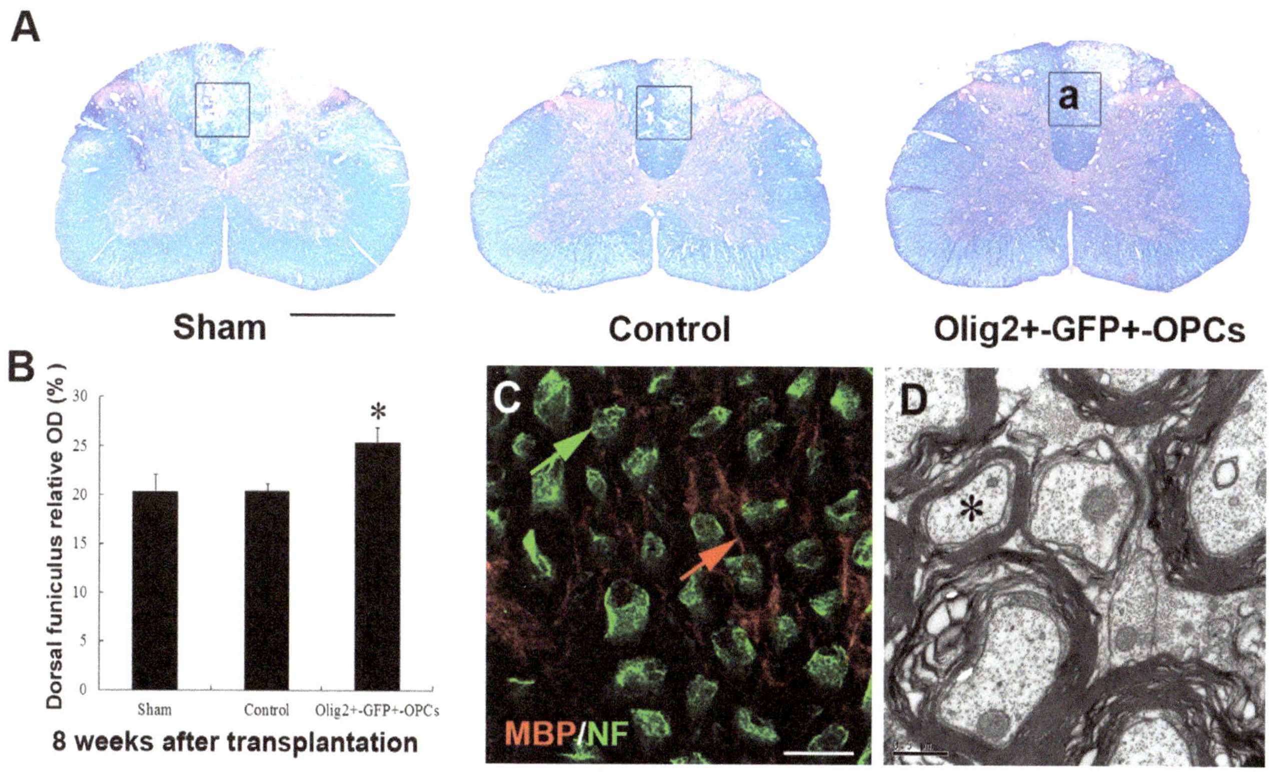

Figure 5. Transplantation of Olig2$^+$-GFP$^+$-OPCs results in a delayed demyelination and cavitation. (A) LFB/H&E staining showed smaller cystic cavitations in the transplanted cord than those in the sham and the control group in the dorsal funiculus. (B) Optical densities of dorsal funiculus in spinal cord was significantly increased in rats grafted with Olig2$^+$-GFP$^+$-OPCs, as compared to the sham and the control group (*$p < 0.05$, n = 12). (C) Enlargement of framed area in part a, illustrated immunostaining of MBP and NF, showing axons (green arrow) with or without myelin (red arrow). (D) Electron microscopy confirmed the structure of axons (asterisk). Bar, 200 μm (A); bar, 35 μm (C); bar, 0.5 μm (D).

adopted a typical OPCs morphology, as characterized by bipolar branches (Fig. 3B), and expressed the OPCs marker NG2 (which marks undifferentiated OPCs) (Fig. 3C), indicating that these grafted cells retain the OPCs identity.

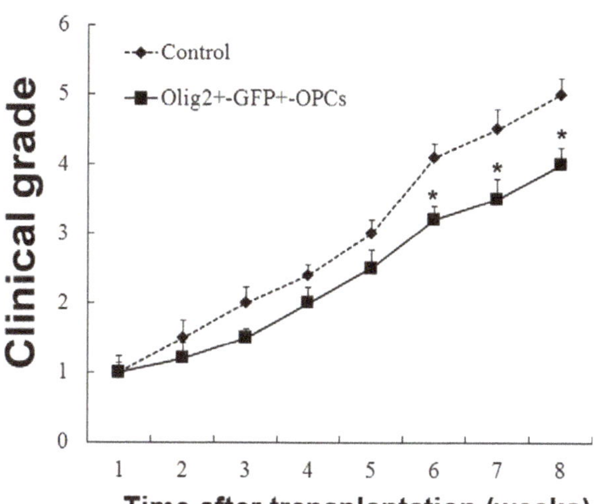

Figure 6. Forelimb locomotion is improved after transplantation of Olig2$^+$-GFP$^+$-OPCs. Locomotion function, as defined using the clinical grade score, was significantly reduced in Olig2$^+$-GFP$^+$-OPCs grafted animals at six to eight weeks after transplantation, as compared to the control group (*$p < 0.05$, n = 12).

Transplanted OPCs Primarily Differentiate into Oligodendrocytes

Eight weeks after transplantation, 15.1±5.53% of the GFP positive cells were double labeled with NG2, a specific protein for precursor cells (Fig. 4A–C, arrows). Around 54.6±10.5% of GFP$^+$ cells expressed APC (Fig. 4D–F, arrows), indicating that the majority of grafted OPCs differentiated into mature oligodendrocytes. About 40.5±3.8% of the grafted cells also expressed MBP, a major constitute of myelin (Fig. 4G–I, arrows). Although several previous studies [30,31] showed that adult OPCs differentiated into Schwann cells after transplantation into the chemically demyelinated spinal cord, our transplanted OPCs did not express p75 (Fig. 4M–O). Other studies suggest that the microenvironment in the injured spinal cord induces grafted neural stem cells to differentiate primarily into astrocytes [14,32]. In the present study, the transplanted OPCs did not differentiate into astrocytes marked by GFAP (Fig. 4J–L). In summation, the staining results revealed that Olig2$^+$-GFP$^+$-OPCs mostly differentiate into mature oligodendrocytes in the injured spinal cord. Over the course of the experiment, tumors, teratomas, or non-neuronal tissue formation were not observed in the transplant recipients.

OPCs Transplantation Attenuated Demyelination after Radiation

Eight weeks after transplantation, irradiated spinal cord exhibited obvious demyelination and cavitation (Fig. 5A). However, the degree of demyelination was significantly decreased by OPCs transplantation as compared to the sham and the control group (Fig. 5B). Immunostainning for MBP and NF indicated numerous clusters of axons that maintained integrity (Fig. 5C). Electron microscopic analysis showed myelinated axons (Fig. 5D).

OPCs Grafts Alleviated the Deterioration of Neurologic Function Following Injury

To determine whether transplantation of OPCs improved recovery of function after injury, locomotion was assessed by using the clinical scoring. Six to eight weeks after transplantation, $Olig2^{+}$-GFP^{+}-OPCs grafted animals exhibited significantly lower clinical scores as compared to the control group (Fig. 6) (all $p<0.05$). The behavioral results showed that transplantation of $Olig2^{+}$-GFP^{+}-OPCs significantly improved forelimb functions.

Discussion

In this study, we have directed mESCs to a purified population of OPCs based on the GFP expression in the Olig2 locus, which differentiate into oligodendrocytes *in vitro* and *in vivo*. More importantly, the oligodendrocytes derived from the $Olig2^{+}$-GFP^{+}-OPCs express MBP, an essential component of myelin sheath, which corresponds to correction of locomotion deficits in rats with irradiation injury of spinal cord. These results raise the prospect of cell-based therapy as a potential treatment for irradiation spinal cord injury.

Cell transplantation has been attempted for the radiation injured spinal cord. Adult rat neural stem cells differentiate predominantly into Schwann-like cells and generated peripheral myelin after transplantation into the irradiation injured spinal cord [14]. Olfactory ensheathing cells appear to migrate within X-irradiated area, they behave similarly as Schwann cells, which survive poorly and are unable to migrate significant distances when transplanted into either intact or X-irradiated spinal cords [16,33]. OPCs are extremely motile and can differentiate into oligodendrocytes and produce myelin [34,35]. Differentiation of oligodendrocytes from mESCs was explored by Billon and colleagues [36]. One of the greatest challenges facing ESCs research is the derivation of high purity target cells from pluripotent ESCs [23]. In the present study, we employed a mESCs line that carries a GFP reporter in the Olig2 locus. The modified differentiation protocol that we used is unique in that it generates highly enriched OPCs. FACS sorting resulted in an enriched population of OPCs (76.79±1.35%) (Fig. 2F). This provided us with a novel tool to investigate the ability of these cells to remyelinate demyelinated regions of irradiation spinal cord injury and determine whether remyelination confers functional benefit.

Most irradiation injury models are made using 40 Gy of X-irradiation which creates acute demyelination in the spinal cord [13,14,16,37,38]. However, the latent period of spinal cord irradiation in human has been reported to vary from 4 months to 4 years after cervical or thoracic irradiation [39]. In experimental animals, irradiation of the spinal cord leads to white matter necrosis within 3–8 months [3]. In the present study, we have used the dosage of 22 Gy to mimic the delayed demyelination of the spinal cord irradiation injury. The demyelination latent period was about 112±14 days, while the white matter necrosis and paralysis that occurred within 6 months of radiation exposure. Therefore, our model is similar to the clinical pathology changes of spinal cord irradiation injury.

Promoting remyelination is an important strategy to treat spinal cord injury. Chronic demyelination predisposes axons to degeneration [40], an irreversible event that is thought to be the major cause of progressive functional decline [41]. Previous studies observed cells with the capacity to myelinate following spinal cord injury [32,34,35,42,43,44,45]. The functional behavioral improvement is correlated with the capacity of the transplanted cells to integrate, differentiate, and myelinate axons at sufficient number [9,46,47]. In our study, we have found that transplanted cells migrate to the injured region and approximately 40% of them differentiate into mature oligodendrocytes expressing MBP. More importantly, immunostaining and electron microscopy analysis reveal the presence of many axons in the areas with $Olig2^{+}$-GFP^{+}-OPCs transplantation, suggesting the protection of axonal integrity by transplanted cells. Further study is needed by immunoelectron microscopy to prove remyelination occurred by transplanted cells.

The increased recovery in the transplantation group may also be explained by mechanisms other than remyelination. CNS neurons require multiple signals for optical survival and maturation, and continued oligodendrocyte-derived signals are necessary to maintain neuronal integrity [48]. In addition to their role in myelinating axons, oligodendrocytes release soluble factors, including insulin-like growth factor (IGF-1), glial-derived neurotrophic factor (GDNF) and brain-derived neurotrophic factor (BDNF), that promote neuronal survival, maintain axonal structure, and support synaptic plasticity in surviving axons [49,50,51,52]. The expression and release of trophic factors offer a platform by which oligodendrocytes interact with neurons to form and maintain functional neural circuits in the injured spinal cord. Therefore, neural protection may be another mechanism by which grafted OPCs promote functional recovery.

Acknowledgments

We are grateful to Ya-Ling Huang and Guo-Ping Zhang (Institutes of Biomedical Sciences, Fudan University) for their technical assistance.

Author Contributions

Conceived and designed the experiments: YWP GPZ. Performed the experiments: YS CCX JL XYG. Analyzed the data: YS CCX JL XYG LG LXM RXL. Contributed reagents/materials/analysis tools: YWP. Wrote the paper: YS CCX GPZ.

References

1. Fowler JF, Bentzen SM, Bond SJ, Ang KK, van der Kogel AJ, et al. (2000) Clinical radiation doses for spinal cord: the 1998 international questionnaire. Radiother Oncol 55: 295–300.
2. Bijl HP, van Luijk P, Coppes RP, Schippers JM, Konings AW, et al. (2003) Unexpected changes of rat cervical spinal cord tolerance caused by inhomogeneous dose distributions. Int J Radiat Oncol Biol Phys 57: 274–281.
3. Okada S, Okeda R (2001) Pathology of radiation myelopathy. Neuropathology 21: 247–265.
4. Wong CS, Van der Kogel AJ (2004) Mechanisms of radiation injury to the central nervous system: implications for neuroprotection. Mol Interv 4: 273–284.
5. Li YQ, Jay V, Wong CS (1996) Oligodendrocytes in the adult rat spinal cord undergo radiation-induced apoptosis. Cancer Res 56: 5417–5422.
6. Atkinson S, Li YQ, Wong CS (2003) Changes in oligodendrocytes and myelin gene expression after radiation in the rodent spinal cord. Int J Radiat Oncol Biol Phys 57: 1093–1100.

7. Chari DM, Huang WL, Blakemore WF (2003) Dysfunctional oligodendrocyte progenitor cell (OPC) populations may inhibit repopulation of OPC depleted tissue. Journal of Neuroscience Research 73: 787–793.
8. Hopewell JW, van der Kogel AJ (1999) Pathophysiological mechanisms leading to the development of late radiation-induced damage to the central nervous system. Front Radiat Ther Oncol 33: 265–275.
9. Franklin RJ, Ffrench-Constant C (2008) Remyelination in the CNS: from biology to therapy. Nat Rev Neurosci 9: 839–855.
10. Schultheiss TE, Kun LE, Ang KK, Stephens LC (1995) Radiation response of the central nervous system. Int J Radiat Oncol Biol Phys 31: 1093–1112.
11. Schultheiss TE, Stephens LC, Peters LJ (1986) Survival in radiation myelopathy. Int J Radiat Oncol Biol Phys 12: 1765–1769.
12. Franklin RJ, Kotter MR (2008) The biology of CNS remyelination: the key to therapeutic advances. J Neurol 255 Suppl 1: 19–25.
13. Rezvani M, Birds DA, Hodges H, Hopewell JW, Milledew K, et al. (2001) Modification of radiation myelopathy by the transplantation of neural stem cells in the rat. Radiat Res 156: 408–412.
14. Mothe AJ, Tator CH (2008) Transplanted neural stem/progenitor cells generate myelinating oligodendrocytes and Schwann cells in spinal cord demyelination and dysmyelination. Exp Neurol 213: 176–190.
15. Chari DM, Gilson JM, Franklin RJM, Blakemore WF (2006) Oligodendrocyte progenitor cell (OPC) transplantation is unlikely to offer a means of preventing X-irradiation induced damage in the CNS. Experimental Neurology 198: 145–153.
16. Lankford KL, Sasaki M, Radtke C, Kocsis JD (2008) Olfactory ensheathing cells exhibit unique migratory, phagocytic, and myelinating properties in the X-irradiated spinal cord not shared by Schwann cells. Glia 56: 1664–1678.
17. Monje ML, Mizumatsu S, Fike JR, Palmer TD (2002) Irradiation induces neural precursor-cell dysfunction. Nat Med 8: 955–962.
18. Zhang SC, Lundberg C, Lipsitz D, O'Connor LT, Duncan ID (1998) Generation of oligodendroglial progenitors from neural stem cells. J Neurocytol 27: 475–489.
19. Avellana-Adalid V, Nait-Oumesmar B, Lachapelle F, Baron-Van Evercooren A (1996) Expansion of rat oligodendrocyte progenitors into proliferative "oligospheres" that retain differentiation potential. J Neurosci Res 45: 558–570.
20. Bain G, Kitchens D, Yao M, Huettner JE, Gottlieb DI (1995) Embryonic stem cells express neuronal properties in vitro. Dev Biol 168: 342–357.
21. Okabe S, Forsberg-Nilsson K, Spiro AC, Segal M, McKay RD (1996) Development of neuronal precursor cells and functional postmitotic neurons from embryonic stem cells in vitro. Mech Dev 59: 89–102.
22. Brustle O, Jones KN, Learish RD, Karram K, Choudhary K, et al. (1999) Embryonic stem cell-derived glial precursors: a source of myelinating transplants. Science 285: 754–756.
23. Evans M (2011) Discovering pluripotency: 30 years of mouse embryonic stem cells. Nat Rev Mol Cell Biol 12: 680–686.
24. Zhou Q, Choi G, Anderson DJ (2001) The bHLH transcription factor Olig2 promotes oligodendrocyte differentiation in collaboration with Nkx2.2. Neuron 31: 791–807.
25. Du ZW, Li XJ, Nguyen GD, Zhang SC (2006) Induced expression of Olig2 is sufficient for oligodendrocyte specification but not for motoneuron specification and astrocyte repression. Molecular and Cellular Neuroscience 33: 371–380.
26. Sharp J, Frame J, Siegenthaler M, Nistor G, Keirstead HS (2010) Human embryonic stem cell-derived oligodendrocyte progenitor cell transplants improve recovery after cervical spinal cord injury. Stem Cells 28: 152–163.
27. Zhang SC, Wernig M, Duncan ID, Brustle O, Thomson JA (2001) In vitro differentiation of transplantable neural precursors from human embryonic stem cells. Nat Biotechnol 19: 1129–1133.
28. Ushio Y, Posner R, Posner JB, Shapiro WR (1977) Experimental spinal cord compression by epidural neoplasm. Neurology 27: 422–429.
29. Delattre JY, Rosenblum MK, Thaler HT, Mandell L, Shapiro WR, et al. (1988) A model of radiation myelopathy in the rat. Pathology, regional capillary permeability changes and treatment with dexamethasone. Brain 111 (Pt 6): 1319–1336.
30. Talbott JF, Cao Q, Enzmann GU, Benton RL, Achim V, et al. (2006) Schwann cell-like differentiation by adult oligodendrocyte precursor cells following engraftment into the demyelinated spinal cord is BMP-dependent. Glia 54: 147–159.
31. Cao Q, He Q, Wang Y, Cheng X, Howard RM, et al. Transplantation of ciliary neurotrophic factor-expressing adult oligodendrocyte precursor cells promotes remyelination and functional recovery after spinal cord injury. J Neurosci 30: 2989–3001.
32. Hofstetter CP, Holmstrom NA, Lilja JA, Schweinhardt P, Hao J, et al. (2005) Allodynia limits the usefulness of intraspinal neural stem cell grafts; directed differentiation improves outcome. Nat Neurosci 8: 346–353.
33. Iwashita Y, Fawcett JW, Crang AJ, Franklin RJ, Blakemore WF (2000) Schwann cells transplanted into normal and X-irradiated adult white matter do not migrate extensively and show poor long-term survival. Exp Neurol 164: 292–302.
34. Keirstead HS, Nistor G, Bernal G, Totoiu M, Cloutier F, et al. (2005) Human embryonic stem cell-derived oligodendrocyte progenitor cell transplants remyelinate and restore locomotion after spinal cord injury. J Neurosci 25: 4694–4705.
35. Cao Q, He Q, Wang Y, Cheng X, Howard RM, et al. (2010) Transplantation of ciliary neurotrophic factor-expressing adult oligodendrocyte precursor cells promotes remyelination and functional recovery after spinal cord injury. J Neurosci 30: 2989–3001.
36. Billon N, Jolicoeur C, Ying QL, Smith A, Raff M (2002) Normal timing of oligodendrocyte development from genetically engineered, lineage-selectable mouse ES cells. J Cell Sci 115: 3657–3665.
37. Franklin RJ, Bayley SA, Blakemore WF (1996) Transplanted CG4 cells (an oligodendrocyte progenitor cell line) survive, migrate, and contribute to repair of areas of demyelination in X-irradiated and damaged spinal cord but not in normal spinal cord. Exp Neurol 137: 263–276.
38. Jeffery ND, Crang AJ, O'Leary M T, Hodge SJ, Blakemore WF (1999) Behavioural consequences of oligodendrocyte progenitor cell transplantation into experimental demyelinating lesions in the rat spinal cord. Eur J Neurosci 11: 1508–1514.
39. Schultheiss TE, Stephens LC (1992) Invited review: permanent radiation myelopathy. Br J Radiol 65: 737–753.
40. Nave KA, Trapp BD (2008) Axon-glial signaling and the glial support of axon function. Annu Rev Neurosci 31: 535–561.
41. Trapp BD, Nave KA (2008) Multiple sclerosis: an immune or neurodegenerative disorder? Annu Rev Neurosci 31: 247–269.
42. Cummings BJ, Uchida N, Tamaki SJ, Salazar DL, Hooshmand M, et al. (2005) Human neural stem cells differentiate and promote locomotor recovery in spinal cord-injured mice. Proc Natl Acad Sci U S A 102: 14069–14074.
43. Karimi-Abdolrezaee S, Eftekharpour E, Fehlings MG (2004) Temporal and spatial patterns of Kv1.1 and Kv1.2 protein and gene expression in spinal cord white matter after acute and chronic spinal cord injury in rats: implications for axonal pathophysiology after neurotrauma. Eur J Neurosci 19: 577–589.
44. Mitsui T, Shumsky JS, Lepore AC, Murray M, Fischer I (2005) Transplantation of neuronal and glial restricted precursors into contused spinal cord improves bladder and motor functions, decreases thermal hypersensitivity, and modifies intraspinal circuitry. J Neurosci 25: 9624–9636.
45. Cao Q, Zhang YP, Iannotti C, DeVries WH, Xu XM, et al. (2005) Functional and electrophysiological changes after graded traumatic spinal cord injury in adult rat. Exp Neurol 191 Suppl 1: S3–S16.
46. Bruce CC, Zhao C, Franklin RJ (2010) Remyelination - An effective means of neuroprotection. Horm Behav 57: 56–62.
47. Jadasz JJ, Aigner L, Rivera FJ, Kury P (2012) The remyelination Philosopher's Stone: stem and progenitor cell therapies for multiple sclerosis. Cell Tissue Res.
48. Goldberg JL, Barres BA (2000) The relationship between neuronal survival and regeneration. Annu Rev Neurosci 23: 579–612.
49. Wilkins A, Majed H, Layfield R, Compston A, Chandran S (2003) Oligodendrocytes promote neuronal survival and axonal length by distinct intracellular mechanisms: a novel role for oligodendrocyte-derived glial cell line-derived neurotrophic factor. J Neurosci 23: 4967–4974.
50. Du Y, Dreyfus CF (2002) Oligodendrocytes as providers of growth factors. Journal of Neuroscience Research 68: 647–654.
51. Dai X, Lercher LD, Clinton PM, Du Y, Livingston DL, et al. (2003) The trophic role of oligodendrocytes in the basal forebrain. J Neurosci 23: 5846–5853.
52. Maier IC, Schwab ME (2006) Sprouting, regeneration and circuit formation in the injured spinal cord: factors and activity. Philos Trans R Soc Lond B Biol Sci 361: 1611–1634.

5

Use of Self-Complementary Adeno-Associated Virus Serotype 2 as a Tracer for Labeling Axons: Implications for Axon Regeneration

Yingpeng Liu, Kathy Keefe, Xiaoqing Tang, Shen Lin, George M. Smith*

Shriners Hospitals Pediatric Research Center, Temple University School of Medicine, Philadelphia, Pennsylvania, United States of America

Abstract

Various types of tracers are available for use in axon regeneration, but they require an extra operational tracer injection, time-consuming immunohistochemical analysis and cause non-specific labeling. Considerable efforts over the past years have explored other methodologies, especially the use of viral vectors, to investigate axon regeneration after injury. Recent studies have demonstrated that self-complementary Adeno-Associated Virus (scAAV) induced a high transduction efficiency and faster expression of transgenes. Here, we describe for the first time the use of scAAV2-GFP to label long-projection axons in the corticospinal tract (CST), rubrospinal tract (RST) and the central axons of dorsal root ganglion (DRG) in the normal and lesioned animal models. We found that scAAV2-GFP could efficiently transduce neurons in the sensorimotor cortex, red nucleus and DRG. Strong GFP expression could be transported anterogradely along the axon to label the numerous axon fibers from CST, RST and central axons of DRG separately. Comparison of the scAAV2 vector with single-stranded (ss) AAV2 vector in co-labeled sections showed that the scAAV2 vector induced a faster and stronger transgene expression than the ssAAV2 vector in DRG neurons and their axons. In both spinal cord lesion and dorsal root crush injury models, scAAV-GFP could efficiently label the lesioned and regenerated axons around the lesion cavity and the dorsal root entry zone (DREZ) respectively. Further, scAAV2-GFP vector could be combined with traditional tracer to specifically label sensory and motor axons after spinal cord lesion. Thus, we show that using scAAV2-GFP as a tracer is a more effective and efficient way to study axon regeneration following injury.

Editor: Simone Di Giovanni, Hertie Institute for Clinical Brain Research, University of Tuebingen., Germany

Funding: This work was funded by a grant from the NIH/National Institute of Neurological Disorders and Stroke R01 NS060784 and the Shriners Hospital for Pediatric Research, grants SHC 84050 and SHC 85200 (GMS). The funders had no role in study design, data collection and analysis, decision to publish, or preparation of the manuscript.

Competing Interests: The authors have declared that no competing interests exist.

* E-mail: george.smith@temple.edu

Introduction

Axonal tracing using tracer molecules such as BDA, CTB or fluorogold has been an essential tool for many years in studying axonal structure and continuity [1], [2]. However, this approach has certain drawbacks. It requires time consuming procedures such as tracer injections and immunohistochemical staining, can cause non-specific labeling, and limits detection to a specific time window [3]. Previous studies showed that AAV2 vectors provide distinct advantages over classic anterograde tracers and these vectors have the ability to transduce neurons efficiently and transport to axon terminals, which allow entire axons to be labeled [4], [5], [6], [7]. Neuronal transduction by conventional AAV vectors has been demonstrated in the cortex, brainstem, and sensory ganglia [5], [4], [8]. However, conventional AAV vectors carry a single-stranded (ss) DNA genome, which must be converted by host-cell-mediated DNA synthesis to double-stranded DNA for transgene expression. This requirement for formation of double-stranded DNA has proven to be an important limiting factor for AAV vector transduction. The recently developed self-complementary AAV (scAAV) vectors provide an invaluable tool in AAV-mediated gene therapy studies for CNS diseases due to their faster expression and high transduction efficiency [9]. The application of scAAV vectors in normal and lesioned axonal labeling in the CST, RST and central axons of the DRG has not been fully investigated. In this study, scAAV serotype 2 vector was used to transfect neurons in the sensorimotor cortex, red nucleus and DRG to anterogradely trace their axons in normal and lesioned animal models. Our aim in this study was to determine whether scAAV2-GFP could serve as a suitable tracer to label long axonal tracts in animal models of CNS or PNS injury. This tracer can also be used in conjunction with other tracers to label multiple axon tracts.

Materials and Methods

Vector Construction and Production

Serotype 2 AAV vector was generated by helper virus-free transfection of 293 T cells with three-plasmid helper-virus free system. 293 T cells from the American Type Culture Collection (ATCC) were grown to 70–80% confluence at which point they were transfected with two packaging plasmids using PEI (Polyethylenimine, linear, MW-25 k, Warrington, PA): one carrying the AAV rep, cap genes and another helper plasmid carrying the adenovirus helper functions. The ssAAV and scAAV were type 2 vectors carrying the enhanced GFP (eGFP) or mCherry gene driven by the chicken beta actin promoter. The self-complementary GFP vector contains both the positive and negative strand of the DNA to be packaged in the vector. Three days after transfection, cell lysates and supernatants were harvested and 40% PEG 8000 was added to precipitate crude virus for 2 hours. Adeno-associated virus from this preparation was purified by double-centrifugation with cesium chloride (CsCl) and the isolated virus was dialyzed in 0.1 M PBS/5% sorbital overnight [10]. The titers of scAAV-GFP and ssAAV-mCherry used in this study were determined by infecting fibroblast cells. Serial dilutions of scAAV2-GFP and ssAAV2-mCherry vectors were added to a 24-well plate, which had been seeded with 0.5×10^5 fibroblast cells per well. After one day, fibroblast cells expressing GFP or mCherry were counted under the fluorescence microscope to determine the vector titer per ml and then converted to genomic copy titer/mL (GC/mL) [10]. The scAAV2-GFP was found to be 1.6×10^{12} GC/mL and the ssAAV2-mCherry was prepared to the same titer.

Animals and Surgical Procedures

A total of twenty-five adult Fischer 344 rats (Harlan) weighing 175–200 g were used in this study. All surgical interventions and postoperative animal care were provided in accordance with the guide for the care and use of laboratory animals, and the guidelines for rodent survival surgery provided and approved by the Institutional Animal Care and Use Committees of Temple University. The rats were anesthetized by intraperitoneal injection of ketamine (67 mg/kg) and xylazine (6.7 mg/kg). To determine whether scAAV2-GFP can label the CST, RST and central DRG axons in an anterograde manner, scAAV-GFP was directly injected into the sensorimotor cortex, red nucleus or dorsal root ganglions, respectively. For the cortex and red nucleus viral injections, the animals were placed into a stereotaxic frame (David Kopf Instruments, Tujunga, CA). After exposure of the skull surface, a burr hole was made in the skull to expose either the sensorimotor cortex or the right red nucleus with a dental drill at the coordinates described previously (Sensorimotor cortex: anteroposterior (AP): 2.0 mm; Lateral (L): 2.0; dorsoventral (DV):1.8 mm; AP: 0 mm; L: 2.0 mm; DV: 1.8 mm; AP: −2.0 mm; L: 2.0 mm; DV: 1.8 mm. Red nucleus: AP: −6.1 mm; L: 0.6 mm; DV: 7.2 mm and AP: −5.88 mm; L: 0.6 mm; DV: 7.2 mm). For DRG AAV injection, the dorsal aspects of cervical levels 5, 6 and 7 spinal cord segments were exposed by performing a cervical laminectomy and associated DRGs were exposed. One microliter of viral vector was injected into each site of the cortex, red nucleus or DRG. Red nucleus injections were performed with a 30 G steel needle that was attached to a 10µl Hamilton syringe (Hamilton, Reno, NV). After the needle was lowered to the appropriate depth, AAV vectors were infused at a rate of 0.40 µl/min. After completion of the injection, the needle was left in place for 5 min to allow for the vector to diffuse away from the injection site. The cortex and DRG injections were performed using a nanoliter injection system (Nanoliter 2000, World Precision Instruments) mounted on a micromanipulator. Beveled tips with diameters of 20 to 40 µm were used for this purpose. AAV vectors were injected at a rate of 0.10 µl/min using a Micro4 microsyringe pump controller (World Precision Instruments) and the pipette was left in place for 5 min before removal to insure good viral diffusion into the tissue.

For evaluation of scAAV2-GFP tracing of lesioned axons after injury, we performed dorsal column lesion and dorsal root crush injury on 12 animals. The animals receiving spinal cord dorsal column lesions underwent a laminectomy at C4 spinal level, and a Kopf microwire knife (Kopf Instruments, Tujunga, CA) was used to make the lesions at 1.5 mm-width and 1.5 mm depth from the dorsal spinal cord surface as previously described [11]. For dorsal root crush injury, the animals underwent a hemilaminectomy at the L1–L2 vertebral segments to expose the lumbar dorsal roots. With the use of #5 Dummond forceps, triple-crush lesions, 10 seconds each, were inflicted at two sites separated by 3 mm along the L4, L5 afferents. All lesions were performed unilaterally on the right side. For dorsal column lesions, scAAV2-GFP was injected into the sensorimotor cortex after injury to anterogradely trace the CST. In the model of dorsal root crush injury, scAAV2-GFP was injected into the DRGs at L4 and L5 after injury to anterogradely trace the central branch of dorsal root axons. To trace both sensory and CST axons in the dorsal column lesion model, we injected scAAV2-GFP into the cervical DRGs to label dorsal column sensory axons and performed dorsal column lesion with Kopf microwire knife (Kopf Instruments, Tujunga, CA). After one week we injected 10% BDA (Molecular Probes, Eugene, OR) into the sensorimotor cortex at the coordinates described above to label CST axons and waited for 2 weeks before euthanizing animals. After surgery, rats were placed on a temperature controlled heating pad to allow the animals to recover. (Figure 1 shows schematic overview of surgical methods).

Tissue Processing and Immunohistochemistry

At the end of the 2–4 week survival period, the animals were sacrificed by injection of Fatal-Plus (Dearborn, MI) and perfused transcardially with 0.9% NaCl, followed by 4% paraformaldehyde (PFA) in 0.1 M phosphate buffer (PB, pH 7.4). The brains, spinal cords, dorsal roots and DRGs were removed, post-fixed in 4% PFA at 4°C overnight and moved to 30% sucrose in 0.1 M PB at 4°C for 2–3 days. Tissue blocks were embedded in M-1 Embedding Matrix (Kalamazoo, MI) and quick frozen on dry-ice. Brains were sectioned into six series at 30 µm coronally using a cryostat, and stained as free floating sections before being mounted onto slides. The spinal cords and DRGs were serially sectioned into five series at 16 µm using a cryostat and mounted directly on slides. To identify the nuclei of neuronal cells or neurons with axons, immunostainings of NeuN and Neurofilament were performed as previously reported [12], [13]. The sections were permeabilized and non-specific antigenic sites blocked with 0.3% Triton X-100/10% normal goat serum in 0.1 M PBS for 30 min at room temperature. Tissues were then incubated with rabbit-anti-NeuN antibody (1:400, Millipore, Temecula, CA), mouse-anti- βIII tubulin (1:1000, Promega) or rabbit-anti-GFAP antibody (1:500, DAKO, Corporation) at 4°C overnight. In order to increase GFP signals, some sections from brain or spinal cord were stained with a mouse-anti-GFP antibody (1:500, from Molecular Probes, Eugene, OR). In most cases, sections were viewed directly for GFP fluorescence.

For BDA reaction, sagittal sections were incubated with ABC reagent (Vector Laboratories) for 30 min and visualized with streptavidin 594 (1:400, Invitrogen). The next day, sections were incubated with Texas red-anti-rabbit IgG, AMCA-anti-rabbit IgG and FITC-anti-mouse IgG (1:400, Jackson ImmunoResearch, West Grove, PA) at room temperature for 60 min. After staining, sections were coverslip-mounted with Fluoromount-G (SouthernBiotech, San Diego, CA) and photographed under a Nikon microscope.

Results

Specific and Stable Neuronal Transduction

The injection of scAAV2-GFP resulted in the transduction of numerous neuronal populations and GFP expression appeared to

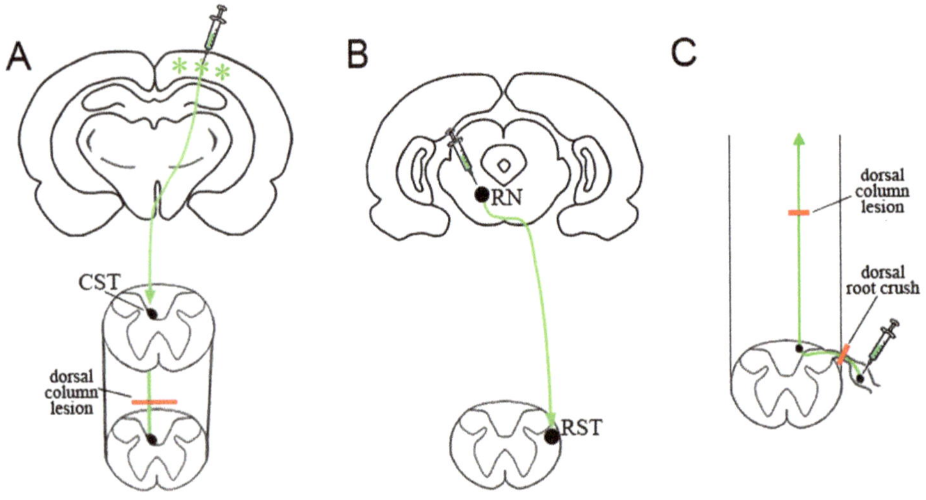

Figure 1. Schematic overview of experimental procedures. Schematic representations show pathways for the CST, RST and central axons of the DRG. A: The CST originates from the sensorimotor cortex, decussates at the medullary level of the brain stem and descends in the deep layer of the dorsal column. scAAV2-GFP vector was injected into sensorimotor cortex (green stars indicate GFP expression). Dorsal column lesion (red line in A) was performed to transect fibers of the CST in the cervical spinal cord. B: The RST runs from the neuronal bodies in the brainstem, crosses to the contralateral side and descends in the lateral white matter of the spinal cord. scAAV2-GFP was injected into the red nucleus (RN) to label the RST. C: Central axons of DRG originate from DRG neurons, pass through the dorsal root entry zone and ascend in the spinal cord dorsal column to reach the brain stem. Red lines in C indicate dorsal root crush and dorsal column lesions that transect the central axons of DRG in the dorsal root and spinal cord respectively. scAAV2-GFP was injected into DRG to anterogradely label central axons of the DRG.

be greatly restricted to neurons in the sensorimotor cortex (Fig. 2A–D), red nucleus (Fig. 2E–H), or DRG (Fig. 2I–L), depending on injection site. To identify if GFP staining co-localized to neurons, Neuronal nuclear protein (NeuN) was used to specifically label neurons. Co-labeling was seen in many scAAV-GFP transduced cells in these three areas (Fig. 2D, H and L). Colabeling also indicated that scAAV-GFP transduced very few non-neuronal cells (data not shown). In order to examine the stability of GFP expression at different time points we compared the GFP expression level 2 weeks and 8 weeks following AAV injection. We found that the numbers of GFP-positive neurons at both time points did not change, demonstrating that GFP expression level was stable over time (data not shown). This neuronal selectivity of scAAV2-GFP demonstrates its use as a powerful tool for targeting neuronal populations for axon regeneration.

Expression of AAV-scGFP in the Sensorimotor Cortex and CST Fibers in the Spinal Cord

Following delivery of scAAV2-GFP to the primary sensorimotor cortex for 4 weeks, GFP expression was detected in the brain and the spinal cord (Fig. 3). For the brain, coronal sections revealed neurons expressing GFP at the injection site (Fig. 3B and C). At high magnification, proximal dendrites and axonal collaterals could be easily identified (Fig. 3C). GFP-labeled cortical fibers were observed along the corpus callosum (Fig. 3D and E). Examination of midbrain (Fig. 3F and G, which received unilateral cortical injections) and cervical spinal cord (Fig. 3H and I, which received bilateral cortical injections) revealed GFP-labeled CST fibers descending within the CST pathway. In the cervical spinal cord, GFP-positive fibers were found at the base of the deep dorsal columns following bilateral cortex injections (Fig. 3H). In sagittal sections numerous GFP-labeled CST fibers were also detected and found parallel to the longitudinal axis of the spinal cord (Fig. 3I).

Transduction of AAV in the Red Nucleus and RST Fiber Labeling in the Spinal Cord

Stereotaxic scAAV2-GFP injections were performed into the right red nucleus and transduction efficiency of scAAV2-GFP in the red nucleus was examined at 2 weeks after AAV injections in coronal sections (Fig. 4). The scAAV2-GFP-transduced cells had a neuronal phenotype and high magnification imaging revealed transduced RN cells with long GFP-positive axons decussating to the contralateral site (Fig. 4B and C). GFP fluorescence was also found within the rubrospinal tract in the midbrain and cervical level 2 weeks after a unilateral scAAV2-GFP injection (Fig. 4E, F and H). In sagittal sections, GFP anterogradely transported to the cervical spinal cord showed straight GFP-labeled RST axons within the lateral funiculus (Fig.4H and I).

Neuronal Transduction and Axonal Labeling After Direct Injection of scAAV2-GFP into the DRG

GFP expression was examined after injecting scAAV2-GFP directly into C5–C7 DRGs. At 1 week post-injection, many neurons were transduced and expressed GFP (data not shown). Four weeks after AAV viral injections, DRG sections were stained with βIII tubulin antibody to label neurons and axons (Fig. 5A–C). GFP fluorescence was observed in cell bodies and axons (Fig. 5A–C). Within the spinal cord, GFP expression was seen in all laminae from lamina I to X and within the cuneate fasciculus (Fig. 5D and E) indicating labeling of both small and large diameter axons. Continuous labeling of the dorsal roots from the DRG cell bodies extending into the dorsal horn of the cervical spinal cord was also clearly observable (Fig. 5F). Sagittal sections at up to two spinal levels from injected DRGs were also examined and revealed GFP fluorescence in a large number of ascending sensory fibers within the dorsal columns (Fig. 5H). GFP fluorescent labeling was also clearly seen in the sciatic nerve innervating DRGs injected with scAAV2-GFP (Fig. 5I). In summary, DRG neuronal transduction

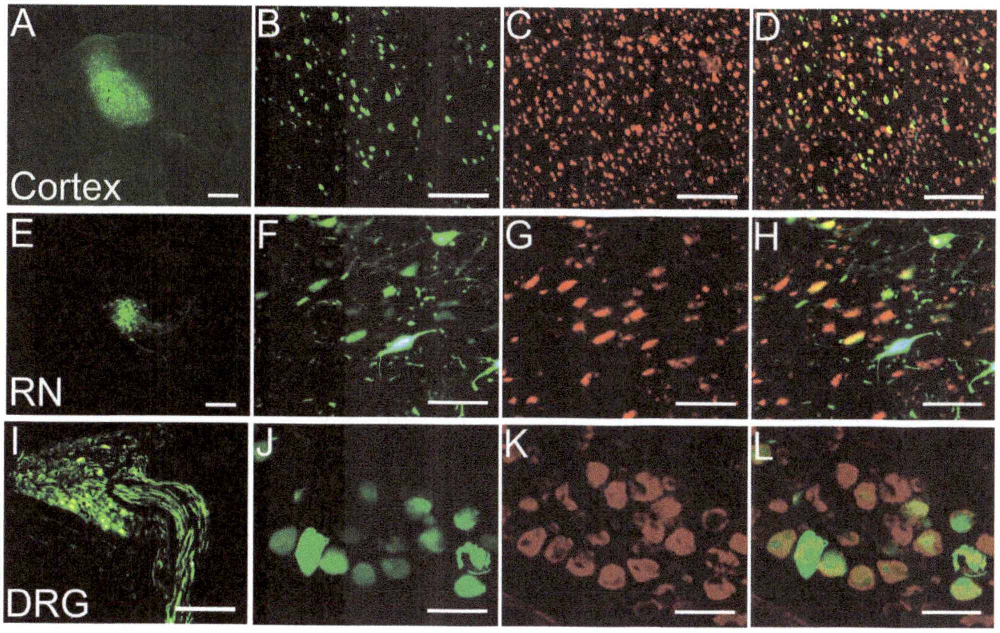

Figure 2. Specific neuronal transduction by recombinant scAAV2-GFP. Following injections of scAAV2-GFP into the sensorimotor cortex (A–D), red nucleus (RN) (E–H) and DRG (I–L), strong expression of GFP (green) was detected. The sections from these three areas were stained for NeuN (red) to specifically label the neurons (C, G and K). Scale Bars: 500 μm (A–E and I) and 200 μm (F–H, J–L).

by scAAV2-GFP results in GFP transport into both the peripheral and central projections of sensory neurons from a single ganglion.

Comparison of Transgene Expression of scAAV2-GFP with ssAAV2-mCherry Vectors in the DRG

To compare self-complementary (sc) and single-stranded (ss) adeno-associated viral vectors for neuronal transduction in the DRG, scAAV2-GFP and ssAAV2-mCherry vectors were prepared to the same titer and equal amounts of scAAV2-GFP and ssAAV2-mCherry viral particles were injected into the same DRGs. Sections of DRG sample were analyzed 1 week after viral delivery and comparison of transgene expression of scAAV2-GFP (Fig. 6A and D) with ssAAV2-mCherry (Fig. 6B and E) was performed on the same sections. Expression of GFP was seen at higher levels in the DRG neurons compared with mCherry expression. Overlaid images showed most DRG neurons were transduced by both vectors (Fig. 6C and F). In high-magnification images, only GFP was expressed independently in some DRG neurons without ssAAV-mCherry expressed (arrowhead) and strong GFP expression, without mCherry expression, was detectable in dorsal root axons (Fig. 6C and F). To control for saturation of GFP in our images, we also injected scAAV2-GFP and ssAAV2-GFP separately into different animals. We found similarly high expression of scAAV2-GFP and low expression of ssAAV2-GFP (data not shown).

Implication of scAAV2-GFP Vector for Tracing Axonal Regeneration in CST Injury Model

To examine whether axonal labeling of scAAV2-GFP could be an appropriate tool for visualizing axonal regeneration after spinal cord injury, we performed a dorsal column lesion to transect fibers of the CST at the cervical level. The dorsal column lesion model has been widely used to investigate axon regeneration [14], [15], [16]. In these animals, scAAV2-GFP was injected into the sensorimotor cortex and GFP expression was examined at the lesion site in sagittal sections. We found that GFP-labeled CST fibers (Fig. 7A and D) labeled all the way to the lesion site, which was localized by GFAP staining (Fig. 7B and E). High magnification images showing the morphology of GFP labeled CST axons in the terminal areas and some axons indicated dieback with swollen terminals apparent at their endpoints (Fig. 7D and F). We did not perform staining to increase the GFP signal. In certain cases, weak GFP expression in individual fibers or higher background may be overcome using a GFP specific antibody.

scAAV2-GFP Vector for Tracing Axonal Regeneration in a Dorsal Root Crush Model

Primary sensory axons injured by a dorsal root crush fail to regenerate into the spinal cord and regenerated axons of dorsal roots stop at the dorsal root entry zone (DREZ), the interface between the CNS and PNS. Many studies have previously examined regeneration of dorsal root axons into the DREZ to identify key molecules involved in axon regeneration [17], [18], [19]. In this experiment, we used this injury model to examine the regeneration of GFP-labeled axons through the DREZ and into the spinal cord after dorsal root crush injury. For these experiments, the dorsal roots were crushed unilaterally at the lumber level and two DRGs (L4, L5) were injected with scAAV2-GFP. In the normal uninjured animal, scAAV2-GFP labeled axons were found in spinal cord laminae I to III transported through the DREZ (Fig. 8A and B, dashed line in B). After a dorsal root crush injury, GFP-expressing axons were found only in the dorsal root, distal to the DREZ and not in the spinal cord (Fig. 8C and D). High-magnification images of a DREZ after crush showed that GFP-labeled axons stopped at the DREZ (Fig. 8D, dashed line).

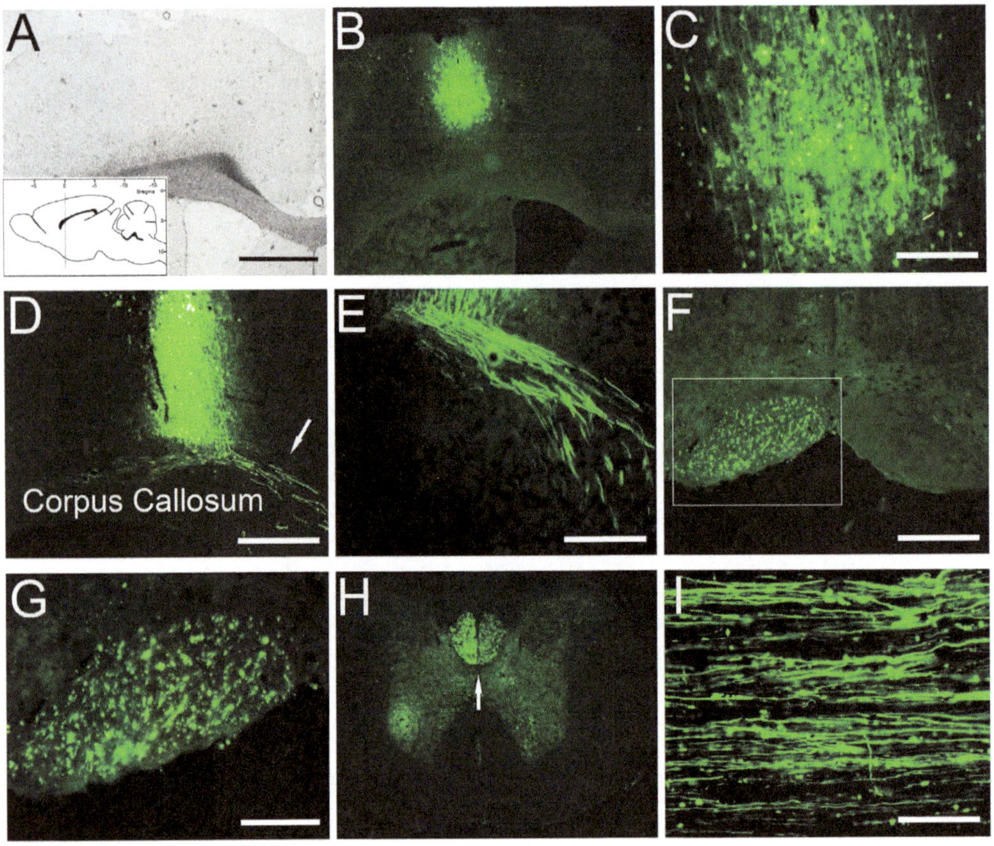

Figure 3. GFP expression in the sensorimotor cortex and anterograde labeling of CST axons. A shows the bright field of low-power image of sensorimotor cortex and corresponding low-power and high-power fluorescence images demonstrate high transduction efficiency of GFP (B and C). The schematic inset in panel A illustrates the coordinates and levels of this section. GFP positive CST fibers were found 4 weeks after viral injections above the corpus callosum (D and E), in the medulla (F and G), in the cervical spinal cord, in coronal (H) and sagittal (I) sections. The frame in the panel F shows a low magnification of the pyramidal tract, box represent high magnification in panel G. Animals used for panels A–E and H–I received bilateral viral injection. Animal for panels F and G received unilateral viral injections. Scale Bars: 500 µm (A, B and H), 200 µm (C, D and F) and 100 µm (E, G and I).

Combination of scAAV2-GFP Viral Vector with BDA Tracer for Labeling of Sensory and Motor Axons

In some studies, such as cell transplantation or drug treatments for spinal cord injury, it would be advantageous to use labels that can distinguish between sensory and motor axons. In this study, we combined the viral tracing method with a traditional tracer to separately identify dorsal sensory axons and CST axons in the same sections. We injected scAAV2-GFP into the DRG and BDA into the sensorimotor cortex. Two weeks after BDA or four weeks after scAAV2-GFP injections, cervical spinal cord sections were examined and stained for BDA and GFP labeling. In the normal animal, numerous GFP-labeled dorsal sensory axons and many BDA-labeled CST fibers were found parallel to the longitudinal axis of the spinal cord (Fig. 9. A–D). After dorsal column lesion in the spinal cord, GFP-labeled dorsal sensory axons (right of the lesion) and BDA labeled CST fibers (left of the lesion) reached and stopped at the lesion site, which is indicated by GFAP staining (Fig. 9E–H). High magnification images showed the morphology of GFP labeled sensory axons with BDA labeled CST axons around the lesion areas (Fig. 9I–L).

Discussion

The AAV vector is one of the most promising viral vectors for human gene therapy. Gene transfer via AAV vectors for the treatment of several CNS disorders, including Parkinson's disease [20], [21], [22], Alzheimer's disease [23], [24], [25] and lysosomal storage diseases [26] demonstrate the potential of human gene therapy applications. Recombinant Adeno-Associated Virus serotype 2 (AAV2) is the most widely used AAV vector, bringing advantages in long-term gene expression in post-mitotic neurons and a minimal immune response reaction, even after administration of high virus doses [27], [28]. In addition, AAV2 vectors can be packaged with capsid proteins from different AAV serotypes. These alternative serotypes can give unique tropisms and improve transduction efficiency depending on the region of interest and the target neuronal subtype [29], [30], [31]. Taken together, these advantages have led to considerable interest in the AAV2 vector as a gene transfer vehicle in axon regeneration after injury. The conventional AAV2 vector containing the single stranded DNA has to be converted to a double-stranded replicative form, which is a rate limiting step in the replicative cycle of AAV vectors [32], [33]. Double-stranded, self-complementary AAV vectors (scAAV) bypass this step and provide the opportunity to achieve more efficient transduction and faster, more prolonged transgene expression [34], [35]. In this study, a scAAV2 was compared to

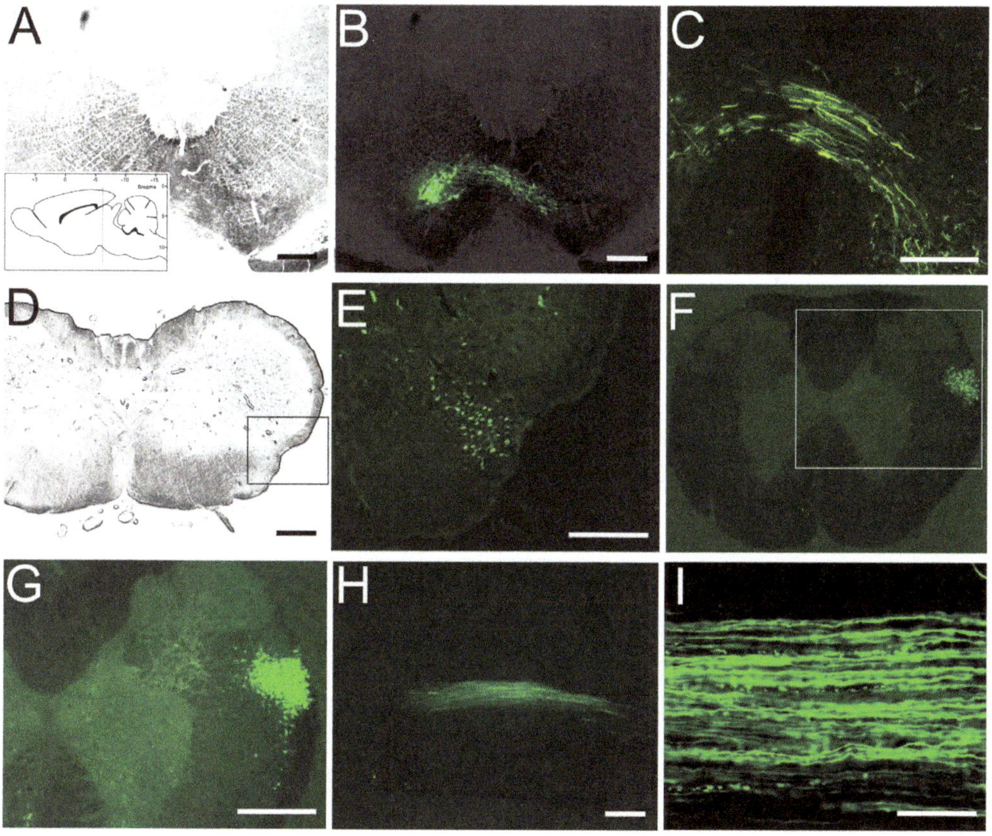

Figure 4. GFP expression in RN and anterograde labeling of RST. GFP expression was observed in the RN following scAAV2-GFP injection, as illustrated in coronal sections (A and B). The schematic inset in panel A illustrates the coordinates and levels of this section. Higher magnification images demonstrate anterograde transport of GFP to the contralateral site (C), midbrain (D and E) and cervical spinal cord in coronal (F and G) and sagittal sections (H and I). The box frames in panels D and F represent the regions magnified in panels E and G, respectively. Scale Bars: 500 μm (AH), 200 μm (I).

traditional single-stranded (ss) AAV2 vector for reporter gene expression in the DRG and shown that scAAV2 transgene expression is faster and stronger compared with that achieved by the equivalent ssAAV2 vector. For small tissues in the CNS, such as DRG, a stronger level of expression may be critical, and scAAV vectors can significantly minimize the vector load required to achieve sustained transgene expression. The use of lower viral titers can also reduce the risk of adverse effects due to immune responses caused by the vector itself.

In addition to high transduction efficiency, transgene expression in specific neurons of the nervous system is very important for axonal tracing and gene therapy. To determine whether scAAV2-GFP specifically transduces neurons, we examined a subset of tissues derived from AAV injected animals. These tissues were sectioned and co-labeled with NeuN, a marker for a neuronal nuclear protein or Neurofilament M, a marker for neurons and axons. Our results demonstrate that scAAV2-GFP showed high selectivity for neuronal cells of the sensorimotor cortex, red nucleus and DRG. We did not compare the temporal expression profile or the cellular tropism of different AAV serotype vectors in our present study. In the past few years, several groups have compared the transduction rate and expression level from different AAV serotypes and their results indicated AAV1 (AAV2 vector packaged with serotype 1 capsid proteins) was the optimal serotype for transducing CST neurons and axons projecting through the dorsal CST of the cervical spinal cord [36]. AAV5 has been shown to have the maximum transduction efficiency following direct injection into the dorsal root ganglia, compared to AAV serotypes 1, 2, 3, 4, 6, and 8, and lentivirus (LV) vectors. The time course of GFP expression showed increasing neuronal transduction rates from 12 weeks after AAV5-GFP injections [8]. For RST, quantification of the ratio of transduced RN neurons and RST fibers revealed that AAV1 and AAV8 transduced the highest ratio of RN neurons and the highest number of RST labeling was found in the AAV1-treated animals at 1 month post-injection [37]. Our future studies will utilize the most favorable scAAV serotype to express GFP combined with the appropriate regulatory promoters [38], [39] to achieve the highest-level of sustained GFP expression for axonal tracing.

To assess the ability of AAV to anterogradely transport and label the long-tract axons from the CST, RST and central axons of the DRG, scAAV2-GFP was injected into the sensorimotor cortex, red nucleus and DRGs, respectively. scAAV2-GFP was successfully transported as shown by labeling of GFP-positive fibers in the appropriate descending or ascending tracts extending to the cervical spinal cord. Furthermore, we examined the GFP labeling of axons in two injury models and our data demonstrate that lesioned or regenerated axons could be clearly visualized and easily identified directly under fluorescent microscopy. For visualization of the RST and dorsal root, two weeks provided enough time for infected neurons to express GFP in both their cell bodies and their axons. If the longer axonal tracts such as those of

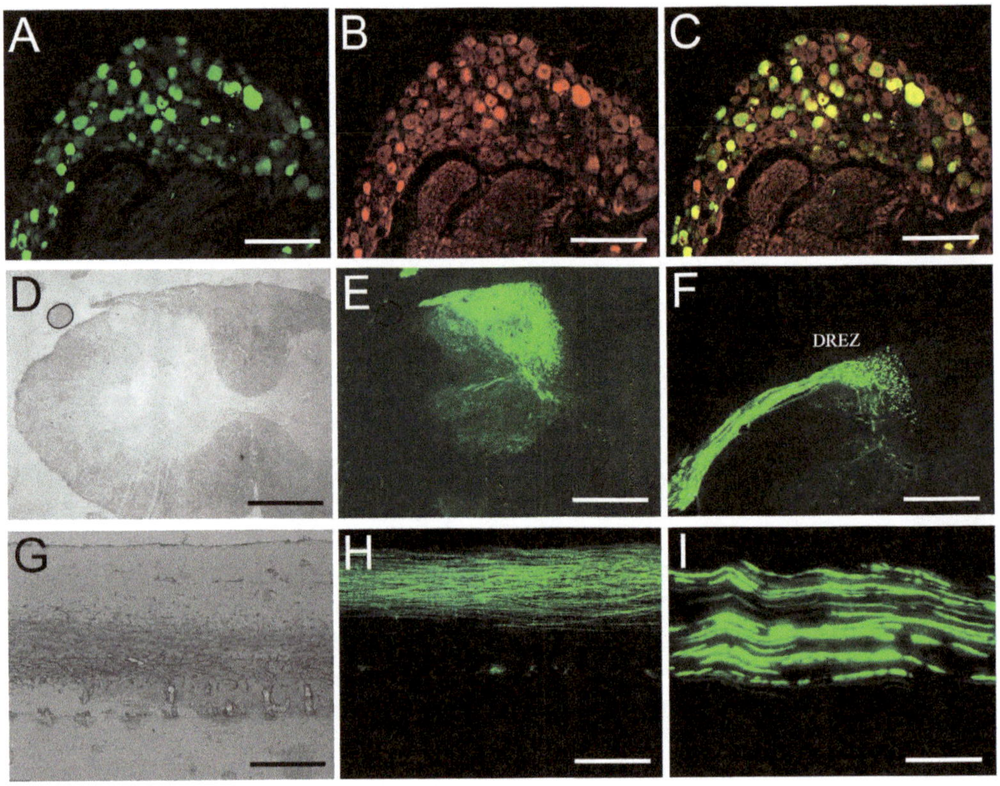

Figure 5. GFP expression in DRG and labeling of central and peripheral axons. GFP expressed in DRG neurons of the cervical spinal cord after scAAV2-GFP intraganglion injections (A–C). βIII-tubulin staining showed labeling in both neurons and axons (B and C). Many GFP positive fibers are visible in the dorsal horn (D and E), the dorsal roots (F), and can be traced over long distances to the cervical level of spinal cord (G and H). The peripheral nerve was also brightly labeled (I). Scale Bars: 200 μm (A–C, F and I), 500 μm (D–E, G–H).

the CST need to be labeled, longer survival times are desired, such as 4 weeks post-injection, as used in the present study. Our observations suggest that scAAV2-GFP is an excellent anterograde tracer for long axonal pathways. In addition to using viral vectors as anterograde labeling, AAV vectors can also retrogradely label axons from their terminals to neuronal bodies. Previous studies

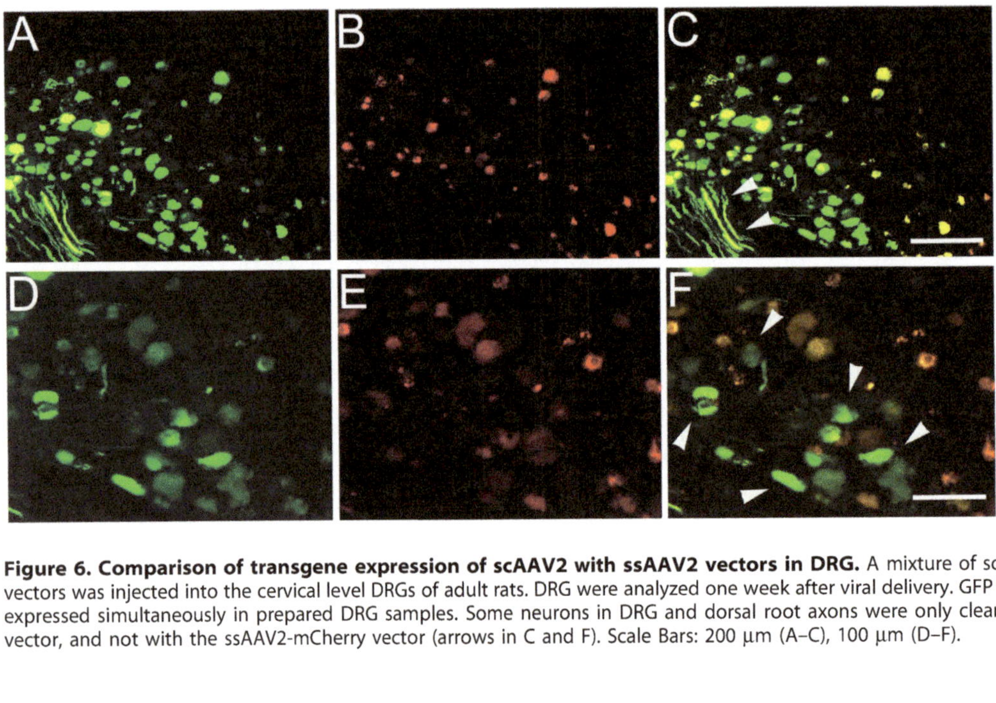

Figure 6. Comparison of transgene expression of scAAV2 with ssAAV2 vectors in DRG. A mixture of scAAV2-GFP and ssAAV2-mCherry vectors was injected into the cervical level DRGs of adult rats. DRG were analyzed one week after viral delivery. GFP (A and D) and mcherry (B and E) expressed simultaneously in prepared DRG samples. Some neurons in DRG and dorsal root axons were only clearly labeled with the scAAV2-GFP vector, and not with the ssAAV2-mCherry vector (arrows in C and F). Scale Bars: 200 μm (A–C), 100 μm (D–F).

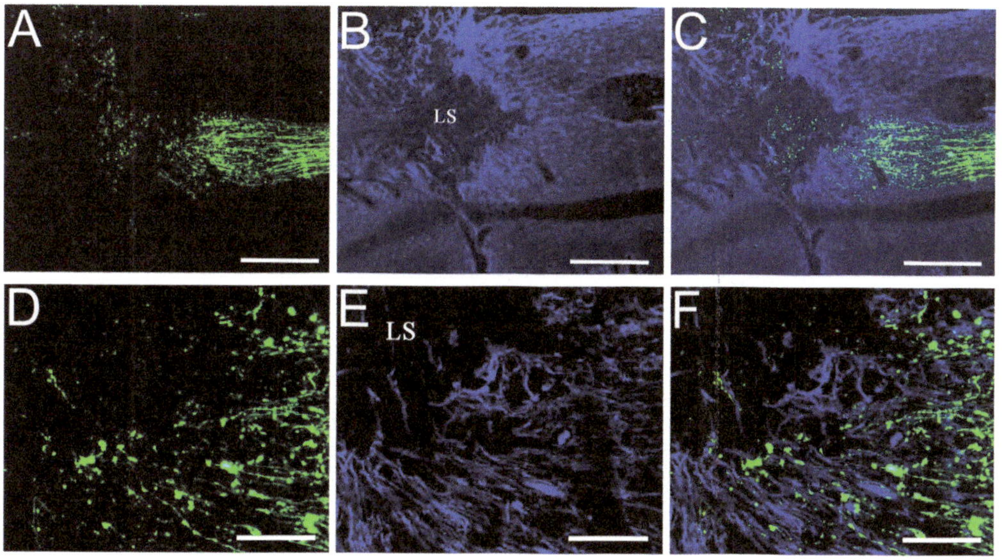

Figure 7. Implication of scAAV2-GFP for labeling CST axons after injury. Dorsal column lesion resulted in a corresponding loss of CST axons, as visualized by anterograde transport of scAAV2-GFP at 4 weeks after viral injection into the sensorimotor cortex (A and C). GFAP staining of the section was to label the lesion site and cavity (B and E). Low magnification images shown in A–B, Corresponding high-magnification images shown in D–F. Scale Bars: 500 μm (A–C), 200 μm (D–F).

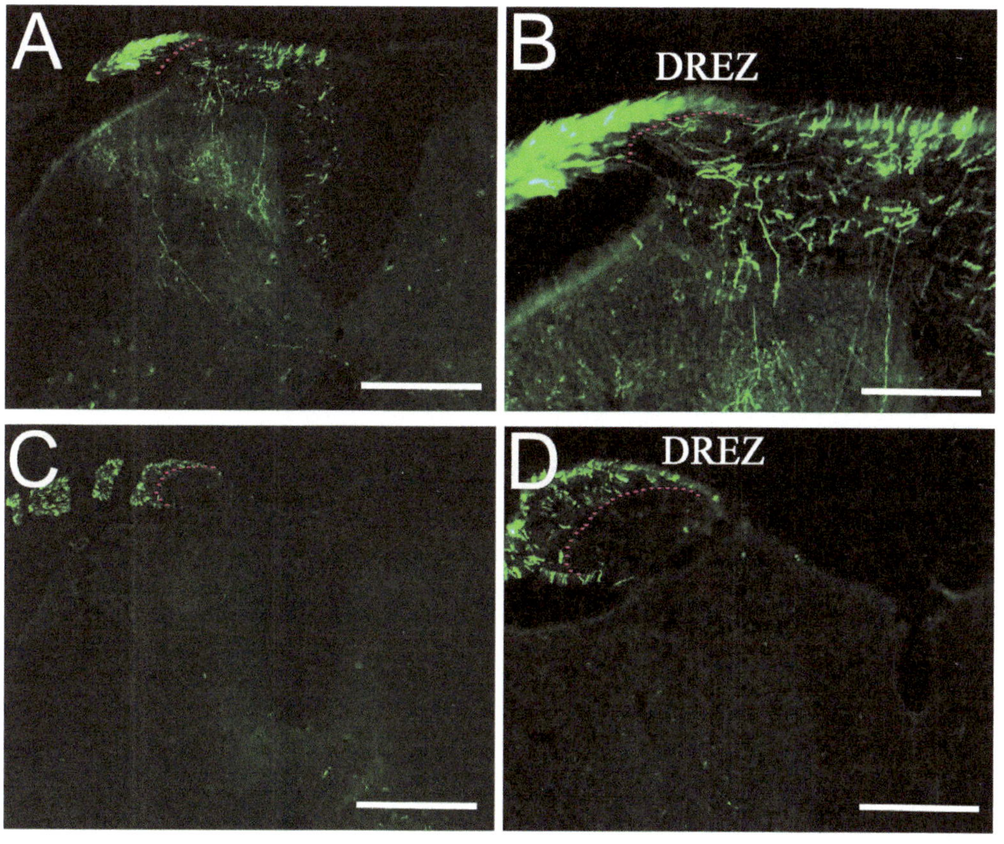

Figure 8. Implications of scAAV2-GFP labeling in dorsal root axons after crush. GFP-labeled axons were examined after dorsal root crush injury. In un-injured animals, GFP-labeled axons enter the spinal cord from the entry zone along with other axons (A and B). After dorsal root crush, cross sections of injured dorsal root with attached spinal cord showing GFP-expressing axons stopped in the DREZ (G and H). DREZ boundary is approximated with a dashed line. Scale Bars: 500 μm (A and C), 200 μm (B and D).

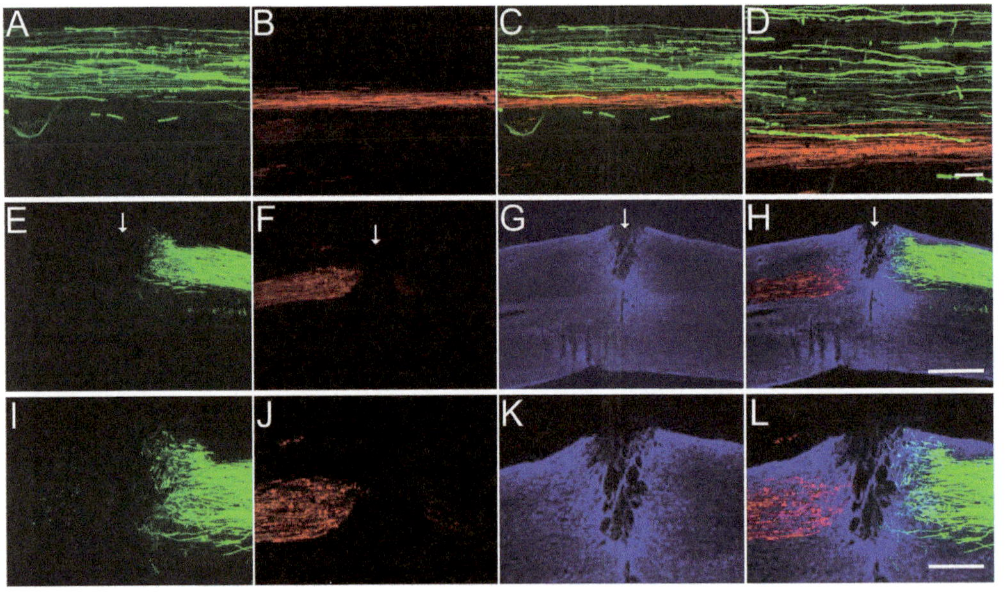

Figure 9. Combining scAAV2-GFP with BDA tracer for labeling sensory and motor axons after injury. Following injections of scAAV2-GFP into the DRG and BDA into the sensorimotor cortex, sections of cervical spinal cord were examined in normal (A–D) and dorsal column lesion animals (E–L). GFAP staining labeling the lesion cavity are shown in blue (G and K). scAAV2-GFP-labeled dorsal sensory axons are shown in green (right of the lesion) (E and I) and BDA labeled CST fibers are shown in red (left of the lesion) (F and J). Scale Bars: 500 μm (A–H), 200 μm (I–L).

indicate that many anterograde tracers also resulted in some retrograde transport. Retrograde infection can occur through active transport of the viral genome from synaptic terminals in the area of injection [40]. In our unpublished data, injection of scAAV2-GFP into the L2 spinal cord retrogradely labeled the RST and their rubrospinal neurons in the brain stem (data not shown). Thus, in the future, the injections of double or triple fluorescence expressing scAAV vectors, such as GFP (green), mCherry (red) and Tomato (red-orange) can be used to provide multiple tracts tracings anterogradely and retrogradely at the same time.

AAV2-mediated gene transfer approaches have been designed for the treatment of spinal cord injury and neurological disorders [16], [20], [21]. Concurrent injection of different AAV2 vectors can co-express therapeutic genes and fluorescent markers like GFP. Because the neuronal cell body of the labeled axons also expresses the therapeutic gene, the resulting regeneration of anterogradely labeled axons will directly demonstrate that this regenerative effect comes from the therapeutic gene [4]. Other studies have shown that GFP labeled axons can be used for the visualization and quantification of sprouting and regeneration of CST axons without tracers. For example, coinjection of AAV8-GFP and AAV8-KLF7 into the sensorimotor cortex was shown to promote CST axonal sprouting and growth [14]. Further, scAAV tract tracing techniques combined with viral-mediated expression of axonal growth promoting genes, such as growth factors [41], [42], [43], mTOR activators [44] or channelrhodopsins (ChRs) [45], [46] will allow axon regeneration to be detected more easily and precisely.

In summary, we report that the development of a recombinant scAAV2 vector carrying a GFP reporter gene can efficiently transduce neurons in the sensorimotor cortex, red nucleus and DRGs, and intensely label their axonal fibers. Following lesions in the dorsal column or dorsal roots, injection of scAAV2-GFP into the sensorimotor cortex or DRGs allows direct visualization of transected or regenerating axons in the lesion site or dorsal root entry zone. The scAAV2-GFP axon tracing technique can also be combined with scAAV2-mediated expression of other genes to directly and precisely assess the transgene effect on axon regeneration.

Author Contributions

Conceived and designed the experiments: YL KK GMS. Performed the experiments: YL KK XT SL. Analyzed the data: YL KK XT GMS. Contributed reagents/materials/analysis tools: YL KK XT GMS. Wrote the paper: YL KK XT SL GMS.

References

1. Raju DV, Smith Y (2006) Anterograde axonal tract tracing. Curr Protoc Neurosci Chapter 1: Unit 1 14.
2. Zhang J, Xi M, Fung SJ, Sampogna S, Chase MH (2012) Projections from the central nucleus of the amygdala to the nucleus pontis oralis in the rat: an anterograde labeling study. Neurosci Lett 525: 157–162.
3. Steward O, Zheng B, Tessier-Lavigne M, Hofstadter M, Sharp K, et al. (2008) Regenerative growth of corticospinal tract axons via the ventral column after spinal cord injury in mice. J Neurosci 28: 6836–6847.
4. Williams RR, Pearse DD, Tresco PA, Bunge MB (2012) The assessment of adeno-associated vectors as potential intrinsic treatments for brainstem axon regeneration. J Gene Med 14: 20–34.
5. Chamberlin NL, Du B, de Lacalle S, Saper CB (1998) Recombinant adeno-associated virus vector: use for transgene expression and anterograde tract tracing in the CNS. Brain Res 793: 169–175.
6. Xiao X, Li J, McCown TJ, Samulski RJ (1997) Gene transfer by adeno-associated virus vectors into the central nervous system. Exp Neurol 144: 113–124.
7. Kells AP, Hadaczek P, Yin D, Bringas J, Varenika V, et al. (2009) Efficient gene therapy-based method for the delivery of therapeutics to primate cortex. Proc Natl Acad Sci U S A 106: 2407–2411.
8. Mason MR, Ehlert EM, Eggers R, Pool CW, Hermening S, et al. (2010) Comparison of AAV serotypes for gene delivery to dorsal root ganglion neurons. Mol Ther 18: 715–724.

9. McCarty DM, Monahan PE, Samulski RJ (2001) Self-complementary recombinant adeno-associated virus (scAAV) vectors promote efficient transduction independently of DNA synthesis. Gene Ther 8: 1248–1254.
10. Ayuso E, Mingozzi F, Montane J, Leon X, Anguela XM, et al. (2010) High AAV vector purity results in serotype- and tissue-independent enhancement of transduction efficiency. Gene Ther 17: 503–510.
11. Lu P, Yang H, Jones LL, Filbin MT, Tuszynski MH (2004) Combinatorial therapy with neurotrophins and cAMP promotes axonal regeneration beyond sites of spinal cord injury. J Neurosci 24: 6402–6409.
12. Hu X, Cai J, Yang J, Smith GM (2010) Sensory axon targeting is increased by NGF gene therapy within the lesioned adult femoral nerve. Exp Neurol 223: 153–165.
13. Liu YP, Zhao HB (2008) Cellular characterization of Connexin26 and Connnexin30 expression in the cochlear lateral wall. Cell Tissue Res 333: 395–403.
14. Blackmore MG, Wang Z, Lerch JK, Motti D, Zhang YP, et al. (2012) Kruppel-like Factor 7 engineered for transcriptional activation promotes axon regeneration in the adult corticospinal tract. Proc Natl Acad Sci U S A 109: 7517–7522.
15. Wang D, Ichiyama RM, Zhao R, Andrews MR, Fawcett JW (2011) Chondroitinase combined with rehabilitation promotes recovery of forelimb function in rats with chronic spinal cord injury. J Neurosci 31: 9332–9344.
16. Liu K, Lu Y, Lee JK, Samara R, Willenberg R, et al. (2010) PTEN deletion enhances the regenerative ability of adult corticospinal neurons. Nat Neurosci 13: 1075–1081.
17. Tan CL, Andrews MR, Kwok JC, Heintz TG, Gumy LF, et al. (2012) Kindlin-1 enhances axon growth on inhibitory chondroitin sulfate proteoglycans and promotes sensory axon regeneration. J Neurosci 32: 7325–7335.
18. Tang XQ, Tanelian DL, Smith GM (2004) Semaphorin3A inhibits nerve growth factor-induced sprouting of nociceptive afferents in adult rat spinal cord. J Neurosci 24: 819–827.
19. Ramer MS, Priestley JV, McMahon SB (2000) Functional regeneration of sensory axons into the adult spinal cord. Nature 403: 312–316.
20. Marks WJ Jr, Bartus RT, Siffert J, Davis CS, Lozano A, et al. (2010) Gene delivery of AAV2-neurturin for Parkinson's disease: a double-blind, randomised, controlled trial. Lancet Neurol 9: 1164–1172.
21. LeWitt PA, Rezai AR, Leehey MA, Ojemann SG, Flaherty AW, et al. (2011) AAV2-GAD gene therapy for advanced Parkinson's disease: a double-blind, sham-surgery controlled, randomised trial. Lancet Neurol 10: 309–319.
22. Kaplitt MG, Feigin A, Tang C, Fitzsimons HL, Mattis P, et al. (2007) Safety and tolerability of gene therapy with an adeno-associated virus (AAV) borne GAD gene for Parkinson's disease: an open label, phase I trial. Lancet 369: 2097–2105.
23. Mandel RJ (2010) CERE-110, an adeno-associated virus-based gene delivery vector expressing human nerve growth factor for the treatment of Alzheimer's disease. Curr Opin Mol Ther 12: 240–247.
24. Ryan DA, Mastrangelo MA, Narrow WC, Sullivan MA, Federoff HJ, et al. (2010) Abeta-directed single-chain antibody delivery via a serotype-1 AAV vector improves learning behavior and pathology in Alzheimer's disease mice. Mol Ther 18: 1471–1481.
25. Azzouz M, Hottinger A, Paterna JC, Zurn AD, Aebischer P, et al. (2000) Increased motoneuron survival and improved neuromuscular function in transgenic ALS mice after intraspinal injection of an adeno-associated virus encoding Bcl-2. Hum Mol Genet 9: 803–811.
26. Fu H, Samulski RJ, McCown TJ, Picornell YJ, Fletcher D, et al. (2002) Neurological correction of lysosomal storage in a mucopolysaccharidosis IIIB mouse model by adeno-associated virus-mediated gene delivery. Mol Ther 5: 42–49.
27. Samulski RJ, Chang LS, Shenk T (1989) Helper-free stocks of recombinant adeno-associated viruses: normal integration does not require viral gene expression. J Virol 63: 3822–3828.
28. Zaiss AK, Muruve DA (2005) Immune responses to adeno-associated virus vectors. Curr Gene Ther 5: 323–331.
29. Burger C, Gorbatyuk OS, Velardo MJ, Peden CS, Williams P, et al. (2004) Recombinant AAV viral vectors pseudotyped with viral capsids from serotypes 1, 2, and 5 display differential efficiency and cell tropism after delivery to different regions of the central nervous system. Mol Ther 10: 302–317.
30. Taymans JM, Vandenberghe LH, Haute CV, Thiry I, Deroose CM, et al. (2007) Comparative analysis of adeno-associated viral vector serotypes 1, 2, 5, 7, and 8 in mouse brain. Hum Gene Ther 18: 195–206.
31. Cearley CN, Vandenberghe LH, Parente MK, Carnish ER, Wilson JM, et al. (2008) Expanded repertoire of AAV vector serotypes mediate unique patterns of transduction in mouse brain. Mol Ther 16: 1710–1718.
32. Ferrari FK, Samulski T, Shenk T, Samulski RJ (1996) Second-strand synthesis is a rate-limiting step for efficient transduction by recombinant adeno-associated virus vectors. J Virol 70: 3227–3234.
33. Hauck B, Zhao W, High K, Xiao W (2004) Intracellular viral processing, not single-stranded DNA accumulation, is crucial for recombinant adeno-associated virus transduction. J Virol 78: 13678–13686.
34. Wang Z, Ma HI, Li J, Sun L, Zhang J, et al. (2003) Rapid and highly efficient transduction by double-stranded adeno-associated virus vectors in vitro and in vivo. Gene Ther 10: 2105–2111.
35. McCarty DM (2008) Self-complementary AAV vectors; advances and applications. Mol Ther 16: 1648–1656.
36. Hutson TH, Verhaagen J, Yanez-Munoz RJ, Moon LD (2012) Corticospinal tract transduction: a comparison of seven adeno-associated viral vector serotypes and a non-integrating lentiviral vector. Gene Ther 19: 49–60.
37. Blits B, Derks S, Twisk J, Ehlert E, Prins J, et al. (2010) Adeno-associated viral vector (AAV)-mediated gene transfer in the red nucleus of the adult rat brain: comparative analysis of the transduction properties of seven AAV serotypes and lentiviral vectors. J Neurosci Methods 185: 257–263.
38. Paterna JC, Bueler H (2002) Recombinant adeno-associated virus vector design and gene expression in the mammalian brain. Methods 28: 208–218.
39. Paterna JC, Moccetti T, Mura A, Feldon J, Bueler H (2000) Influence of promoter and WHV post-transcriptional regulatory element on AAV-mediated transgene expression in the rat brain. Gene Ther 7: 1304–1311.
40. Wang X, Smith GM, Xu XM (2011) Preferential and bidirectional labeling of the rubrospinal tract with adenovirus-GFP for monitoring normal and injured axons. J Neurotrauma 28: 635–647.
41. Smith GM, Falone AE, Frank E (2012) Sensory axon regeneration: rebuilding functional connections in the spinal cord. Trends Neurosci 35: 156–163.
42. Jin Y, Ziemba KS, Smith GM (2008) Axon growth across a lesion site along a preformed guidance pathway in the brain. Exp Neurol 210: 521–530.
43. Romero MI, Rangappa N, Garry MG, Smith GM (2001) Functional regeneration of chronically injured sensory afferents into adult spinal cord after neurotrophin gene therapy. J Neurosci 21: 8408–8416.
44. Park KK, Liu K, Hu Y, Smith PD, Wang C, et al. (2008) Promoting axon regeneration in the adult CNS by modulation of the PTEN/mTOR pathway. Science 322: 963–966.
45. Depuy SD, Kanbar R, Coates MB, Stornetta RL, Guyenet PG (2011) Control of breathing by raphe obscurus serotonergic neurons in mice. J Neurosci 31: 1981–1990.
46. Alilain WJ, Li X, Horn KP, Dhingra R, Dick TE, et al. (2008) Light-induced rescue of breathing after spinal cord injury. J Neurosci 28: 11862–11870.

6

Age-Dependent Transcriptome and Proteome Following Transection of Neonatal Spinal Cord of *Monodelphis domestica* (South American Grey Short-Tailed Opossum)

Norman R. Saunders[1]*, Natassya M. Noor[1], Katarzyna M. Dziegielewska[1], Benjamin J. Wheaton[1], Shane A. Liddelow[1,2], David L. Steer[3], C. Joakim Ek[4], Mark D. Habgood[1], Matthew J. Wakefield[5,6], Helen Lindsay[5,7], Jessie Truettner[8], Robert D. Miller[9], A. Ian Smith[3], W. Dalton Dietrich[8]

1 Department of Pharmacology & Therapeutics, The University of Melbourne, Victoria, Australia, **2** Department of Neurobiology, Stanford University, Stanford, California, United States of America, **3** Department of Biochemistry and Molecular Biology, Monash University, Clayton, Victoria, Australia, **4** Department of Neuroscience and Physiology, University of Gothenburg, Gothenburg, Sweden, **5** Walter & Eliza Hall Institute of Medical Research, Victoria, Australia, **6** Department of Genetics, The University of Melbourne, Victoria, Australia, **7** Institute of Molecular Life Sciences, University of Zurich, Zurich, Switzerland, **8** The Miami Project to Cure Paralysis, University of Miami, Miller School of Medicine, Miami, Florida, United States of America, **9** Center for Evolutionary & Theoretical Immunology, Department of Biology, University of New Mexico, Albuquerque, New Mexico, United States of America

Abstract

This study describes a combined transcriptome and proteome analysis of *Monodelphis domestica* response to spinal cord injury at two different postnatal ages. Previously we showed that complete transection at postnatal day 7 (P7) is followed by profuse axon growth across the lesion with near-normal locomotion and swimming when adult. In contrast, at P28 there is no axon growth across the lesion, the animals exhibit weight-bearing locomotion, but cannot use hind limbs when swimming. Here we examined changes in gene and protein expression in the segment of spinal cord rostral to the lesion at 24 h after transection at P7 and at P28. Following injury at P7 only forty genes changed (all increased expression); most were immune/inflammatory genes. Following injury at P28 many more genes changed their expression and the magnitude of change for some genes was strikingly greater. Again many were associated with the immune/inflammation response. In functional groups known to be inhibitory to regeneration in adult cords the expression changes were generally muted, in some cases opposite to that required to account for neurite inhibition. For example myelin basic protein expression was reduced following injury at P28 both at the gene and protein levels. Only four genes from families with extracellular matrix functions thought to influence neurite outgrowth in adult injured cords showed substantial changes in expression following injury at P28: Olfactomedin 4 (*Olfm4*, 480 fold compared to controls), matrix metallopeptidase (*Mmp1*, 104 fold), papilin (*Papln*, 152 fold) and integrin α4 (*Itga4*, 57 fold). These data provide a resource for investigation of *a priori* hypotheses in future studies of mechanisms of spinal cord regeneration in immature animals compared to lack of regeneration at more mature stages.

Editor: Michelle L. Baker, CSIRO, Australia

Funding: This project was supported by the Victoria Neurotrauma Initiative. The funders had no role in study design, data collection and analysis, decision to publish, or preparation of the manuscript.

Competing Interests: The authors have declared that no competing interests exist.

* E-mail: n.saunders@unimelb.edu.au

Introduction

The studies of Aguayo and colleagues in the 1980s [1,2], which repeated an old experiment of Tello [3] using implants and bridges of sciatic nerve to promote regeneration of the central nervous system (CNS) resulted in a concentrated effort to understand the mechanisms underlying the failure of the adult mammalian spinal cord to exhibit regenerative recovery following injury. Since then several such inhibitory mechanisms have been described including myelin inhibitory factors [4,5] and proteoglycans [6–8]. So far no effective therapy has emerged and disappointingly, attempts to replicate apparently promising animal studies have been mostly unsuccessful (e.g., [9–13]). One reason for this may simply be that the responses of the injured CNS are so complex that a repair strategy based on modifying only one aspect of this process is unlikely to be successful. A strong indication of the complexity of the response of the spinal cord to injury came first from the microarray study by Aimone and colleagues [14]. Similarly complex findings following brain injury have been reported [15]. Verhaagen et al. [16] provided an overview of 25 gene expression profiling studies (over the period of 2001 to 2009, see [16]) of spinal cord injury in rodents. The sites examined were at or around the lesion, which were mainly a contusion in the thoracic spinal cord. The studies used microarrays (generally Affymetrix) to investigate gene expression over a wide range of post injury times (30 min to 90 days). One of these studies involved embryonic spinal cord, which was uninjured but compared to adult injured spinal cord [17]. To date, only one RNA-Seq dataset of injured spinal cord has been published [18] although additional information may perhaps be gleaned from an RNA-Seq study that examined the effects of transplanted progenitor/stem cells following spinal cord injury [19].

Verhaagen et al. [16] reported that the observed changes in gene expression across this large number of studies were "remarkably consistent" and summarized the results under 8 functional categories that showed changed expression. Genes in some of these groups were generally upregulated: immediate early genes, proinflammatory genes, phagocytosis & induction of the complement system, neuronal genes (some implicated in neurite outgrowth or synaptic plasticity). Other groups showed a mixture of up- and downregulation: genes related to apoptosis, angiogenesis. Some showed predominantly downregulation: genes encoding neurotransmitter synthesis and other aspects of synaptic function, ion channels. Surprisingly, no mention was made of genes that generate various extracellular matrix factors such as proteoglycans, as this family of proteins has been implicated in several studies to be involved in the failure of neurite outgrowth following injury (see [20]).

In contrast to the lack of functional recovery from severe spinal cord injury in adult mammals, immature animals show a significant degree of recovery. This has been demonstrated in two species of marsupial opossum, where substantial growth of axons across a lesion was observed. Some of these axons were shown to be regenerating and some were growing as a part of normal development [21–23]. This response to injury appears to be age dependent [23–25] providing an opportunity to compare gene regulation in a mammalian species at a stage of development when regeneration and axon growth occurs and one when it does not [25,26]. To undertake a similar study in rodents would require *in utero* transection of the spinal cord at around E15 (permissive stage, [27]) and at a stage that was non-permissive but with bodyweight bearing locomotion (probably E19–20).

Some preliminary studies in developing spinal cord have been carried out using human microarrays [28], mouse microarrays [24] and tammar wallaby microarrays [29] as well as different forms of polymerase chain reaction methods [24,30]. These showed that there is indeed substantial age-dependent gene regulation in the response of the spinal cord to injury [24,28–30]. The most comprehensive study of these responses was that by Mladinic et al., [29] using a combination of microarray (tammar wallaby, a marsupial species) and qRT-PCR for specific genes of interest. These authors divided the genes identified into categories relating to whether changes in expression (up- or downregulation) might be expected to be contributing to successful growth of axons across a lesion made at P8, but not at P13. However, these studies used *in vitro* preparations of isolated *Monodelphis* spinal cord at 25°C, which may have had an influence on some aspects of the response to injury (see General Discussion).

With the recent sequencing of the opossum genome [31] and the advent of high throughput RNA sequencing (RNA-Seq) it is now possible to examine overall gene expression changes in response to injury in this species. In the present study we investigated both the transcriptome and the proteome in the segment of cord rostral to the site of injury following a complete spinal cord transection in opossums at an age when axonal growth across a lesion and substantially normal locomotor development occur (postnatal day 7, P7) and compared this with an older age when no axon growth can be seen, but nevertheless a demonstrable body weight-bearing locomotion is present (P28, [25]). A study of changes in the spinal cord proteome caudal to the site of injury following spinal cord transection in *Monodelphis* at these two ages has been previously published [32].

Materials and Methods

Animals used

Monodelphis domestica were obtained from a colony based at the University of Melbourne Medical Sciences Animal House Facility, Melbourne, Australia. Procedures were performed according to National Health and Medical Research Council guidelines, with the approval of the University of Melbourne Animal Ethics Committee (Ethics #0707108). Pups of both sexes were used. Day of birth was designated as postnatal day zero, P0 (see [25,26]).

The pups were assigned to two age groups and spinal cord injuries (SCIs) were performed at either P7 or P28. At P7, whole litters (6–7 pups) were operated on. Separate litters of pups were kept as controls as there is no consistent way to mark these very young animals without increasing the risk of cannibalisation by the mother [22]. Injuries at P28 were usually made on half the pups in a litter, since at P28 their ears can be marked. The remaining pups from these litters were anaesthetised but remained uninjured and were used as controls. For RNA-Seq and proteomic analyses experimental and control pups were collected at 24 h (+24 h) post surgery. For morphological studies, animals were collected as unoperated controls and at 0 h and 24 h post injury in both age groups. The total number of animals used in the transcriptomic study was: P8 control ($n = 24$), P7+24 h ($n = 24$), P29 control ($n = 12$), P28+24 h ($n = 12$). These were obtained from several separate litters. In the proteomic study the number of animals and weights of tissues used are shown in Table 1. For the morphological studies at least 3 pups at each age were used, usually from different litters [32,33].

Spinal cord transection

At P7, *Monodelphis* pups are still attached to the mothers' teats [34]. The female adult *Monodelphis* were anaesthetized with 2–3% isofluorane; the same anaesthetic was administered to the P7 pups via a small facemask during the surgical procedure. Pups at P28 are no longer attached to the mother and were separately anaesthetized with isofluorane throughout the surgical procedure [25].

Complete spinal cord transection was performed at thoracic level 10 (T10) using sharp sterilized fine scissors. Skin was closed using surgical grade glue (Vetbond, 3 M, St. Paul, MN, USA). Animals were returned to their cages and allowed to recover for 24 hours (+24 h) post injury. At the end of the experimental period, control and injured animals were terminally anaesthetized with an overdose of isofluorane and spinal cords were dissected out.

The cords were separated into two segments, the upper (rostral to the injury) and lower (caudal to the injury) divided at T10 (site of transection), or corresponding segments from control animal spinal cords. Samples were stored at −80°C until used. Rostral segments of the cords were used in the present study. For morphological studies spinal cords were dissected out, fixed in Bouin's fixative and paraffin embedded as described previously [32,33].

RNA extraction

Samples of rostral cord were homogenized using Qiashredder columns (Qiagen, Valencia, CA, USA) and total RNA was extracted using the RNeasy Plus Mini Kit (Qiagen) according to standard supplier protocol. Total RNA samples were quantified using a NanoDrop ND-100 UV-VIS spectrophotometer (Thermo Scientific, Wilmington, DE, USA) and quality checked on an RNA chip using and Agilent 2100 Bioanalyzer (Agilent, Santa Clara,

Table 1. Number, tissue weight and protein concentration of spinal cord tissue used for proteomic analysis in this study.

Age group	Number of cords	Tissue weight (mg)	Total protein concentration (µg/µl)
P7+24 h transected	11	37.7	4.7
P8 control	11	27.8	5.14
P28+24 h transected	4	66.5	6.97
P29 control	4	87	8.74

Samples rostral to the site of injury (T10) were used in proteomic analysis for control and transected spinal cords of *Monodelphis domestica* at P7 or P28. Note that individual cords were pooled from more than one litter.

CA, USA). Only samples with an RNA Integrity Number close to 9 were kept for further sequencing experiments.

RNA sequencing

RNA sequencing was performed at the Australian Genome Research Facility (Melbourne, Australia). A cDNA library was prepared from 10 µg of total RNA from pools of two individuals using the RNA-Seq Sample Preparation Kit (Illumina, San Diego, CA, USA) according to the standard manufacturer protocol. Quality of the library was verified using a DNA 1000 chip using the Agilent 2100 Bioanalyzer (Agilent) and quantified by fluorimetry. The library was subjected to 100 bp single end read cycles of sequencing on an Illumina Genome Analyzer IIx (Illumina) as per manufacturer protocol. Cluster generation was performed on a c-Bot (Illumina) with a single read cluster generation kit. Sequencing was performed using a 36-cycle sequencing kit v4. In total 16 separate sequencing lanes were run on the platform. Two separate runs were conducted from separately collected samples, which were: rostral spinal cords from P8 control, P7+24 h injury, P29 controls and P28+24 h injury.

Statistical analysis of RNA-Seq data

Gene expression level analysis. Short reads were trimmed to remove ambiguous bases from the start and segments with low quality scores from the end. Trimmed reads were mapped with Bowtie2 version 2.0.4 [35] to the Ensembl *Monodelphis domestica* genome, release 69 [36]. The number of reads mapped to nuclear genes was determined with HTSeq [37], using the default "union" counting option.

An average of 4.6 M mapped reads were obtained per sample. Raw data are available at: Gene Expression Omnibus (http://www.ncbi.nlm.nih.gov/geo/) under accession code GSE54805. Differential expression between the adult and embryonic samples was detected using an exact test in the Bioconductor [38] 6dger package version 2.6.12 [39]. Genes considered to be significantly differentially expressed were those with a p-value of less than 0.05 after false discovery rate correction. Changes in expression were considered significant where there was a fold change greater than 2.00 and an adjusted p-value of less than 0.05. Gene targets with fold changes less than 2.00 were considered unchanged. Genes that showed changes according to the above criteria are shown Table S1 (P7+24 h) and Table S2 (P28+24 h).

Gene ontology level analysis. Gene Ontology (GO) analysis was completed using GOSeq software [40]. Differentially expressed genes were split into up- and down-regulated groups and a separate GOSeq enrichment test was applied for each set. A final Benjamini-Hochberg correction was applied to adjust for multiple tests.

Illumina RNA sequencing data have been deposited with the Gene Expression Omnibus http://www.ncbi.nlm.nih.gov/geo/) under accession code GSE54805.

Proteomics

Methods for the 2-dimensional separation of proteins, selection of protein bands and mass spectrometry have been published previously [32] but are described here in full.

Sample preparation for proteomic analysis. Spinal cord segments rostral to the site of injury performed at P7 or P28 were collected 24 hours after transection (P7+24 h or P28+24 h) together with corresponding segments from age-matched controls. Tissue was pooled from several pups (n = 4–20) in order to obtain a total of a minimum of 30 mg (wet tissue weight) per sample (Table 1). Pooled tissue samples were homogenized 1:10 w/v in homogenization buffer containing 0.32 mM sucrose, 25 mM Tris, 1 mM MgCl2, pH 7. This was done by passing the samples through 20 Gauge (G), 21 G, 25 G and 27 G needles until the suspension offered no more resistance. Samples were centrifuged at 2000×g for 2 minutes at 4°C and supernatants retained for further analysis. Total protein concentration was estimated using the Bradford Assay [40] with a protein standard (Sigma-Aldrich, St Louis, MO, USA) to ensure the consistency of the extraction process as all samples were normalized weight to volume. The same volume for all samples was used throughout the study (Table 1).

The clean-up step. Contaminants were removed from 50 µl aliquots of each sample using the 2-dimensional (2D) clean-up kit (GE Healthcare Bio-Sciences Corp., Piscataway, NJ, USA) as detailed in the Manufacturer's Protocol (Procedure B). Fifty µl aliquots of each sample were used for the clean-up. Samples were centrifuged for 10 minutes at 8000×g and wash buffer was removed without disturbing the pellet. Acetone present in the wash buffer was evaporated before moving to the next step. Six clean-up samples were prepared for each age group,

Off-gel Fractionator. An Off-gel Fractionator 3100 (Agilent Technologies, Santa Clara, CA, USA) was used in accordance with the Manufacturer's Protocol. Immobilized pH gradient (IPG) strips (12 cm, pH 3–10, Linear, Agilent Technologies, Santa Clara, CA, USA) were used for this separation. A total of 150 µl from cleaned-up sample (see above) was rehydrated (as specified by Manufacturer's Protocol) and prepared for each lane together with IPG strips (also rehydrated with the Off-gel buffer prior to sample loading). Each sample was run in duplicate on two separate IEF lanes. The fractionator was set to run under the default Manufacturer's settings until the current was reduced to zero. Samples from each well were collected and the Bradford assay [40] was performed on each sample. Variation in protein concentrations between the duplicates was within ±10%. For further analysis duplicates of each sample fraction were combined and all

Off-gel fractions were used. Aliquots (25 µl) from each fraction were subjected to a further clean-up step as described above. Again, duplicates were prepared for each sample. In the final step, the wash buffer was carefully decanted without disturbing the pellet before pellets were dried at 37.5°C in a heat block for 10 minutes to fully evaporate any wash buffer residue.

Lithium dodecyl sulfate –polyacrylamide gel electrophoresis (LDS-PAGE). The obtained dried pellet was re-suspended in 5 µl LDS sample buffer (Invitrogen, Carlsbad, CA, USA) [23], 2 µl reducing agent (Invitrogen, Carlsbad, CA, USA) and 13 µl deionized water. The mixture was heated in a 37.5°C heat block for 10 minutes. Pre-cast 4–12% NuPage Bis-Tris 10 well Mini Gels (Invitrogen, Carlsbad, CA, USA) were used with 2-(N-morpholino) ethanesulfonic acid (MES)-SDS running buffer (Invitrogen, Carlsbad, CA, USA) diluted 1:20. Samples from each fraction from injured and control animals were loaded as duplicates. One lane of each gel contained a molecular weight standard (NovexH Sharp pre-stained standard, Invitrogen, Carlsbad, CA, USA). Gels were run at 200 V constant voltage for approximately 35 minutes.

Silver Staining and Densitometric Gel Analysis. Separated protein bands were visualised using silver stain. Gels were stained for 10–15 min (Silver Stain Plus Kit, Bio-Rad Laboratories, Hercules, CA, USA) according to the Manufacturer's Protocol. Silver stained gels were scanned on a flatbed scanner (Agfa Duoscan, Mortsel, Belgium) and analysed using 1D gel analysis software, GeneTools V4.01.02 (Syngene, Synoptics Ltd, Cambridge, England). The number of bands visible in each lane was counted and consistency between duplicates in each lane was checked. Protein profiles from injured spinal cord samples were compared to those from controls for each fraction. Differences in band intensity, staining pattern or molecular weight changes were recorded. A relative change threshold of ±0.5 compared to control (set as 1) was accepted to identify proteins that changed their expression following spinal injury. This threshold was set after evaluation of technical variability of the methods employed [32,41]. As is usually the case for such proteomic studies it was not possible to make a sufficient number of biological replicates for a statistical analysis to be applied. The results are therefore presented as an increase or decrease compared to controls.

Mass Spectrometry

Tryptic digestion. Each protein band of interest was individually and manually excised from gels and de-stained in 50 mM ammonium bicarbonate with 50% acetonitrile. Obtained gel pieces were washed and dehydrated in 50 mM ammonium bicarbonate and acetonitrile in alternating wash steps until completely dehydrated. Once dehydrated, gel pieces were subsequently rehydrated in 0.5 µg trypsin (Promega corp., Madison, WI, USA) and 20 mM ammonium bicarbonate solution for in-gel digestion by incubating at 37°C overnight and sonicated (Health Sonics, Livermore CA, USA) for 10 minutes prior to analysis.

LC-MS/MS. Tryptic digests were analysed by LC-MS/MS using the HCT ULTRA ion trap mass spectrometer (Bruker Daltonics, Bremen, Germany) coupled online with nanoflow HPLC (Ultimate 3000, Thermo Scientific, Breman, germany). Samples injected onto a pepmap100, 75 µm id, 100 Å pore size, reversed phase nano column with 95% buffer A (0.1% Formic acid) at a flow rate of 300 nl/minute. The peptides were eluted over a 30-minute gradient to 70% B (80% Acetonitrile 0.1% formic acid). The eluant is nebulised and ionised using the Bruker ESI electrospray source via the nanoflow ESI sprayer with a capillary voltage of 4000 V, dry gas at 200°C and flow rate of 5.0l/minute and nebuliser gas at 6psi. Peptides are selected for MSMS analysis in autoMSn mode with smart parameter settings selected with a target mass of 900 m/z and active exclusion released after 1 minute. Data obtained from LC-MS/MS were searched against a custom database downloaded from the National Center for Biotechnology Information (NCBI) ftp site and Swiss-Prot databases using the MASCOT search engine (version 2.1, Matrix Science Inc., London, UK) with all taxonomy selected.

Identified proteins were categorized by relevance to spinal cord injury, obtained from search of relevant literature published in PubMed (http://www.ncbi.nlm.nih.gov/pubmed).

Morphology and Immunohistochemistry

Bouin's-fixed, paraffin embedded spinal cords from P8, P7+24 h, P29 and P28+24 h animals (n = 3–4) were obtained from previous studies [32,33] with some additional material collected specifically for this project. All sections were cut in either coronal or sagittal plane at 5 µm thickness. Ten consecutive sections were placed on each glass slide. Routine hematoxylin and eosin (H&E) staining was performed on every 10th slide for general morphology. Immunocytochemistry using the PAP (peroxidase-anti-peroxidase) detection method [32,42] was applied to map the cellular distribution of individual proteins. Briefly, sections were dewaxed in histolene (Fronine, Australia) followed by rehydration in ethanol of decreasing concentration and final wash in phosphate buffered saline with 0.2% Tween20 (PBS/Tween). After blocking non-specific binding sites with Peroxidase and Protein Blockers (DAKO) sections were incubated with primary antibodies (rabbit anti- human IL-1β, Endogen, USA). This was followed by consecutive incubations with appropriate secondary antibodies (swine anti rabbit, DAKO, 1:200 dilution and rabbit PAP, Sigma, 1:200 dilution) and developed with DAKO DAB+ detection kit. Finally the stained sections were dehydrated through graded alcohol and histolene and mounted with Ultramount (Fronine, Australia). Control sections did not contain the primary antibody and these always appeared blank.

The presence of myelin was detected in paraffin sections by the histological stain Luxol Fast Blue as described in detail previously [25].

Results and Discussion

General Morphology of the injury site of *Monodelphis* spinal cord injured at P7 or P28

The morphological appearance of the spinal cord of *Monodelphis* after injury is illustrated in H&E stained sections in Fig. 1. Note the completeness of the transections at P7 and P28 (Fig. 1A&B) and the obvious bleeding into the wound site in the P28 spinal cord (Fig. 1B). It was noticeable that at the time of injury bleeding was more prominent in the P28 spinal cords than at P7. It is likely that bleeding occurred in some of the P7 injured cords collected for RNA-Seq analysis, but the P28 cords were probably more contaminated, which may account for the presence of upregulated blood-related genes at P28 but not P7 following injury (see below). Note also that the gap between the rostral and caudal ends of the transected spinal cord at 24 h post injury was much greater in the P28 (Fig. 1D) cord compared to the P7 cord (Fig. 1C). A similar difference between P7 and P14 transected cords was reported previously [24]. This difference was attributed to greater arching of the back in the P14 *Monodelphis*. The even larger gap in transected spinal cords of older opossum may contribute to the lack of neurite growth across the site of injury in P28 pups. Nevertheless at both ages 24 h after injury the cut ends of the

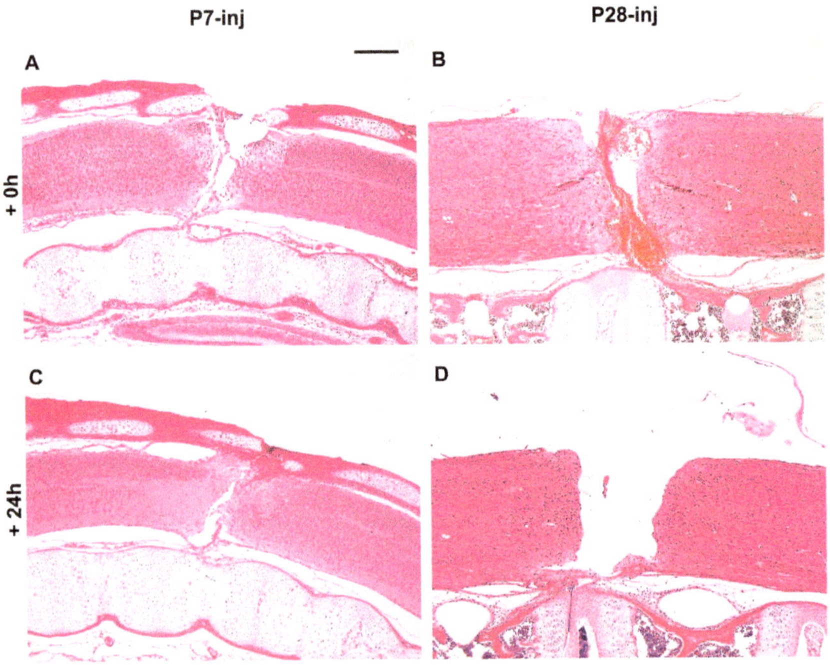

Figure 1. ***Monodelphis domestica*** **spinal cords injured at P7 or P28.** Longitudinal sections (hematoxylin & eosin staining) of spinal cords injured at P7 or P28 shown immediately after complete spinal transection at T10 (A, B) or 24 hours later (C, D). Note obvious bleeding into the injury site at P28 (B), which was more pronounced than at P7 (A) One day after transection (+24 h) the gap between severed ends of the cord was larger in P28 injured animals (D) than in P7 injured animals (C). Rostral end is to the left, caudal to the right, dorsal is uppermost. Scale bar is 500 μm.

spinal cord were clearly sealed without showing much cellular damage in the surrounding spinal cord tissue.

Transcriptomic analysis of postnatal *Monodelphis* spinal cord following transection

The gene expression responses to injury have been examined in the segment of spinal cord rostral to a complete spinal transection (T10) at two postnatal ages: P7 when substantial axon growth occurs across the lesion site and P28 when no such axon growth occurs [25]. Gene expression patterns were investigated using high throughput RNA-Seq analysis at 24 h after injury. Genes were assigned to functional categories based on published information on function, taking account of studies of gene expression changes in injured adult spinal cord (e.g., [16,17,20,43]) as well as those we deduce might have effects on neurite outgrowth at P7 and P28, 24 h after spinal cord transection (Fig. 2 and Tables S2 and S3). Only a single assignment was made for each gene (Tables 2–4, S5), although many appear to have multiple functions.

Changes in gene ontology

There was a striking difference in the number of genes that changed their expression level at the two ages; many more were changed at P28 than at P7 following injury and the magnitude of many gene expression changes at P28 was much greater (Fig. 2). In addition at P7 no genes were downregulated (>-2 fold) in response to injury in contrast to many at P28. It is also striking that at P7 almost all of the genes affected were immune/inflammatory related. Only four genes identified in the P7 injury group were categorized in the other functional groups.

Twenty-four hours following injury at P28 about half as many genes were upregulated as were downregulated and the largest category upregulated was also immune/inflammatory while the largest category of downregulated genes was enzymes & metabolism. However, nearly all categories identified in the P28 injury group contained genes that were both up- and downregulated. These gene expression changes following injury at the two ages are summarized in Fig. 2.

Gene expression in postnatal *Monodelphis* spinal cord 24 h following transection at P7

At P7+24 h only 40 genes showed a significant expression change of ≥2 fold (Fig. 3 and Table S1); all of these were upregulated, none was downregulated. The gene descriptions and details of the statistical analysis are shown in Table S1 and illustrated in Fig. 3. Thirty-six of these genes were in the immune/inflammatory group (Table S1); the highest expressed of these were interleukin 1β, which was 54 fold higher than uninjured control spinal cord and a *novel* gene (C-C motif chemokine similar to *Ccl8* and *Ccl13*) which was 33 fold higher than uninjured control spinal cord. The four non immune-related genes upregulated at this age (green in Fig. 3) were the metalloproteinase inhibitor *Timp* (3.2 fold), one novel gene related to cell proliferation and apoptosis (similar to *Samd9/Samd9l* sterile alpha motif domain 9), which was upregulated 4 fold, the syntaxin binding protein *Stxbp2* was upregulated 2.7 fold and a novel gene similar to MT3 Metallothionein 3, upregulated 2 fold. It has been shown before that in adult spinal cord injury, one of the main functional groups of genes to show regulatory changes soon after injury is the inflammatory group (e.g., [16]). The finding that almost all of the gene expression changes identified at 24 h after spinal cord injury at P7 were immune/inflammatory genes with only single members of other gene families shown to have marked expression changes, suggests that the overwhelming inflammatory response at this age may reflect a general response to injury. It does itself appear to affect the outgrowth of neurites, which has previously been shown to be profuse at this age [21,22]. The absence of an immune/

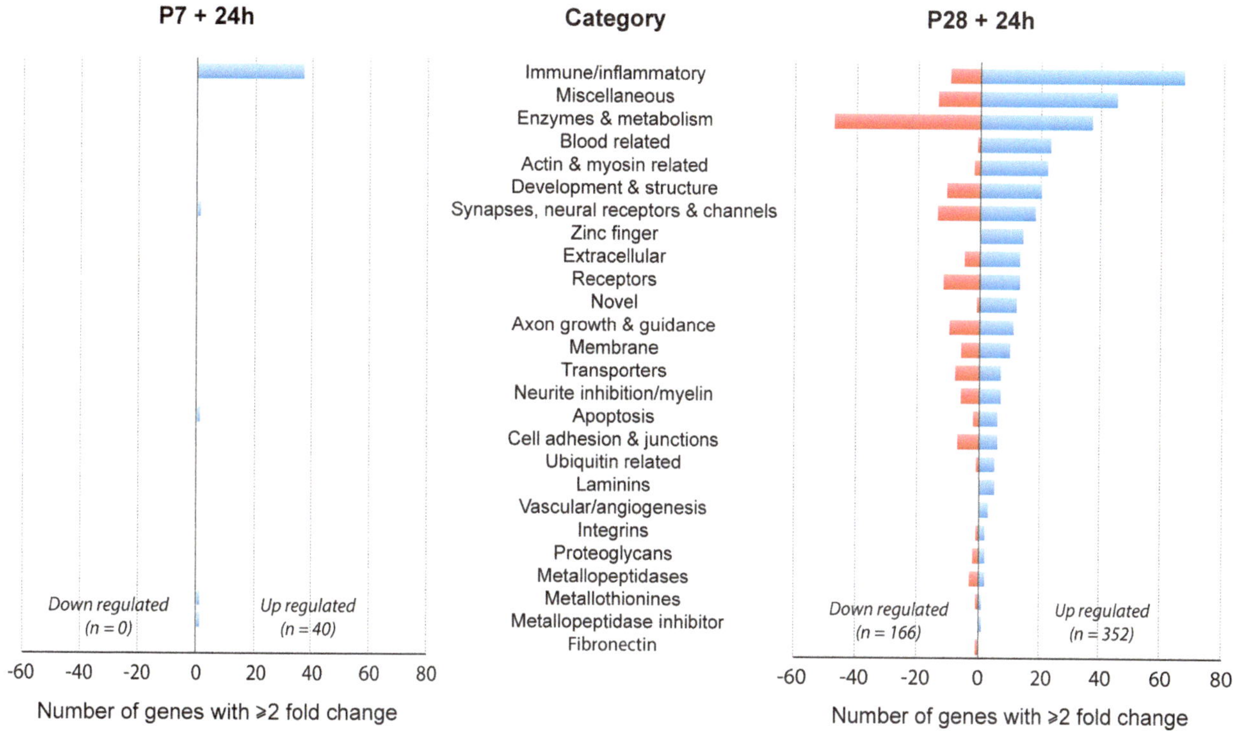

Figure 2. Changes in gene expression in spinal cord 24 h following transection at P7 or P28 in *Monodelphis domestica*. Numbers of genes in each functional category that showed ±≥2 fold change compared to uninjured aged matched controls. Note dominance of immune/inflammatory genes particularly at P7. Also note that at P28 many more genes showed expression changes (both up and down). See Tables S1 and S2 for gene descriptions, fold change and p values.

inflammatory response to injury in isolated postnatal *Monodelphis* spinal cord [28,29] supports this conclusion; this is discussed further below. Given the successful growth of axons across the lesion site at this age it would appear that the injury does little to interfere with the process, because most of the known genes associated with axon growth or inhibition were unaffected.

The immature state of the immune system at the end of the first week of postnatal life in *Monodelphis* may help to explain the complexity of immune/inflammatory genes upregulated at this time, compared with P28 (see below). That the majority of immune/inflammatory genes are upregulated is consistent with responses that are generally associated with non-specific or innate cell types, and with the early stage of development at P7/P8. At the end of the first week of postnatal life in the opossum, the αβ T cell receptor (*Tcr*) is present, although the thymus itself is still relatively immature [44]. T cells expressing the *γδTcr*, a lineage that has been implicated in playing a role in wound healing, are first detectable at P8 [44,45]. The ontogeny of antibody producing B cells is similarly at an early transitional point. Cells committed to the B cell lineage are found in prenatal embryos and within the first 24 postnatal hours B cells that have rearranged their heavy chain antibody genes are detected [46]. But the first wave of light chain gene rearrangements necessary for developing mature B cells is not detected until P7 at the earliest. T and B cells at this stage are fairly limited in their diversity, most likely consistent with low numbers of cells. Given the immature state of the adaptive side of the immune system it may not be surprising that components of the innate immune system such as complement components *C1q* and *Factor B* are upregulated.

Upregulated transcripts such as those encoding Sialic acid-binding immunoglobulin-type lectins (*Siglecs*) and *Vsig4* have been implicated in inhibitory regulation of inflammation and adaptive immune responses through regulation of B and T cells. *Siglecs* are involved in the cell adhesion and phagocytosis, among other things, and are expressed on a variety of immune system cells including macrophages. They have been implicated in binding pathogen associated molecular patterns (*Pamps*), transmitting inhibitory signals and participating in B cell tolerance (reviewed in [47]). Likewise, *Vsig4* is a receptor for the complement component 3 fragments, *C3b* and *iC3b* and has been implicated in being a negative regulator of T cells [48]. We were only able to obtain antibody cross-reactivity for one of the protein products of the large number of genes that showed upregulation (Il-1β). Its distribution in P7 and P28 spinal cord 24 h after injury is illustrated in Fig. 4 (for description see below).

Only two genes at P7 that might be expected to be related to a neural response to injury were upregulated >2 fold (Table S1). These were metallopepetidase inhibitor 1 (*Timp1*, 3.2 fold) and syntaxin binding protein 2 (*Sxbp2*, 2.7 fold). As these were also similarly upregulated following injury at P28 (Fig. 5) it seems unlikely that they account for successful neurite outgrowth at P7, which was lacking at P28.

Gene expression in postnatal *Monodelphis* spinal cord 24 h following transection at P28, including comparison with injury at P7

Examination of the whole gene list shows that at P28+24 h there were 332 genes that increased their expression by 2 fold or more (Table S2); 149 genes reduced their expression by 2 fold or more. This contrasts with the response at P7 when no genes were found to be downregulated (Fig. 2 and Fig. 3, Table S1). For comparison of the response at 24 h after injury, all 40 genes that

Table 2. Change in expression of neurite inhibitory and axon growth/guidance genes 24 h following spinal cord injury at P28.

SYMBOL	GENE DESCRIPTION	FOLD
NEURITE INHIBITION/MYELIN		
Efna4	ephrin-A4	5.0
Arhgap6	Rho GTPase activating protein 6	3.1
Gmip	GEM interacting protein encodes a member of the ARHGAP family of Rho/Rac/Cdc42-like GTPase activating proteins.	3.0
Novel	similar to SMPD3 sphingomyelin phosphodiesterase	2.4
Novel	similar to OPHN1 oligophrenin 1,encodes Rho-GTPase-activating protein	2.3
Mpz	myelin protein zero	1.8
Rtn4	Nogo, myelin inhibitory factor	1.2
Mog	myelin oligodendrocyte glycoprotein	−1.7
Mag	myelin associated glycoprotein	−1.8
Arhgef10	Rho guanine nucleotide exchange factor (GEF) 10	−2.0
Arhgap35	Rho GTPase activating protein 35	−2.1
Mbp	myelin basic protein	−2.2
Plp1	proteolipid protein 1	−2.4
AXON GROWTH & GUIDANCE		
Hhipl2	HHIP-like 2, hedgehog interacting protein-like 2	6.5
Sgsm3	small G protein signaling modulator 3	4.5
Slit3	slit homolog 3 (Drosophila) interacts with Robo; axon repellent	4.0
Novel	similar to DNAH7 dynein, axonemal, heavy chain	3.1
Robo3	roundabout, axon guidance receptor, homolog 3 (Drosophila)	3.0
Mical1	microtubule assoc monoxygenase, calponin & LIM domain containing 1	2.3
Serpinf1	serpin peptidase inhib, clade F α-2 antiplasmin, pigment epithelium factor)	2.3
Tgfb3	transforming growth factor, β 3, regulator of ECMs and integrins	2.2
Ntn5	netrin 5	2.1
Tcerg1l	transcription elongation regulator 1-like	2.0
Elmo3	engulfment and cell motility 3	2.0
Cntn2	contactin 2 (axonal) [Source:HGNC Symbol;Acc:2172]	−2.0
Sema4f	sema domain, immunoglobulin domain (Ig), transmembrane domain (TM)	−2.0
Astn1	astrotactin 1, neuronal adhesion molecule required for glial-guided migration of young postmitotic neuroblasts, previously described in developing brain	−2.1
Olig2	oligodendrocyte lineage transcrip factor 2, enhances myelination after SCI	−2.1
Pak7	p21 protein (Cdc42/Rac)-activated kinase 7	−2.3
Plekhb1	pleckstrin homology domain containing, family B (evectins) member 1	−2.4
Sema5a	sema domain, seven thrombospondin repeats (type 1 and type 1-like), transmembrane domain TMand short cytoplasmic domain, (semaphorin) 5A	−2.4
Sema3e	sema domain, immunoglobulin domain (Ig), short basic domain, secreted	−2.5
Pak2	p21 protein (Cdc42/Rac)-activated kinase 2	−2.9
Gas7	growth arrest-specific 7, neurite outgrowth in some cultured neurons	−7.7

Change in expression of neurite inhibitory and axon growth/guidance genes in rostral spinal cord 24 h following spinal cord injury at P28. Note that most of the myelin inhibitory factor genes have not changed their expression in response to injury (fold <2).

showed a change in expression at P7+24 h (Table S1) are compared with the top 40 genes that increased in expression at P28+24 h (from Table S2 as shown in Fig. 5). It is noteworthy that several genes upregulated following injury at both ages showed a much greater change at P28+24 h than even the top gene at P7+24 h (Fig. 5 and Cf Tables S1 and S2). Genes that changed expression 24 h following spinal transection at P28 are listed by functional category in Table S3 and are next considered.

Immune-inflammatory genes. Seventy-four genes were classified as immune-inflammatory at P28 (Fig. 2 and Table S3); of these 66 were upregulated and the remaining 8 were downregulated. Twenty-three of the immune/inflammatory genes upregulated following injury at P28 were also upregulated following injury at P7 (Fig. 5) however, only 2 were upregulated substantially more than following injury at P7 (a novel C-C motif chemokine similar to *Ccl8* and *Ccl13*, 322 compared to 33.4 fold and C type lectin/mannose receptor similar to *Mrc1*, 9.3 compared to 3.6 fold); the others were either upregulated to a similar extent or only marginally more than at P7 (Fig. 5).

The difference in the response between P7 and P28 is in the complexity. The much greater P28 response in immune/inflammatory genes may be a reflection of the state of

Table 3. Change in expression of extracellular matrix factor genes in 24 h following spinal cord injury at P28.

SYMBOL	GENE DESCRIPTION	FOLD
EXTRACELLULAR MATRIX		
Olfm4	olfactomedin 4, also OlfD, hOlfD, ECM glycoprotein that facilitates cell adhesion.	480
Mgp	matrix Gla protein	5.1
Col21a1	collagen, type XXI, alpha 1	4.8
Novel	similar to AMY cluster collagen COL25A1	4.3
Col24a1	collagen, type XXIV, alpha 1	3.5
Lox	lysyl oxidase	3.4
Ecm1	extracellular matrix protein 1	3.2
Pxdn	peroxidasin homolog (Drosophila)	2.9
Col7a1	collagen, type VII, alpha 1	2.9
Sod3	superoxide dismutase 3, extracellular	2.6
Srrm4	serine/arginine repetitive matrix 4	2.4
Fbn3	fibrillin 3	2.3
Col27a1	collagen, type XXVII, alpha 1	2.0
Col15a1	collagen, type XV, alpha 1	−2.0
Dag1	dystroglycan 1 (dystrophin-associated glycoprotein 1)	−2.0
Emilin2	elastin microfibril interfacer 2	−2.1
Nfasc	neurofascin, L1 family immunoglobulin cell adhesion molecule with multiple IGcam and fibronectin domains: neurite outgrowth, neurite fasciculation	−2.2
Nid2	nidogen 2 (osteonidogen) binds collagens I and IV and laminin	−2.2
FIBRONECTIN		
Elfn2	extracellular leucine-rich repeat and fibronectin type III domain containing 2	−2.9
METALLOPEPTIDASES		
Adam11	ADAM metallopeptidase domain 11	3.0
Adamts10	ADAM metallopeptidase with thrombospondin type 1 motif, 10	2.5
Ermp1	endoplasmic reticulum metallopeptidase 1	−2.0
Adam17	ADAM metallopeptidase domain 17	−2.1
Cndp1	carnosine dipeptidase 1 (metallopeptidase M20 family)	−2.2
METALLOPEPTIDASE INHIBITOR		
Timp1	TIMP metallopeptidase inhibitor 1	4.4
METALLOTHIONINES		
Mmp1	matrix metallopeptidase 1 (interstitial collagenase)	104
Mmp15	matrix metallopeptidase 15 (membrane-inserted)	−2.4
PROTEOGLYCANS		
Papln	papilin, proteoglycan-like sulfated glycoprotein	152
Bcan	brevican	2.1
Novel	similar to HS2ST1 heparan sulfate 2-O-sulfotransferase 1	−2.6
Extl1	exostoses (multiple)-like 1	−3.0
LAMININS		
Lamc3	lamin gamma 3	4.8
Lamb2	lamini beta 2	2.6
Lamc2	laminin gamma 2	2.4
Lamc1	laminin gamma 1	2.2
Lama4	laminin alpha 4	2.0
INTEGRINS		
Itgb1bp2	integrin beta 1 binding protein (melusin) 2	6.2
Itga2b	integrin, alpha 2b (platelet glycoprotein IIb of IIb/IIIa complex, antigen CD41)	6.1
Itga4	integrin, alpha 4 (antigen CD49D, alpha 4 subunit of VLA-4 receptor)	−57

Change in expression of extracellular matrix (ECM) factor genes 24 h following spinal cord injury at P28, subdivided into ECM, metallopeptidases, inhibitors, proteoglycans, laminins and integrins.

development of the immune system. By P28 the opossum immune system is fully mature in cellular composition [46,49]. There were 44 additional immune/inflammatory genes upregulated after injury at P28 and 9 that were downregulated (Table S3); none of these showed detectable expression changes at P7. The distribution of Il-1β immunostaining in P28 spinal cord 24 h after injury is illustrated in Fig. 4. In P7 injured cords no immunoreactivity for the cytokine could be detected in the cord but was clearly visible in the connective tissue and forming bone surrounding the spinal cord, confirming cross-species cross-reactivity (Fig. 4A). In contrast in P28 injured cords Il-1β immunoreactivity was detected in several cells of monocytic appearance mostly in close proximity to the central canal (Fig. 4B&C). These cells were present in spinal segments both rostral (Fig. 4B&C) and caudal to the site of the injury. They were not visible in control cords nor were they present in P7 injured tissue.

Blood-related. At P28, 24 h after injury 25 genes in this functional group were upregulated between 2 fold (von Willebrand factor precursor) and 99 fold (novel, haptoglobin-related protein; see Table S5). Only 2 genes in this category were upregulated following injury at P7: a *novel* gene (Similar to Gp6 glycoprotein VI (platelet)) was upregulated 7.8 fold compared to 2.3 fold at P28 and *Trem3* (triggering receptor expressed on myeloid cells 2) which was upregulated 12.4 fold at P7 but was unchanged at P28. One gene in this group was downregulated at P28: *Thbs2* (-4 fold). The observation that bleeding following operation on the cords at P28 was greater than at P7 (Fig. 1) perhaps accounts for the presence of some of the much greater number of genes with changed regulation at P28 (see Fig. 2).

Neurite inhibitory, growth/guidance and extracellular matrix genes. Studies of spinal cord injury in adult animals have shown upregulation of genes with protein products that inhibit neurite outgrowth following axonal injury by a variety of mechanisms. Many of these have been targets for therapies aimed at improving function following spinal cord injury. The main groups are:

(i) Those associated with myelin and the ephrin genes (e.g., [20,50–52]).
(ii) Extracellular matrix genes, including metallopeptidases and proteoglycans [20].
(iii) RhoA activation by myelin associated inhibitors and chondroitin sulphate proteoglycans [43].
(iv) Genes involved in axon growth and guidance [53].

Only *Timp1* (tissue inhibitor of metalloproteinase) in this category was found to change expression following injury at P7 (3.2 fold, Table S1). Genes that increased or decreased their expression in this category at P28 are listed in Table 2.

Many inhibitory factors converge on Rho, an intracellular GTPase. These include myelin-derived inhibitory factors, semaphorins, chondroitin sulphate proteoglycans (CPSGs), ephrins, netrins and repulsive guidance molecules (RGMs; see [43]). Neither *Rho* nor its downstream effector Rho kinase (*Rock*) changed expression by 24 h after spinal cord injury at P28. Four Rho family members were identified that change expression level after injury at P28. Amongst other Rho family members, two were upregulated 3 fold (*Arhgap6, Gmip*) and 2 were downregulated 2 fold (*Arhgef10, Arhgap35*) see Table 2. Thus even if any of the numerous upstream neurite inhibitory factors changed expression after injury, it seems unlikely they would be effective in influencing neurite outgrowth. In fact, very few were found to change expression. Following injury at P28, none of the seven myelin-associated genes identified was upregulated. Five did not change expression (*Rtn4* also known as *Nogo, Mpz, Mag, Mog, Ngr*) and only two were marginally downregulated (*Mbp, Plp1*). These findings are consistent with the morphological observation that myelination is not complete at this stage of spinal cord development (Fig. 6).

Luxol Fast Blue stain for myelin demonstrated that the process of myelination in the thoracic region of *Monodelphis* spinal cord does not begin until about 3 weeks of age. There was no myelin staining at P8 (Fig. 6A). By P28 the distinctive myelin staining was apparent; however, the thickness of the myelinated white matter was still smaller than in the adult (compare Fig. 6B with Fig. 6A in [25]). From preliminary studies we have established that myelination is relatively rapid after P28 and by P35 the staining pattern of the thoracic cord is very similar to that in the adult (unpublished observations).

Of seven ephrin and nine ephrin receptor genes identified, only Ephrin-A4 (*Eph4a*) was upregulated (5 fold). *Eph4A* -/- mutant mice have been suggested to show greater axon growth after spinal cord injury [54] but others have not confirmed this [55]. Even if *Eph4A* is involved in inhibition of axon growth the lack of change in *Rho/Rock* expression suggests it would not have contributed in the present experiments. Equally, myelin inhibition is unlikely to have contributed to the failure of axons to grow across a lesion made at P28.

Twenty-one genes associated with axon growth and guidance during spinal cord development were identified as having changed expression levels following injury at P28 (Table 2). Eight were downregulated 2 to 3 fold and could therefore have possibly contributed to the lack of axon growth. The others were upregulated (Table 2) including *Hhipl2* (hedgehog interacting protein-like- 2, 6.5 fold) and *Sgsm3* (small G protein signalling modulator 3) and are thus unlikely to have contributed to lack of axon growth at P28. Amongst six netrin genes identified, only *Ntn5* was marginally upregulated (2.1 fold) and amongst seven CSPGs only one was marginally upregulated (Brevican, *Bcan*, 2 fold). Neither of the repulsive guidance molecules, *Rgma, Rgmb*, changed expression following injury.

Thirty-nine genes with extracellular matrix products, including fibronectin, metallopeptidases, metallothionines, laminins, integrins and proteoglycans showed changed expression following injury at P28 (Table 3). Of these, twenty-six were upregulated 2 to 480 fold and thirteen were downregulated (2 to 3 fold) except for *Itga4* which showed expression levels 57 fold less than controls). The most strikingly upregulated were olfactomedin 4 (*Olfm4*, 480 fold), papilin, proteoglycan-like sulfated glycoprotein (*Papln* 152 fold, see below) and matrix metallopepetidase 1 (*Mmp1*, 104 fold). *Olfm4* is a member of the 4-member olfactomedin family. Originally identified as the human granulocyte colony-stimulating factor stimulated clone-1 (hGC-1; [56]), *Olfm4* has been suggested to be specifically expressed in gut and pancreas [57] in contrast to *Olfm1*, which was reported to be specifically expressed in brain [58]. It is an extracellular matrix glycoprotein that facilitates cell adhesion by binding to cadherin and lectins [57], although it is not clear if this is its function in the spinal cord. *Olfm4* has been implicated in suppressing inflammation. Mice deficient in *Olfm4* have a stronger anti-bacterial response including enhanced inflammation to *Helicobacter pylori* [59]. However, it may be that its function in the extracellular matrix of the spinal cord may be more relevant to the present study.

Using western blotting and immunocytochemistry MMP1 has been found to be increased 24 h following spinal cord injury in rats, [60] and in human postmortem studies using immunocytochemistry [61]. Its gene expression does not appear to have been studied. The protein has been localized in macrophages and

Table 4. Change in expression of channel, synapse, neural receptor, actin, myosin and related genes 24 h following spinal cord injury at P28.

SYMBOL	GENE DESCRIPTION	FOLD
SYNAPSES, NEURAL RECEPTORS & CHANNELS		
Gpr26	G protein-coupled receptor 26	6.6
Trpc7	transient receptor potential cation channel, subfamily C, member 7	4.6
Hcrt	hypocretin (orexin) neuropeptide precursor	3.8
Novel	Similar to UNC80 unc-80 homolog (C. elegans)	3.7
Sytl1	synaptotagmin-like 1	3.0
Fchsd1	FCH and double SH3 domains 1	3.0
Adora2a	adenosine A2a receptor	3.0
Fam40b	family with sequence similarity 40, member B, correct symbol STRIP2	3.0
Clcn2	chloride channel, voltage-sensitive 2	2.6
Bzrap1	benzodiazapine receptor (peripheral) associated protein 1	2.6
Mast1	microtubule associated serine/threonine kinase 1	2.4
Trpt1	tRNA phosphotransferase 1	2.4
Stxbp2	syntaxin binding protein 2	2.3
Mcoln1	mucolipin 1	2.3
C10orf10	chromosome 10 open reading frame 10	2.3
Ano8	anoctamin 8	2.1
Cacnb3	calcium channel, voltage-dependent, beta 3 subunit	2.1
Adrbk2	adrenergic, beta, receptor kinase 2	2.0
Camkk1	calcium/calmodulin-dependent protein kinase 1α, modulation of neuron survival	2.0
Syt2	synaptotagmin II	−1.8
Trpc4ap	transient receptor potential cation channel, subfamily C, member 4 assoc prot	−2.1
Gprc5b	G protein-coupled receptor, family C, group 5, member B	−2.1
Ncs1	neuronal calcium sensor 1	−2.1
Kif1b	kinesin family member 1B	−2.2
Gab1	GRB2-associated binding protein 1	−2.2
Kcnj10	potassium inwardly-rectifying channel, subfamily J, member 10	−2.3
Shroom2	shroom family member 2	−2.5
Syn3	synapsin III	−2.5
Gpr17	G protein-coupled receptor 17	−2.6
Gabrb1	gamma-aminobutyric acid (GABA) A receptor, beta 1	−2.9
Gpr75	probable G-protein coupled receptor 75	−2.9
Kcnj12	potassium inwardly-rectifying channel, subfamily J, member 12	−5.8
Novel	similar to CLCNKA/CLCNKB chloride channel	−27
ACTIN, MYOSIN & RELATED		
Trdn	triadin	206
Myl1	myosin, light chain 1, alkali; skeletal, fast	139
Mylpf	myosin light chain, phosphorylatable, fast skeletal muscle	22
MYH4	myosin, heavy chain 4, skeletal muscle	18
Acta1	actin, alpha 1, skeletal muscle	8.6
Mybpc3	myosin binding protein C, cardiac	4.8
Parvg	parvin, gamma	4.7
Novel	LOC100015891 Similar to Myosin heavy chain	4.6
Pgam2	phosphoglycerate mutase 2 (muscle)	4.3
Myof	myoferlin	4.2
Nexn	nexilin (F actin binding protein)	4.0
Myo19	myosin XIX	3.7
Tpm2	tropomyosin 2 (beta) member of the actin filament binding protein family	3.1
Miox	myo-inositol oxygenase	2.9

Table 4. Cont.

SYMBOL	GENE DESCRIPTION	FOLD
Speg	SPEG complex locus	2.8
Novel	similar to actinin alpha, F-actin cross-linking protein	2.8
Tagln	transgelin 22 kDa actin-binding protein	2.7
Ryr3	ryanodine receptor 3 brain ryanodine receptor-calcium release channel	2.7
Ttll9	tubulin tyrosine ligase-like family, member 9	2.6
Neb	nebulin	2.6
Myo1f	myosin IF	2.6
Novel	LOC100014836 similar to ACTA1 actin, alpha 1, skeletal muscle	2.2
Popdc3	popeye domain containing 3	−2.2
Kif13b	kinesin family member 13B	−2.3

Change in expression of channel, synapse, neural receptor, actin, myosin and related genes 24 h following spinal cord injury at P28. Note that myosin and actin genes are important structural and functional components of synapses.

astrocytes in the human study [61] but also in neurons in the rat study [60]. MMPs are a family of peptidases that degrade extracellular matrix proteins. Early increased expression of for example *Mmp-9* is thought to have deleterious effects whereas the later upregulation of MMP-2 may be beneficial as part of the repair process [62]. The role of MMP-1 following spinal cord injury is unknown but given its early and substantial upregulation in P28 *Monodelphis* spinal cord following injury described here, it may be contributing to the lack of neurite outgrowth at this age.

Proteoglycans, particularly chondroitin sulphate proteoglycans (CSPGs) are known to be upregulated following injury to adult spinal cord and are thought to be a major component of neurite inhibition following injury [20]. These proteoglycans were not found to be upregulated in the current study (see above). However, a novel gene similar to papilin, *Papln* proteoglycan-like sulfated glycoprotein was upregulated 152 fold; this gene has not previously been identified in spinal cord but perhaps it also has neurite inhibitory properties as in the case of CSPGs. Several collagens have been identified in the post injury scar that restricts neurite outgrowth following spinal cord injury in the adult [20]. In the present study three collagen genes were upregulated (Table 3) and may have contributed to the lack of neurite outgrowth at P28, as collagen is an important component of the glial scar [20]; one was marginally downregulated (-2 fold). It seems unlikely that the rather modest changes in expression of metalloproteinase genes, some of which increased and others decreased (Table 3), would

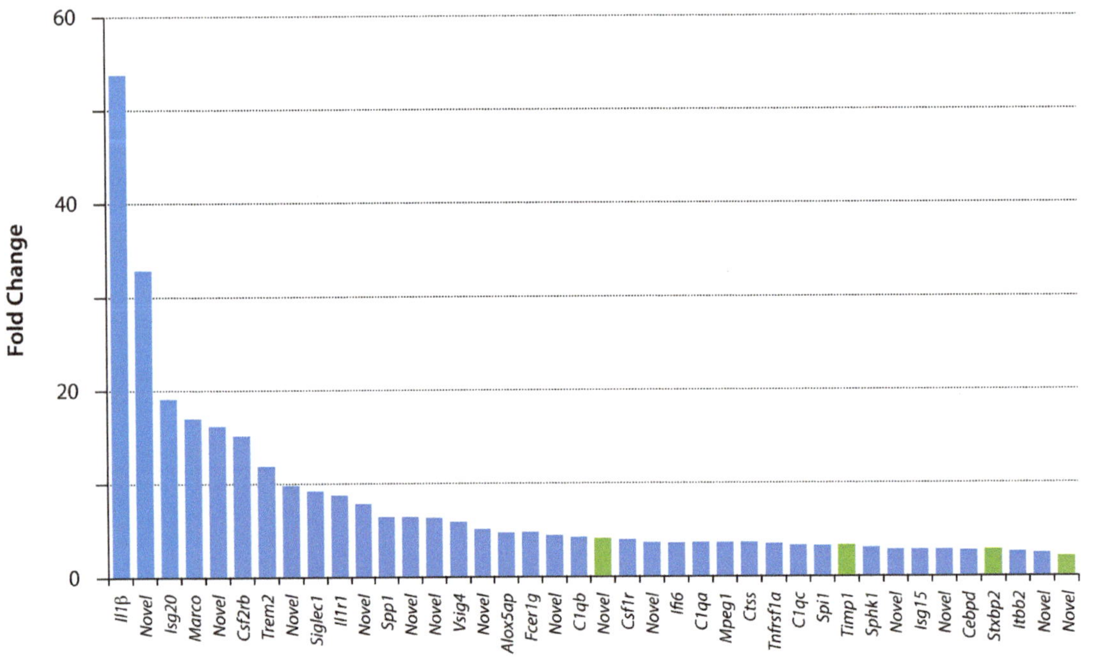

Figure 3. Changes in gene expression 24 h following spinal transection at P7. Only 40 genes changed their expression levels by ≥2 fold. All were upregulated. See Table S1 for gene descriptions and statistics. There were 12 "novel" genes; search of GO categories showed that these have immune/inflammatory properties. Note that only four of the genes in this figure (green bars) are not in the immune/inflammatory category (blue bars).

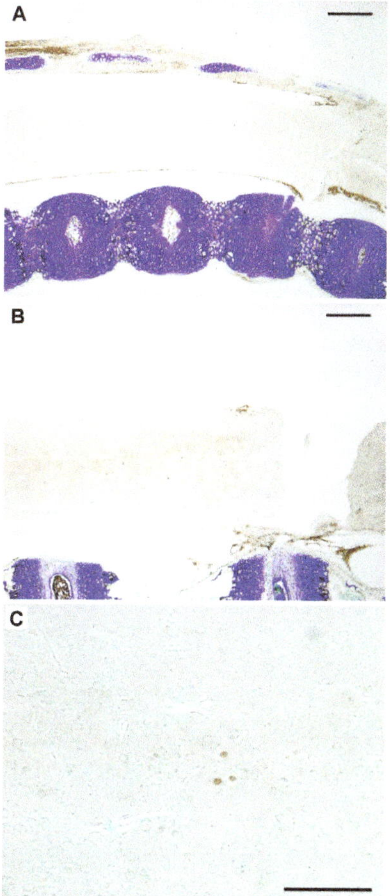

Figure 4. Interleukin-1β in *Monodelphis* spinal cord 24 hours after a complete transection at P7 or P28. In the segment of the cord rostral to the site of injury Il-1β was detected using cross-reacting antibodies to the human cytokine. Note strong immunopositive signal in the tissue surrounding the cords at P7-injured (A) and P28 (B) but lack of significant staining within the spinal tissue especially at P7 (A). One day following injury at P28 a few immunopositive cells with the general morphology of monocytes were detected, especially in segments of the cord more rostral to the injury (C). Scale bars A, B = 500 μm, C = 100 μm.

have contributed to the lack of neurite outgrowth at P28. Of 13 laminins, 5 were upregulated 2.0–4.8 fold (Table 3).

Integrins are an important receptor family promoting axon growth during development and regeneration following injury to peripheral nerves. They interact with the extracellular matrix factors described above (e.g. collagen, laminin, tenascin, vitronectin). Integrins are cell surface proteins. They bind to molecules in the extracellular matrix and transduce extrinsic cues that regulate the cytoskeleton leading to modulation of axon growth (for references see [63]). In contrast to their activity in developing nervous system and peripheral nerve regeneration, there appears to be little change in integrin expression following injury to the adult central nervous system [63]. Integrins are also present on the surface of leukocytes; for example, antibodies to integrin α4vβ1 reduced neutrophil and monocyte/macrophage influx into adult spinal cord following injury [64]. In the present study there was a substantial reduction (57 fold) in expression of *Itga4* (integrin α4) following injury at P28. Lane et al. [24] reported a small infiltration of granulocytes at 24 h following spinal cord transection in *Monodelphis* at P7. At P14 the infiltration was 2–3 times larger but was delayed compared to P7 injuries. This may explain why we do not see many granulocytes 24 hours after injury in the P28 spinal cords. However, we observe some monocytic cells as illustrated in Fig. 4. Only two other integrins (*Itgibp2, Itga2b*) showed a change in expression, increasing about 6 fold in both cases. However, these integrins have not previously been identified in spinal cord so their possible role in lack of neurite outgrowth is unclear.

Rho signaling proteins regulate the dynamics of cytoskeleton and cell motility [65]. Rho appears to be the common target of the main mechanisms that limit neurite outgrowth following spinal cord injury: myelin inhibitors, CSPGs, and guidance inhibitors [43]. Given the rather small and opposing changes in expression of Rho family genes and of many of the genes that target Rho following injury in adult spinal cords (see above) it seems unlikely that Rhos and inhibitory factors that target them contribute to the lack of axon growth following injury at P28. However, many of the axons passing through the site of injury have their cell bodies of origin in the brainstem, where changes in Rho genes might be expected to be manifest. Changes in brainstem gene expression will be the subject of a separate report (Saunders *et al.*, in preparation) but preliminary examination of the RNA-Seq data suggests that here too changes in expression of Rho-related genes following spinal cord injury are also marginal.

Cell adhesion and intercellular junctions. There were twelve genes in this functional category (S3). Only four were upregulated (2.2. to 3 fold). The other seven decreased their expression (-2 to -3 fold). Most of these genes have not previously been identified in spinal cord. *Pdch1* appears to play a role in spinal cord development in the mouse [66] and *Pdch18* in chick and zebrafish developing spinal cord [67,68]. *Gjc2* encodes the gap junction protein connexin-47; a mutation of this gene has been associated with hypomyelination [69]. Of all the genes identified in this group only *Icam-1* has been found to change expression in injured adult spinal cord. Thus its expression has been found to increase following spinal cord injury in rats; endothelial cell upregulation of *Icam1* was suggested to increase adhesion and extravasation of leukocytes 1–2 days following injury [70]. The possible importance of ICAM-1 in the response to injury is indicated by the report that intravenous injection of ICAM-1 monoclonal antibody 30 min after spinal cord injury in rats reduced motor disturbance and enhanced recovery [71].

Channels, synapses and neural receptors. In previous studies of adult spinal cord it has been reported that some ion channel genes, including those for sodium, potassium and calcium are downregulated shortly after injury [16]. In the present study four channel genes were downregulated (Table 4), including one potassium channel (*Kcnj12*, -5.8 fold) and one chloride channel (a novel gene, similar to *Clcnka/Clcnkb* chloride channel) that was markedly downregulated (27 fold). In addition three channel genes were upregulated (*Trpc7, Clcn2, Cacnb3*, Table 4).

In reviewing a large number of microarray studies of adult rodent spinal cord Verhaagen *et al.* [16] also reported genes encoding enzymes involved in neurotransmitter synthesis and genes encoding proteins involved in synaptic vesicle transport and docking as well as expression of glutamate receptors, which were generally downregulated following spinal cord injury. In our dataset in this category, there were five genes that were upregulated (2 to 3 fold) and six that were downregulated (2.1 to 2.9 fold) see Table 4. Myosin and actin are important for normal structure and function of neural synapses [72–74]. Genes related to these protein products have been listed separately in Table 4. Twenty-three were identified with significant changes in expression; all but one (*Popdc*, -2.2 fold) was upregulated. Of those

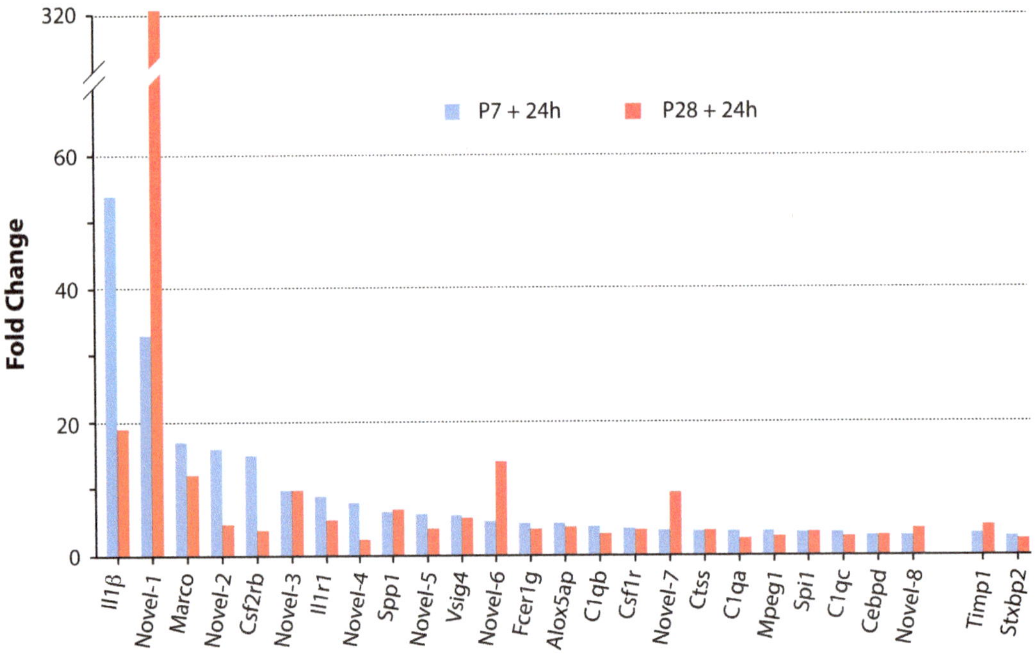

Figure 5. Comparison of expression levels of the twenty-six genes that changed expression in spinal cord 24 h following transection at both P7 and P28. All but two of these genes (Timp1 and Stxbp2) were in the immune/inflammatory category. The magnitude of the expression changes was generally similar at the two ages, but more genes (six: IL1β, MARCO, novel-2, CSF2RB, IL1-R1, novel-4) showed greater upregulation at P7 than at P28 (three: novel-1, novel-6, novel-7). A search of Ensembl, NCBI "Gene" and GO categories showed that all of these novel genes are involved in immune/inflammatory functions (see Tables S1 and S2).

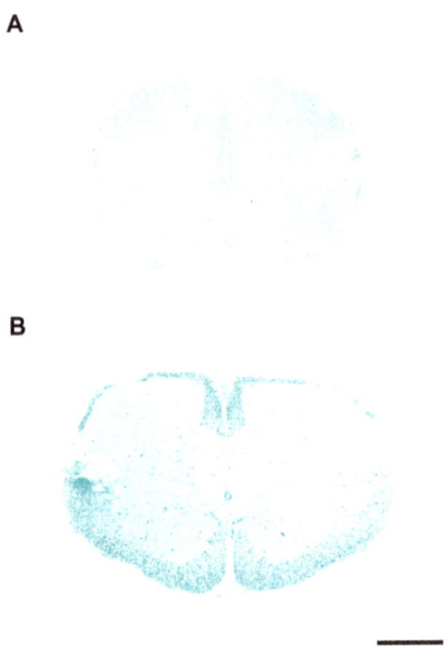

Figure 6. Myelin staining in the developing spinal cord of *Monodelphis domestica*. Transverse sections through thoracic spinal cord of P8 (A) and P29 (B) spinal cord stained with Luxol fast blue (LFB). There was no LFB stained myelin at P8 (A) but relatively well- developed myelin was present at P28 (B). However even at P28 the myelination is only beginning to appear (first detected between P21 and P28) and does not reach adult levels until several weeks later (not illustrated). Dorsal is uppermost. Scale bar is 500 μm.

upregulated, some increased their expression very substantially: *Triadin* (206 fold), *Myl1* (139 fold), *Mylpf* (22 fold) and a *novel* gene *LOC100027326*, myosin-4-like (18 fold). Triadin was first discovered as an important intrinsic membrane glycoprotein in the sarcoplasmic reticulum of skeletal muscle [75]. Although initially thought to be exclusive to skeletal muscle, according to Dulhunty *et al.*, [76] it has been found in a range of tissues. However, it does not seem to have been identified previously in spinal cord, but there is one report of Triadin 2 (the cardiac isoform) in mouse brain [77] together with the intracellular calcium channel proteins ryanodine receptors (RyR) 1 and 3. *Ryr3* was upregulated in the present study (Table 4). Ryanodine receptors and Triadin are essential components of sarcoplasmic Ca^{2+} transduction in skeletal muscle [76]. Their presence in spinal cord suggests that they may have a role in Ca^{2+} storage and release there too. *Myl1* and the *novel* gene (*myosin-4-like*) have not been identified in spinal cord previously. *Mylpf* a gene involved in muscle contraction has been found to be downregulated in the spinal cord in response to acrylamide [78]. These genes and those listed in Table 4 show changes in expression following injury that is presumably related to changes in synaptic function at later stages after the injury. They may reflect some of the changes in gene expression and neural circuits in opossum spinal cord caudal to the injury site following injury at P28 [26]. These may be important for the weight bearing locomotion displayed by these animals when adult, in spite of the lack of axonal growth across the lesion (25). However, it seems unlikely that these changes in synapse-related genes are contributing to this lack of axon growth following injury at P28.

Apoptosis and ubiquitin. Only one apoptosis-related gene was upregulated at P7 following injury: a *novel* gene, related to *Samd9*. In contrast, five genes with products that are involved in apoptosis were upregulated 3 to 6 fold in the P28 injured cords:

Dnajb13 (*Hsp40* homologue), three *novel* genes and *Plac8* (Table S3). *Faim2*, a gene for Fas apoptotic inhibitory molecule was downregulated (−2.3 fold) as was the apoptosis-associated tyrosine kinase *Aatk* (Table S3). This suggests a degree of apoptotic activity that was not present following injury at P7. Lane *et al.* [24] reported a large increase in pyknotic cells 3 h after spinal cord transection in P7 and P14 *Monodelphis*. This returned to control levels by 24 h, which may account for the limited expression changes in apoptotic-related genes at P7 and P28 in the present study conducted 24 hours after injury (Tables S1, S2 and S3).

Four ubiquitin-related genes increased expression (4.0 to 7.6 fold, Table S3). Only one was downregulated (a novel gene similar to *Ubr3*, -2 fold). These genes, *Wsb1*, *Cul7*, *Cul9* and *Ubr3* are all genes for different E3 ubiquitin ligases that ubiquitinate various target proteins, signaling them for protein degradation. WSB1 is a hedgehog inducible ubiquitin ligase socs-box-containing WD-40 protein. Currently, there is no evidence for this process following spinal cord injury; however, it is an E3 ubiquitin ligase for thyroid hormone-activating type 2 iodothyronine deiodinase [79], which is a HIPK2-interacting protein [80]. The cullin family of genes codes for *cullin E3 ligase* scaffold protein, which interacts with *Rbx1*. In this study, we identified two cullin family members with >2 fold change, *Cul7* and *Cul9*. CUL7 has only been shown to bind with FBXW8 [81]. However, there is some evidence that this protein heterodimerizes with CUL1, facilitating polyubiquitination of target proteins [81]. The specific function of CUL7 in the spinal cord is otherwise unknown; however, CUL1 [82] and CUL3 [83] have been shown to be important during embryonic development through interaction with cyclin E. *Cul7* knockout-mice also show neonatal lethality [84]. CUL9, previously known as PARC on the other hand has been shown to bind and promote p53-dependent apoptosis [85]. The last of the E3 protein ligase genes identified is *Ubr3*, ubiquitin protein ligase E3 component n-recognin 3. This gene codes for a ligase that specifically targets the N-terminal residues for degradation [86]. Although its role has not been previously described in spinal cord injury, this ligase has been shown to play a role in olfactory and tactile sensory systems [86].

Vascular/angiogenesis and transporters. Three genes with vascular/angiogenic properties were upregulated 2.5 to 3.8 fold (Table S3). Of fifteen transporter genes seven were upregulated (3 to 12 fold) and eight were downregulated (−2 to −5 fold). Only two have previously been identified in spinal cord (*Sclc18a3*, vesicular acetylcholine transporter and *Atp2a1*, both downregulated). There was only one efflux transporter gene (*Abcc5*, *Mrp5*, upregulated 4.5 fold). Most of the influx transporters were ion carriers, some upregulated, others downregulated. Of two monocarboxylic transporters one (*Slc16a4*) was upregulated (8 fold) and one (*Slc16a1*) downregulated (−2 fold). The highest change in expression was that of the vitamin C transporter *Slc23a3* (12 fold). It seems unlikely that any of these changes are directly related to the lack of axon growth following injury at P28.

Development and structure. Thirty-one genes were classified as development and structure related genes (Table S3). Of these, twenty were upregulated, 2.1 to 21 fold and eleven were downregulated, (−2 to −11 fold). Several of these genes have important roles in neural development. For example *Fuz*, which was upregulated 21 fold, is a planar polarity gene, mutations of which are associated with neural tube defects [87]. *Hoxb1* (12 fold) and *Hoxb3* (2.4 fold) are transcription factors involved in patterning of the caudal central nervous system [88,89]. *Hoxd4* (2.4 fold) does not appear to have been identified previously in spinal cord but *Hoxd10* has been implicated in determining motor neuron numbers and spinal nerve trajectories in lumbar spinal cord of mice [90]. There were two insulin growth factor-like genes, one upregulated (*Igf2bp2*, 2.5 fold) and one downregulated (*Igfbpl1*, −11 fold); there was also one IGF-like receptor (*Igflr1*, 5.2 fold). None of these have previously been identified in spinal cord. Only five of the remaining genes have been identified previously in spinal cord (*Tube1*, *Notch3*, *Rhou*, *Sort1*, *Vim*). Of these, tubulin protein has been reported in spinal cord injury, where it was upregulated 2.7 fold [91] compared with a 4.5 fold in gene expression, and vimentin (*Vim*) was upregulated [92]. Given that many of these genes are of unclear function in normal or injured spinal cord it cannot be concluded whether they contribute to the lack of neurite outgrowth following injury at P28, although this seems unlikely.

Proteomic analysis in postnatal *Monodelphis* spinal cord following transection

The changes in proteomic expression have been examined in the segment of the cord rostral to the lesion compared to age-matched controls. Proteins identified from gel bands that showed changes in the density were classified under the same functional categories as those used in the RNA-Seq analysis (see above).

Protein expression in postnatal *Monodelphis* spinal cord 24 h following transection at P7

Compared to P8 age-matched controls, in cords injured at P7 and analysed 24 h later there were only four proteins with increased band intensity (upregulated). Almost all of the rest of the proteins identified at this age (twenty-six) showed reduced band intensity (downregulated); one protein was identified with both an increased and a decreased density that depended on the fraction in which the protein was separated (Tables S4 and S6). The identity of these proteins and their classification into functional categories are shown in Table S4. Four of the functional groups: Neurite Inhibition, Guidance & Extracellular; Apoptosis & Ubiquitin; Synapses, Neural Receptors & Channels and Development & Structure are illustrated in Fig. 7.

Neurite inhibition, guidance and extracellular proteins. One neurite inhibitory protein, myelin basic protein, was upregulated, whereas a protein that interacts with the myelin inhibitory protein, NOGO (Ubiquinol-cytochrome c reductase core protein II, see [93]) was downregulated. Three tubulin proteins were also downregulated (Fig. 7A and Table S4).

Apoptosis and ubiquitin-related. All six of the proteins in this group were downregulated. Three were ubiquitin-related, two were peroxiredoxins with an antioxidant protective role [94] and one was an immunoproteasome protein, which also is involved in processing of class 1 MHC peptides (http://www.ncbi.nlm.nih.gov/gene/5689). This is illustrated in Fig. 7B (data in Table S4).

Synapses, neural receptors and channels. Six of the seven proteins in this group were down regulated. Their functions appear to relate to intracellular structure, motility and transport. The one protein that was upregulated was a vesicle transport and fusion protein (valosin).

All of the proteins assigned to the development and structure and the metabolic-associated protein groups were downregulated; two stress response genes changed in opposite directions (Fig. 7C and Table S4).

Development and structure

Four proteins in this group (glial fibrillary acidic protein, transgelin-2, peptidylprolyl isomerase A-like and phosphatidylethanolamine-binding protein 1) were downregulated. None was upregulated (Fig. 7D and Table S4).

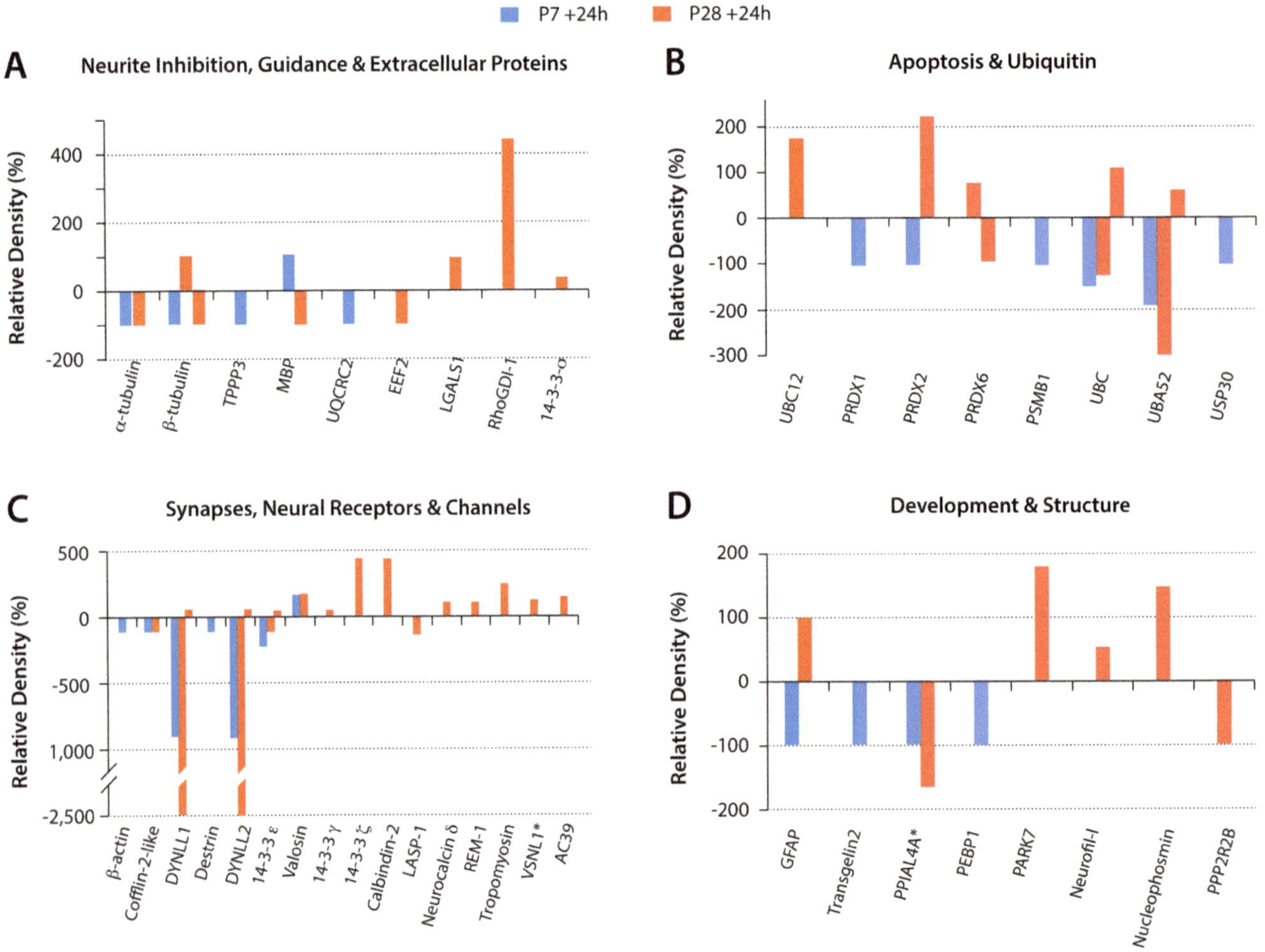

Figure 7. Proteins by functional groups with changed expression levels after spinal transection at P7 or P28. Estimates of protein expression levels from densitometry measurements. Values are expressed as % change from control values (100%). y axis: Relative Density (%). Proteins grouped by functions as listed in Tables S4 and S5. Abbreviations: TPPP3-Brain specific protein; UQCRC2-Ubiquinol-cytochrome c reductase core protein II; EEF2-Elongation factor 2 isoform 1; LGALS1-galactin1; MBP–Myelin basic protein; PRDX1-peroxiredoxin1; PRDX2–peroxiredoxin 2; PRDX6–peroxiredoxin 6; PSMB1-Proteasome subunit β type 1; UBC–Ubiquitin C; UBA52-Ubiquitin A-52; USP30-Ubiquitin specific peptidase 30 phosphoglycerate kinase; BC12-NEDD8-conjugating enzyme UBC12; DYNLL1- Cytoplasmic dynein light chain 1; DYNLL2-Dynein light chain LC8 type 2; VSLN1-Visinin like-1; AC39-AC39/physophilin; GFAP–glial fibrillary acidic protein; TAGLN2-transgelin 2; PPIAL4A - Peptidylprolyl isomerase A-like PEBP1 - Phosphatidylethanolamine-binding protein 1; PARK7 - Parkinson protein 7; Neurofil-L – Neurofilament-L subunit; PPP2R2B - Protein phosphatase 2 regulatory subunit B. Two proteins, VSNL1 and PPIAL4A (marked with *) are mean values as their expression levels changes were detected in more than one fraction (see Table S4 and S5 for individual changes). Note also that a few of the proteins listed showed both up- and downregulation but only in P28 injury group.

Blood-related proteins. Two hemoglobin proteins, hemoglobin-α and hemoglobin subunit β-M showed changes in band density; hemoglobin-α was increased in Off gel fraction 12 and reduced in fraction 9 (Table S4), hemoglobin subunit β-M was increased. Neither of these proteins has been identified previously in spinal cord. It is possible that their presence was due to blood contamination in the injured cords (see Fig. 1).

Protein expression in postnatal *Monodelphis* spinal cord 24 h following transection at P28

Following injury at P28 (P28+24 h) compared to P29 controls twenty eight protein bands were identified with increased intensity, fourteen protein bands with reduced intensity and thirteen that showed both increased or decreased intensity depending on the Off-gel fraction in which they were present (Fig. 8, Table S6) most likely reflecting changes in post-translational modifications [31]. The variability in the proteome following injury at P28 is in contrast to the response to injury at P7 when almost all of the proteins identified were downregulated (Fig. 7).

Immune-inflammatory proteins. In contrast to the very large number of genes in this functional category that changed their regulation at P28 following injury, only three proteins were identified here (Table S5). One was *Anxa2* (annexin a2), which showed decreased expression, although the expression of its gene was unchanged. Annexin2 is involved in recruitment and activation of immune cells [95]. A protein that is likely to have immune related functions was also identified (immunoglobulin lambda-like polypeptide 5-like) and found to be upregulated (Table S5). However, its actual function appears to be unknown. A third protein was Melanocortin 1 Receptor, which is said to have anti-inflammatory and immunomodulatory effects [96]. The discrepancy between the large number of identified genes and

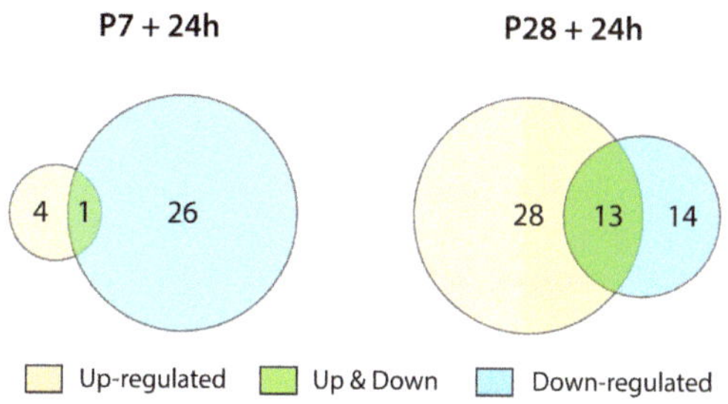

Up	Down	Up & Down
13%	84%	3%

Up	Down	Up & Down
51%	25%	24%

Figure 8. Summary of numbers of proteins that changed expression levels 24 h following spinal transection at P7 or P28. All but five of the proteins identified at P7 as showing a change in expression after injury were downregulated. At P28 half of the proteins were upregulated.

small number of proteins is most likely to be due to the sensitivity of detection methods: proteomic analysis is not likely to detect molecules within relatively low concentration range as is the case for most cytokines. It is also possible that some of the genes detected by RNA-Seq. analysis were not yet translated into their protein products within the time frame used in this study (24 hours).

Neurite inhibition and guidance proteins. Unlike results following injury at P7, at P28 myelin basic protein was downregulated (Fig. 7A). On the other hand Rho GTPase activating protein, through which many of the neurite inhibitory factors act (see above) was increased. Two other proteins that have been suggested to influence neurite outgrowth (Elongation Factor 2 Isoform 1 [97] and Lectin, galactoside-binding, soluble 1 (Galectin 1) [98,99]) changed in opposite directions (Fig. 7A, Table S5). Galectin-1 has also been described in neutrophils at the site of a spinal cord injury made 24 h earlier and in macrophages/ microglia at 3 days post injury [100]. This increase in Galectin-1 protein was not accompanied by a change in transcript expression (Table S6).

Apoptosis and ubiquitin. Five of the eight proteins in this category were upregulated in contrast to P7 injured spinal cord when the proteins in this group were all downregulated (Fig. 7B). However, there were three proteins in this group, which were identified as a band in a different fraction that showed decreased density (periredoxin-6, ubiquitin c and ubiquitin A52, Fig. 7B, Table S5). Detailed studies of the apoptotic activity in *Monodelphis* spinal cord after injury have not been conducted, mostly due to the lack of cross-reactivity of commercially available antibodies commonly used as markers for this process.

Synapses, receptors and channels. There were twelve proteins in this category, including three members of 14-3-3 proteins (ε, γ, ξ) that were upregulated. These are involved in tyrosine 3-monooxygenase/tryptophan 5-monooxygenase activation signal transduction. Seven proteins involved in synaptic structure and function were upregulated, but only two (Cofilin and LIM & SH3 protein) were downregulated (Fig. 7C, Table S5). It seems unlikely that these proteins would play a role in the lack of neurite outgrowth following injury at P28, but they may indicate an early aspect of synaptic reorganisation in the injured spinal cord.

Development and structure. There were eight proteins identified as changing their expression in this category, including glial fibrillary acidic protein (GFAP). All but two (PPIAL4A, PPP2R2B) were upregulated (Fig. 7D, Table S5). However two of the upregulated proteins also appeared as bands in other fractions that indicated downregulation. These changes may be a reflection of developmental reorganization of spinal cord tissue rather than involvement in blocking neurite outgrowth at P28.

Stress response proteins. Five proteins with changed expression were identified in this category (Table S5). Two were upregulated (heat shock proteins HSP84b and HSP90B1), two were downregulated (glucose regulated heat shock protein 70kDa, protein 5; novel heat shock protein) and one (heat shock protein 90) was both increased or decreased depending on the fraction. Heat shock proteins are highly expressed cellular proteins in all species examined so far [101]. Stressors of various kinds generally result in an increase in the levels of these proteins e.g., HSP70 and HSP90 [101]. Several authors have reported this effect early after spinal cord injury in adult animals [102,103]. However, down-regulation of some heat shock proteins by various drug treatments has been reported in spinal cord injury (see [104] for references). It has therefore been suggested that both up- and down-regulatory changes in heat shock proteins may have neuroprotective effects, reflecting a complex role in protective responses to injury [104].

Blood-related proteins. As observed following P7 injury two hemoglobins showed a change in regulation. However, following injury at P28 hemoglobin α was decreased whereas at P7 different fractions showed either a decrease or/and an increase (Cf Tables S4 and S5). For hemoglobin β, the changes were the opposite; that is at P7 this protein was increased but at P28 different fractions showed opposite changes. In addition to these two hemoglobins, two other proteins showed an increase following injury at P28: the plasma carrier protein albumin and NADPH-flavin reductase, which is involved in heme metabolism. As suggested for P7 it may be that these blood-related proteins originate from blood contamination of the spinal cord as a consequence of the injury (see Fig. 1).

Comparison of gene and protein expression

Based on the proteins identified, we searched for corresponding genes or family of genes associated with these proteins. Table S6 shows the matches of proteins and genes identified from RNA-Seq analysis that were up- or downregulated (proteins ± 0.5 band density, genes ± 2 fold change). A few proteins did not have IDs that corresponded to a gene in our RNA-Seq dataset. This may be due to incompleteness of the annotation of the opossum genome. Most of the genes corresponding to up- or downregulated proteins that we identified as changing their expression following injury at either P7 or P28 did not show changes in the RNA-Seq analysis. In only two cases did both gene and protein changed both at P28. (i) Hemoglobin beta M was identified in three different fractions. In two of these the protein was upregulated and in the third it was decreased. The corresponding gene is a *novel* opossum gene (LOC100019389) that was upregulated 2.2 fold. (ii) A second upregulated gene (*Blvrd*) corresponded to an upregulated protein (NADPH-flavin reductase) that is involved in heme metabolism. The protein products of these genes may perhaps be explained by blood contamination in the injured spinal cord. However, this would not explain the presence of these genes. Erythrocytes are no longer nucleated in opossums after birth and hemoglobin transcripts have been identified in cerebral endothelial cells of neonatal mice [105], which may thus explain the changes in gene expression found in the present study.

There are several reasons why there were so many more genes that showed changes in expression that was the case for the proteins. The main one is likely to be that the protein extraction method used was favorable for soluble cytoplasmic proteins, whereas many of the products of genes identified are associated with cell membranes and intracellular structures such as microtubules and actin filaments. It is also possible that the increased expression of some of the genes had not yet resulted in increased protein synthesis within the 24 h period following injury. In addition, as mentioned earlier, the sensitivity of the two methods is very different and many proteins whose genes showed changes are not present in cord tissue in concentrations high enough to be detected by silver staining of separated bands. In addition we have identified previously that some of the observed changes in the bands intensity are due to post translational modifications rather than changes in corresponding gene expression [32,33].

General Discussion

The most striking observation from this study is the large number of genes and proteins that change their level of expression within 24h after spinal cord injury in the neonatal opossum. The number of these changes was much greater following injury at P28 compared to P7, particularly when considering transcriptome changes. At P7 there were no genes that showed significant decrease (i.e., ≥−2 fold) in expression. In contrast most of (84%) of the proteins that changed expression at P28 were downregulated. This could in part be due to tissue loss following injury, thus reducing the amount of protein-containing tissue sampled but is also likely to be a reflection of the timing of these experiments: early tissue loss is followed by a later adaptation of the cellular response, as reflected by transcriptome changes detected.

The comparatively muted response to injury at P7 may indicate that the injury was introduced at an age when substantial spinal cord growth occurs as part of normal development and that this was little impaired by the trauma. Whereas by P28, when many of the spinal cord tracts are established, the response is more "adult-like" in the inability of the injured spinal cord to display a regenerative response [25]. By far the largest category of genes to respond to injury was the immune/inflammatory group. There were twenty-four genes that changed expression after injury at both ages, all increasing their expression. Nineteen changed to a similar extent at both ages (< two times difference between the ages). More genes in this category showed a larger increase in expression at P7 than at P28; only three novel genes at P28 showed substantially higher increases (322, 14 and 9.3 fold) in expression than at P7 (Fig. 5).

In vivo compared to *in vitro* opossum spinal cord injury experiments

Several previous studies have assessed the importance of the developmental stage and the consequences of spinal cord injury on patterns of gene expression in the opossum [28–30]. In these investigations, changes in specific families of genes associated with axonal growth as well as inhibitory molecules were emphasized. In contrast, more extensive changes in gene expression were documented in the present study. There are several possibilities for these differences that relate to the experimental design of the studies. At a technical level the coverage of RNA Sequencing is potentially much greater than that of a microarray chip. In papers in which an isolated spinal cord preparation was used [29,30] the tissues were bathed in a room temperature solution (24–25°C; [28]) during and after the spinal cord injury. Mild levels of hypothermia are known to be neuroprotective after brain and spinal cord injury and may alter specific secondary injury mechanisms including alterations in gene expression [106–109]. Thus, the hypothermic conditions that were used in the isolated opossum spinal cord preparation may have influenced some injury-induced gene expression changes compared to *in vivo* spinal cord injury preparations conducted at normal body temperature (31–34°C in the opossum [110]). In addition, because these opossum studies used an isolated spinal cord preparation, the involvement of acute systemic responses to spinal cord injury would also be expected to differ in comparison to *in vivo* injury conditions, due to the lack of blood circulation. Thus the well-described inflammatory response to spinal cord injury involving infiltration of different types of immune cells after experimental and clinical neurotrauma [111–113] would not occur in the absence of a circulation. These injury-modeling conditions may therefore help explain some differences in patterns of gene expression between the *in vitro* versus *in vivo* spinal cord injury studies. The relative contributions of lower temperature and absence of immune cell infiltration are hard to judge. The lower temperature of the *in vitro* preparations does not appear to have suppressed other aspects of the response to injury compared to the absence of an immune/inflammatory response. Since there was a lack of neurite growth across the lesion both at P13 *in vitro* and P28 *in vivo* it seems unlikely that the large number of additional immune/inflammatory genes that changed their expression at P28 compared to P7 *in vivo* was a major factor in this lack of neurite outgrowth. Also it is apparent from the Supplementary data in Mladinic *et al.*, [29] that only a few immune genes were detected and they changed little in response to injury at either age. This would suggest that the lack of a circulation in the *in vitro* preparations might have been the main factor in the absence of much of an inflammatory response in these isolated preparations. In addition, it is clear from studies of injured adult spinal cord that changes in expression of immune and inflammatory genes and proteins are mainly of significance in relation to secondary injury that follows the primary injury with a time course that has been variously estimated to be days to weeks (see [114,115]).

To what extent may the observed changes in gene and protein expression account for the lack of neurite outgrowth at P28 following injury?

Twenty-nine of thirty-four genes suggested to influence neurite growth (Table 2) only changed their expression to a limited extent in the range +3 to −3 fold change, with equal numbers up- and downregulated. In addition, key inhibitory genes either did not change their expression (*Nogo, Mag, Mog*) or were downregulated (*Mbp, Plp1*), rather than upregulated. Thus it seems unlikely that the explanation for the lack of neurite outgrowth is accounted for by inhibitory activity of the protein products of these genes. There were similar numbers of opposing changes in protein expression for this functional group after injury at P28 (Fig. 7, Table S5) and myelin basic protein was downregulated as was its gene. Most extracellular matrix genes (Table 3) also showed relatively small and opposing changes in expression, but there were some notable exceptions. Three genes showed very large increases in expression: olfactomedin 4 (480 fold), *Mmp1* (104 fold) and *Papln* (*papilin*, proteoglycan-like sulfated glycoprotein, 152 fold). One gene in this category showed a marked decrease in expression: integrin α4 (−57 fold). Overall, there were some thirty-four genes that increased their expression by >10 fold following injury at P28 and only four that showed reduced expression of >10 fold. Of the upregulated genes almost half were in the immune and blood-related functional categories, which for reasons outlined above were probably not contributing to the lack of neurite outgrowth. Only three of the substantially upregulated genes (*Olfm4, Mmp-1, Papln*) and one markedly downregulated gene (*Itga4*) are in a functional category (see Table 5) in which there is evidence for effects on neurite outgrowth. Proteoglycans generally seem to have inhibitory effects on neurite outgrowth [20]. *Mmp-1* has been reported to be increased by one day after injury in adult spinal cord, but MMPs as a group appear to have rather complex effects following spinal cord injury, some deleterious and others beneficial [116,117]. It is not known what the function of olfactomedin-4 may be in spinal cord injury, but it binds to cadherins and lectins [57]. Olfactomedin-1 promotes neurite outgrowth by binding to the Nogo A receptor complex (NgR1) and inhibiting the growth cone collapse induced by myelin inhibitors [118]. Several integrins (α6, α7, α9 and β1) have been implicated in promoting axon growth during development and in the response of the peripheral nervous system to injury [63]. Integrin α4β1 is expressed by leukocytes that invade spinal cord tissue following injury [64]. However, it has also been described as having a role in regenerating growth cones following injury to sensory neurons where it provides a signaling pathway for re-expression of fibronectin (for references see [119]). Thus its downregulation could be contributing to the lack of neurite outgrowth in P28 injured spinal cord, particularly if combined with inhibitory effects of MMP1 and papilin.

An additional possibility is that changes in the growth potential of brainstem neurons with axons that project to the spinal cord may be reduced by P28 in opossums. This is an aspect of the failure of neural regeneration in injured adult spinal cord that has been little studied. However, its importance is suggested by the experiments of Kobayashi et al. [120] who showed that infusion of BDNF and NT-4/5 prevented atrophy of rat rubrospinal axons after cervical axotomy. This treatment evoked upregulation of a number of regeneration-associated genes, which they considered correlated with an increased regenerative capacity of axotomized rubrospinal neurons.

Comparing proteome results from segments of spinal cord rostral and caudal to the transection

The present study reports on the changes in gene and protein expression in the segment of spinal cord rostral to the site of transection of the spinal cord. These changes would be expected to affect centrally projecting neurites from sensory neurons, should they regenerate following injury. There is only limited information about changes in gene expression in the segment of cord caudal to the site of injury in postnatal opossums [24]. That study used a combination of a mouse microarray of genes encoding cytokines and chemokines with some qPCR validation, as discussed above. However, we have previously published a proteomic analysis of the spinal cord segment caudal to the injury in the same animals that have been used in the present study for the segments of cord rostral to the lesion [32].

There were ten proteins in the P7 injured spinal cords that were common to the two segments of cord (Table 6). All but two of these had bands that were decreased in density compared to the controls. Cofilin and peptidylprolyl isomerase A-like proteins were reduced in the rostral spinal cord and increased in the caudal segment. In the P28 injured spinal cord there were fourteen proteins that were common to both segments of cord (Table 7). All but four of the proteins had bands that changed in the same direction in both cord segments, but several of these proteins had bands that increased or decreased in different fractions. As observed at P7, cofilin and peptidylprolyl isomerase a-like decreased in the rostral segment but increased in the caudal segment. Annexin-A2 decreased in the rostral cord but increased in the caudal segment. Tropomyosin on the other hand increased in the rostral segment but decreased caudally. There were more proteins that were identified as changing their regulation only in one segment or the other. These are listed in Tables S7A & S7B for P7+24 h and Tables S7C & S7D for P28+24 h. As we discussed in detail previously [32] some of the observed changes in identified proteins were more likely to be due to post-translational modifications than changes in the expression of their coding genes.

Limitations of the Study

This study was restricted to the changes in gene and protein expression that could be identified 24 h after injury at P7 or at P28 in the cord segment rostral to the transection (T10). Further changes in gene and protein expression may well occur at later times following injury as suggested by studies in injured adult spinal cord [16,103].

This study was initiated early in the adoption of RNA-Seq and involved a small number of samples. Although technical variability is low, a large degree of biological variability was observed, consistent with level of manipulation required in the experimental preparation of samples. This variability is likely to have reduced the number of genes observed to be statistically significantly differentially expressed. This reduced power necessitated the simplification of the analytical design to exclude direct modeling of interaction between development and injury.

In presenting the data we have concentrated on functional categories that previous work in the injured adult spinal cord suggested to be important for the characteristic failure of neurites to grow following injury to the adult spinal cord. This is something that has been known since the time of Ramon y Cajal [121]. Our description has tended to emphasize the genes that showed the largest changes in expression, many of which had not previously been implicated in the failure of neurite outgrowth following spinal cord injury. Since little is known about the functions of some of these genes (e.g., olfactomedin 480 fold; triadin 206 fold and several novel opossum genes, see Table S3) their role in failure of neurite outgrowth is speculative, as was considered in the General Discussion above.

An alternative possibility is that relatively small changes in expression of a large number of key genes may account for the lack of neurite outgrowth. This has been considered in the General Discussion, above.

An important limitation on providing an overall functional view of the large number of expression changes in both genes and proteins is that we were unsuccessful in attempts at pathway analysis, with identified pathways consisting of small number of genes with only one differentially expressed member. We hypothesize that this was primarily because of limitations in the functional annotation of the opossum genome. We also eschewed the use of heat maps for presenting our data in favour of a numerical approach of presenting data in graphs and tables. The visual approach of heat maps puts undue emphasis on expression differences by using colour coding which, although eye catching, may give a misleading impression of the statistical validity of differences in gene expression.

The number of antibodies available that cross react with opossum material is very limited. At this stage it is therefore not possible to define in which cell populations these genes and their protein products are expressed. In future studies it is planned to localize some of the key genes using *in situ* hybridisation.

It may be considered by some that the lack of overlap between the genes we have identified in RNA-Seq analysis and the protein gene products identified in the proteomic part of the study may indicate a fault in the experimental design. There are several reasons for this lack of overlap. The most obvious one is the difference in the sensitivity of the two methods as detection of the

Table 5. Genes that changed most in expression (±≥10 FOLD) 24 h following spinal cord injury at P28.

SYMBOL	GENE DESCRIPTION	FOLD
MOST UPREGULATED GENES		
IMMUNE & INFLAMMATORY		
Novel	C-C motif chemokine similar to CCL8 and CCL13	322
Dok3	docking protein 3	266
Novel	C-C motif chemokine similar to CCL2, CCL7, CCL8, CCL11 and CCL13	197
Pstpip1	proline-serine-threonine phosphatase interacting protein 1	167
Lrrc33	leucine rich repeat containing 33 Official name NRROS	160
Novel	similar to TARM1 T cell-interacting, activating receptor on myeloid cells 1	22
Il1b	interleukin 1, β	20
Vav1	VAV1 guanine nucleotide exchange factor	17
Osmr	oncostatin M receptor	14
Lgals4	lectin, galactoside-binding, soluble, 4	14
Amh	anti-Mullerian hormone	12
Marco	macrophage receptor with collagenous structure	12
Igsf22	immunoglobulin superfamily, member 22	12
Novel	LOC100020928 C-C motif chemokine similar to CCL3 and CCL4	10
BLOOD-RELATED		
Novel	similar to HPR, haptoglobin-related protein	99
Novel	similar to TARM1 T cell-interacting, activating receptor on myeloid cells 1	22
EXTRACELLULAR MATRIX		
Olfm4	olfactomedin 4, ECM glycoprotein that facilitates cell adhesion.	480
METALLOTHIONINE		
Mmp1	matrix metallopeptidase 1 (interstitial collagenase)	104
PROTEOGLYCAN		
Papln	papilin, proteoglycan-like sulfated glycoprotein	152
ACTIN, MYOSIN & RELATED		
Trdn	triadin	206
Myl1	myosin, light chain 1, alkali; skeletal, fast	139
Mylpf	myosin light chain, phosphorylatable, fast skeletal muscle	22
Myh4	myosin, heavy chain 4, skeletal muscle	18
TRANSPORTERS		
Slc23a3	solute carrier family 23, sodium-dependent vitamin C transporter 3	12
DEVELOPMENT & STRUCTURE		
fuz	fuzzy homolog (Drosophila) cell polarity, ciliogenesis & cell movement.	21
hoxb1	homeobox B1, transcription factor role in morphogenesis	12
des	desmin	12
MEMBRANE		
Novel	novel protein with potential transmembrane domains	254
Novel	novel protein with potential transmembrane domains	241
Tmem106a	transmembrane protein 106A	157
ENZYMES & METABOLISM		
Pstpip1	proline-serine-threonine phosphatase interacting protein 1	167
Novel	similar to ATP13A5 ATPase type 13A5	23
MISCELLANEOUS		
Ttc40	tetratricopeptide repeat domain 40	89
ZINC FINGER		
Novel	similar to ZC3H13 zinc finger CCCH-type containing 13	352
MOST DOWN REGULATED GENES		
Itga4	integrin, α 4 (antigen CD49D, alpha 4 subunit of VLA-4 receptor)	−57
Novel	similar to CLCNKA/CLCNKB chloride channel	−27

Table 5. Cont.

SYMBOL	GENE DESCRIPTION	FOLD
Igfbpl1	insulin-like growth factor binding protein-like 1	−11
Gxylt2	glucoside xylosyltransferase 2	−16

protein by even silver staining is several orders of magnitude less than that for RNA. The second main difference is the timing of the extraction protocol—many genes are transcribed much earlier than the translation of their products. Our study was performed at one time point only (24 h post injury). The third, and most biologically relevant possibility is that proteomic analysis identifies not only changes in the concentration levels of individual proteins but also in their post-translational modifications. This would be difficult to detect at the transcriptome level. That this may be the case has been suggested in our earlier proteomic study in which RT-qPCR was used to examine the expression levels of the genes of some of the proteins identified as changing following injury. Many of the identified proteins showed changes in their isoelectric mobility but not in their gene expression [32]. This is important because it indicates that analysis of the transcriptome alone may in fact not provide a comprehensive overall picture of changes occurring in the whole tissue in response to injury.

Despite these limitations the unique nature of these data provide a valuable resource for the investigation of the *a priori* hypotheses of mechanisms of spinal cord regeneration and as a foundation for future studies.

Conclusions

Morphological repair and functional recovery following spinal cord injury requires a complex but coordinated set of cellular responses; they are particularly complicated because they involve sites close to the injury (local) as well as distant locations such as neuronal cells bodies of axotomised axons. The very large number of genes that changed their expression level significantly following injury, particularly in the more mature spinal cord at P28, is very striking. It reinforces microarray studies of injured adult spinal cord that also show expression changes in a large number of genes [16] indicating just how complicated the response of the spinal cord to injury is. It seems unlikely that the preoccupation of most studies of trying to identify a single gene or protein will provide a therapy for patients with spinal cord injuries, unless key upstream regulatory genes and their proteins can be identified.

In the present study we report on the changes detected in transcript and protein expression that follow complete spinal cord transection at two different ages (P7 and P28) in postnatal *Monodelphis domestica*. P7 pups were chosen because at this age the animals show substantial axon growth across the lesion. This axon growth is partly regenerative from injured axons and partly due to axon growth that occurs as continued postnatal development of the spinal cord [21]. When these animals reach adulthood their locomotor behavior is essentially normal [25]. P28 animals were chosen for comparison because following a similar complete transection there is no axon growth across the lesion although the animals, when adult, exhibit weight-bearing locomotion [25]. The present study was designed to see whether short-term changes in gene and protein expression that occur after a complete spinal transection at T10 might account for these differences in axon growth and subsequent behaviour. Although some immune/inflammatory genes were highly upregulated (Table S3), comparison of the results presented in this study together with previously published work on *Monodelphis* spinal cord *in vitro* suggests that immunological/inflammatory genes may not be involved in the differential response to primary injury we observe at the two ages. However, as we discuss above, they are more likely to be important in the secondary phase of the process.

From the analysis of known functional groups of genes and proteins presented here we conclude that there appear to be at

Table 6. Proteins that changed level 24 h following spinal cord injury at P7 in *Monodelphis* in segments rostral and caudal to site of transection.

Protein	Rostral SC	Caudal SC
14-3-3	↓	↑↓
cofilin	↓	↑
destrin	↓	↓
Hemoglobin α	↑↓	↓
Hemoglobin subunit β M	↑	↑↓
Peptidylprolyl isomerase a-like	↓	↑
Pyruvate dehydrogenase	↓	↓
Tubulin α	↓	↓
Tubulin β	↓	↓
ubiquitin	↓	↓

↑increased band density, ↓ decreased band density. Some proteins showed an increase or decrease in different fractions (↑↓).

Table 7. Proteins that changed level 24 h following spinal cord injury at P28.in *Monodelphis* in segments rostral and caudal to site of transection.

Protein	Rostral SC	Caudal SC
14-3-3 protein	↑	↑↓
albumin	↑	↑↓
Alpha enolase	□	↑↓
Annexin-a2	↓	↑
ATP synthase subunit β, mitochondrial	↑	↑↓
cofilin	↓	↑
GFAP	↑	↑
Glyceraldehyde 3 phosphate dehydrogenase	↑↓	↑↓
Hemoglobin subunit β M	↑↓	↑↓
Neurofilament L subunit	↑	↓
Peptidylprolyl isomerase A-like	↓	↑
Tropomyosin	↑	↓
Tubulin α	↑↓	↑↓
ubiquitin	↑↓	↑

↑increased band density, ↓ decreased band density. Some proteins showed an increase or decrease in different fractions (↑↓).

least three not mutually exclusive general mechanisms that may be involved in the age-related response to injury and in particular the lack of neurite outgrowth following injury at P28:

(i) Changes in expression of genes and proteins that are known to be involved in axon guidance and inhibition (Table 2). However, these were not significant at P7 and at P28 they were relatively small and many were in opposing directions. One example is two of the key *Rho* activating genes (*Arhgap6*, 3.1 fold; *Arhgef10*, −2.1 fold) that are central to control of many of the downstream neurite inhibitory factors. In addition, almost all of the myelin-associated genes and their proteins were either unchanged or downregulated (Tables 2 and 6) which perhaps makes this explanation less likely.

(ii) Down regulation of essential neurotrophic genes in brain stem neurons with axonal projections to the spinal cord. This will be the subject of a separate study (Saunders et al., in preparation).

(iii) Major changes in expression of a few genes at P28 that produce extracellular matrix proteins (Table 3). Most of these have not previously been described in studies of adult spinal cord injury, but they are members of gene families that have been implicated. These seem to be plausible candidates to explain the failure of neurite growth following injury that will be worthy of further study.

This study provides a large database of changes in expression of genes and proteins at 24 h after spinal cord injury at two ages in postnatal *Monodelphis*. We have provided a detailed analysis based on functional groups thought to be important in the response of the spinal cord to injury. There were several novel genes that showed strikingly large changes in expression following injury at P28. Their identity and function will need to be determined before their roles in the response to injury can be considered.

Supporting Information

Table S1 Data used for analysis of gene expression changes 24 h following spinal cord transection at P7. Gene symbols, description and ENSEMBL ID shown. Log2F-C = Log_2 fold change. These values were derived by comparing expression at P7+24 h with P8 control. See Methods for details of statistical analysis used. Updated 13 May 2013.

Table S2 Data used for analysis of gene expression changes 24 h following spinal cord transection at P28. Gene symbols, description and ENSEMBL ID shown. Log2F-C = Log_2 fold change. These values were derived by comparing expression at P28+24 h with P29 control. See Methods for details of statistical analysis used. Updated 13 May 2014.

Table S3 Gene expression P28+24 h following spinal cord transection. Genes categorized by function with their ID and description included. FC = Fold Change compared to P29 controls. Updated 13 May 2014.

Table S4 Proteins that changed expression level 24 h following spinal cord injury at P7 in *Monodelphis domestica*. Arrows indicate direction of change in gel band density (upregulation ↑or downregulation ↓). Relative change is densitometry value of gel band at P7+24 h compared to P8 control. Gene name symbol or provisional ID in genome and protein function are included.

Table S5 Proteins that changed expression level 24 h following spinal cord injury at P28 in *Monodelphis domestica*. Arrows indicate direction of change in gel band density (upregulation ↑ or downregulation ↓). Relative change is densitometry value of gel band at P28+24 h compared to P29 control. Gene name, symbol or provisional ID in genome and protein function are included.

Table S6 Proteomic results of identified proteins in different fractions and bands compared with expression of their respective genes in the transcriptome. ***Column A*** shows fraction in which protein was identified, ***Column B*** shows band in gel in which protein was identified. Note that some proteins were identified in more than one fraction or band. ***Column C*** is ENSEMBL protein ID, where known. ***Column D*** is protein name. ***Column E*** and ***F*** show whether protein band density was increased ≥0.5 compared to age-matched controls 24 h following spinal cord injury at P7 or P28. ***Column G*** shows corresponding gene symbol or name. ***Column H*** shows ENSEMBL gene ID. ***Column I*** and ***J*** show gene expression level 24 h following injury at P7 or P28. Note the relative lack of correlation between identified changes in the transcriptome and the proteome. Updated 13 May 2014

Table S7 A. Proteins that were identified as changing expression level in the spinal cord *rostral* but not caudal to the site of transection 24 h after injury at P7. ↑ increased band density, **↓** decreased band density. Some proteins showed an increase or decrease in different fractions (**↑↓**). **B. Proteins that were identified as changing in expression level in the spinal cord *caudal* but not rostral to the site of transection 24 h after injury at P7. ↑** increased band density, **↓** decreased band density. Some proteins showed an increase or decrease in different fractions (**↑↓**). **C.** *Monodelphis* spinal cord. Proteins that were identified in the spinal cord *rostral* but not caudal to the site of transection 24 h after injury at P28. **↑** increased band density, **↓** decreased band density. Some proteins showed an increase or decrease in different fractions (**↑↓**). **D:** *Monodelphis* spinal cord. Proteins that were identified in the spinal cord *caudal* but not rostral to the site of transection 24 h after injury at P28. **↑** increased band density, **↓** decreased band density. Some proteins showed an increase or decrease in different fractions (**↑↓**).

Author Contributions

Conceived and designed the experiments: NRS NMN KMD BJW SAL DLS CJE MDH MW HL JT RDM AIS WDD. Performed the experiments: NRS NMN KMD BJW SAL DLS CJE MDH MW HL JT RDM AIS WDD. Analyzed the data: NRS NMN KMD BJW SAL DLS CJE MDH MW HL JT RDM AIS WDD. Contributed reagents/materials/analysis tools: NRS NMN KMD BJW SAL DLS CJE MDH MW HL JT RDM AIS WDD. Wrote the paper: NRS NMN KMD BJW SAL DLS CJE MDH MW HL JT RDM AIS WDD.

References

1. Aguayo AJ, David S, Bray GM (1981) Influences of the glial environment on the elongation of axons after injury: transplantation studies in adult rodents. The Journal of experimental biology 95: 231–240.
2. David S, Aguayo AJ (1981) Axonal elongation into peripheral nervous system "bridges" after central nervous system injury in adult rats. Science 214: 931–933.
3. Tello F (1911) La influencia del neurotropismo en la regeneracion de los centros nerviosos. Trab Laborator Invest Biol University Madrid 9: 123–159.
4. Akbik F, Cafferty WB, Strittmatter SM (2011) Myelin associated inhibitors: A link between injury-induced and experience-dependent plasticity. Experimental neurology.
5. Buchli AD, Schwab ME (2005) Inhibition of Nogo: a key strategy to increase regeneration, plasticity and functional recovery of the lesioned central nervous system. Annals of medicine 37: 556–567.
6. Bradbury EJ, Carter LM (2011) Manipulating the glial scar: chondroitinase ABC as a therapy for spinal cord injury. Brain research bulletin 84: 306–316.
7. Fawcett JW (2006) Overcoming inhibition in the damaged spinal cord. Journal of neurotrauma 23: 371–383.
8. Galtrey CM, Fawcett JW (2007) The role of chondroitin sulfate proteoglycans in regeneration and plasticity in the central nervous system. Brain research reviews 54: 1–18.
9. Hurtado A, Marcillo A, Frydel B, Bunge MB, Bramlett HM, et al. (2012) Anti-CD11d monoclonal antibody treatment for rat spinal cord compression injury. Experimental neurology 233: 606–611.
10. Pinzon A, Marcillo A, Pabon D, Bramlett HM, Bunge MB, et al. (2008) A re-assessment of erythropoietin as a neuroprotective agent following rat spinal cord compression or contusion injury. Experimental neurology 213: 129–136.
11. Pinzon A, Marcillo A, Quintana A, Stamler S, Bunge MB, et al. (2008) A re-assessment of minocycline as a neuroprotective agent in a rat spinal cord contusion model. Brain research 1243: 146–151.
12. Sharp KG, Flanagan LA, Yee KM, Steward O (2012) A re-assessment of a combinatorial treatment involving Schwann cell transplants and elevation of cyclic AMP on recovery of motor function following thoracic spinal cord injury in rats. Experimental neurology 233: 625–644.
13. Steward O, Sharp K, Yee KM, Hofstadter M (2008) A re-assessment of the effects of a Nogo-66 receptor antagonist on regenerative growth of axons and locomotor recovery after spinal cord injury in mice. Experimental neurology 209: 446–468.
14. Aimone JB, Leasure JL, Perreau VM, Thallmair M (2004) Spatial and temporal gene expression profiling of the contused rat spinal cord. Experimental neurology 189: 204–221.
15. Crack PJ, Gould J, Bye N, Ross S, Ali U, et al. (2009) The genomic profile of the cerebral cortex after closed head injury in mice: effects of minocycline. Journal of neural transmission 116: 1–12.
16. Verhaagen J, Van Kesteren RE, Bossers KA, Macgillavry HD, Mason MR, et al. (2012) Molecular target discovery for neural repair in the functional genomics era. Handbook of clinical neurology 109: 595–616.
17. Gris P, Murphy S, Jacob JE, Atkinson I, Brown A (2003) Differential gene expression profiles in embryonic, adult-injured and adult-uninjured rat spinal cords. Molecular and cellular neurosciences 24: 555–567.
18. Chen K, Deng S, Lu H, Zheng Y, Yang G, et al. (2013) RNA-seq characterization of spinal cord injury transcriptome in acute/subacute phases: a resource for understanding the pathology at the systems level. PloS one 8: e72567.
19. Kumamaru H, Ohkawa Y, Saiwai H, Yamada H, Kubota K, et al. (2012) Direct isolation and RNA-seq reveal environment-dependent properties of engrafted neural stem/progenitor cells. Nature communications 3: 1140.
20. Fawcett JW, Schwab ME, Montani L, Brazda N, Muller HW (2012) Defeating inhibition of regeneration by scar and myelin components. Handbook of clinical neurology 109: 503–522.
21. Fry EJ, Stolp HB, Lane MA, Dziegielewska KM, Saunders NR (2003) Regeneration of supraspinal axons after complete transection of the thoracic spinal cord in neonatal opossums (Monodelphis domestica). J Comp Neurol 466: 422–444.
22. Saunders NR, Kitchener P, Knott GW, Nicholls JG, Potter A, et al. (1998) Development of walking, swimming and neuronal connections after complete spinal cord transection in the neonatal opossum, Monodelphis domestica. J Neurosci 18: 339–355.
23. Wang XM, Terman JR, Martin GF (1998) Regeneration of supraspinal axons after transection of the thoracic spinal cord in the developing opossum, Didelphis virginiana. J Comp Neurol 398: 83–97.
24. Lane MA, Truettner JS, Brunschwig JP, Gomez A, Bunge MB, et al. (2007) Age-related differences in the local cellular and molecular responses to injury in developing spinal cord of the opossum, Monodelphis domestica. Eur J Neurosci 25: 1725–1742.
25. Wheaton BJ, Callaway JK, Ek CJ, Dziegielewska KM, Saunders NR (2011) Spontaneous development of full weight-supported stepping after complete spinal cord transection in the neonatal opossum, Monodelphis domestica. PloS one 6: e26826.
26. Wheaton BJ, Noor NM, Whish SC, Truettner JS, Dietrich WD, et al. (2013) Weight-bearing locomotion in the developing opossum, Monodelphis domestica following spinal transection: remodeling of neuronal circuits caudal to lesion. PloS one 8: e71181.
27. Saunders NR, Balkwill P, Knott G, Habgood MD, Mollgard K, et al. (1992) Growth of axons through a lesion in the intact CNS of fetal rat maintained in long-term culture. Proc Biol Sci 250: 171–180.
28. Farlow DN, Vansant G, Cameron AA, Chang J, Khoh-Reiter S, et al. (2000) Gene expression monitoring for gene discovery in models of peripheral and central nervous system differentiation, regeneration, and trauma. Journal of cellular biochemistry 80: 171–180.
29. Mladinic M, Lefevre C, Del Bel E, Nicholls J, Digby M (2010) Developmental changes of gene expression after spinal cord injury in neonatal opossums. Brain research 1363: 20–39.
30. Mladinic M, Wintzer M, Del Bel E, Casseler C, Lazarevic D, et al. (2005) Differential expression of genes at stages when regeneration can and cannot

occur after injury to immature mammalian spinal cord. Cellular and molecular neurobiology 25: 407–426.
31. Mikkelsen TS, Wakefield MJ, Aken B, Amemiya CT, Chang JL, et al. (2007) Genome of the marsupial Monodelphis domestica reveals innovation in non-coding sequences. Nature 447: 167–177.
32. Noor NM, Steer DL, Wheaton BJ, Ek CJ, Truettner JS, et al. (2011) Age-dependent changes in the proteome following complete spinal cord transection in a postnatal South American opossum (Monodelphis domestica). PloS one 6: e27465.
33. Noor NM, Mollgard K, Wheaton BJ, Steer DL, Truettner JS, et al. (2013) Expression and cellular distribution of ubiquitin in response to injury in the developing spinal cord of Monodelphis domestica. PloS one 8: e62120.
34. Saunders NR, Adam E, Reader M, Mollgard K (1989) Monodelphis domestica (grey short-tailed opossum): an accessible model for studies of early neocortical development. Anat Embryol (Berl) 180: 227–236.
35. Langmead B, Salzberg SL (2012) Fast gapped-read alignment with Bowtie 2. Nature methods 9: 357–359.
36. Flicek P, Amode MR, Barrell D, Beal K, Brent S, et al. (2011) Ensembl 2011. Nucleic acids research 39: D800–806.
37. Anders A (2011) HTSeq: Analysing high-throughput sequencing data with Python. Available: http://www.huber.embl.de/users/anders/HTSeq. Accessed 2014, May 14.
38. Gentleman RC, Carey VJ, Bates DM, Bolstad B, Dettling M, et al. (2004) Bioconductor: open software development for computational biology and bioinformatics. Genome biology 5: R80.
39. McCarthy DJ, Chen Y, Smyth GK (2012) Differential expression analysis of multifactor RNA-Seq experiments with respect to biological variation. Nucleic acids research 40: 4288–4297.
40. Young MD, Wakefield MJ, Smyth GK, Oshlack A (2010) Gene ontology analysis for RNA-seq: accounting for selection bias. Genome biology 11: R14.
41. Gerner C, Frohwein U, Gotzmann J, Bayer E, Gelbmann D, et al. (2000) The Fas-induced apoptosis analyzed by high throughput proteome analysis. The Journal of biological chemistry 275: 39018–39026.
42. Dziegielewska KM, Daikuhara Y, Ohnishi T, Waite MP, Ek J, et al. (2000) Fetuin in the developing neocortex of the rat: distribution and origin. J Comp Neurol 423: 373–388.
43. McKerracher L, Ferraro GB, Fournier AE (2012) Rho signaling and axon regeneration. International review of neurobiology 105: 117–140.
44. Parra ZE, Baker ML, Lopez AM, Trujillo J, Volpe JM, et al. (2009) TCR mu recombination and transcription relative to the conventional TCR during postnatal development in opossums. Journal of immunology 182: 154–163.
45. Jameson J, Ugarte K, Chen N, Yachi P, Fuchs E, et al. (2002) A role for skin gammadelta T cells in wound repair. Science 296: 747–749.
46. Wang X, Sharp AR, Miller RD (2012) Early postnatal B cell ontogeny and antibody repertoire maturation in the opossum, Monodelphis domestica. PloS one 7: e45931.
47. Pillai S, Netravali IA, Cariappa A, Mattoo H (2012) Siglecs and immune regulation. Annual review of immunology 30: 357–392.
48. Vogt L, Schmitz N, Kurrer MO, Bauer M, Hinton HI, et al. (2006) VSIG4, a B7 family-related protein, is a negative regulator of T cell activation. The Journal of clinical investigation 116: 2817–2826.
49. Miller RD (2010) Those other mammals: the immunoglobulins and T cell receptors of marsupials and monotremes. Seminars in immunology 22: 3–9.
50. Duffy P, Wang X, Siegel CS, Tu N, Henkemeyer M, et al. (2012) Myelin-derived ephrinB3 restricts axonal regeneration and recovery after adult CNS injury. Proceedings of the National Academy of Sciences of the United States of America 109: 5063–5068.
51. Pernet V, Schwab ME (2012) The role of Nogo-A in axonal plasticity, regrowth and repair. Cell and tissue research 349: 97–104.
52. Goldshmit Y, Spanevello MD, Tajouri S, Li L, Rogers F, et al. (2011) EphA4 blockers promote axonal regeneration and functional recovery following spinal cord injury in mice. PloS one 6: e24636.
53. Hollis ER II, Zou Y (2012) Expression of the Wnt signaling system in central nervous system axon guidance and regeneration. Frontiers in molecular neuroscience 5: 5.
54. Goldshmit Y, Galea MP, Wise G, Bartlett PF, Turnley AM (2004) Axonal regeneration and lack of astrocytic gliosis in EphA4-deficient mice. J Neurosci 24: 10064–10073.
55. Cruz-Orengo L, Figueroa JD, Torrado A, Puig A, Whittemore SR, et al. (2007) Reduction of EphA4 receptor expression after spinal cord injury does not induce axonal regeneration or return of tcMMEP response. Neurosci Lett 418: 49–54.
56. Zhang J, Liu WL, Tang DC, Chen L, Wang M, et al. (2002) Identification and characterization of a novel member of olfactomedin-related protein family, hGC-1, expressed during myeloid lineage development. Gene 283: 83–93.
57. Liu W, Chen L, Zhu J, Rodgers GP (2006) The glycoprotein hGC-1 binds to cadherin and lectins. Experimental cell research 312: 1785–1797.
58. Kulkarni NH, Karavanich CA, Atchley WR, Anholt RR (2000) Characterization and differential expression of a human gene family of olfactomedin-related proteins. Genetical research 76: 41–50.
59. Liu W, Yan M, Liu Y, Wang R, Li C, et al. (2010) Olfactomedin 4 down-regulates innate immunity against Helicobacter pylori infection. Proceedings of the National Academy of Sciences of the United States of America 107: 11056–11061.
60. Xu J, Kim GM, Ahmed SH, Yan P, Xu XM, et al. (2001) Glucocorticoid receptor-mediated suppression of activator protein-1 activation and matrix metalloproteinase expression after spinal cord injury. The Journal of neuroscience: the official journal of the Society for Neuroscience 21: 92–97.
61. Buss A, Pech K, Kakulas BA, Martin D, Schoenen J, et al. (2007) Matrix metalloproteinases and their inhibitors in human traumatic spinal cord injury. BMC neurology 7: 17.
62. Zhang H, Adwanikar H, Werb Z, Noble-Haeusslein LJ (2010) Matrix metalloproteinases and neurotrauma: evolving roles in injury and reparative processes. The Neuroscientist: a review journal bringing neurobiology, neurology and psychiatry 16: 156–170.
63. Eva R, Andrews MR, Franssen EH, Fawcett JW (2012) Intrinsic mechanisms regulating axon regeneration: an integrin perspective. International review of neurobiology 106: 75–104.
64. Fleming JC, Bao F, Chen Y, Hamilton EF, Relton JK, et al. (2008) Alpha4beta1 integrin blockade after spinal cord injury decreases damage and improves neurological function. Experimental neurology 214: 147–159.
65. Hall A, Lalli G (2010) Rho and Ras GTPases in axon growth, guidance, and branching. Cold Spring Harbor perspectives in biology 2: a001818.
66. Redies C, Heyder J, Kohoutek T, Staes K, Van Roy F (2008) Expression of protocadherin-1 (Pcdh1) during mouse development. Developmental dynamics: an official publication of the American Association of Anatomists 237: 2496–2505.
67. Kubota F, Murakami T, Tajika Y, Yorifuji H (2008) Expression of protocadherin 18 in the CNS and pharyngeal arches of zebrafish embryos. The International journal of developmental biology 52: 397–405.
68. Lin J, Wang C, Redies C (2012) Expression of delta-protocadherins in the spinal cord of the chicken embryo. The Journal of comparative neurology 520: 1509–1531.
69. Biancheri R, Rosano C, Denegri L, Lamantea E, Pinto F, et al. (2013) Expanded spectrum of Pelizaeus-Merzbacher-like disease: literature revision and description of a novel GJC2 mutation in an unusually severe form. European journal of human genetics: EJHG 21: 34–39.
70. Isaksson J, Farooque M, Holtz A, Hillered L, Olsson Y (1999) Expression of ICAM-1 and CD11b after experimental spinal cord injury in rats. Journal of neurotrauma 16: 165–173.
71. Hamada Y, Ikata T, Katoh S, Nakauchi K, Niwa M, et al. (1996) Involvement of an intercellular adhesion molecule 1-dependent pathway in the pathogenesis of secondary changes after spinal cord injury in rats. Journal of neurochemistry 66: 1525–1531.
72. Hirokawa N, Niwa S, Tanaka Y (2010) Molecular motors in neurons: transport mechanisms and roles in brain function, development, and disease. Neuron 68: 610–638.
73. van den Berg R, Hoogenraad CC (2012) Molecular motors in cargo trafficking and synapse assembly. Advances in experimental medicine and biology 970: 173–196.
74. Kneussel M, Wagner W (2013) Myosin motors at neuronal synapses: drivers of membrane transport and actin dynamics. Nature reviews Neuroscience 14: 233–247.
75. Knudson CM, Stang KK, Moomaw CR, Slaughter CA, Campbell KP (1993) Primary structure and topological analysis of a skeletal muscle-specific junctional sarcoplasmic reticulum glycoprotein (triadin). The Journal of biological chemistry 268: 12646–12654.
76. Dulhunty A, Wei L, Beard N (2009) Junctin - the quiet achiever. The Journal of physiology 587: 3135–3137.
77. Li C, Dong S, Wang H, Hu Y (2011) Microarray analysis of gene expression changes in the brains of NR2B-induced memory-enhanced mice. Neuroscience 197: 121–131.
78. Seale SM, Feng Q, Agarwal AK, El-Alfy AT (2012) Neurobehavioral and transcriptional effects of acrylamide in juvenile rats. Pharmacology, biochemistry, and behavior 101: 77–84.
79. Dentice M, Bandyopadhyay A, Gereben B, Callebaut I, Christoffolete MA, et al. (2005) The Hedgehog-inducible ubiquitin ligase subunit WSB-1 modulates thyroid hormone activation and PTHrP secretion in the developing growth plate. Nature cell biology 7: 698–705.
80. Choi DW, Seo YM, Kim EA, Sung KS, Ahn JW, et al. (2008) Ubiquitination and degradation of homeodomain-interacting protein kinase 2 by WD40 repeat/SOCS box protein WSB-1. The Journal of biological chemistry 283: 4682–4689.
81. Ponyeam W, Hagen T (2012) Characterization of the Cullin7 E3 ubiquitin ligase—heterodimerization of cullin substrate receptors as a novel mechanism to regulate cullin E3 ligase activity. Cellular signalling 24: 290–295.
82. Dealy MJ, Nguyen KV, Lo J, Gstaiger M, Krek W, et al. (1999) Loss of Cul1 results in early embryonic lethality and dysregulation of cyclin E. Nature genetics 23: 245–248.
83. Singer JD, Gurian-West M, Clurman B, Roberts JM (1999) Cullin-3 targets cyclin E for ubiquitination and controls S phase in mammalian cells. Genes & development 13: 2375–2387.
84. Arai T, Kasper JS, Skaar JR, Ali SH, Takahashi C, et al. (2003) Targeted disruption of p185/Cul7 gene results in abnormal vascular morphogenesis. Proceedings of the National Academy of Sciences of the United States of America 100: 9855–9860.

85. Pei XH, Bai F, Li Z, Smith MD, Whitewolf G, et al. (2011) Cytoplasmic CUL9/PARC ubiquitin ligase is a tumor suppressor and promotes p53-dependent apoptosis. Cancer research 71: 2969–2977.
86. Tasaki T, Sohr R, Xia Z, Hellweg R, Hortnagl H, et al. (2007) Biochemical and genetic studies of UBR3, a ubiquitin ligase with a function in olfactory and other sensory systems. The Journal of biological chemistry 282: 18510–18520.
87. Seo JH, Zilber Y, Babayeva S, Liu J, Kyriakopoulos P, et al. (2011) Mutations in the planar cell polarity gene, Fuzzy, are associated with neural tube defects in humans. Human molecular genetics 20: 4324–4333.
88. Jungbluth S, Bell E, Lumsden A (1999) Specification of distinct motor neuron identities by the singular activities of individual Hox genes. Development 126: 2751–2758.
89. Yau TO, Kwan CT, Jakt LM, Stallwood N, Cordes S, et al. (2002) Auto/cross-regulation of Hoxb3 expression in posterior hindbrain and spinal cord. Developmental biology 252: 287–300.
90. Lin AW, Carpenter EM (2003) Hoxa10 and Hoxd10 coordinately regulate lumbar motor neuron patterning. Journal of neurobiology 56: 328–337.
91. Afjehi-Sadat L, Brejnikow M, Kang SU, Vishwanath V, Walder N, et al. (2010) Differential protein levels and post-translational modifications in spinal cord injury of the rat. Journal of proteome research 9: 1591–1597.
92. Xiao L, Ma ZL, Li X, Lin QX, Que HP, et al. (2005) cDNA microarray analysis of spinal cord injury and regeneration related genes in rat. Sheng li xue bao: [Acta physiologica Sinica] 57: 705–713.
93. Hu WH, Hausmann ON, Yan MS, Walters WM, Wong PK, et al. (2002) Identification and characterization of a novel Nogo-interacting mitochondrial protein (NIMP). Journal of neurochemistry 81: 36–45.
94. Zhu H, Santo A, Li Y (2012) The antioxidant enzyme peroxiredoxin and its protective role in neurological disorders. Experimental biology and medicine 237: 143–149.
95. Swisher JF, Khatri U, Feldman GM (2007) Annexin A2 is a soluble mediator of macrophage activation. Journal of leukocyte biology 82: 1174–1184.
96. Catania A (2008) Neuroprotective actions of melanocortins: a therapeutic opportunity. Trends in neurosciences 31: 353–360.
97. Iketani M, Iizuka A, Sengoku K, Kurihara Y, Nakamura F, et al. (2013) Regulation of neurite outgrowth mediated by localized phosphorylation of protein translational factor eEF2 in growth cones. Developmental neurobiology 73: 230–246.
98. McGraw J, Oschipok LW, Liu J, Hiebert GW, Mak CF, et al. (2004) Galectin-1 expression correlates with the regenerative potential of rubrospinal and spinal motoneurons. Neuroscience 128: 713–719.
99. McGraw J, Gaudet AD, Oschipok LW, Kadoya T, Horie H, et al. (2005) Regulation of neuronal and glial galectin-1 expression by peripheral and central axotomy of rat primary afferent neurons. Experimental neurology 195: 103–114.
100. Kurihara D, Ueno M, Tanaka T, Yamashita T (2010) Expression of galectin-1 in immune cells and glial cells after spinal cord injury. Neuroscience research 66: 265–270.
101. Lindquist S, Craig EA (1988) The heat-shock proteins. Annual review of genetics 22: 631–677.
102. Chen A, McEwen ML, Sun S, Ravikumar R, Springer JE (2010) Proteomic and phosphoproteomic analyses of the soluble fraction following acute spinal cord contusion in rats. Journal of neurotrauma 27: 263–274.
103. Yan X, Liu J, Luo Z, Ding Q, Mao X, et al. (2010) Proteomic profiling of proteins in rat spinal cord induced by contusion injury. Neurochemistry international 56: 971–983.
104. Reddy SJ, La Marca F, Park P (2008) The role of heat shock proteins in spinal cord injury. Neurosurgical focus 25: E4.
105. Daneman R, Zhou L, Agalliu D, Cahoy JD, Kaushal A, et al. (2010) The mouse blood-brain barrier transcriptome: a new resource for understanding the development and function of brain endothelial cells. PloS one 5: e13741.
106. Chatzipanteli K, Yanagawa Y, Marcillo AE, Kraydieh S, Yezierski RP, et al. (2000) Posttraumatic hypothermia reduces polymorphonuclear leukocyte accumulation following spinal cord injury in rats. Journal of neurotrauma 17: 321–332.
107. Kinoshita K, Chatzipanteli i K, Vitarbo E, Truettner JS, Alonso OF, et al. (2002) Interleukin-1beta messenger ribonucleic acid and protein levels after fluid-percussion brain injury in rats: importance of injury severity and brain temperature. Neurosurgery 51: 195–203; discussion 203.
108. Truettner JS, Alonso OF, Bramlett HM, Dietrich WD (2011) Therapeutic hypothermia alters microRNA responses to traumatic brain injury in rats. Journal of cerebral blood flow and metabolism: official journal of the International Society of Cerebral Blood Flow and Metabolism 31: 1897–1907.
109. Truettner JS, Suzuki T, Dietrich WD (2005) The effect of therapeutic hypothermia on the expression of inflammatory response genes following moderate traumatic brain injury in the rat. Brain research Molecular brain research 138: 124–134.
110. Kraus DB, Fadem BH (1987) Reproduction, development and physiology of the gray short-tailed opossum (Monodelphis domestica). Lab Anim Sci 37: 478–482.
111. Alexander JK, Popovich PG (2009) Neuroinflammation in spinal cord injury: therapeutic targets for neuroprotection and regeneration. Progress in brain research 175: 125–137.
112. Bethea JR, Dietrich WD (2002) Targeting the host inflammatory response in traumatic spinal cord injury. Current opinion in neurology 15: 355–360.
113. Fleming JC, Norenberg MD, Ramsay DA, Dekaban GA, Marcillo AE, et al. (2006) The cellular inflammatory response in human spinal cords after injury. Brain: a journal of neurology 129: 3249–3269.
114. Ek CJ, Habgood MD, Callaway JK, Dennis R, Dziegielewska KM, et al. (2010) Spatio-temporal progression of grey and white matter damage following contusion injury in rat spinal cord. PLoS One 5: e12021.
115. Ek CJ, Habgood MD, Dennis R, Dziegielewska KM, Mallard C, et al. (2012) Pathological changes in the white matter after spinal contusion injury in the rat. PloS one 7: e43484.
116. Veeravalli KK, Dasari VR, Rao JS (2012) Regulation of proteases after spinal cord injury. Journal of neurotrauma 29: 2251–2262.
117. Veeravalli KK, Dasari VR, Tsung AJ, Dinh DH, Gujrati M, et al. (2009) Human umbilical cord blood stem cells upregulate matrix metalloproteinase-2 in rats after spinal cord injury. Neurobiology of disease 36: 200–212.
118. Nakaya N, Sultana A, Lee HS, Tomarev SI (2012) Olfactomedin 1 interacts with the Nogo A receptor complex to regulate axon growth. The Journal of biological chemistry 287: 37171–37184.
119. Gardiner NJ (2011) Integrins and the extracellular matrix: key mediators of development and regeneration of the sensory nervous system. Developmental neurobiology 71: 1054–1072.
120. Kobayashi NR, Fan DP, Giehl KM, Bedard AM, Wiegand SJ, et al. (1997) BDNF and NT-4/5 prevent atrophy of rat rubrospinal neurons after cervical axotomy, stimulate GAP-43 and Talpha1-tubulin mRNA expression, and promote axonal regeneration. The Journal of neuroscience: the official journal of the Society for Neuroscience 17: 9583–9595.
121. Ramon y Cajal S (1928) Degeneration and regeneration of the nervous system. May RM, translator; De Felipe J, Jones EG, editors: Oxford University Press.

7

Stem Cell Therapy and Curcumin Synergistically Enhance Recovery from Spinal Cord Injury

D. Ryan Ormond[1], Craig Shannon[1], Julius Oppenheim[1], Richard Zeman[2], Kaushik Das[1], Raj Murali[1], Meena Jhanwar-Uniyal[1]*

1 Department of Neurosurgery, New York Medical College, Valhalla, New York, United States of America, **2** Department of Cell Biology and Anatomy, New York Medical College, Valhalla, New York, United States of America

Abstract

Acute traumatic spinal cord injury (SCI) is marked by the enhanced production of local cytokines and pro-inflammatory substances that induce gliosis and prevent reinnervation. The transplantation of stem cells is a promising treatment strategy for SCI. In order to facilitate functional recovery, we employed stem cell therapy alone or in combination with curcumin, a naturally-occurring anti-inflammatory component of turmeric (*Curcuma longa*), which potently inhibits NF-κB. Spinal cord contusion following laminectomy (T9–10) was performed using a weight drop apparatus (10 g over a 12.5 or 25 mm distance, representing moderate or severe SCI, respectively) in Sprague-Dawley rats. Neural stem cells (NSC) were isolated from subventricular zone (SVZ) and transplanted at the site of injury with or without curcumin treatment. Functional recovery was assessed by BBB score and body weight gain measured up to 6 weeks following SCI. At the conclusion of the study, the mass of soleus muscle was correlated with BBB score and body weight. Stem cell therapy improved recovery from moderate SCI, however, it had a limited effect on recovery after severe SCI. Curcumin stimulated NSC proliferation *in vitro*, and in combination with stem cell therapy, induced profound recovery from severe SCI as evidenced by improved functional locomotor recovery, increased body weight, and soleus muscle mass. These findings demonstrate that curcumin in conjunction with stem cell therapy synergistically improves recovery from severe SCI. Furthermore, our results indicate that the effect of curcumin extends beyond its known anti-inflammatory properties to the regulation of stem cell proliferation.

Editor: Cesar V. Borlongan, University of South Florida, United States of America

Funding: This work was funded from the American Association of Neurological Surgeons NREF/Medtronic Research Fellowship grant. The funders had no role in study design, data collection and analysis, decision to publish, or preparation of the manuscript.

Competing Interests: The authors have declared that no competing interests exist.

* E-mail: meena_jhanwar@nymc.edu

Introduction

Acute traumatic spinal cord injury (SCI) occurs at an estimated annual incidence of 15–40 cases per million [1]. The prevalence of SCI is estimated at 1.275 million people (0.4% of the population) in the United States alone [2]. Much of the morbidity associated with SCI occurs due to the limited intrinsic ability of the spinal cord to recover following transection or contusion. The pathophysiology of SCI is considered biphasic in nature. Primary injury results from mechanical force injuring the spinal cord, tearing axons, blood vessels, and causing cell membrane disruption. Secondary injury occurs via the subsequent edema, ischemia, inflammation, cytokine production, free radical damage, glial scar formation, apoptosis and necrosis that ensue. Perilesional astrocytes alter their phenotype and over the weeks following SCI form the glial scar composed of astrocytes and a dense extracellular matrix [3]. Therapeutic modalities that promote recovery could be better understood by elucidating the pathophysiology of SCI. Necrosis, apoptosis, and inflammation play critical roles in defining neuronal cell death and formation of the glial scar implicated in limiting SCI recovery. In addition, secreted inflammatory cytokines and growth factors generally up-regulate pro-survival molecules, such as NF-κB [4]. Thus, the major hurdles in complete recovery from SCI are mostly due to the upregulation of certain inflammatory molecules after injury that result in gliosis. Curcumin (diferuloylmethane), the active ingredient in turmeric (*Curcuma longa*), is a highly pleiotropic molecule with potent anti-inflammatory properties. The pleiotropic activities attributed to curcumin because of its chemical structure appear to influence multiple signaling pathways activated in SCI [5,6,7]. Some of these signaling pathways include phospholipase, lipooxygenase, cyclooxygenase 2, leukotrienes, thromboxane, prostaglandins, nitric oxide, collagenase, elastase, hyaluronidase, monocyte chemoattractant protein-1 (MCP-1), interferon-inducible protein, tumor necrosis factor (TNF), interleukin-12 (IL-12), and NF-κB [6,7,8]. It has also been shown to reduce the inflammatory cascade and may help prevent plaque deposition and protein oxidation in neurodegenerative conditions [6]. Curcumin's benefits in SCI have been recently reported in the literature, and this benefit may be due to a reduction in secondary injury to the spinal cord [9–16]. Furthermore, a study using curcumin with other dietary compounds showed enhancement of sensorimotor function, especially after exercise [15]. This suggests that curcumin added to the diet has a beneficial effect on recovery. In addition, the molecular mechanism underlying curcumin as a dietary supplement with Omega-3 fatty acids (DHA) has suggested that secondary injury can be prevented with such a treatment [16].

Stem cell therapies offer a promising way to replace neurons and oligodendrocytes lost to necrosis or apoptosis, help remyelinate axons, and increase the availability of neurotrophic factors to aid in local recovery [17–26]. Furthermore, stem cell therapy provides support to the surrounding milieu after injury to enhance axonal regeneration and/or neuroprotection. Transplantation of *in vitro* expanded NSC into rat spinal cord after contusion injury induced their differentiation into neurons or oligodendrocytes, and promoted functional recovery of limb movement [23,26]. Also, restoration of neurotrophic factors seen in stem cells may aid in supporting the surrounding milieu after injury in order to enhance axonal regeneration and neuroprotection [27]. Stem cell therapy has been explored in animal models as an aid to recovery following SCI. Curcumin, a potent anti-inflammatory compound, has been shown to improve functional recovery from SCI [5–14]. However the use of curcumin with stem cell therapy has not been well defined. The purpose of this study is to investigate stem cell therapy with or without curcumin in treatment of moderate as well as severe SCI. Herein we provide evidence that the combined use of stem cell therapy with curcumin aid in recovery after thoracic SCI in an animal model.

Materials and Methods

Animals

Animal work was performed with the approval of the New York Medical College IACUC under approval number: 137-1-1210.1. Adult female Sprague-Dawley rats (200–250 grams; Charles River, Troy, NY) were maintained on a routine 12:12 hour light/dark cycle with *ad libitum* access to food and water. The main purpose of using female rats in this study was that one of the common sequelae of SCI is neurogenic bladder. This results in overflow incontinence and loss of voluntary bladder control. Bladder distention and subsequent rupture is more common, and has a higher mortality rate, in males.

Neural Stem Cells

NSC were extracted from the subventricular zone (SVZ) of female Sprague-Dawley rat brains (Fig. 1A). Brain was removed following craniectomy from a euthanized animal and was placed in dissecting media. Brain was sectioned in multiple coronal sections approximately 3–4 microns thick rostral to the optic chiasm. The SVZ area was microdissected using the micropunch technique described previously [28] and areas micropunched as shown in Fig. 1A. The microdissected specimens were then digested using an enzyme digestion solution for 1–3 hrs at 37°C in a water bath. Following enzymatic digestion, the cells were resuspended in a specialized serum-free stem cell media containing growth factors such as epidermal growth factor, fibroblast growth factor, etc., and plated onto 12-well plates. The cells were incubated at 37°C in a 5% CO_2 chamber. Neurospheres formed in 5–6 days and the expansion was performed as previously described [29]. Neurospheres were stained for the stem cell marker nanog for authenticity, as shown in Fig. 1C.

Effect of Curcumin on Stem Cell Proliferation (*in Vitro*)

NSC were grown in stem cell media in the presence or absence of curcumin (500 nM or 1 uM). DMSO treated NSCs were used as controls. After 24 hours, neurosphere proliferation was determined by measuring the diameter of each neurosphere.

Spinal Cord Injury

Surgery was performed as described previously [14,30–32]. Briefly, aseptic T9–T10 laminectomy under anesthesia (pentobarbital sodium; dose 50–80 mg/kg IP; Hospira, Lake Forest, IL) was performed. Spinal cord contusion was induced using a weight-drop apparatus, where a guided 10 g rod was dropped 12.5 or 25 mm onto the exposed dura mater, representing moderate or severe SCI, respectively. Following contusion, the incision was closed with wound clips. The rats received 0.02% amoxicillin in the drinking water to prevent infection throughout the duration of the experiment. Body temperature of 37°C during anesthesia was maintained by a temperature-controlled heating pad and recorded with a rectal thermometer. During the recovery, urine was expressed manually twice daily to assist in urination until intrinsic function returned to normal.

Stem Cell Transplant

Rats in the stem cell treatment group underwent repeat surgery one week after injury. Under pentobarbital anesthesia (as described above) and sterile conditions, the original incision was reopened and the dura overlying the site of contusion was exposed. 1×10^6 neural stem cells in 20 ul of sterile PBS were then microinjected directly into the injured spinal cord. Stem cell injections were performed manually over ten minutes using a 30-guage needle. Injections were performed 1 mm into the spinal cord at the site of contusion injury. The incision was then closed in layers.

Treatments

Rats were randomized into the 3 (moderate SCI) or 4 (Severe SCI) treatment groups as shown in Table 1. The schemas of treatments/protocols for moderate or severe SCI used in this study are described in Fig. 1A.

Moderate SCI. Within 30 minutes following the contusion, rats were given either curcumin (60 mg/ml/kg BW in DMSO), or DMSO (1 ml/kg BW) via percutaneous, intramuscular injection near the site of injury. These injections were continued weekly for six weeks. Stem cell transplantation occurred one week following injury via direct injection into the spinal cord at the site of injury as described above. Rats were given either NSC or combinational treatment (NSC+curcumin) (Fig. 1A). Rats were given curcumin alone following this same protocol in a study previously reported by our laboratory [14].

Severe SCI. Within 30 minutes following the contusion, rats were given either curcumin (60 mg/ml/kg BW in DMSO), or DMSO (1 ml/kg BW) via percutaneous-intramuscular injection at the site of injury. Rats were given NSC, curcumin, or combinational treatment (NSC+curcumin). Rats given curcumin monotherapy continued to receive weekly injections at 60 mg/ml/kg BW in DMSO. Rats given stem cell transplant, following the initial dose of DMSO or high dose curcumin (60 mg/ml/kg in DMSO), then received daily IP injections of low dose curcumin (0.5 mmol/ml/kg BW), or an equivalent dose of DMSO alone, for two weeks following stem cell transplant. Stem cell transplant occurred one week following SCI.

Basso, Beattie and Bresnahan Score

Functional tests were performed before the injury and then weekly after the treatment. Locomotor activity was evaluated using the Basso, Beattie and Bresnahan (BBB) scores for hindlimb rat motor function and was recorded weekly [33]. Testing involved placing the rat on a large open field where a natural aversion to open spaces forced the rat to move towards the edges of the field.

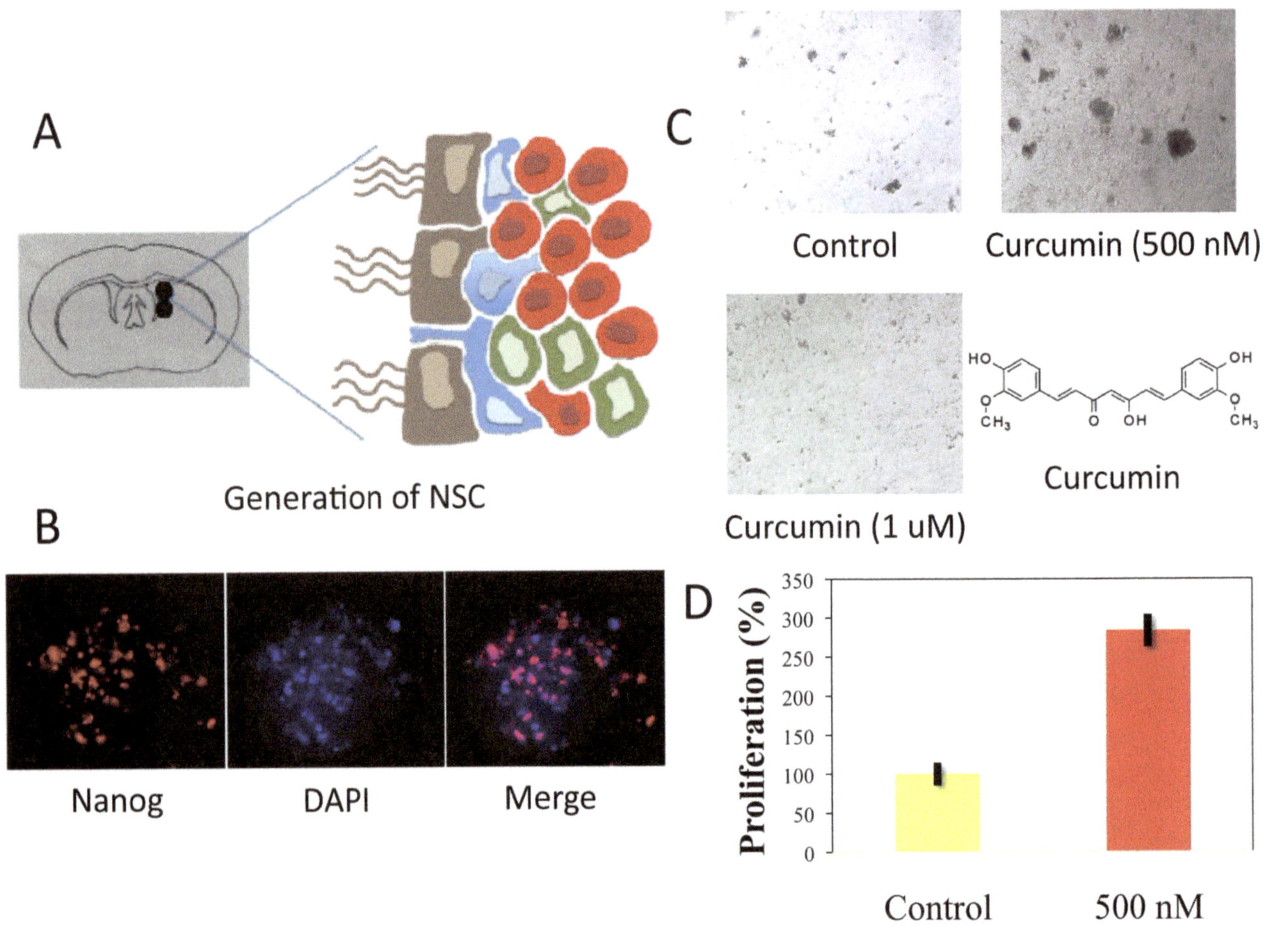

Figure 1. Curcumin enhances stem cell proliferation of NSC derived from SVZ in low doses, however it induces apoptosis at high doses. A: Schematic presentation of treatments timeline used in moderate and severe SCI. **B:** Micropunched area of the subventricular zone (SVZ), depicting the presence of ependymal cells (brown), astrocytes (blue), transit amplifying cells (green) and neuroblasts (red). **C:** Immunofluorescence analysis demonstrates the presence of stem cell marker nanog in neurospheres and DAPI staining for DNA. **D, E:** Effect of curcumin on neurosphere formation. At a low concentration of 500 nM, curcumin treatment stimulated proliferation of NSC in 24 hr. At higher concentrations (1 uM), curcumin caused autolysis and neurosphere fragmentation. The chemical structure of curcumin is also displayed.

Two independent blinded examiners observed hind-limb movements and assessed the rats' locomotor function [33]. Rats that demonstrated any functional recovery of limb movement within 72 hours of contusion injury were excluded from the study, allowing a more uniform cohort [33]. Rats falling more than two standard deviations above or below the mean were excluded from final statistical review. Data used for analysis included both left and right limb movements, which were recorded separately, but averaged in the final analysis. Body weight was also recorded weekly.

Table 1. Experimental cohorts: number of animals per cohort.

SCI severity	Control (DMSO)	Curcumin	NSC	NSC+Curcumin
Moderate	6	*	7	6
Severe	12	10	9	13

*Published [14].

Soleus Muscle Dissection

After 6 weeks, rats were sacrificed under pentobarbital anesthesia (100 mg/kg IP), and were then perfused with formalin prior to dissection. Perfusion fixation occurred in the following manner: a 5 cm incision rostral to caudal down the sternum was made followed by a 3 cm incision medial to lateral in order to cut the diaphragm. Afterwards, a needle attached to a vacuum-pump system was inserted through the apex of the left ventricle into the ascending aorta whereby formalin fixative was perfused into the rodent. Following fixation, a 1 cm incision was made in both posterior hindlimbs to retrieve soleus muscles. First, the Achilles' tendon was dissected out, and then the gastrocnemius muscle was elevated to expose the soleus muscle. This was identified, removed *en bloc*, and the weight of each soleus muscle was separately recorded, and averaged for final analysis.

Histopathological Analysis

Spinal cords at the region of injury were fixed in formalin and placed in paraffin blocks. Six μm axial sections were cut and placed onto the slides. The sections were then stained with Lox Blue staining. Spinal cord atrophy was evaluated by determining the epicenter using an Axiovert Zeiss microscope (Carl Zeiss

Microscopy, Thornwood, New York) with the AxioVision software. The spinal cord photographs were then measured utilizing ImageJ software to determine the spared tissue area as well as total spinal cord area. The peak contusion site (epicenter) was recorded as the area with the least amount of spared spinal cord tissue. Five different measurements were taken for each rat, which included one for the epicenter and two from either side of the epicenter (cranial and caudal). Total spinal cord values were also recorded for each section, and percentage of spared area in relation to total area was used for final analysis. The presented values are an average for each rat ± SEM (standard error of the mean).

Statistical Analysis

Data are presented as a mean ±SEM. BBB scores and body weight were analyzed by two-way analysis of variance (2-ANOVA) between groups over time followed by two-tailed t-test. Soleus muscle was analyzed using the two-tailed t-test. A correlation between the BBB scores and body weight and between BBB score and soleus muscle weight was established using the Pearson method. Statistical significance was determined at $p \leq 0.05$. For histopathological analysis, the statistical analysis was done using the two-tail T-test between DMSO treated versus other treatments individually.

Results

The Effect of Curcumin on NSC Proliferation

The effect of curcumin on NSC proliferation was examined in a cell culture model. NSC, as represented by neurospheres and staining positive with nanog, were grown in stem cell media in the presence or absence of curcumin. At a low concentration, curcumin (500 nM) caused a significant increase in neurosphere proliferation by over 180% in comparison to control. However, curcumin at higher doses (1 uM) caused widespread apoptosis and neurosphere fragmentation (Fig. 1 D, E).

BBB Score after Moderate SCI

Animals undergoing NSC transplant, or with combined treatment using NSC+curcumin, were tested after moderate SCI. Rats treated with NSC transplant demonstrated a significant improvement starting at week three. A significant difference in BBB score between cohorts was seen with the scores of 12.14±0.65 and 9.33±0.99 ($p = 0.028$) at week five and 12.86±0.93 and 9.67±1.02($p = 0.029$) at week six, for NSC treated and control rats, respectively. Combinational treatment with high dose curcumin and NSC transplant significantly improved the BBB score as compared to control. However, between combinational treatment and NSC alone, there was no noticeable difference in improvement based on BBB score (Fig. 2A). Curcumin monotherapy showed significant improvement in recovery from SCI in comparison to control, as we have previously reported [14].

BBB Score after Severe SCI

Curcumin and NSC treatment demonstrated similar results, in that they both initially demonstrated significant improvement at week two, but this significance was lost through the remainder of the experiment in comparison to controls (Fig. 2B). Rats undergoing combined NSC transplantation and curcumin showed consistent significant improvement in BBB score as compared to controls. This improvement began at week one, where BBB scores were 1.15±0.33 vs. 0.33±0.19 for combinational treatment and control, respectively ($p = 0.037$), and persisted through week six. While control rats continued to show some improvement over time, the combined NSC/curcumin cohort displayed more rapid and elevated BBB scores in comparison to controls. In fact, by week six, animals continued this significant difference with BBB scores of 8.81±0.82 and 4.75±0.78, for combinational treatment and control, respectively ($p = 0.0001$). Statistical analysis of combined NSC/curcumin treatment also demonstrated significant improvement in comparison to NSC or curcumin treatment alone.

Body Weight Gain after Moderate SCI

Weekly body weight is presented as a percent change from initial body weight recorded immediately prior to SCI. Many animals initially lost weight after SCI, but then began to increase in weight in a manner that often correlated with recovery. Body weight gain became statistically significant in NSC treated rats at week three and remained significant through week 5 (Fig. 3A). Combined treatment of NSC and curcumin in high doses after moderate SCI showed no statistically significant benefit in body weight gain in comparison to control. Correlation analysis once weight gain resumed (starting week two) demonstrated a linear relationship between BBB score and body weight after moderate SCI (Fig. 3B), suggesting a strong correlation between body weight gain and BBB score.

Body Weight Gain after Severe SCI

Weekly body weight changes are presented in Figure 3C, where the initial values are set equal to 100, as recorded at the time of contusion. All rats showed a decrease in body weight at week one, as expected, immediately following injury. Combinational treatment showed significance in comparison to control by week five ($p = 0.029$), curcumin alone showed a trend toward significance ($p = 0.20$), and NSC treatment showed no significance ($p = 0.55$). Correlation analysis demonstrated a linear relationship between body weight gain after week one in comparison to BBB score (Fig. 4D).

Soleus Muscle Mass after Moderate SCI

Soleus muscle weight (mg) was taken at the conclusion of the experiment. Values are reported as a percentage of the control = 100 (see Fig. 4). Rats treated after moderate SCI were not significantly different across cohorts (Fig. 4A). However, NSC treated rats showed higher soleus muscle weight in comparison to control or combined treatment. Specifically, rats had a soleus muscle weight of 100±6.01, 107.12±7.95, and 101.58±13.52 for control, NSC, and combined groups, respectively ($p = 0.48$ and $p = 0.92$ for NSC and combinational groups, respectively). Soleus muscle weight correlated with BBB score, implying that higher soleus muscle weight was associated with higher BBB score (Fig. 4B).

Soleus Muscle Mass after Severe SCI

After severe SCI, control animals had a soleus muscle weight of 100±7.09. Soleus muscle weight was higher in all groups in comparison to control, but only reached significance in the combined treatment cohort. Curcumin had a soleus muscle weight of 105.3±9.46. NSC transplant animals had a soleus weight of 115.54±8.51. Combinational therapy produced a soleus weight of 125.86±5.09. Importantly, soleus muscle weight was significantly better in combined treatment (NSC+curcumin) in comparison to control or in comparison to curcumin or NSC cohorts ($p = 0.005$, 0.03, and 0.046, respectively) (Fig. 4C). Correlation analysis demonstrated a linear relationship between BBB score and soleus

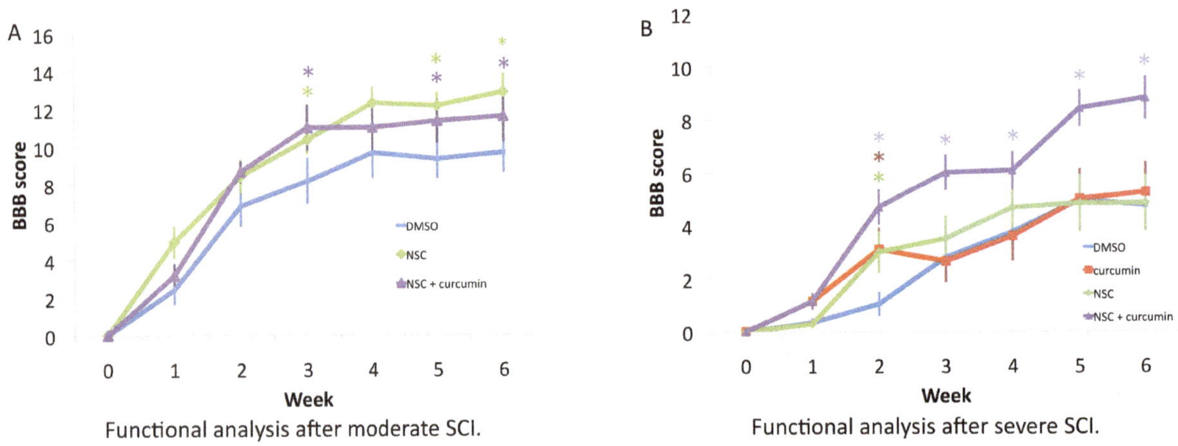

Figure 2. Stem cell therapy in conjunction with low-dose curcumin had a synergistic effect in recovery from severe SCI, as demonstrated by improved BBB score. A: Functional analysis (BBB) after moderate SCI showed that stem cell therapy with a high dose of curcumin rendered BBB scores, which were statistically significant as compared to control rats (DMSO), starting from week 3. **B:** In severe SCI, rats undergoing combined NSC transplantation and curcumin showed consistent improvement in BBB score as compared to DMSO treated controls. Statistical analysis of combined NSC+curcumin treatment also demonstrated significant improvement in comparison to NSC or curcumin treatment alone.

weight (Fig. 4D), demonstrating that the groups showing the most improved BBB score had the greatest soleus muscle mass.

Histopathological Analysis (Severe SCI)

Spared tissue in relation to the total area of NSC+Curcumin-, Curcumin-, and NSC-treated rats were presented along with control rats treated with DMSO (Fig. 5A). The rats treated with NSC+Curcumin and NSC monotherapy-treated rats showed better recovery as shown by the spared as compared to the total area.

The statistical analysis using the One Way ANOVA and post test analysis demonstrated no significant difference between the groups ($F(3,16) = 1.19$; NS), however, it should be noted that curcumin treated rats had the least spared area of the total area as shown in Fig. 5B.

Discussion

The data presented here demonstrate that NSC transplantation with curcumin synergistically enhanced recovery from severe SCI in a rat model. Recovery from SCI was demonstrated by improvement in parameters including BBB score, body weight, and soleus muscle weight. Stem cell therapies have been shown to be a promising way to regenerate neurons and oligodendrocytes lost during SCI, and have demonstrated efficacy in multiple animal studies [21–23,26,27]. This is an emerging field in spinal cord injury research, with several human studies currently being conducted worldwide [34]. Our findings differentiate the beneficial effects of NSC transplant by severity of injury. Although NSC treatment alone was sufficient to induce statistically significant recovery after moderate SCI, it could not induce significant recovery after severe injury except in combination with curcumin.

The rationale behind combinational therapy using stem cells and curcumin originates from the idea that curcumin, an anti-inflammatory compound, could reduce gliosis, while stem cells aid in reinervation by increasing the availability of neurotrophic factors at the site of injury. In addition, stem cells may also contribute oligodendrocytes, glia, and neurons to aid in recovery [21,22,23,26,27]. We have previously demonstrated the benefit of curcumin in moderate SCI where curcumin-treated rats showed marked improvement in functional recovery as early as the first week [14]. Consistently, this study demonstrated that after severe SCI there also was an initial benefit using curcumin. However, this effect was unsustained beyond week two (Fig. 3). Interestingly, combined stem cell treatment with low dose curcumin (0.5 mM/IP daily) significantly improved functional recovery starting from week 2, resulting in many animals recovering to weight bearing status even after severe SCI (Fig. 2B). It should be noted here that this effect of curcumin with stem cell transplant might not be attributable to its anti-inflammatory effect alone. A recent study demonstrated that low dose curcumin treatment increased the number of BrdU-labeled cells in mouse hippocampus, suggesting an enhanced proliferative effect *in vitro*, as well as *in vivo* [35]. Consistent with these findings, we observed curcumin in low doses induced stem cell proliferation *in vitro* (Fig. 1D). Curcumin, however, in higher doses (1 uM) caused apoptosis of stem cells. This proliferative effect may be one reason there is a synergistic effect of combinational treatment on SCI recovery. The lack of benefit of high dose curcumin in combination with stem cell transplant in the moderate injury cohort may also be explained by these findings, where the NSC+high dose curcumin cohort recovered less well than NSC treatment alone (Fig. 3A). Thus, it is possible that curcumin may not only aid the local cellular microenvironment, but also cause proliferation of transplanted stem cells in low doses.

Body weight and soleus muscle weight were used as surrogate markers of recovery following moderate or severe SCI. There was a decrease in body weight during the first week following SCI, however an increase in body weight began starting the second week in a manner that often correlated with functional recovery [14,30–33]. Combinational treatment with curcumin in high doses also demonstrated similar results after moderate injury, and did not significantly differ from controls. Combinational treatment improved body weight gain in a statistically significant manner following severe SCI. These data all correlate well with BBB score findings. Soleus muscle weight has also been used in previous studies as a surrogate marker of recovery of hindlimb motor function [14,30–33]. Following SCI, muscle atrophy is more pronounced in paralyzed muscles that contain a large proportion of slow fatigue-resistant muscle fibers, such as the soleus muscle,

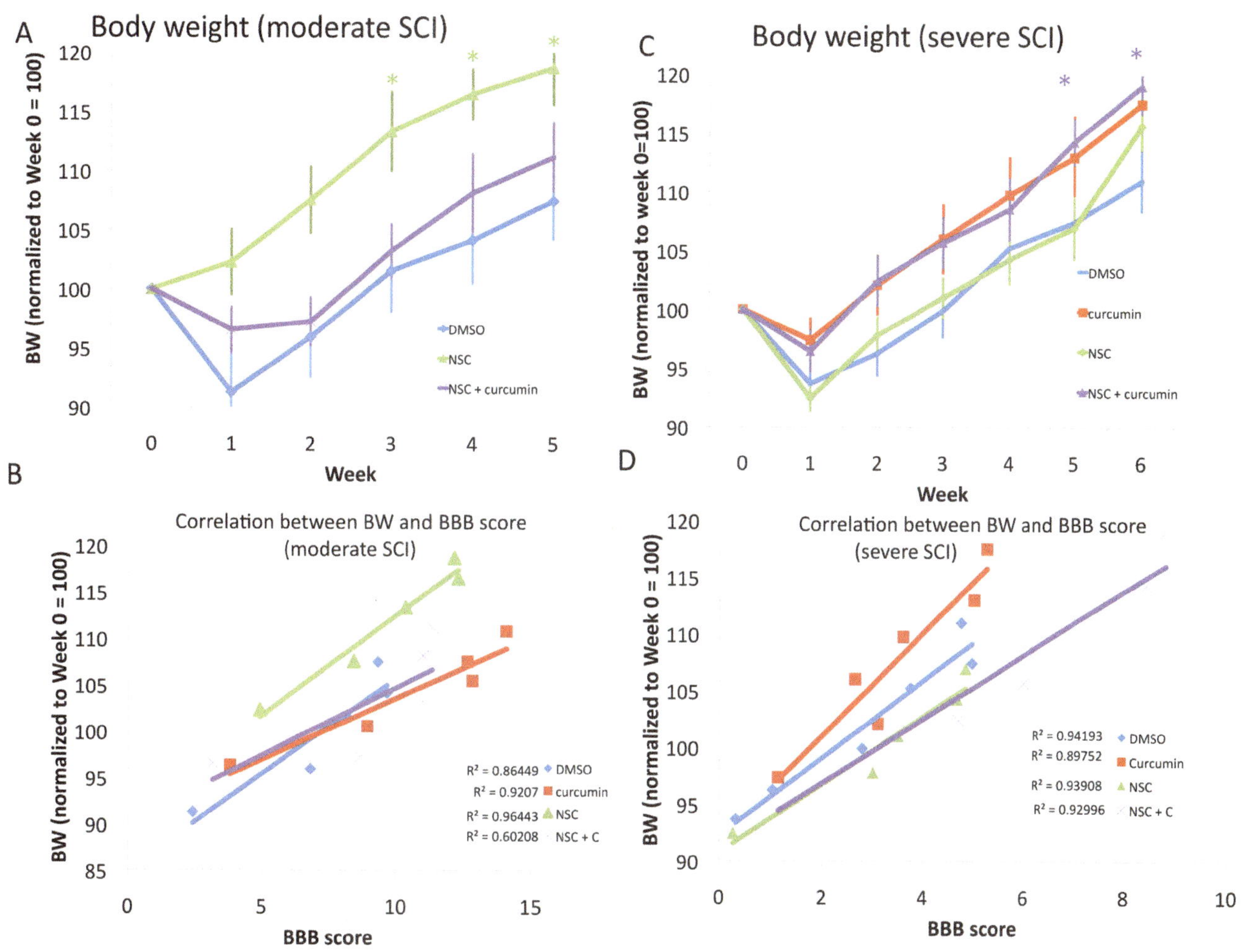

Figure 3. Stem cell therapy in conjunction with curcumin synergistically improves recovery from moderate or severe SCI, as demonstrated by improved body weight gain, which correlated with BBB score. A: Stem cell transplanted animals showed improved body weight gain in comparison to combinational treatment or DMSO treated controls. **B:** A positive correlation exists between body weight gain and improved BBB score in moderate SCI. R^2 values are listed next to their respective cohort. **C:** Combination of NSC therapy with curcumin treatment showed significant improvement in body weight gain in comparison to DMSO control. Curcumin treated rats showed a trend toward significance in BW gain. **D:** Correlation of BBB scores with body weight after severe SCI. R^2 values are listed next to their respective cohort.

that are largely responsible for maintaining posture and bearing weight [36]. Therefore, soleus muscle atrophies more quickly and recovers more slowly than other hindlimb muscles [37]. It also is anatomically simple to isolate and remove completely for assessing its mass [14,30–33,46]. Additionally, functional recovery following SCI, frequently measured by the BBB score, has been positively correlated to soleus muscle changes including improvement in muscle mass, MRI T2 changes, electrophysiological testing parameters, and a change in the proportion of slow Type 1 fibers [14,30–33,36–40]. This implies that enhanced locomotor activity leads to an improvement in muscle mass. In our study, soleus muscle mass also demonstrated improvement in stem cell transplanted animals after severe SCI in a statistically significant manner (Fig. 5). Correlation data also demonstrated significant correlation between BBB score and soleus muscle mass or body weight, adding credibility to the findings of significant synergistic improvement after severe SCI (Fig. 4–5).

Histopathology data somewhat correlated with functional outcomes. Combined treatment, with the best functional outcome, also had the largest spared tissue. NSC transplant monotherapy also fared better than control, although functional outcomes were not significantly different. Of note, curcumin monotherapy had the least spared tissue among the severe SCI cohorts, but functionally showed similar outcomes to control and NSC transplant alone. It should be emphasized that multiple previous studies have found no relation between functional outcome and the amount of spared tissue at the site of injury [42–44]. In general, these data serve to corroborate findings of BBB score, body weight, and soleus muscle weight, supporting the conclusion that improved functional outcomes have a physiologic correlation.

Various types of stem cells have been used for transplantation after SCI. These cell types most commonly include embryonic and adult NSC, fate-restricted neural-glial precursor cells, olfactory ensheathing glial cells, Schwann cells, mesenchymal stem cells, and bone-marrow stromal cells [20]. Adult NSC have been previously characterized in mammalian brain, and are abundant in the SVZ and dentate gyrus [27,45–48]. Endogenous NSC have even been found to exist in the spinal cord, although oligodendrocyte differentiation of these cells has not proven sufficient to promote remyelination after SCI [21–23,47]. This remains true even following infusion of exogenous growth factors [49–50]. More recently, however, studies have provided evidence of

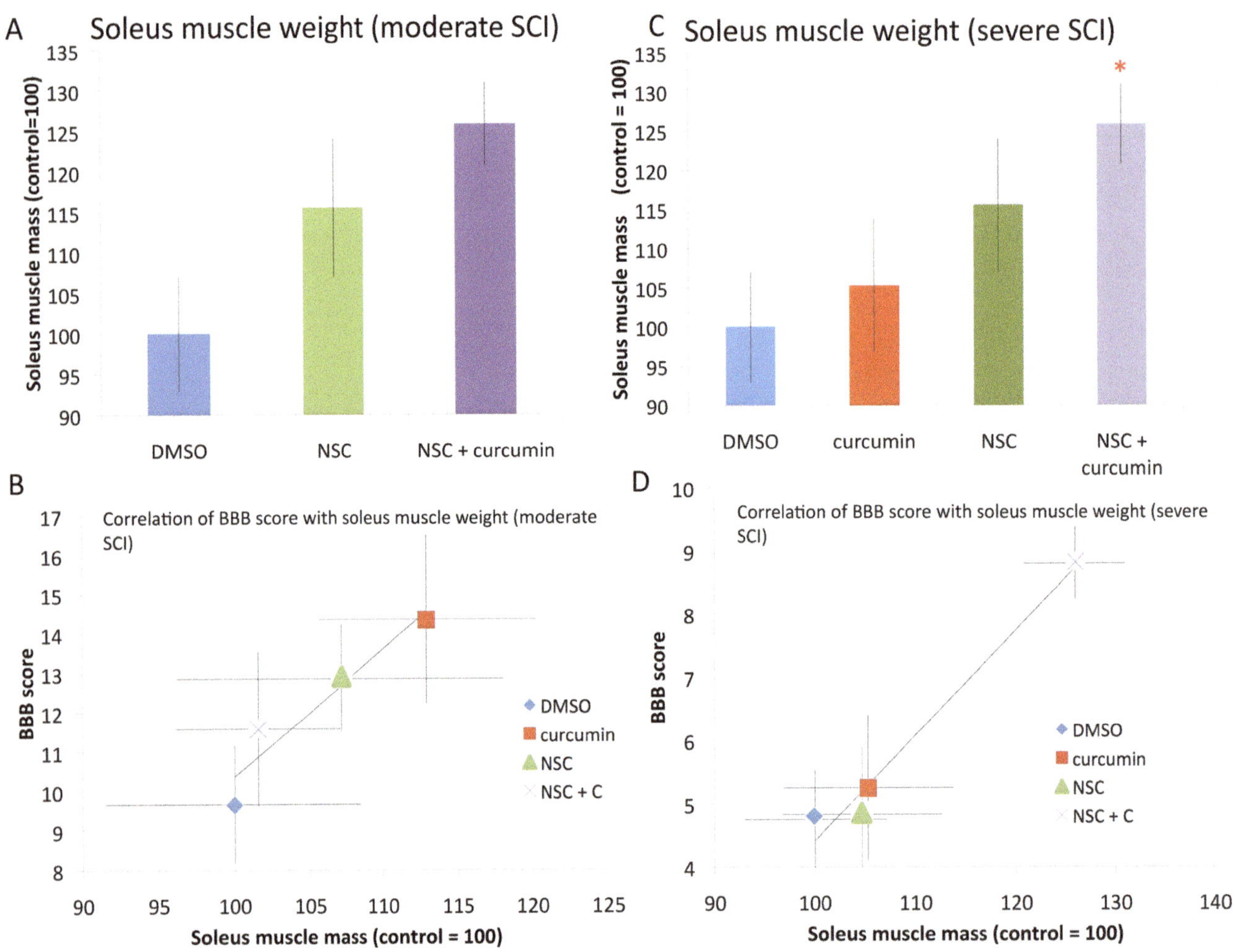

Figure 4. Soleus muscle weight as an indicator of recovery after moderate and severe SCI, and correlated with BBB score. A: Rats with greater recovery of hindlimb motor function have better soleus muscle weight at necropsy. While stem cell transplanted animals and combinational treatments had improved soleus muscle weight in comparison to DMSO controls, this did not reach statistical significance. **B:** Correlation of BBB score with soleus muscle weight after moderate SCI demonstrates strong correlation (0.97). Values presented are mean ± SEM. $*p<0.05$. **C:** Soleus muscle weight after severe SCI showed that all cohorts had larger soleus muscle mass compared to DMSO treated controls, however curcumin or stem cell monotherapy showed only a trend towards significance. NSC plus curcumin treatment improved soleus muscle weight significantly in comparison to DMSO controls. **D:** Correlation of BBB score with soleus muscle weight after severe SCI demonstrated a strong correlation ($r^2=0.91$). Values presented are mean ± SEM. $*p<0.05$.

functional motor recovery after transplantation of ependymal stem progenitor cells that were derived from adult rat spinal cord with a traumatic lesion [51]. In this study, cells were propagated and differentiated *in vitro* into oligodendrocyte precursor cells (OPCs) and engrafted after cell transplantation. Endogenous or transplanted NSCs can differentiate into oligodendrocytes and astrocytes, contributing to remyelination of axons and aiding in recovery [52]. While recruitment of these endogenous NSCs can occur as a part of spontaneous recovery, transplantation of NSCs provides an improved strategy for a faster and better recovery after SCI.

Adult neural stem cells are most commonly derived from the SVZ of the brain and have been found to differentiate to neurons, glia, and oligodendrocytes, although neuronal marker expression is generally rare [20]. This may be due to the local microenvironment at the site of injury, that may affect the differentiation of transplanted NSC. These adult NSC have been found to generate compact myelin in the injured spinal cord, although this has been somewhat inconsistently reported [20–23]. The choice of using adult NSC is due to their decreased risk of tumorigenesis [20–22], their ability to differentiate along a neural lineage with great consistency [18,20–23,26,53,54], and their repeated benefit to recovery using a thoracic contusion model with behavioral recovery evaluated with the open field BBB score [21–23,55–57]. All but one of these studies delivered stem cells directly to the injured spinal cord, similar to what was performed in this study [20,56].

Secondary damage to the spinal cord following SCI is induced primarily by inflammation and ischemia/reperfusion injury. White matter is especially susceptible to ischemic damage, especially by lipid peroxidation [58,59]. Oligodendrocytes are also vulnerable to superoxide produced during ischemia because these cells only contain low levels of superoxide antagonists like Mu-superoxide and catalase [58,60]. Apoptosis also occurs due, in part at least, to the inflammatory cascade, influx of calcium, and the activation of the caspase cascade [58,61,62]. A number of agents have been used to reduce ischemia/reperfusion injury to the spinal cord with varying degrees of success including statins, calcium channel

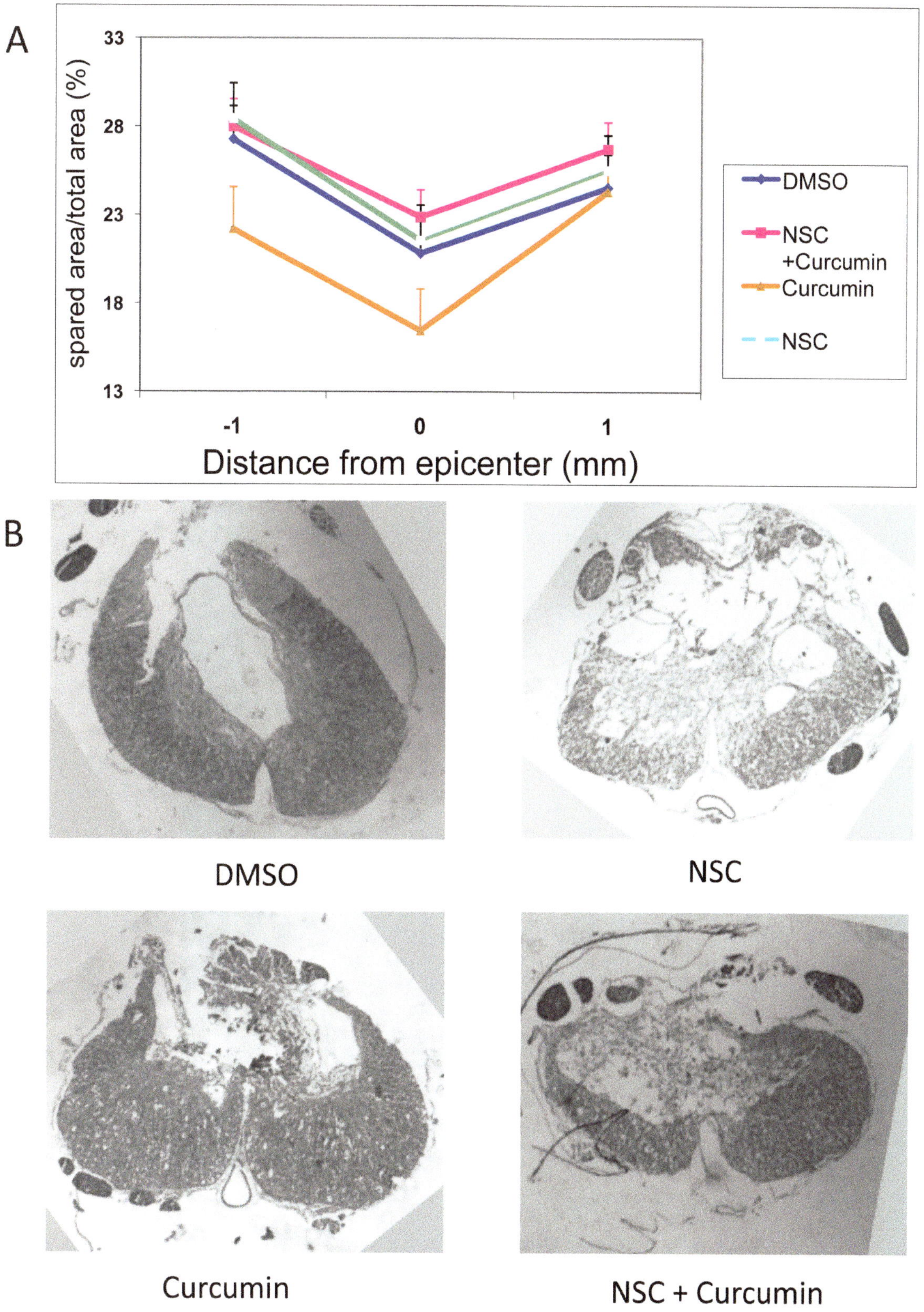

Figure 5. Histopathological examination after severe SCI. A: NSC plus curcumin and NSC all displayed enhanced spared area relative to the total area suggesting an improvement in recovery. DMSO treated rats also demonstrated increased spared area of the spinal cord, but somewhat less than the NSC plus curcumin, or NSC treatments. Curcumin-treated rats demonstrated less spared area than the other three treatments. **B:** Photomicrographs of representative samples of spinal cord sections across the area of contusion stained with Lox blue.

blockers, and caspase inhibitors, among others [58,61,62]. These studies demonstrate the risk of further SCI secondary to ischemia/reperfusion, and the possible benefits of using agents for their neuroprotective effects.

Curcumin is a potent antioxidant and free radical scavenger, and has been shown to improve ischemia-reperfusion injury in multiple studies [63–66]. Curcumin has a potent inhibitory effect on the NF-kB pathway in settings where it is activated [67–69]. NF-kB has been demonstrated to be highly upregulated in SCI, and is associated with glial scar formation [70–71]. Curcumin may exert its benefit in SCI recovery via inhibition of this pathway [9–12,14]. Absorbtion of curcumin in the GI tract has been debatable, and once absorbed into the blood stream, detectable levels are transient and require very high oral doses to achieve [72]. In order to alleviate the difficulties of poor bioavailability of curcumin, we dissolved curcumin in DMSO as a solvent to increase the rate of transfer across membranes, and administered it by IP injection or locally at the site of injury. Side effects of curcumin are limited, with no side effects noted in our animals [73]. It is noteworthy that despite the previously noted studies demonstrating curcumin's benefit after SCI, this study extends the findings by demonstrating that this benefit appears to be limited depending on the severity of injury [9–12,14]. For example, in severe injury, curcumin only benefitted recovery following combinational therapy with NSC. Limitations to recovery with existing therapies are not completely surprising, and have been noted in SCI studies in the past with other agents [74–76].

Our study demonstrates some of the limitations not only of curcumin, but also stem cell monotherapy, on recovery from SCI. While curcumin's bioavailability is limited, this may be useful where it is used in combinational therapy [35,73–74]. There is evidence, for example, that only very low concentrations of curcumin following IP injection cross the blood brain barrier [35,73–74]. However, it is precisely this low dose of curcumin that creates the synergistic effect seen in our study. A higher dose of curcumin in combination with NSC had a less significant effect than either therapy alone (Fig. 2A). These results emphasize that the synergistic effect of curcumin with stem cell therapy in severe SCI may occur via dual action of curcumin, i.e. it reduces the inflammation at the local SCI region induced by secondary injury and may also induce proliferation of stem cells required for faster regeneration. With the great interest in stem cell transplant after SCI, it is important to know what adjunctive agents may serve to enhance their effect. This is the first study to demonstrate significant functional recovery from severe SCI in animals treated with curcumin in combination with NSC transplant. Many of these animals regained independent ambulatory function even after severe SCI, a feat not accomplished with either therapy alone. Curcumin and NSC transplant appear to be a safe and effective treatment to improve recovery from SCI. Future studies would include the analysis of discrete biomarkers associated with inflammation and recovery after curcumin treatment.

Conclusions

The results of this study provide a strong basis for stem cell therapy in conjunction with curcumin in the treatment and management of SCI in humans.

Acknowledgments

We are thankful for Dr. Hong Peng for her help with histology.

Author Contributions

Conceived and designed the experiments: DRO MJ RZ. Performed the experiments: DRO CS JO. Analyzed the data: DRO CS JO MJ RZ RM KD. Contributed reagents/materials/analysis tools: DRO MJ RZ RM KD. Wrote the paper: DRO CS JO MJ RZ KD RM.

References

1. Sekhon LH, Fehlings MG (2001) Epidemiology, demographics, and pathophysiology of acute spinal cord injury. Spine 26(24 Suppl): S2–12.
2. Christopher & Dana Reeve Foundation (2009) One Degree of Separation: Paralysis and Spinal Cord Injury in the United States. Christopher & Dana Reeve Foundation.
3. Renault-Mihara F, Okada S, Shibata S, Nakamura M, Toyama Y, et al. (2008) Spinal cord injury: emerging beneficial role of reactive astrocytes' migration. Int J Biochem Cell Biol 40(9): 1649–53.
4. Ghosh S, Hayden MS (2008) New regulators of NF-kappaB in inflammation. Nat Rev Immunol 8(11): 837–48.
5. Aggarwal BB, Sung B (2009) Pharmacological basis for the role of curcumin in chronic diseases: an age-old spice with modern targets. Trends Pharmacol Sci 30(2): 85–94.
6. Begum AN, Jones MR, Lim GP, Morihara T, Kim P, et al. (2008) Curcumin structure-function, bioavailability, and efficacy in models of neuroinflammation and Alzheimer's disease. J Pharmacol Exp Ther 326(1): 196–208.
7. Chainani-Wu N (2003) Safety and anti-inflammatory activity of curcumin: a component of tumeric (Curcuma longa). J Altern Complement Med 9(1): 161–8.
8. Aggarwal BB, Harikumar KB (2009) Potential therapeutic effects of curcumin, the anti-inflammatory agent, against neurodegenerative, cardiovascular, pulmonary, metabolic, autoimmune and neoplastic diseases. Int J Biochem Cell Biol 41(1): 40–59.
9. Lin MS, Lee YH, Chiu WT, Hung KS (2011) Curcumin provides neuroprotection after spinal cord injury. J Surg Res 166: 280–289.
10. Lin MS, Sun YY, Chiu WT, Hung CC, Chang CY, et al. (2011) Curcumin attenuates the expression and secretion of RANTES after spinal cord injury in vivo and lipopolysaccharide-induced astrocyte reactivation in vitro. J Neurotrauma 28: 1259–1269.
11. Lee SG, Su ZZ, Emdad L, Sarkar D, Franke TF, et al. (2008) Astrocyte elevated gene-1 activates cell survival pathways through PI3K-Akt signaling. Oncogene 27(8): 1114–21.
12. Cemil B, Topuz K, Demircan MN, Kurt G, Tun K, et al. (2010) Curcumin improves early functional results after experimental spinal cord injury. Acta Neurochir (Wien) 152: 1583–1590.
13. Sahin Kavaklı H, Koca C, Alici O (2011) Antioxidant effects of curcumin in spinal cord injury in rats. Ulus Travma Acil Cerrahi Derg 17: 14–18.
14. Ormond DR, Peng H, Zeman R, Das K, Murali R, et al. (2012) Recovery from spinal cord injury using naturally occurring antiinflammatory compound curcumin. J Neurosurg Spine. 16(5): 497–503.
15. Joseph MS, Ying Z, Zhuang Y, Zhong H, Wu A, et al. (2012) Effects of Diet and/or Exercise in Enhancing Spinal Cord Sensorimotor Learning. PLoS ONE 7(7): 1–10.
16. Holly LT, Blaskiewicz D, Wu A, Feng C, Ying Z, et al. (2012) Dietary therapy to promote neuroprotetion in chronic spinal cord injury. J Neurosurg Spine 17(2): 134–140.
17. Teng YD, Lavik EB, Qu X, Park KI, Ourednik J, et al. (2002) Functional recovery following traumatic spinal cord injury mediated by a unique polymer scaffold seeded with neural stem cells. Proc Natl Acad Sci USA 99(5): 3024–9.
18. Vroemen M, Aigner L, Winkler J, Weidner N (2003) Adult neural progenitor cell grafts survive after acute spinal cord injury and integrate along axonal pathways. Eur J Neurosci 18(4): 743–51.
19. Ruff CA, Wilcox JT, Fehlings MG (2012) Cell-based transplantation strategies to promote plasticity following spinal cord injury. Exp Neurol. 235(1): 78–90.
20. Tetzlaff W, Okon EB, Karimi-Abdolrezaee S, Sparling JS, Plemel JR, et al. (2011) A Systematic Review of Cellular Transplantation Therapies for Spinal Cord Injury. J of Neurotrauma 28: 1611–1682.
21. Parr AM, Kulbatski I, Zahir T, Wang X, Yue C, et al. (2008) Transplanted adult spinal cord-derived neural stem/progenitor cells promote early functional recovery after rat spinal cord injury. Neuroscience 155(3): 760–70.
22. Parr AM, Kulbatski I, Wang XH, Keating A, Tator CH (2008) Fate of transplanted adult neural stem/progenitor cells and bone marrow-derived mesenchymal stromal cells in the injured adult rat spinal cord and impact on functional recovery. Surg Neurol 70(6): 600–7.
23. Karimi-Abdolrezaee S, Eftekharpour E, Wang J, Morshead CM, Fehlings MG (2006) Delayed transplantation of adult neural precursor cells promotes remyelination and functional neurological recovery after spinal cord injury. J Neurosci 26(13): 3377–89.
24. Yan J, Welsh AM, Bora SH, Snyder EY, Koliatsos VE (2004) Differentiation and tropic/trophic effects of exogenous neural precursors in the adult spinal cord. J Comp Neurol 480(1): 101–14.
25. Miller RH, Bai L (2012) Translating stem cell therapies to the clinic. Neurosci Lett. 519(2): 87–92.

26. Parr AM, Kulbatski I, Tator CH (2007) Transplantation of adult rat spinal cord stem/progenitor cells for spinal cord injury. J Neurotrauma 24(5): 835–45.
27. Temple S, Alvarez-Buylla A (1999) Stem cells in the adult mammalian central nervous system. Curr Opin Neurobiol 9(1): 135–41.
28. Jhanwar-Uniyal M, Beck B, Jhanwar YS, Burlet C, Leibowitz SF (1993) Neuropeptide Y projection from arcuate nucleus to parvocellular division of paraventricular nucleus: specific relation to the ingestion of carbohydrate. Brain Res 631(1): 97–106.
29. Marshall GP, Ross HH, Suslov O, Zheng T, Steindler DA, et al. (2008) Production of neurospheres from CNS tissue. Methods Mol Biol 438: 135–50.
30. Zeman RJ, Feng Y, Peng H, Etlinger JD (1999) Clenbuterol, a beta(2)-adrenoceptor agonist, improves locomotor and histological outcomes after spinal cord contusion in rats. Exp Neurol 159(1): 267–73.
31. Zeman RJ, Feng Y, Peng H, Visintainer PF, Moorthy CR, et al. (2001) X-irradiation of the contusion site improves locomotor and histological outcomes in spinal cord-injured rats. Exp Neurol 172(1): 228–34.
32. Zeman RJ, Peng H, Feng Y, Song H, Liu X, et al. (2006) Beta2-adrenoreceptor agonist-enhanced recovery of locomotor function after spinal cord injury is glutathione dependent. J Neurotrauma 23(2): 170–80.
33. Basso DM, Beattie MS, Bresnahan JC (1996) Graded histological and locomotor outcomes after spinal cord contusion using the NYU weight-drop device versus transection. Exp Neurol 139(2): 244–56.
34. Fehlings MG, Vawda R (2011) Cellular Treatments for Spinal Cord Injury: The Time is Right for Clinical Trials 8(4): 704–720.
35. Kim SJ, Son TG, Park HR, Park M, Kim MS, et al. (2008) Curcumin stimulates proliferation of embryonic neural progenitor cells and neurogenesis in the adult hippocampus. J Biol Chem 283(21): 14497–505.
36. Liu M, Stevens-Lapsley JE, Jayaraman A, Ye F, Conover C, et al. (2010) Impact of treadmill locomotor training on skeletal muscle IGF1 and myogenic regulatory factors in spinal cord injured rats. Eur J Appl Physiol 109(4): 709–20.
37. Liu M, Bose P, Walter GA, Anderson DK, Thompson FJ, et al. (2006) Changes in muscle T2 relaxation properties following spinal cord injury and locomotor training. Eur J of Appl Physiol 97(3): 355–61.
38. Lee Y, Lin C, Calozzo VJ, Robertson RT, Yu J, et al. (2007) Repair of spinal cord transection and its effects on muscle mass and myosin heavy chain isoform phenotype. J of Appl Physiol 103(5): 1808–1814.
39. Dupont-Versteegden EE, Houlé JD, Gurley CM, Peterson CA (1998) Early changes in muscle fiber size and gene expression in response to spinal cord transection and exercise. Am J Physiol. 275(4 Pt 1): C1124–33.
40. Landry E, Frenette J, Guertin PA (2004) Body weight, limb size, and muscular properties of early paraplegic mice. J Neurotrauma. 21(8): 1008–16.
41. Singh A, Balasubramanian S, Murray M, Lemay M, Houle J (2011) Role of spared pathways in locomotor recovery after body-weight-supported treadmill training in contused rats. J Neurotrauma. 28(12): 2405–16.
42. Rabchevsky AG, Streit WJ (1997) Grafting of cultured microglial cells into the lesioned spinal cord of adult rats enhances neurite outgrowth. J Neurosci Res 47(1): 34–48.
43. Guízar-Sahagún G, Ibarra A, Espitia A, Martínez A, Madrazo I, et al. (2005) Glutathione monoethyl ester improves functional recovery, enhances neuron survival, and stabilizes spinal cord blood flow after spinal cord injury in rats. Neuroscience. 130(3): 639–49.
44. Jakeman LB, Wei P, Guan Z, Stokes BT (1998) Brain-derived neurotrophic factor stimulates hindlimb stepping and sprouting of cholinergic fibers after spinal cord injury. Exp Neurol. 154(1): 170–84.
45. Weiss S, Dunne C, Hewson J, Wohl C, Wheatley M, et al. (1996) Multipotent CNS stem cells are present in the adult mammalian spinal cord and ventricular neuroaxis. J Neurosci. 16(23): 7599–609.
46. Johansson CB, Momma S, Clarke DL, Risling M, Lendahl U, et al. (1999) Identification of a neural stem cell in the adult mammalian central nervous system. Cell. 96(1): 25–34.
47. Namiki J, Tator CH (1999) Cell proliferation and nestin expression in the ependyma of the adult rat spinal cord after injury. J Neuropathol Exp Neurol. 58(5): 489–98.
48. Horner PJ, Power AE, Kempermann G, Kuhn HG, Palmer TD, et al. (2000) Proliferation and differentiation of progenitor cells throughout the intact adult rat spinal cord. J Neurosci. 20(6): 2218–28.
49. Kojima A, Tator CH (2002) Intrathecal administration of epidermal growth factor and fibroblast growth factor 2 promotes ependymal proliferation and functional recovery after spinal cord injury in adult rats. J Neurotrauma. 19(2): 223–38.
50. Martens DJ, Seaberg RM, van der Kooy D (2002) In vivo infusions of exogenous growth factors into the fourth ventricle of the adult mouse brain increase the proliferation of neural progenitors around the fourth ventricle and the central canal of the spinal cord. Eur J Neurosci. 16(6): 1045–57.
51. Moreno-Manzano V, Rodriguez-Jimenez FJ, Garcia-Rosello M, Lainez S, Erceq S, et al. (2009) Activated Spinal Cord Ependymal Stem Cells Rescue Neurological Function. Stem Cells 27: 733–743.
52. Barnabé-Heider F, Frisen J (2008) Stem cells for spinal cord repair. Cell Stem Cell 3: 16–24.
53. Cao Q, Benton RL, Whittemore SR (2002) Stem cell repair of central nervous system injury. J Neurosci Res. 68(5): 501–10.
54. Pfeifer K, Vroemen M, Blesch A, Weidner N (2004) Adult neural progenitor cells provide a permissive guiding substrate for corticospinal axon growth following spinal cord injury. Eur J Neurosci. 20(7): 1695–704.
55. Hofstetter CP, Holmström NA, Lilja JA, Schweinhardt P, Hao J, et al. (2005) Allodynia limits the usefulness of intraspinal neural stem cell grafts; directed differentiation improves outcome. Nat Neurosci. 8(3): 346–53.
56. Bottai D, Madaschi L, Di Giulio AM, Gorio A (2008) Viability-dependent promoting action of adult neural precursors in spinal cord injury. Mol Med. 14(9–10): 634–44.
57. Ziv Y, Avidan H, Pluchino S, Martino G, Schwartz M (2006) Synergy between immune cells and adult neural stem/progenitor cells promotes functional recovery from spinal cord injury. Proc Natl Acad Sci USA. 103(35): 13174–9.
58. Saito T, Tsuchida M, Umehara S, Kohno T, Yamamoto H, et al. (2011) Reduction of Spinal Cord Ischemia/Reperfusion Injury with Simvastatin in Rats. Neuroscience in Anesthesiology and Perioperative Medicine 113(3): 565–71.
59. Morell P, Quarles RH (1999) Myelin formation, structure and biochemistry: In: Siegel GJ, Agranoff BW, Fisher SK, Albers RW, Uhler MD, eds. Basic Neurochemistry: Molecular, Cellular and Medical Aspects. 6th edition. New York: Lippincott-Raven, 69–94.
60. Bernardo A, Greco A, Levi G, Minghetti L (2003) Differential lipid peroxidation, Mn superoxide, and bcl-2 expression contribute to the maturation-dependent vulnerability of oligodendrocytes to oxidative stress. J Neuropathol Exp Neurol 62: 509–19.
61. Fansa I, Altug ME, Melek I, Ucar E, Kontas T, et al. (2009) The Neuroprotective and Anti-inflammatory Effects of Diltiazem in Spinal Cord Ischaemia–Reperfusion Injury. The Journal of International Medical Research 37: 520–533.
62. Dolgun H, Sekerci Z, Turkoglu E, Kertmen H, Yilmaz ER, et al. (2010) Neuroprotective effect of mesna (2-mercaptoethane sulfonate) against spinal cord ischemia/reperfusion injury in rabbits. J Clin Neurosci. 17(4): 486–9.
63. Avci G, Kadioglu H, Sehirli AO, Bozkurt S, Guclu O, et al. (2012) Curcumin protects against ischemia/reperfusion injury in rat skeletal muscle. J Surg Res. 172(1): e39–46.
64. Pogue AI, Percy ME, Cui JG, Li YY, Bhattacharjee S, et al. (2011) Up-regulation of NF-kB-sensitive miRNA-125b and miRNA-146a in metal sulfate-stressed human astroglial (HAG) primary cell cultures. J Inorg Biochem. 105(11): 1434–7.
65. Barzegar A, Moosavi-Movahedi AA (2011) Intracellular ROS protection efficiency and free radical-scavenging activity of curcumin. PLoS One. 6(10): e26012.
66. Kuo CP, Lu CH, Wen LL, Cherng CH, Wong CS, et al. (2011) Neuroprotective effect of curcumin in an experimental rat model of subarachnoid hemorrhage. Anesthesiology. 115(6): 1229–38.
67. Ammon HP, Wahl MA (1991) Pharmacology of Curcuma longa. Planta Med 57: 1–7.
68. Satoskar RR, Shah SJ, Shenoy SG (1986) Evaluation of anti-inflammatory property of curcumin (diferuloyl methane) in patients with postoperative inflammation. Int J Clin Pharmacol Ther Toxicol 24: 651–654.
69. Shankar TN, Shantha NV, Ramesh HP, Murthy IA, Murthy VS (1980) Toxicity studies on turmeric (Curcuma longa): acute toxicity studies in rats, guineapigs & monkeys. Indian J Exp Biol 18: 73–75.
70. Brambilla R, Hurtado A, Persaud T, Esham K, Pearse DD, et al. (2009) Transgenic inhibition of astroglial NF-kappa B leads to increased axonal sparing and sprouting following spinal cord injury. J Neurochem 110: 765–778.
71. Rafati DS, Geissler K, Johnson K, Unabia G, Hulsebosch C, et al. (2008) Nuclear factor-kappaB decoy amelioration of spinal cord injury-induced inflammation and behavior outcomes. J Neurosci Res 86(3): 566–80.
72. Anand P, Kunnumakkara AB, Newman RA, Aggarwal BB (2007) Bioavailability of curcumin: problems and promises. Mol Pharm 4: 807–818.
73. Sharma RA, Steward WP, Gescher AJ (2007) Pharmacokinetics and pharmacodynamics of curcumin. Adv Exp Med Biol 595: 453–70.
74. Sharma S, Zhuang Y, Ying Z, Gomez-Pinilla F (2009) Dietary Curcumin Supplementation Counteracts reduction in levels of Molecules involved in Energy Homeostasis after Brain Trauma. Neuroscience 161(4): 1037–44.
75. Nesathurai S (1998) Steroids and spinal cord injury: revisiting the NASCIS 2 and NASCIS 3 trials. J Trauma 45(6): 1088–93.
76. Bracken MB, Shepard MJ, Holford TR, Leo-Summers L, Aldrich EF, et al. (1997) Administration of methylprednisolone for 24 or 48 hours or tirilazad mesylate for 48 hours in the treatment of acute spinal cord injury. Results of the Third National Acute Spinal Cord Injury Randomized Controlled Trial. National Acute Spinal Cord Injury Study. JAMA. 277(20): 1597–604.

8

Central Canal Ependymal Cells Proliferate Extensively in Response to Traumatic Spinal Cord Injury but Not Demyelinating Lesions

Steve Lacroix[2], Laura K. Hamilton[1], Alexandre Vaugeois[1], Stéfanny Beaudoin[1], Christian Breault-Dugas[1], Isabelle Pineau[2], Sébastien A. Lévesque[2], Catherine-Alexandra Grégoire[1], Karl J. L. Fernandes[1]*

1 Department of Neurosciences, Faculty of Medicine, Centre de recherche du Centre hospitalier de l'Université de Montréal (CRCHUM), and Groupe de recherche sur le système nerveux central (GRSNC), Université de Montréal, Quebec, Canada, **2** Centre de recherche du Centre hospitalier universitaire (CHU) de Québec – CHUL et Département de médicine moléculaire, Faculté de médecine, Université Laval, Québec, Canada

Abstract

The adult mammalian spinal cord has limited regenerative capacity in settings such as spinal cord injury (SCI) and multiple sclerosis (MS). Recent studies have revealed that ependymal cells lining the central canal possess latent neural stem cell potential, undergoing proliferation and multi-lineage differentiation following experimental SCI. To determine whether reactive ependymal cells are a realistic endogenous cell population to target in order to promote spinal cord repair, we assessed the spatiotemporal dynamics of ependymal cell proliferation for up to 35 days in three models of spinal pathologies: contusion SCI using the Infinite Horizon impactor, focal demyelination by intraspinal injection of lysophosphatidylcholine (LPC), and autoimmune-mediated multi-focal demyelination using the active experimental autoimmune encephalomyelitis (EAE) model of MS. Contusion SCI at the T9–10 thoracic level stimulated a robust, long-lasting and long-distance wave of ependymal proliferation that peaked at 3 days in the lesion segment, 14 days in the rostral segment, and was still detectable at the cervical level, where it peaked at 21 days. This proliferative wave was suppressed distal to the contusion. Unlike SCI, neither chemical- nor autoimmune-mediated demyelination triggered ependymal cell proliferation at any time point, despite the occurrence of demyelination (LPC and EAE), remyelination (LPC) and significant locomotor defects (EAE). Thus, traumatic SCI induces widespread and enduring activation of reactive ependymal cells, identifying them as a robust cell population to target for therapeutic manipulation after contusion; conversely, neither demyelination, remyelination nor autoimmunity appears sufficient to trigger proliferation of quiescent ependymal cells in models of MS-like demyelinating diseases.

Editor: Norbert Weidner, Heidelberg University Hospital, Germany

Funding: This investigation was supported by grants from the Canadian Institutes of Health Research (grant no. 111095) and the Multiple Sclerosis Society of Canada. Salary support was provided by the Fonds de recherche du Québec en Santé (SL), a postdoctoral fellowship from the Multiple Sclerosis Society of Canada (SAL), and a Canada Research Chair (KF). The funders had no role in study design, data collection and analysis, decision to publish, or preparation of the manuscript.

Competing Interests: The authors have declared that no competing interests exist.

* E-mail: karl.jl.fernandes@umontreal.ca

Introduction

Ependymal cells (EpCs) of the adult spinal cord are an enigmatic population of ciliated cells lining the central canal. They are comprised of multiple morphologically identifiable subtypes, including cuboidal EpCs and radial tanycytic EpCs [1–5], and are descended developmentally from embryonic neuroepithelial stem cells located in the ventral neural tube [6–8]. In lower vertebrates, such as certain types of fish, amphibians and reptiles, EpCs play a central role in the remarkable regeneration observed following spinal cord transection [9–11]. However, in the adult mammalian spinal cord, which is notable for its lack of regenerative ability, EpCs are thought to primarily serve endocrinological and protective roles [4], and exhibit relatively low basal mitotic activity [2,12–14].

Despite the limited anatomical and functional regeneration observed following damage to the adult mammalian spinal cord [15,16], recent studies indicate that reactive mammalian EpCs re-express neural stem cell properties following spinal cord injury (SCI) [1,17,18]. Mechanical damage to the central canal triggers a robust increase in EpC proliferation [12,19,20], and an upregulation in expression of the neuroepithelial stem cell marker Nestin [19,21]. This is followed by migration of EpC-derived progeny to the site of injury [12,20], where they exhibit multi-lineage differentiation into both astrocytes and oligodendrocytes [1,17,22]. Consistent with a latent neural stem cell potential, tissue culture and fate-mapping experiments have revealed that virtually all stem-like cells that can be isolated from the intact or injured spinal cord using the colony-forming neurosphere assay are derived from the EpC population [17].

The induction of stem cell properties in reactive EpCs raises the fascinating possibility of targeting these endogenous cells to promote spinal cord repair. For example, reactive EpCs could be targeted to modulate their astrocytic contribution to the glial scar; to increase the size of the oligodendrocyte progenitor pool; or to potentially generate interneurons capable of relaying impulses across the injury site. However, important questions remain unanswered, including the timing, location and extent of EpC reactions to an injury, and the types of damage to spinal cord tissue that are capable of inducing EpC reactions. In the present study, we have investigated in detail the pattern of EpC activation in response to spinal cord pathologies. We first examined the spatiotemporal dynamics of injury-induced EpC proliferation using the Infinite Horizon (IH) impactor, a clinically relevant model of spinal cord contusion injury [23]. We then asked whether non-traumatic spinal cord pathologies are capable of eliciting EpC activation, focusing on the lysophosphatidylcholine (LPC, also called lysolecithin) model of focal demyelination and the experimental autoimmune encephalomyelitis (EAE) model of multi-focal demyelination. Our findings provide insights relevant to the development of potential therapeutic strategies for using endogenous EpCs to promote repair of the injured or diseased spinal cord.

Materials and Methods

Animals

A total of 165 adult female C57BL/6 mice were used in this study. Mice were purchased from Charles River Laboratories (St-Constant, QC, Canada) and had free access to food and water. All surgical procedures were approved by the Laval University Animal Care Committee and followed Canadian Council on Animal Care guidelines. The distribution of mice used among the three different models of spinal pathologies and time points at which animals were sacrificed are reported in Table 1.

Spinal Cord Injury (SCI)

C57BL/6 (N = 46) mice were anesthetized with isoflurane and underwent a laminectomy at vertebral level T9–10, which corresponds to spinal segment T10–11. Briefly, the vertebral column was stabilized and a contusion of 50 kdyn (moderate injury) was performed using the IH SCI device (Precision Systems & Instrumentation, Lexington, KY), typically resulting in a spinal cord displacement of 400 to 500 μm. Overlying muscular layers were then sutured and cutaneous layers stapled. Post-operatively, animals received manual bladder evacuation twice daily to prevent urinary tract infections. SCI mice were sacrificed by perfusion at 1, 3, 7, 14, 21, and 35 days post-contusion. Naive (N = 4) and sham-operated mice were used as controls.

Table 1. Overview of the number of mice included in experiments.

Group	Time of sacrifice (days)						
	0	1	3	7	14	21	35
SCI (n = 50)							
1. Naive	4						
2. Sham		4				4	
3. SCI		10	6	6	6	5	5
LPC (n = 92)							
1. PBS-injected			4	12	4	9	8
2. LPC-injected			9	19	9	9	9
EAE (n = 23)							
1. Naive	5						
2. Immunized				5	4	5	4

Lysophosphatidylcholine (LPC)-induced Demyelination

A laminectomy was done to expose the spinal cord at vertebral level T9–10, and 1 μl of either L-α-LPC (L-α-lysolecithin, catalog # L-1381; Sigma-Aldrich Canada, Oakville, ON, Canada) at a concentration of 1 μg/μl or PBS injected into the dorsal column or dorsolateral funiculus (DLF) white matter using a glass micropipette with a tip diameter of 40 μm, as previously described [24]. Mice (N = 92) were sacrificed at 3, 7, 14, 21, and 35 days post-injection.

Experimental Autoimmune Encephalomyelitis (EAE)

Induction of EAE in C57BL/6 mice (N = 18) was used as a model for multiple sclerosis (MS). EAE was induced by subcutaneous injections of 100 μg of myelin oligodendrocyte glycoprotein (MOG_{35-55}; MEVGWYRSPFSRVVHLYRNGK, AnaSpec Inc., Fremont, CA) in complete Freund's adjuvant (incomplete Freund's adjuvant containing 4 mg/ml of heat-inactivated *Mycobacterium tuberculosis* H37Ra; BD Biosciences, Mississauga, ON, Canada). An intravenous injection of 200 ng of pertussis toxin (PTX; List Biological Laboratories Inc., Campbell, CA) was also administered on days 0 and 2 of the immunization. The severity of EAE was scored daily using a grading scale of 0–5, following recommendations of Stromnes and Goverman [25]: 0 = unaffected, 0.5 = partially limp tail, 1 = paralyzed tail, 2 = hind limb paresis and loss in coordinated movement, 2.5 = one hind limb paralyzed, 3 = both hind limbs paralyzed, 3.5 = hind limbs paralyzed and weakness in forelimbs, 4 = forelimbs paralyzed, and 5 = moribund/death. Animals were sacrificed at 7, 14, 21, and 35 days post-immunization. Naive mice (N = 5) were used as controls.

Tissue Processing and Histology

Spinal cords were collected and prepared as previously described [26,27]. Briefly, mice were overdosed with a mixture of ketamine-xylazine and transcardially perfused with 4% paraformaldehyde (PFA), pH 7.4, in PBS. Spinal cords were dissected out, post-fixed for 2 days at 4°C, and then transferred for 2 days into PBS containing 30% sucrose. For each SCI mouse, a spinal cord segment of 12 mm centered over the lesion site was cut in 12 series of 30-μm-thick coronal sections using a cryostat. In addition, a 4-mm spinal segment corresponding to the C4–6 level was isolated and processed for each SCI animal. Cervical, thoracic and lumbar spinal segments corresponding to the same levels, respectively C4–6, T5–12 and L1–4 levels, were isolated from the spinal cord of LPC-injected and EAE mice as well as control animals. All sections were collected directly onto Surgipath X-tra microslides having a permanent positive charged surface (Leica Microsystems Canada, Concord, ON, Canada) and stored at −20°C until use. To identify the site of SCI and visualize demyelinating lesions, one series of adjacent sections was stained with cresyl violet (CV) and/or Luxol Fast blue (LFB).

Immunohistochemistry

Primary antibodies used in this study were mouse anti-human Ki67 (1:200, BD Biosciences), chicken anti-Vimentin polyclonal (1:1000, Millipore, Billerica, MA), rabbit anti-mouse Olig2 monoclonal (1:250, Millipore). Brightfield immunohistochemistry for Ki67 was performed using a biotinylated anti-mouse secondary antibody (Jackson ImmunoResearch, West Grove, PA) in conjunction an avidin-biotin-peroxidase amplification system

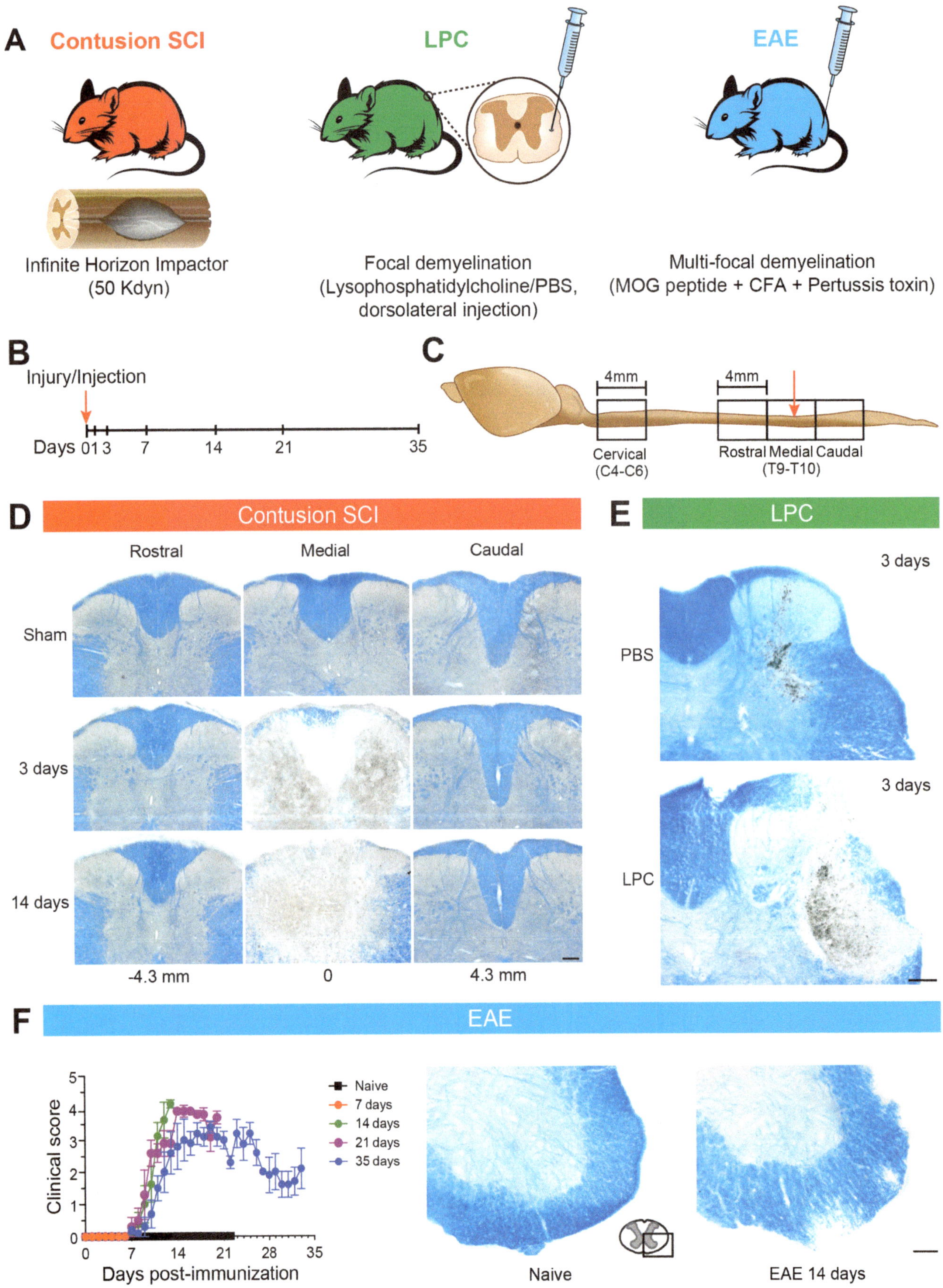

A
Contusion SCI
LPC
EAE
Infinite Horizon Impactor
(50 Kdyn)
Focal demyelination
(Lysophosphatidylcholine/PBS,
dorsolateral injection)
Multi-focal demyelination
(MOG peptide + CFA + Pertussis toxin)
B
Injury/Injection
Days 0 1 3 7 14 21 35
C
4mm
4mm
Cervical
(C4-C6)
Rostral Medial Caudal
(T9-T10)
D
Contusion SCI
Rostral
Medial
Caudal
Sham
3 days
14 days
-4.3 mm
0
4.3 mm
E
LPC
3 days
PBS
3 days
LPC
F
EAE
Clinical score
Days post-immunization
Naive
7 days
14 days
21 days
35 days
Naive
EAE 14 days

Figure 1. Description of SCI, LPC and EAE models of spinal cord pathologies. (**A**) Models of spinal cord pathologies. (**B**) Time course of mouse sacrifices. Day 0 is the time of contusion SCI, intraspinal injection of lysophosphatidylcholine (LPC) or PBS, or peripheral injection of EAE-inducing MOG/CFA/Pertussis toxin. Only SCI and LPC mice were sacrificed at days 1 and 3, due to the slow onset of EAE following immunization. (**C**) Spinal cord segments harvested for sectioning and analysis. The red arrow points to the lesion epicenter. (**D**) Gross histology of the low thoracic spinal cord following contusion SCI. Shown are representative examples of Luxol Fast blue (LFB)-stained sections taken from the Rostral segment (left column), Medial segment (middle column) and Caudal segment (right column) of a sham-operated mouse (sacrificed at day 21) and SCI mice at 3 and 14 days post-injury. Approximate distances (in millimeters) are shown from the lesion epicenter at the middle of the Medial segment (0). (**E**) Gross histology of the T9–10 thoracic spinal cord injection of PBS (upper panel) or LPC (lower panel) in the dorsolateral funiculus. Luxol Fast blue stains the white matter myelin, and reveals the large zone of demyelination already evident at 3 days after LPC injection. (**F**) Clinical scores and histopathology of EAE mice. Note the rapid increase in clinical scores between 1 and 21 days after immunization, reflecting declining locomotor function that stabilizes and slightly improves between 21 and 35 days after immunization (left). See Methods for description of clinical scores. Luxol Fast blue staining documented the presence of demyelinating plaques spread in the spinal cord white matter of EAE mice at 14 days post-immunization (right). Scale bars: **D–F** 100 µm.

(VectaStain ABC Kit, Vector Laboratories, Burlington, ON, Canada) and 3,3-diaminobenzidine (DAB). Brightfield sections were counterstained with CV. Multilabel immunofluorescence was performed by co-incubating cryostat sections with Ki67, Olig2 and Vimentin primary antibodies and detecting them with Alexa 555 goat anti-mouse (1:1000), Alexa 488 goat anti-rabbit (1:1000) and Dylight donkey anti-chicken (1:500) secondary antibodies (Jackson ImmunoResearch). Immunofluorescence sections were counter-stained with Hoechst 33342 (0.2 µM, Sigma-Aldrich Canada).

Microscopy

Brightfield images were captured using an Olympus BX43F microscope equipped with an Olympus DP-21 color camera. Immunofluorescence images were captured using an Olympus IX81 motorized microscope equipped with a Retiga 2000RV black and white CCD camera (Q-Imaging, Surrey, BC, Canada) and a Metamorph image acquisition/analysis software (Molecular Devices Corporation, Sunnyvale, CA). Co-localization of immunofluorescence signals were confirmed using Z-stacks, which were subsequently processed using a 2D deconvolution function and flattened by Maximum projection for presentation. Images were

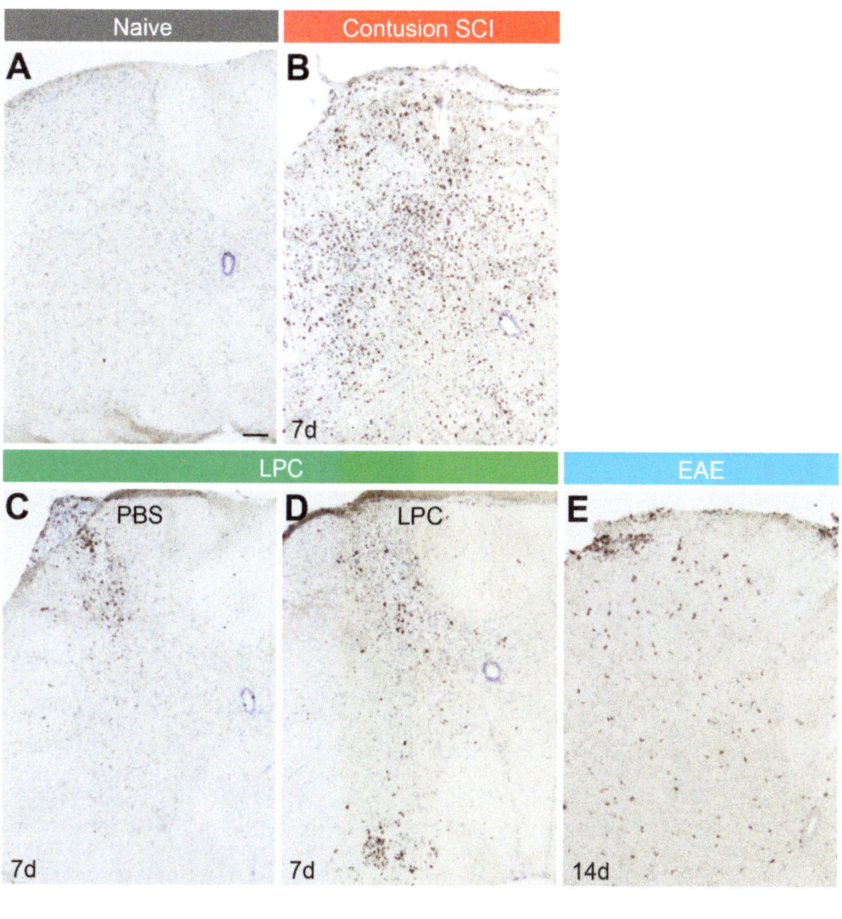

Figure 2. Distinct proliferative reactions in the spinal cord following SCI, LPC and EAE. (**A–E**) Low magnification images of the spinal cord following immunohistochemistry for the cell proliferation marker Ki67 in a naive mouse (**A**), 7 days following contusion SCI (**B**), 7 days following intraspinal injection of PBS (**C**) or LPC (**D**), or 14 days following peripheral immunization in EAE mice (**E**). Scale bar: **A–E**, 80 µm.

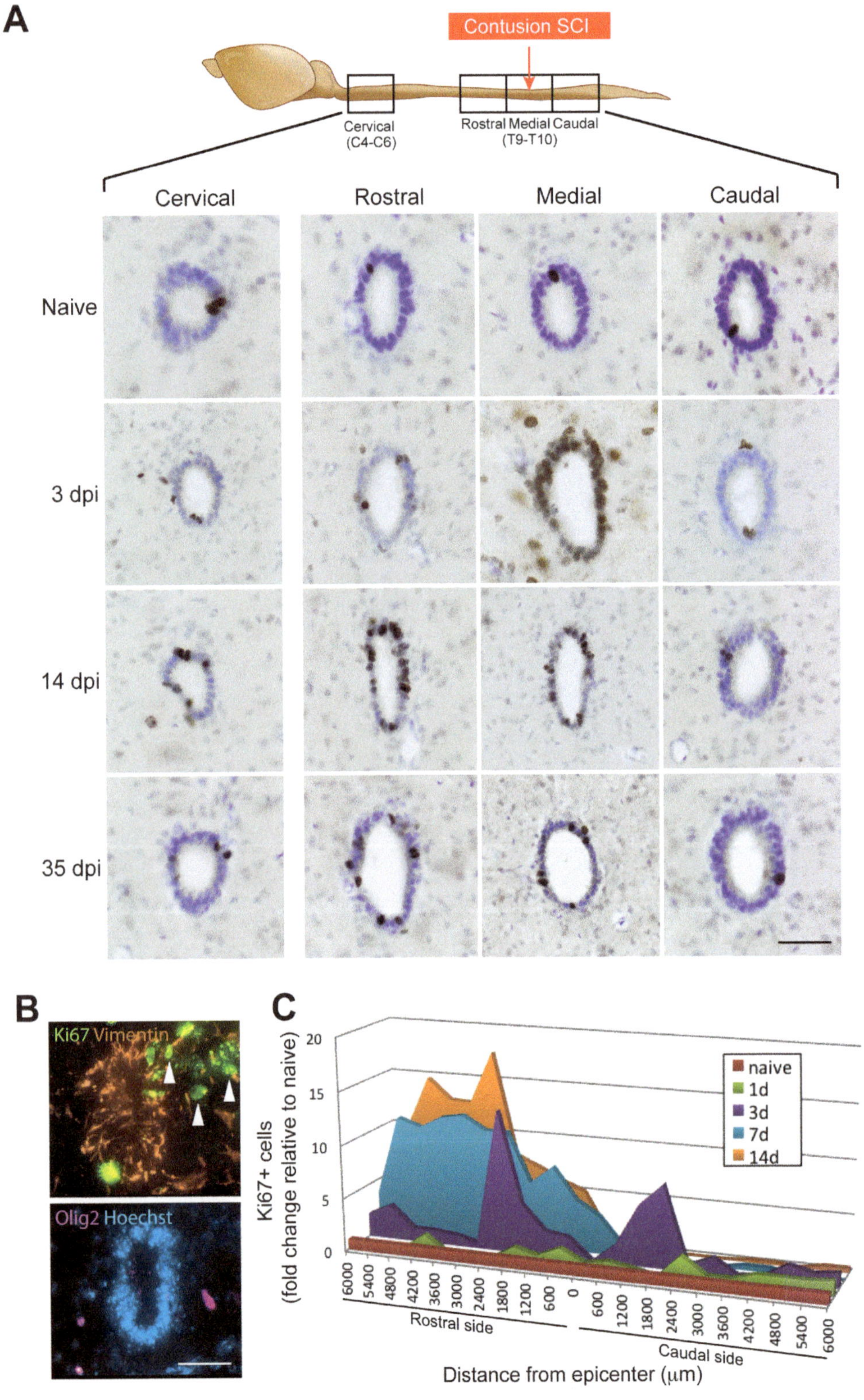

Figure 3. Changes in ependymal zone proliferation following contusion SCI. (**A**) Immunohistochemistry for Ki67-positive (+) proliferating cells in each harvested segment of the spinal cord of naive mice and 3, 14, or 35 days post-injury (dpi). Sections are counterstained with cresyl violet. Note the increased cell proliferation in the ependymal zone of the Medial, Rostral and Cervical spinal cord segments in SCI mice compared to naive animals. (**B**) Multilabel fluorescence immunostaining of the ependymal zone at 7 dpi. Upper panel shows immunostaining for Vimentin (orange) and Ki67 (green) while lower panel shows the same field labeled with Olig2 (fucia) and Hoechst counterstaining (blue). Note that Vimentin+/Ki67+ proliferating EpCs can be seen leaving the central canal ependymal zone (arrowheads). (**C**) Graph of the spatial and temporal progression of changes in ependymal zone proliferation following contusion SCI. Scale bars: **A**, 40 µm; **B**, 35 µm.

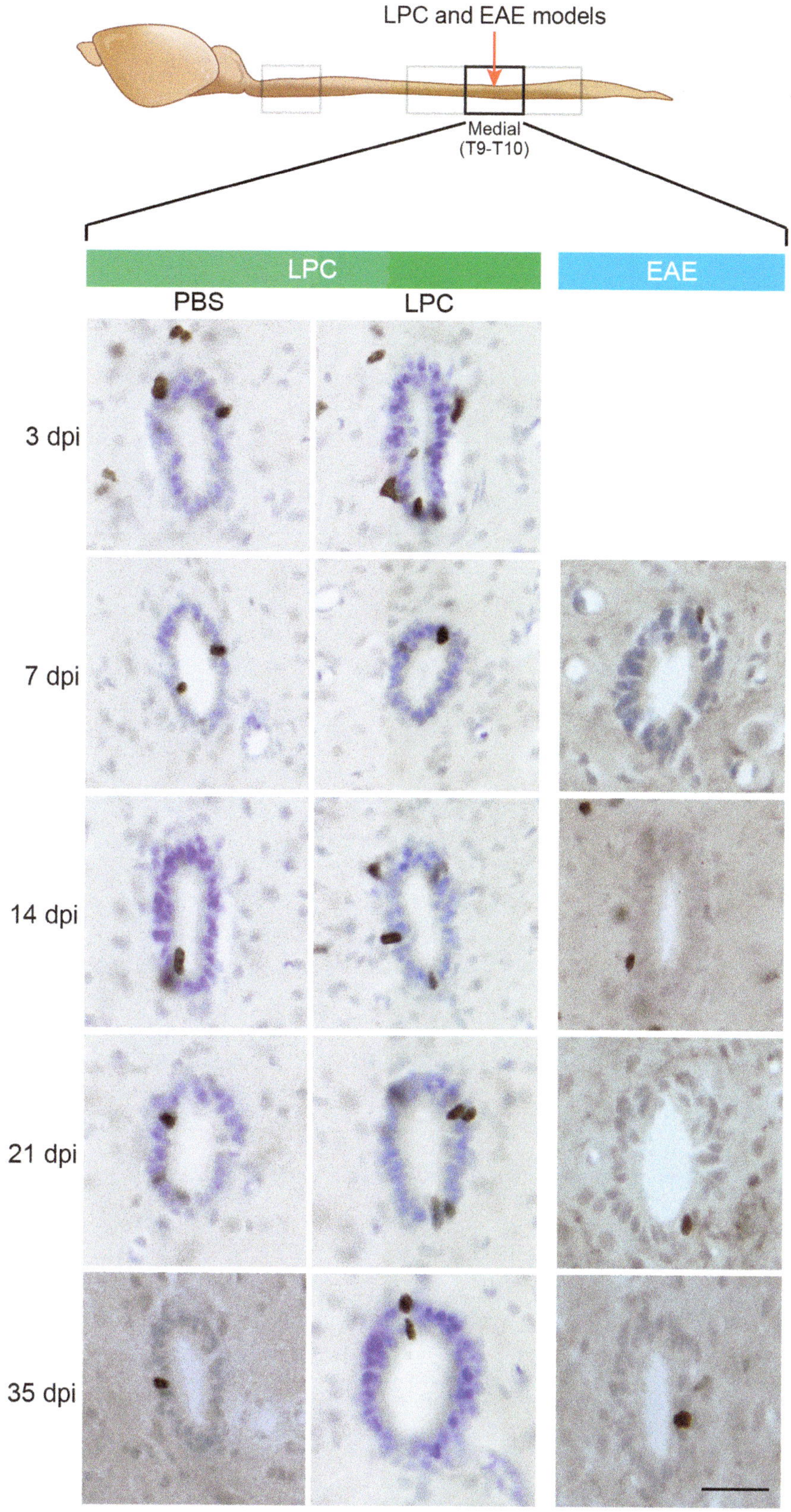

Figure 4. Ependymal cells do not proliferate in response to LPC and EAE models of demyelination. Immunohistochemistry for Ki67-positive (+) ependymal zone cells in the Medial segment of mice injected intraspinally with PBS (left column) or lysophosphatidylcholine (LPC, middle column), or injected peripherally to induce EAE (right column). Images are from mice sacrificed 3, 7, 14, 21, or 35 days post injection/immunization (dpi). Scale bar = 35 μm.

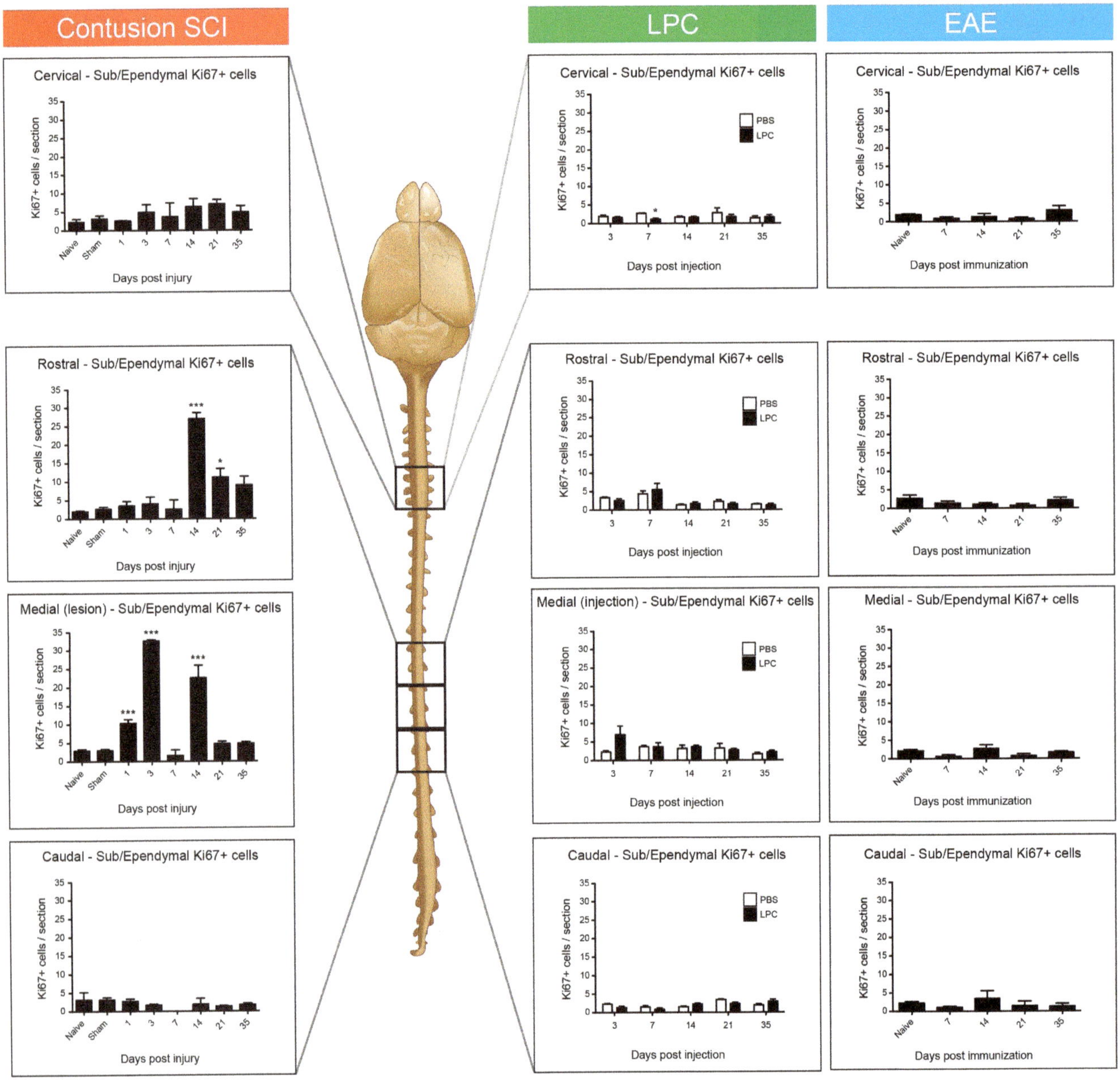

Figure 5. Comparison of spatiotemporal changes in ependymal proliferation after contusion SCI, intraspinal LPC injection or MOG immunization to induce EAE. Complete summary of Ki67+ cell quantifications from the Cervical and three thoracic (Rostral, Medial, Caudal) segments of the spinal cord in all three models of spinal cord pathologies.

colorized and merged using Adobe Photoshop (v. CS5). Figures were assembled using Adobe Illustrator (v. CS5).

Quantification and Statistical Analysis

Counts of Ki67+ cells within the central canal ependymal zone were made using a 40x objective at a total magnification of 400x. Ki67+ cells were quantified from each of the four tissue blocks (cervical, rostral, medial, caudal) of every animal. Proliferation as a function of distance from the lesion epicenter was assessed by 7 cryostat sections located at 500–600-µm intervals in each block. Mean Ki67+ cells/section in each tissue block were obtained by averaging the cell counts from all sections of a block.

Statistical analyses of Ki67 cell counts were made using the Graph-Pad Prism software for Windows, version 5.0a (GraphPad Software Inc., San Diego, CA). In the SCI model, differences between the group means were tested by 1-way ANOVA followed by comparison against the Sham group using Dunnett's post-hoc test. In the LPC model, LPC and PBS conditions were compared against each other at each time point by t-test. In the EAE model, differences between group means were compared by 1-way ANOVA. A p value <0.05 was considered as statistically significant. Error bars represent the standard error of the mean (SEM) of each group.

Results

Experimental Animal Models and Design

Previous studies have shown that proliferation of central canal EpCs is induced in various rodent models of SCI. To better understand EpC reactions to different forms of tissue injury, we compared their responses in three distinct models of traumatic and non-traumatic spinal cord pathologies (Fig. 1A). As a clinically-relevant model of traumatic SCI, we used the IH impactor model of spinal cord contusion, which generates highly reproducible lesions that recapitulate key pathological features of human SCI [27,28]. A medium-impact 50 kdyn IH force was used in order to preserve as much as possible the cytoarchitecture of the ependymal layer and limit motor deficits. In parallel, we used two non-traumatic models of MS-type demyelination. To create focal demyelination, we injected LPC into spinal cord white matter. Following intraspinal injection of LPC, myelin breakdown is rapidly induced in a restricted zone and damaged myelin sheaths are phagocytosed by immune cells within only a few days [24,29]. Importantly, demyelination occurs in the LPC model while axons and neighboring cells remain relatively intact, thus allowing for remyelination [30]. As an MS-like model of autoimmune-mediated, multi-focal demyelination, we performed peripheral injections of MOG_{35-55} emulsified in complete Freund's adjuvant and Pertussis toxin to generate EAE. MOG-induced EAE is a slow onset, autoimmune-mediated process that results in widespread CNS demyelinating lesions and development of quantifiable locomotor deficits [25]. SCI, LPC, and EAE mice were sacrificed at intervals up to 35 days post-spinal cord contusion/intraspinal injection/peripheral immunization (Fig. 1B). Following perfusion fixation, a 12-mm long segment encompassing the mid thoracic and upper lumbar regions of the spinal cord was removed (in the case of SCI and LPC models, centered on the T9/10 contusion or LPC/PBS injection site) and divided into three 4 mm segments (Rostral, Medial and Caudal) (Fig. 1C). In addition, a 4-mm long segment of the mid-cervical (Cervical) spinal cord was harvested for examination of possible changes distant to the injury site (Fig. 1C).

Histopathology of Contusion SCI, LPC and EAE Models

Contusion SCI. Tissue sections at regular intervals across the three thoracic tissue blocks were stained with LFB to examine gross changes in tissue morphology (Fig. 1D). Extensive tissue damage was apparent at the lesion site at 3 days post-injury (dpi), extending ventrally from the dorsal surface and, at the very center of the lesion, often resulting in disappearance of the central canal. Importantly, however, the central canal was preserved both rostral and caudal to the lesion epicenter (even within the Medial block). At 3–14 dpi, edema was particularly pronounced in the caudal direction from the epicenter and was focused within the dorsal column white matter, extending ventrally to the perimeter of the central canal (Fig. 1D). Smaller pockets of blood were intermittently found rostral to the lesion epicenter as well. Interstitial blood was no longer apparent by 14 dpi, and at the lesion epicenter, there was extensive reactive gliosis in the dorsal half of the spinal cord (data not shown). These observations confirmed that the 50 kdyn contusion paradigm would sufficiently spare the central canal to enable further analyses.

LPC-induced focal demyelination. To create a focal zone of rapid demyelination in a specific white matter location, separate mice were injected intraspinally with 1 µl of LPC using a fine glass micropipette with an outer diameter of <40 µm. Our initial experiments were focused on injections into the dorsal column, but over-insertion of the micropipette due to breathing movement was sometimes observed to result in traumatic disturbance of the central canal. We thus decided to opt for a model in which injections were performed in the DLF. A representative example of focal demyelination observed at 3 days after injection is shown in Fig. 1E, as visualized using LFB staining. No demyelination was detected in the DLF of PBS-treated animals. Histological observations revealed that demyelination was considerable on days 3, 7, 14 and 21 post-LPC injection and that remyelination was well advanced by 35 days. Importantly, the cytoarchitecture of the central canal was always preserved with the DLF injections.

EAE-induced multi-focal demyelination. To generate an immune response leading to a more disseminated pattern of demyelinating lesions in the spinal cord, reminiscent of MS plaques, a third series of mice was immunized with MOG in complete Freund's adjuvant. Evaluation of the EAE clinical scores was performed on a daily basis and results are reported in Fig. 1F (left panel). On average, disease onset (i.e. appearance of first signs of paralysis) was observed at day 9.2±0.4. At the peak of disease (day 13.5±0.8), the mean clinical score for EAE mice was 4.0±0.1. Histological staining with LFB at day 14 (peak of disease) confirmed the presence of many demyelinating plaques in the spinal cord of EAE mice, but not in control naive mice (Fig. 1F, right panels).

Gross Proliferative Changes in the Spinal Cord

Distinct macroscopic patterns of proliferative changes were observed in the spinal cords across these three types of pathologies (Fig. 2). Similar to previous studies [2,14], naive animals possessed only rare cells expressing the proliferation-associated antigen Ki67, and these could be found in the white matter, grey matter and/or ependymal zone (Fig. 2A). Seven days following contusion SCI, large numbers of Ki67+ cells were evident in the lesion segment; these cells were concentrated in, but not limited to, the affected dorsal half of the spinal cord (Fig. 2B). At the same 7 day time-point following intraspinal injection of LPC or PBS control (Fig. 2C–D), Ki67+ cells were likewise increased in the spinal cord compared to non-injected controls (naive); however, these cells were largely restricted to the tissue along the needle tract. At 14 days following EAE induction, corresponding to the approximate peak of locomotor deficits, increased numbers of Ki67+ cells were detectable and were distributed throughout the dorso-ventral extent of the spinal cord (Fig. 2E). Thus, increases in overall cell proliferation occurred in all three models of spinal cord pathology, but with distinct spatial patterns.

Robust, Long-distance, and Asymmetric Increase in Proliferation in the Ependymal Zone Following Contusion SCI

We next focused on the proliferative changes occurring in the ependymal zone in the contusion model of SCI (Fig. 3). Naive (non-injured) mice averaged 1–3 proliferating cells/30-µm diameter coronal section in the ependymal zone at cervical, thoracic and lumbar levels of the spinal cord. Following contusion SCI, characteristic patterns of proliferative changes were observed within each tissue block (Fig. 3A). In the lesioned Medial segment, ependymal zone proliferation rapidly increased, peaking at 3 dpi and subsequently declining before peaking again at 14 dpi. Within this Medial segment, the central canal was ablated at the lesion epicenter, but proliferation in the ependymal zone was identifiable within 600 µm rostral and caudal to the injury, and peaked at a distance of approximately 1800 µm (Fig. 3C). In the adjacent Rostral segment, proliferation increased more gradually, peaking at 14 dpi and remaining increased at 21–35 dpi (Fig. 3A).

Although not statistically significant, a trend toward an increase in the proliferation of EpCs was observed at greater distances rostral to the lesion site, as a smaller and slower increase in ependymal zone proliferation was detected in the Cervical block (Fig. 3A), which peaked at 21 dpi (not shown). In marked contrast to the Medial, Rostral and Cervical blocks, ependymal zone proliferation in the segment Caudal to the lesion segment did not increase at any time-point following contusion injury.

Fluorescence immunohistochemistry confirmed that Ki67+ cells surrounding the traumatically injured central canal expressed the EpC markers Sox2 (not shown) and Vimentin (Fig. 3B). Ki67+ cells that were weakly Vimentin+ could occasionally be observed migrating away from the central canal after SCI (Fig. 3B), consistent with previous lineage tracing data [1]. Olig2+ oligodendrocyte progenitors, the principle proliferating cell type in the non-injured spinal cord, were not found to express Ki67+ surrounding the injured central canal (Fig. 3B).

Limited Ependymal Responses in LPC and EAE Models of Demyelination

In the LPC model of focal demyelination, ependymal zone proliferation was assessed using time point-matched injections of LPC versus PBS into the dorsal columns (Fig. 4). In contrast to SCI, there was no detectable LPC-induced increase in ependymal Ki67+ cells (compared to PBS) in any segment or at any time point examined. While quantification showed that PBS injection did by itself cause a small baseline increase in ependymal zone proliferation within the Medial and Rostral segments (Fig. 5), this was attributable to a localized needle-induced traumatic perturbation of the central canal, as histological examination revealed the central canal was occasionally damaged by the injection needle penetrating too deeply through the dorsal columns (not shown). Consistent with this, additional mice were injected with LPC or PBS into the DLF white matter, thereby avoiding central canal damage, and these showed no increase in ependymal zone proliferation (not shown). This finding, when combined with the observation that the remyelination process is well advanced or even completed at 35 days post-LPC treatment, suggests that the proliferation of EpCs is not critical for remyelination in this particular model.

Mice in the EAE model of autoimmune-induced multi-focal demyelination also did not show any increase in numbers of ependymal Ki67+ cells (Figs. 4–5), despite displaying widespread increases in cell proliferation across the spinal cord (Fig. 2E), decreases in LFB-stained white matter (Fig. 1F), and significant functional deficits in locomotor behavior (Fig. 1F).

Quantification and summary comparison of changes in Ki67+ ependymal zone cells in the SCI, LPC and EAE models is shown in Figure 5. Following SCI, the injured Medial segment exhibited a peak in EpC proliferation at 3 dpi at approximately 33 cells/section, in the Rostral segment at 14 dpi at 27 cells/section, and the Cervical segment at 21 dpi at 7 cells/section. No increase was detected in the Caudal segment, and interestingly, a slight depression in proliferation was observed in both the Medial and Caudal segments at 7 dpi. In contrast to SCI, neither chemically-induced nor autoimmune-mediated demyelination resulted in proliferative activation of central canal EpCs.

Discussion

EpCs surrounding the central canal of the adult spinal cord express neural stem cell properties when isolated *in vitro* and after SCI *in vivo*. While directing the responses of reactive EpCs is an attractive potential approach for improving the spinal cord's intrinsic repair mechanisms, neither the extent of EpC proliferation following SCI nor the generality of such proliferative responses in cases of non-traumatic spinal cord pathologies is currently well understood. In the present study, we assessed the spatio-temporal characteristics of EpC proliferative reactions in the IH contusion model of SCI, and then performed a side-by-side comparison of EpC proliferative reactions following SCI, chemically-mediated focal demyelination, and MS-like autoimmune-mediated multifocal demyelination. As discussed below, our data help provide a more complete picture of the extent to which latent EpCs are activated by diverse types of spinal cord pathologies.

Dynamics of Ependymal Cell Reactions in the IH Contusion Model

The IH contusion model provides an excellent experimental approximation of human SCI, and has been endorsed by the Reeve Foundation and most experts in the field as the gold standard for SCI research. The model recapitulates key aspects of human SCI-associated pathology, including inflammation, blood-spinal cord barrier disruption, neuronal and glial cell death, glial scarring, and myelin loss [26–28,31,32]. Importantly, this device generates remarkably similar lesions between animals, and the intensity of the lesions (i.e. impact force) correlates well with lesion volumes and observed motor and behavioral deficits [27,28,31].

Three main conclusions can be made concerning the spatio-temporal kinetics of EpC reactions to the IH contusion model. First, EpC proliferation is rapidly induced in the immediate vicinity of the lesion, and the peak of this proliferation extends away from the injury site in a time-dependent manner. Second, the magnitude of this wave of ependymal proliferation diminishes at greater distances from the lesion, but an approximate 5-fold increase in EpC proliferation still occurs at the cervical level following a low thoracic (T9–10) injury. Third, ependymal proliferation outside of the site of injury is asymmetric, peaking at 3 days within the lesion block, 14 days in an adjacent rostral tissue block, and 21 days at a more distant cervical location, but is absent in a more caudal direction from the lesion segment.

The observation of long-distance and prolonged EpC proliferation in the IH model supports the concept of targeting reactive EpCs to enhance the spinal cord's intrinsic repair capacity. While we did not trace the fate of the proliferating EpCs, previous fate-mapping studies have shown that, at least in the vicinity of the lesion site, the vast majority of EpC progeny adopt an astrocytic fate after SCI, with small numbers of oligodendrocytes also being generated [1,17,22]. Potential therapeutic goals involving endogenous EpCs include modulating their astrocytic contribution to the glial scar, enhancing their rate of oligodendrogenesis, and stimulating their production of replacement or bridge neurons, as such mechanisms are believed to contribute to the functional benefits occurring following neural stem cell transplantation [33,34]. Interestingly, although reactive EpCs spontaneously generate astrocytes and oligodendrocytes following SCI *in vivo*, new neurons have never convincingly been shown to be produced within the adult spinal cord. Since cultured EpCs can spontaneously differentiate into all three of these neural cell types *in vitro*, it appears that the post-SCI environment is dominated by pro-proliferative, pro-astrocytic, and anti-neurogenic factors.

Absence of Ependymal Cell Responses in Non-traumatic Demyelinating Models

We assessed EpC proliferation in two distinct models of non-traumatic demyelinating conditions. LPC injection in mice is characterized by a rapid and focal demyelination at the site of its administration, with a subsequent remyelination that is already well manifested by 35 days. EAE is characterized by an autoimmune reaction directed against myelin proteins (in this case, MOG) that results in multifocal demyelination in the spinal cord and brain. Surprisingly, considering that hundreds of studies have used EAE as an experimental model of MS, the real extent of remyelination occurring spontaneously in MOG-induced chronic EAE in C57BL/6 mice has remained elusive. Despite the possibility that remyelination is scanty or absent in this model, several groups have reported the proliferation of oligodendrocyte progenitors and their differentiation into myelin-producing cells in the damaged CNS of MOG-induced EAE mice [35–37]. The combination of both the LPC and EAE mouse models should therefore be able to cover a broad range of biological responses occurring in MS, including demyelination and remyelination.

The main conclusion that can be drawn regarding these demyelination models is that neither model elicits an increase in EpC proliferation. A recent lineage tracing study likewise found no evidence for increased EpC proliferation in EAE [38]. Our negative finding in the LPC and EAE ependyma is despite the fact that both of the models were associated with increased overall proliferation (with distinct spatial and temporal characteristics) within the spinal cord (Fig. 2). The absence of EpC proliferation is further surprising in light of the fact that EpCs represent a major proliferative population in both the normal and traumatically injured spinal cord. The lack of EpC proliferation in these models indicates that neither the demyelination/remyelination process nor the complex immunological responses associated with autoimmunity is sufficient, by itself, to provide a proliferative trigger for EpCs. To the contrary, in EAE, baseline EpC proliferation tended towards a decrease.

It should be noted that the absence of EpC proliferation does not rule out the possibility of non-proliferative EpC recruitment in non-traumatic spinal cord pathology models. In this regard, there is some evidence of enhanced EpC migration in a transgenic mouse model of amyotrophic lateral sclerosis (ALS) in which motoneurons degenerate [39].

Implications for the Signals Activating Proliferation of Latent Ependymal Cells

The differential proliferation of EpCs following traumatic SCI versus non-traumatic spinal cord demyelination may be linked to the distinct gliogenic responses observed in each case. Following SCI, EpCs primarily produce $Sox9^+$ $GFAP^-$ astrocyte-like cells [1,18] that synthesize CNTF, HGF and IGF-1, and recent work from the lab of Jonas Frisén indicates that these cells are an important component of the protective astroglial scar [18]. In EAE, although astrocytic barriers reminiscent of those induced upon SCI have also been described, these occur on a much smaller scale and are restricted to areas in close proximity to blood vessels [40]. The absence of EpC proliferation during EAE suggests that EpCs only contribute minimally to the scar-like perivascular barriers that restrict leukocyte entry and spread during EAE, and that EAE is not a strong inducer of astrogliogenic signals in the central canal microenvironment. In future work, it would therefore be interesting to determine whether $Sox9^+$ $GFAP^-$ astrocyte-like cells are present in models of EAE and LPC. Rigorous testing of this hypothesis would require the use of an inducible and ependymal-specific transgenic fate-mapping model, enabling tracking of migrating ependymal cell progeny. Unlike the pro-astrogliogenic environment occurring after SCI, the environment found in both the LPC and EAE models involves extensive demyelination and, in the case of LPC, remyelination. Thus, neither demyelination nor remyelination supplies proliferative signals for ependymal cells.

Perspectives

The greatly differing proliferative responses of EpCs in traumatic SCI versus non-traumatic demyelination models highlights the necessity of deciphering the molecular signals controlling activation of latent EpCs. The physiological sources of such activation signals could be diverse, such as: the distinct immune reactions associated with each model; cellular stress and/or cytotoxicity; and the influx of blood-derived factors and/or cells following disruption of the blood-spinal cord barrier. Future work will focus on identifying the endogenous regulators of EpC reactions to tissue injury, in order to develop the potential of harnessing endogenous EpCs to promote spinal cord repair.

Acknowledgments

The authors are grateful to Anne Aumont, Nadia Fortin and Nicolas Vallières for their invaluable technical assistance.

Author Contributions

Conceived and designed the experiments: S. Lacroix LH SB IP KF. Performed the experiments: S. Lacroix LH SB CD IP S. Lévesque CAG. Analyzed the data: S. Lacroix LH AV SB S. Lévesque CD KF. Wrote the paper: S. Lacroix KF.

References

1. Meletis K, Barnabe-Heider F, Carlen M, Evergren E, Tomilin N, et al. (2008) Spinal cord injury reveals multilineage differentiation of ependymal cells. PLoS Biol 6: e182.
2. Hamilton LK, Truong MK, Bednarczyk MR, Aumont A, Fernandes KJ (2009) Cellular organization of the central canal ependymal zone, a niche of latent neural stem cells in the adult mammalian spinal cord. Neuroscience 164: 1044–1056.
3. Bruni JE, Reddy K (1987) Ependyma of the central canal of the rat spinal cord: a light and transmission electron microscopic study. J Anat 152: 55–70.
4. Bruni JE (1998) Ependymal development, proliferation, and functions: a review. Microsc Res Tech 41: 2–13.
5. Rafols JA, Goshgarian HG (1985) Spinal tanycytes in the adult rat: a correlative Golgi gold-toning study. Anat Rec 211: 75–86.
6. Yu K, McGlynn S, Matise MP (2013) Floor plate-derived sonic hedgehog regulates glial and ependymal cell fates in the developing spinal cord. Development 140: 1594–1604.
7. Fu H, Qi Y, Tan M, Cai J, Hu X, et al. (2003) Molecular mapping of the origin of postnatal spinal cord ependymal cells: evidence that adult ependymal cells are derived from Nkx6.1+ ventral neural progenitor cells. J Comp Neurol 456: 237–244.
8. Masahira N, Takebayashi H, Ono K, Watanabe K, Ding L, et al. (2006) Olig2-positive progenitors in the embryonic spinal cord give rise not only to motoneurons and oligodendrocytes, but also to a subset of astrocytes and ependymal cells. Dev Biol 293: 358–369.
9. Ferretti P, Zhang F, O'Neill P (2003) Changes in spinal cord regenerative ability through phylogenesis and development: lessons to be learnt. Dev Dyn 226: 245–256.
10. McHedlishvili L, Mazurov V, Grassme KS, Goehler K, Robl B, et al. (2012) Reconstitution of the central and peripheral nervous system during salamander tail regeneration. Proc Natl Acad Sci U S A 109: E2258–2266.
11. Tanaka EM, Ferretti P (2009) Considering the evolution of regeneration in the central nervous system. Nat Rev Neurosci 10: 713–723.
12. Johansson CB, Momma S, Clarke DL, Risling M, Lendahl U, et al. (1999) Identification of a neural stem cell in the adult mammalian central nervous system. Cell 96: 25–34.
13. Alfaro-Cervello C, Soriano-Navarro M, Mirzadeh Z, Alvarez-Buylla A, Garcia-Verdugo JM (2012) Biciliated ependymal cell proliferation contributes to spinal cord growth. J Comp Neurol 520: 3528–3552.
14. Horner PJ, Power AE, Kempermann G, Kuhn HG, Palmer TD, et al. (2000) Proliferation and differentiation of progenitor cells throughout the intact adult rat spinal cord. J Neurosci 20: 2218–2228.

15. David S, Lacroix S (2003) Molecular approaches to spinal cord repair. Annu Rev Neurosci 26: 411–440.
16. Rossignol S, Frigon A (2011) Recovery of locomotion after spinal cord injury: some facts and mechanisms. Annu Rev Neurosci 34: 413–440.
17. Barnabe-Heider F, Goritz C, Sabelstrom H, Takebayashi H, Pfrieger FW, et al. (2010) Origin of new glial cells in intact and injured adult spinal cord. Cell Stem Cell 7: 470–482.
18. Sabelstrom H, Stenudd M, Reu P, Dias DO, Elfineh M, et al. (2013) Resident neural stem cells restrict tissue damage and neuronal loss after spinal cord injury in mice. Science 342: 637–640.
19. Namiki J, Tator CH (1999) Cell proliferation and nestin expression in the ependyma of the adult rat spinal cord after injury. J Neuropathol Exp Neurol 58: 489–498.
20. Mothe AJ, Tator CH (2005) Proliferation, migration, and differentiation of endogenous ependymal region stem/progenitor cells following minimal spinal cord injury in the adult rat. Neuroscience 131: 177–187.
21. Frisen J, Johansson CB, Torok C, Risling M, Lendahl U (1995) Rapid, widespread, and longlasting induction of nestin contributes to the generation of glial scar tissue after CNS injury. J Cell Biol 131: 453–464.
22. Sabelstrom H, Stenudd M, Frisen J (2013) Neural stem cells in the adult spinal cord. Exp Neurol.
23. Scheff SW, Rabchevsky AG, Fugaccia I, Main JA, Lumpp JE, Jr. (2003) Experimental modeling of spinal cord injury: characterization of a force-defined injury device. J Neurotrauma 20: 179–193.
24. Ghasemlou N, Jeong SY, Lacroix S, David S (2007) T cells contribute to lysophosphatidylcholine-induced macrophage activation and demyelination in the CNS. Glia 55: 294–302.
25. Stromnes IM, Goverman JM (2006) Active induction of experimental allergic encephalomyelitis. Nat Protoc 1: 1810–1819.
26. Pineau I, Lacroix S (2007) Proinflammatory cytokine synthesis in the injured mouse spinal cord: multiphasic expression pattern and identification of the cell types involved. J Comp Neurol 500: 267–285.
27. Basso DM, Fisher LC, Anderson AJ, Jakeman LB, McTigue DM, et al. (2006) Basso Mouse Scale for locomotion detects differences in recovery after spinal cord injury in five common mouse strains. J Neurotrauma 23: 635–659.
28. Nishi RA, Liu H, Chu Y, Hamamura M, Su MY, et al. (2007) Behavioral, histological, and ex vivo magnetic resonance imaging assessment of graded contusion spinal cord injury in mice. J Neurotrauma 24: 674–689.
29. Ousman SS, David S (2000) Lysophosphatidylcholine induces rapid recruitment and activation of macrophages in the adult mouse spinal cord. Glia 30: 92–104.
30. Blakemore WF, Franklin RJ (2008) Remyelination in experimental models of toxin-induced demyelination. Curr Top Microbiol Immunol 318: 193–212.
31. Ghasemlou N, Kerr BJ, David S (2005) Tissue displacement and impact force are important contributors to outcome after spinal cord contusion injury. Exp Neurol 196: 9–17.
32. Lee JY, Kim HS, Choi HY, Oh TH, Yune TY (2012) Fluoxetine inhibits matrix metalloprotease activation and prevents disruption of blood-spinal cord barrier after spinal cord injury. Brain 135: 2375–2389.
33. Lu P, Wang Y, Graham L, McHale K, Gao M, et al. (2012) Long-distance growth and connectivity of neural stem cells after severe spinal cord injury. Cell 150: 1264–1273.
34. Hofstetter CP, Holmstrom NA, Lilja JA, Schweinhardt P, Hao J, et al. (2005) Allodynia limits the usefulness of intraspinal neural stem cell grafts; directed differentiation improves outcome. Nat Neurosci 8: 346–353.
35. Picard-Riera N, Decker L, Delarasse C, Goude K, Nait-Oumesmar B, et al. (2002) Experimental autoimmune encephalomyelitis mobilizes neural progenitors from the subventricular zone to undergo oligodendrogenesis in adult mice. Proc Natl Acad Sci U S A 99: 13211–13216.
36. Aharoni R, Herschkovitz A, Eilam R, Blumberg-Hazan M, Sela M, et al. (2008) Demyelination arrest and remyelination induced by glatiramer acetate treatment of experimental autoimmune encephalomyelitis. Proc Natl Acad Sci U S A 105: 11358–11363.
37. Girolamo F, Ferrara G, Strippoli M, Rizzi M, Errede M, et al. (2011) Cerebral cortex demyelination and oligodendrocyte precursor response to experimental autoimmune encephalomyelitis. Neurobiol Dis 43: 678–689.
38. Guo F, Maeda Y, Ma J, Delgado M, Sohn J, et al. (2011) Macroglial plasticity and the origins of reactive astroglia in experimental autoimmune encephalomyelitis. J Neurosci 31: 11914–11928.
39. Chi L, Ke Y, Luo C, Li B, Gozal D, et al. (2006) Motor neuron degeneration promotes neural progenitor cell proliferation, migration, and neurogenesis in the spinal cords of amyotrophic lateral sclerosis mice. Stem Cells 24: 34–43.
40. Voskuhl RR, Peterson RS, Song B, Ao Y, Morales LB, et al. (2009) Reactive astrocytes form scar-like perivascular barriers to leukocytes during adaptive immune inflammation of the CNS. J Neurosci 29: 11511–11522.

The Asparaginyl Endopeptidase Legumain Is Essential for Functional Recovery after Spinal Cord Injury in Adult Zebrafish

Liping Ma[1], Yan-Qin Shen[2,3], Harsh P. Khatri[1], Melitta Schachner[1,2]*

1 W. M. Keck Center for Collaborative Neuroscience and Department of Cell Biology and Neuroscience, Rutgers University, Piscataway, New Jersey, United States of America, 2 Center for Neuroscience, Shantou University Medical College, Shantou, Guangdong Province, People's Republic of China, 3 Department of Basic Medicine, Jiangnan University Medical School, Wuxi, Jiangsu Province, People's Republic of China

Abstract

Unlike mammals, adult zebrafish are capable of regenerating severed axons and regaining locomotor function after spinal cord injury. A key factor for this regenerative capacity is the innate ability of neurons to re-express growth-associated genes and regrow their axons after injury in a permissive environment. By microarray analysis, we have previously shown that the expression of *legumain* (also known as asparaginyl endopeptidase) is upregulated after complete transection of the spinal cord. *In situ* hybridization showed upregulation of *legumain* expression in neurons of regenerative nuclei during the phase of axon regrowth/sprouting after spinal cord injury. Upregulation of Legumain protein expression was confirmed by immunohistochemistry. Interestingly, upregulation of *legumain* expression was also observed in macrophages/microglia and neurons in the spinal cord caudal to the lesion site after injury. The role of legumain in locomotor function after spinal cord injury was tested by reducing Legumain expression by application of anti-sense morpholino oligonucleotides. Using two independent anti-sense morpholinos, locomotor recovery and axonal regrowth were impaired when compared with a standard control morpholino. We conclude that upregulation of legumain expression after spinal cord injury in the adult zebrafish is an essential component of the capacity of injured neurons to regrow their axons. Another feature contributing to functional recovery implicates upregulation of legumain expression in the spinal cord caudal to the injury site. In conclusion, we established for the first time a function for an unusual protease, the asparaginyl endopeptidase, in the nervous system. This study is also the first to demonstrate the importance of legumain for repair of an injured adult central nervous system of a spontaneously regenerating vertebrate and is expected to yield insights into its potential in nervous system regeneration in mammals.

Editor: Peter Hitchcock, University of Michigan, United States of America

Funding: This work was supported by grants from the New Jersey Commission on Spinal Cord Research (05-3048-SCR-E-0 and 08-3079-SCR-E-0, http://www.state.nj.us/health/spinalcord/). The funders had no role in study design, data collection and analysis, decision to publish, or preparation of the manuscript.

Competing Interests: The authors have declared that no competing interests exist.

* E-mail: schachner@stu.edu.cn

Introduction

In adult mammals, spinal cord injury (SCI) most often causes permanent disabilities due to failure to regenerate. In contrast to mammals, adult zebrafish regenerate successfully after SCI. Features leading to successful regeneration are the innate ability of neurons to re-express growth-associated genes, regrow their axons and adjust their synaptic connections in a permissive CNS tissue environment [1]. Thus, zebrafish have developed into a powerful model to elucidate the molecular mechanisms underlying not only spinal cord regeneration, but also regeneration of the adult CNS in general, raising the hope that the findings from zebrafish may lead to therapeutic approaches in mammals.

To identify novel regeneration-conducive molecules, we have performed mRNA microarray expression profiling of the nucleus of the medial longitudinal fascicle (NMLF), a brainstem nucleus containing neurons capable of axonal regeneration after injury, hypothesizing that genes that are upregulated in expression after SCI contribute to successful recovery of locomotor functions. One of the molecules upregulated in neurons capable of axonal regeneration after SCI was legumain [2], the function of which in regeneration and in nervous system functions in general, is unknown.

Since proteases play important roles in all aspects of nervous system development, tissue remodeling during learning/memory and after injury [3–4], we chose to investigate the unusual proteolytic enzyme legumain among the upregulated molecules. As a member of the C13 family of cysteine proteases, legumain/asparaginyl endopeptidase cleaves protein substrates at the C-terminus of asparagine [5]. Legumain was first observed to be located in the endosome/lysosome systems [6], has since been detected in the nucleus [7–8], at the cell surface [9] and in the extracellular matrix [10–13]. Legumain is involved in many physiological and pathological processes, such as antigen processing [14], cell migration [9] and proliferation [7], regulation of biosynthesis of lysosomal proteins [15], extracellular matrix turnover [12], as well as osteoclast formation and bone resorption [10]. Upregulation of legumain expression has been reported in various solid tumors, positively correlating with their invasive and metastatic potential [9,16–17]. Legumain also functions as a carboxypeptidase [18].

The role of legumain in nervous system function has yet to be determined, particularly in recovery after injury. Here we report a novel function of legumain in the nervous system, and in particular in regeneration of the adult zebrafish CNS. Legumain expression is upregulated after SCI not only in regenerative brainstem neurons, but also in the spinal cord caudal to the lesion site. Inhibition of this expression reduces locomotor recovery, thus identifying legumain as a novel protease that is an important contributor to functional recovery after injury in the adult zebrafish CNS.

Materials and Methods

Spinal cord injury in adult zebrafish

Adult zebrafish (*Danio rerio*, male, age >6 months) were obtained from Aquatica Tropicals Inc. (Plant City, FL, USA). The fish were maintained at 28°C on a 14-h light and 10-h dark cycle. SCI was performed as described [2,19–23]. Briefly, fish were put in phosphate-buffered saline (PBS, pH 7.4) containing 0.033% aminobenzoic acid ethylmethylester (MS222; Sigma, St Louis, MO, USA) for 5 min. To expose the vertebral column, a longitudinal incision at the left side of the fish was made. Then, a complete cut of the spinal cord was performed between the eighth and ninth vertebrae, 3.5 mm caudal to the brainstem-spinal cord junction. The sham-injured control fish (CON) received similar surgical procedures without cutting the spinal cord. The incision was sealed with Histoacryl (B. Braun, Melsungen, Germany) and fish were returned to their rearing tank. Fish were killed by an overdose of MS222 at the appropriate time points. All animal experiments were approved by the Rutgers University Institutional Animal Use and Care Committee (permit number: 10010), which conforms to NIH guidelines.

Quantitative real-time polymerase chain reaction and microarray data

Four millimeters of whole spinal cord tissue caudal to the lesion site was collected at 1 day, 3 days, and 11 days after surgery from SCI or sham-injured fish. Spinal cords from 6 fish were pooled for each group. Total RNA was extracted using Qiagen RNeasy Micro Kit (Qiagen, Hilden, Germany) and a total of 200 ng RNA was used for first-strand cDNA synthesis using Superscript^{TM} II reverse transcriptase (Invitrogen, Carlsbad, CA, USA) according to the manufacturer's instructions. Quantitative real-time polymerase chain reaction (qPCR) was carried out with Power SYBR Green PCR Master Mix (Applied Biosystems, Foster City, CA, USA) and the comparative cycle threshold Ct method ($\Delta\Delta$Ct method) was applied for data analysis as described [24]. No amplified product was observed when the cDNA template was replaced either by RNA sample without reverse transcription or by water. Results are expressed relative to sham-injured fish 1 day after SCI. The primers used were as follows: zebrafish legumain (forward: 5′-GGCGTTCCAGGGTAGCTCTA-3′; reverse: 5′-GACACTGGCTCCACTGCCTT-3′) and zebrafish ribosomal protein P0 (forward: 5′-TCGGCTACCCAACTCTTGCT-3′; reverse: 5′-TGTTTCGACAGTGACAGCCAG-3′).

Microarray analysis was performed and analyzed as described [2]. Please refer to previous publication for detailed information [2]. Data files for this microarray analysis have been deposited in the NIH Gene Expression Omnibus repository. The accession number is GSE28470 and the link is https://www.ncbi.nlm.nih.gov/projects/geo/query/acc.cgi?acc = GSE28470.

In situ hybridization

PCR product for zebrafish *legumain* (NM_214759, 628–1043 bp of coding sequence) was cloned into pGEM-T Easy vector, with which digoxigenin-labeled RNA sense and antisense probes were transcribed *in vitro* using the Megascript^{TM} system (Ambion, Austin, TX, USA) according to the manufacturer's protocol. In situ hybridization was carried out as described [2,25–26]. Briefly, 25-µm-thick coronal brain sections or 20-µm-thick sagittal spinal cord sections were incubated with 0.1 N HCl for 10 min. After three washes in PBS, pH 7.4, the sections were treated with 10 µg/mL proteinase-K (Roche, Indianapolis, IN, USA) for 10 min at room temperature. Then, the sections were hybridized with sense or antisense probes at 55°C overnight. Alkaline phosphatase-coupled anti-digoxigenin antibody (Roche) was used to label the hybridized probes and the signal was developed with NBT/BCIP (nitro-blue tetrazolium and 5-bromo-4-chloro-3-indolyl phosphate, Roche). The same procedure was used for sections from fish that were not injured, sham-injured or spinal cord-injured. In situ hybridization with the sense control probe and the antisense probe was performed in parallel. No significant signal was observed for the sense probe. The NMLF (medial longitudinal fascicle) and IMRF (intermediate reticular formation) can be located according to the atlas of zebrafish brain [27] and the neurons with large cell body size (13–23 µm diameter) [20] are distinguishable from small glial cells [25]. Total positively stained neurons in the NMLF or the IMRF from each fish were counted. For profile measurements of spinal cord sections, cells in fifteen 10× fields, 5 from each animal, were counted. The intensity of each cell, in a total of 60 cells for each treatment, was measured using ImageJ.

Immunohistochemistry and double staining for *in situ* hybridization and immunohistochemistry

Sections from brain (25-µm-thick coronal) or spinal cord (20-µm-thick, sagittal, 0–4 mm caudal to lesion site) were blocked with 1% bovine serum albumin and 3% donkey serum in PBS containing 0.2% Triton-X-100 for 1 hour at room temperature, followed by primary antibody incubation. Primary antibodies used were: goat anti-human legumain (AF2199, 1:200, R&D Systems, Minneapolis, MN, USA), rabbit anti-glial fibrillary acidic protein (GFAP) (1:500, Dako, Carpinteria, CA, USA), mouse anti-NeuN (1:150, A-60, Millipore, Billerica, MA, USA), and mouse 4C4 antibody (92092321, 7.4.C4, 1:60, Health Protection Agency Culture Collection). Legumain protein contains 433 amino acids, and the legumain antibody used here was raised against the human Legumain sequence of amino acids 18–433. The identity of these amino acids between human and zebrafish is 67%. The specificity of the legumain antibody in recognizing zebrafish Legumain was verified by Western blot analysis (Figure S1). Alexa Fluor secondary antibodies (Molecular Probes) were used at a dilution of 1:600. Non-immune mouse or goat IgGs were used in place of primary antibodies at the same concentrations as isotype controls.

The immunohistochemical detection of the expression of NeuN (neuronal marker neuronal nuclei) in *legumain* mRNA positive cells (*in situ* hybridization) was carried out after completion of *in situ* hybridization. After three washes in PBS, the sections were treated with 10 mM citrate buffer (pH 6.0) at 95°C for 15 min for antigen retrieval as described [2,28]. After cool down to room temperature, the sections were washed three times with PBS and blocked with PBS containing 1% bovine serum albumin and 3% goat serum. Then, the sections were incubated with mouse anti-NeuN antibody at 4°C overnight, followed by incubation with secondary antibody Alexa Fluor 555 (1:600, Invitrogen).

Application of morpholinos and biocytin

Two non-overlapping antisense morpholinos (MOs) for zebrafish *legumain* (NM_214759) (*legumain* MO1: 5'-GGCTCATTTCTGCAATTTACAGCTA -3'; *legumain* MO2: 5'-GTACACGACGCCCGAGCTGCCTGTA -3', Gene Tools, LLC, Philomath, OR, USA) were used in this study. Both *legumain* MOs, tagged with carboxyfluorescein at the 3' end, were designed to block translation. The specificity and efficacy of these two *legumain* MOs to knockdown Legumain expression was demonstrated by immunohistochemistry using an antibody against Legumain. The standard control MO (5'- CCTCTTACCT-CAGTTACAATTTATA-3') was also tagged with carboxyfluorescein at the 3' end. MOs were prepared in Danieau solution (58 mM NaCl, 0.7 mM KCl, 0.4 mM $MgSO_4$, 0.6 mM $Ca(NO_3)_2$, 5 mM HEPES, pH 7.6, as described [2,19,21–23].

Five hundred nanograms MO (approximately 0.2 µL, carried by Gelfoam (Upjohn, Kalamazoo, MI, USA)) was applied at the lesion site immediately after transection. Then, the fish were allowed to survive up to 6 weeks. The efficiency of this MO dose (500 ng per fish) was shown in our publication [19] and was confirmed thereafter [2,21–23,29–31]. In order to detect the neurons with regenerated axons, at 6 weeks after the MO treatment, biocytin (Sigma) (50 mg/mL, approximately 0.2 µL, absorbed in Gelfoam) was applied to a secondary lesion site, which was 3.5 mm caudal to the first spinal lesion site for MO treatment, i.e. 7 mm caudal to the brainstem–spinal cord junction. One day afterwards, the brains were dissected and biocytin was detected with the Vectastain ABC-DAB kit (Vector Laboratories, Burlingame, CA, USA) as described [2,19,22]. For cell body profile counting, all positively stained neurons in the NMLF and IMRF of each animal were counted.

Locomotor analysis

To examine locomotor recovery, the total distance swum by the MO-treated fish was measured at 6 weeks after MO treatment. Freely moving fish was tracked as described [2,19,21–23]. Briefly, each fish was placed in a glass tank (50×30 cm) containing aquarium water (5 cm deep). The moving of the fish was recorded for 5 min by a camera mounted above the tank. Ethovision XT software (Noldus, Wageningen, The Netherlands) was used to track and calculate swim paths.

Statistical analysis

A two-tailed Student's *t*-test was used to evaluate the results from microarray analysis of *legumain* mRNA expression in spinal cord, *legumain*-positive neuronal profiles in different regenerative nuclei after SCI, legumain immunostaining intensity in small cells, and numbers of legumain-immunopositive small cells after SCI. One-way ANOVA followed by Tukey's *post hoc* test, when appropriate, was used for analysis of Legumain protein expression profiles after MO treatment, locomotor recovery after MO application, evaluation of fluorescein-positive cell profiles after MO application and of neuronal profiles retrogradely labeled after MO application in two nuclei with innate capacity for regeneration. Two-way ANOVA followed by Tukey's *post hoc* test, when appropriate, was used for evaluation of the qPCR results of *legumain* expression in the caudal part of the spinal cord. The level of significance was set at $P<0.05$ for all analyses. Data are shown as mean values ±SEM. Statistical analyses were performed using R2.12.2 software (http://www.r-project.org).

Results

Legumain expression is upregulated in the nucleus of the medial longitudinal fascicle after SCI

To gain insights into the molecular mechanisms underlying successful spinal cord regeneration after SCI in adult zebrafish, we had performed microarray analysis to detect gene expression profile changes after SCI, when compared to sham-injured fish [2]. For the microarray analysis, RNA samples were prepared from tissue microdissected from the anatomically well defined NMLF nucleus. This analysis showed that *legumain* mRNA expression does not change during early phases after axotomy, i.e. 4 h (1.038±0.067 (SCI) versus 1.000±0.118 (CON), two-tailed *t*-test, $P>0.05$) and 12 h (0.954±0.120 (SCI) versus 1.000±0.089 (CON), two-tailed *t*-test, $P>0.05$) when compared to sham-injured fish, which were generally taken as controls. However, a significant upregulation of *legumain* mRNA expression was observed at 11 days (1.745±0.171 (SCI) versus 1.000±0.089 (CON), two-tailed *t*-test, $P<0.05$), a time point when tissue remodeling begins to lead to locomotor improvement. The expression of *legumain* mRNA in individual neurons in the NMLF and intermediate reticular formation (IMRF), another nucleus capable of innate regenerating lesioned axons, was studied by *in situ* hybridization. With the sense probe, no significant signal was observed when staining was performed in parallel using the antisense probe (Fig. 1A). Positive signal for *legumain* mRNA was observed in the NMLF neurons, which can easily be identified by their location and large cell body size (>13 µm in diameter) (Figs. 1A, 2A). The neuronal cell identity of these cells expressing *legumain* mRNA in the NMLF and IMRF was further validated by double labeling of *legumain* mRNA (*in situ* hybridization) and the neuronal marker NeuN (immunohistochemistry) (Fig. 2A). Consistent with our microarray analysis, the number of *legumain*-positive neuronal profiles was considerably increased in the NMLF at 11 days after SCI (Fig.1A, B). In the IMRF, upregulation of *legumain* mRNA expression was identified by increased numbers of positive neurons 11 days after SCI (Fig. 1A, C). Upregulation of *legumain* mRNA in these regenerative nuclei after SCI suggests that legumain contributes to successful regeneration.

In addition to investigating the nuclei with neurons capable of axonal regrowth, expression of *legumain* mRNA was also examined in neurons with no or limited capacity for innate regeneration, such as Mauthner neurons [20]. Unlike the findings in the NMLF or IMRF, no significant signal was observed in Mauthner neurons in sections from fish with or without SCI (data not shown). This indicates that upregulation of *legumain* mRNA is characteristic of neurons with regenerative capacity.

Microarray analysis showed no change for *legumain* mRNA expression at 4 h and 12 h after SCI in the NMLF. At 1 day after SCI, no change in *legumain* expression was observed in the NMLF (Fig. 1B) or IMRF (Fig. 1C). However, a slight but significant increase in *legumain* mRNA levels was observed at 3 days after SCI in both the NMLF (Fig. 1B) and IMRF (Fig. 1C), suggesting that upregulation of *legumain* expression as measured by *in situ* hybridization occurs at an early time point, but not immediately after axotomy. Upregulation of Legumain expression in the NMLF and IMRF was also seen at the protein level by immunohistochemistry using an antibody against human Legumain, which detects zebrafish Legumain (Fig. 2B). This upregulation of legumain expression by regenerative supraspinal neurons during axon regrowth/sprouting suggests that legumain contributes to regeneration after injury.

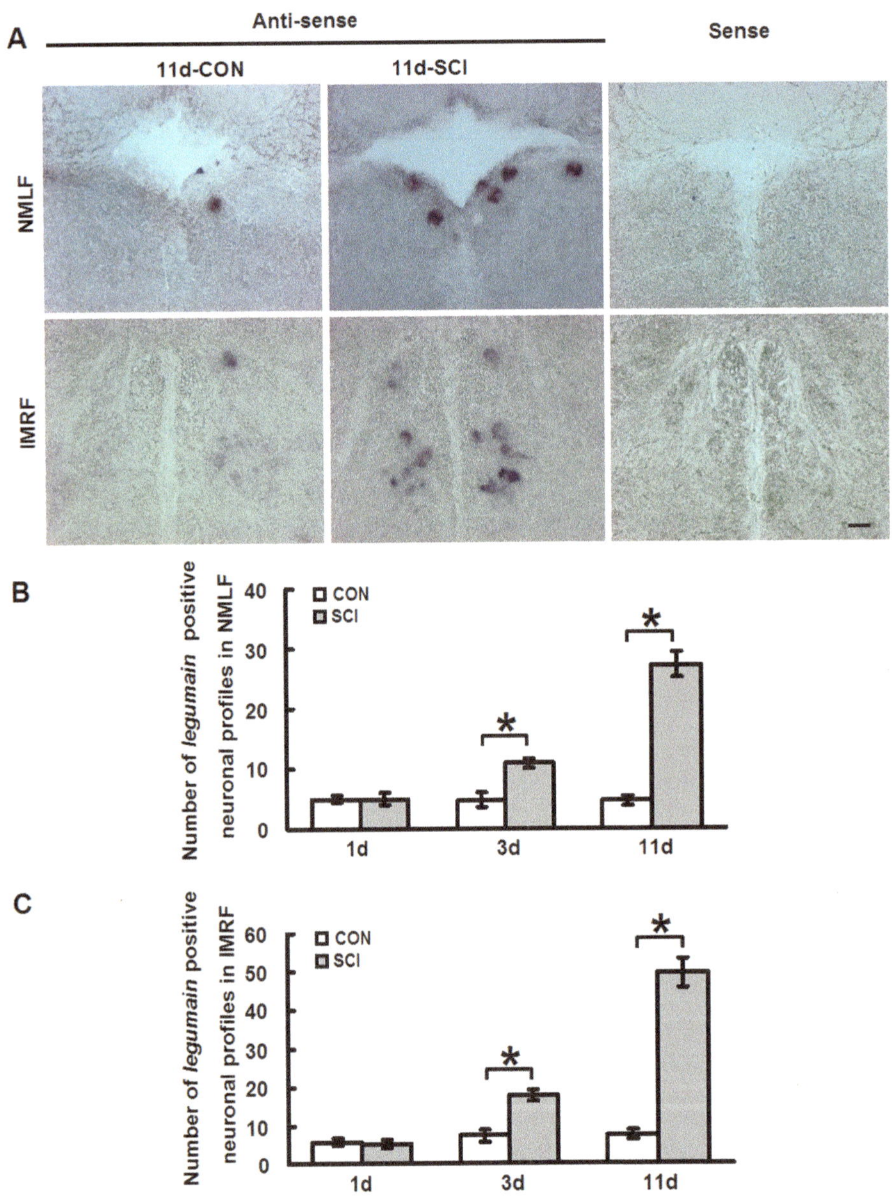

Figure 1. *Legumain* mRNA expression is upregulated in brainstem neurons during the axonal regrowth phase after SCI. (A) *In situ* hybridization was performed to study the expression of *legumain* in the NMLF and IMRF. Representative images depict *legumain*-positive cells in the NMLF and IMRF 11 days after SCI. More positive cells for *legumain* mRNA are observed in the NMLF and IMRF after SCI when compared with sham-injured control. With the sense control probe, no signal is observed. (B, C) Quantification shows that *legumain* mRNA expression is slightly upregulated in the NMLF and IMRF at 3 days and highly upregulated at 11 days after SCI. The expression patterns of *legumain* in the NMLF and IMRF are similar. Dorsal is up. NMLF, $n=6$ fish; IMRF, $n=3$ fish. * $P<0.05$, two-tailed *t*-test; mean values ±SEM are shown. Scale bar, 50 μm.

Legumain expression is upregulated in the caudal spinal cord after SCI

In addition to brainstem neurons which are capable to regrow their axons after SCI, the caudal part spinal cord is another key factor for successful regeneration [19,21,29–33]. It is hypothesized that the caudal spinal cord, into which regenerating axons project, should be permissive for axonal regeneration, and that the cellular rearrangements in the caudal spinal cord also contribute essentially to regeneration. Levels of *legumain* mRNA in the caudal spinal cord were studied by qPCR at 1 day, 3 days and 11 days after SCI, in parallel with cells from the brainstem. Levels of *legumain* mRNA in the caudal spinal cord were not changed 1 day after SCI (Fig. 3A), but considerably increased at 3 days (Fig. 3A). Upregulation was also seen at 11 days after SCI (Fig. 3A), although less so than at 3 days after SCI.

To investigate the expression pattern of *legumain* in the caudal part of the injured spinal cord, *in situ* hybridization was performed. Two regions of the spinal cord were investigated: the tissue immediately caudal to the lesion site (approximately 50–80 μm in length) (Fig. 3B) and the remaining caudal spinal cord tissue (Fig. 3B). The reason for this analysis was that the two regions showed different *legumain* expression patterns by *in situ* hybridization after SCI. In the sham-injured control group, the two spinal cord regions showed a similar expression pattern of *legumain* (Fig. 3B).

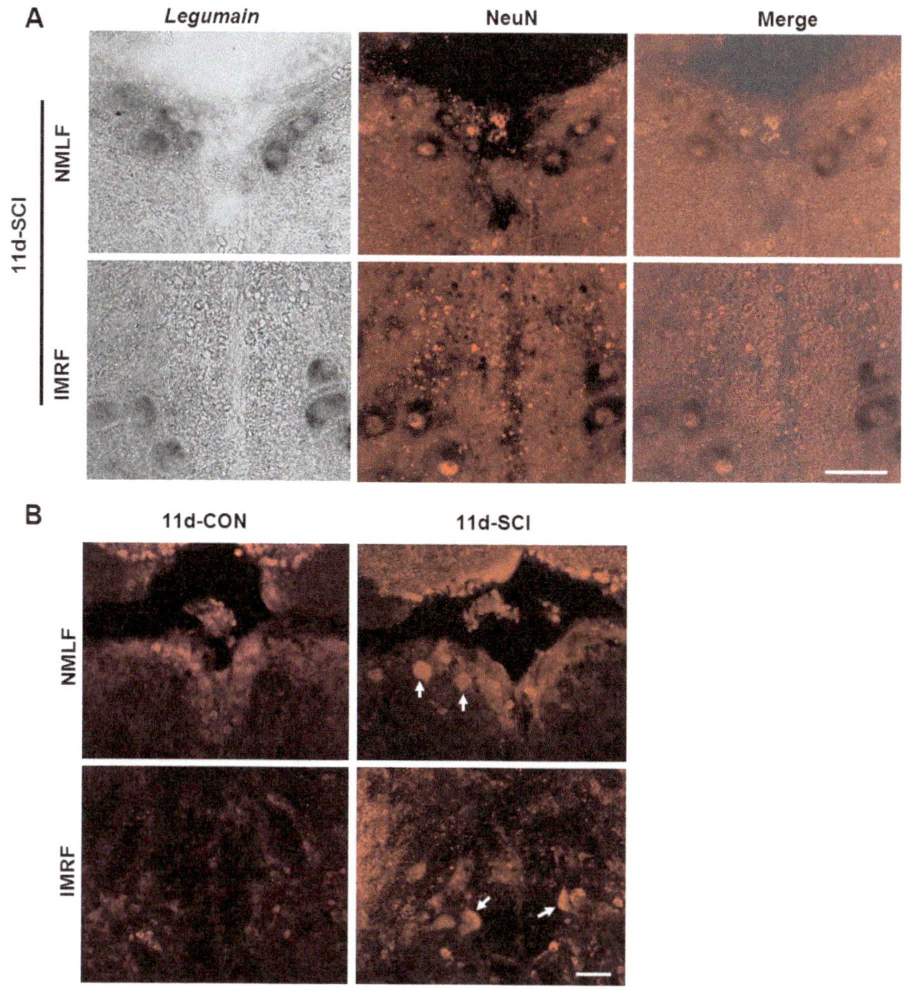

Figure 2. Upregulation of legumain expression in brainstem neurons at 11 days after SCI. (A) Double staining of *legumain* mRNA (*in situ* hybridization) and NeuN (immunohistochemistry) was performed to determine the identity of *legumain*-positive cells. The signal for NeuN locates in the nucleus and *legumain* mRNA locates in the neuronal cytoplasm in the NMLF and IMRF. (B) Immunohistochemistry for Legumain shows more Legumain positive neurons (arrows) in the NMLF and IMRF at 11 days after SCI when compared to the sham-injured control. Dorsal is up. A, $n=3$ experiments; B, $n=3$ fish. Scale bar, 50 μm.

In the non-injured spinal cord, *in situ* hybridization signals were mainly observed in a few neurons with large round cell bodies (> 13 μm in diameter) in the gray matter. These cells were identified as neurons by double immunolabeling with the neuronal marker NeuN (see below). When compared to non-injured fish, positive signals in the 1 day sham-injured control spinal cord was also seen in many small cells with irregular shapes (identified as macrophages/microglia by double immunolabeling with 4C4 antibody, see below) localized in both gray and white matter along the entire length of the caudal spinal cord, indicating that sham-injury induces *legumain* expression. In comparison to the sham-injured group, more intense signals in these small cells were observed in the spinal cord caudal to the lesion site after SCI (Fig. 3B, 1d-CON, 100±8.55%; 1d-SCI, 186.11±6.24 (normalized to 1d-CON), $n=3$ fish, two-tailed *t*-test, $P=0.001$). No difference in the numbers of these small cells was found between the sham-injured and SCI groups (data not shown), indicating that the increased expression of *legumain* 1 day after SCI is due to increased expression intensity by the small cells. At the lesion site, at 1 day, 3 days and 11 days after SCI, many intensely *legumain* positive small cells were observed (Fig. 3B).

Interestingly, the *in situ* hybridization signal for *legumain* in the small cells in 3 days sham-injured control group was no longer detectable, and a positive signal was only seen in neurons as seen in the non-injured spinal cord. However, many small cells with strong signal for *legumain* were observed at 3 days after SCI. Furthermore, when compared to the signal at 1 day after SCI, more small cells were found in the spinal cord caudal to the injury site at 3 days after SCI (Fig. 3B, 1d-SCI, 100±5.02%; 3d-SCI, 149.42±12.03% (normalized to 1d-SCI), $n=3$ fish, two-tailed *t*-test, $P=0.02$), also with a more staining intense signal (Fig. 3B, 1d-SCI, 100±3.354%; 3d-SCI, 124.71±1.16% (normalized to 1d-SCI), $n=3$ fish, two-tailed *t*-test, $P=0.002$). Similar to the findings at 1 day after SCI, no significant differences of *legumain* expression in neurons were found between the sham-injured and SCI groups at 3 days. Thus, increased expression of *legumain* at 3 days after SCI is due to both the increased number of positive cells and expression intensity of *legumain* in the small cells compared to 1 day after SCI.

The expression pattern of *legumain* in the sham-injured group at 11 days was similar to that of the 3 day sham-injured group, i.e. only neurons with a large cell body (>13 μm in diameter) express

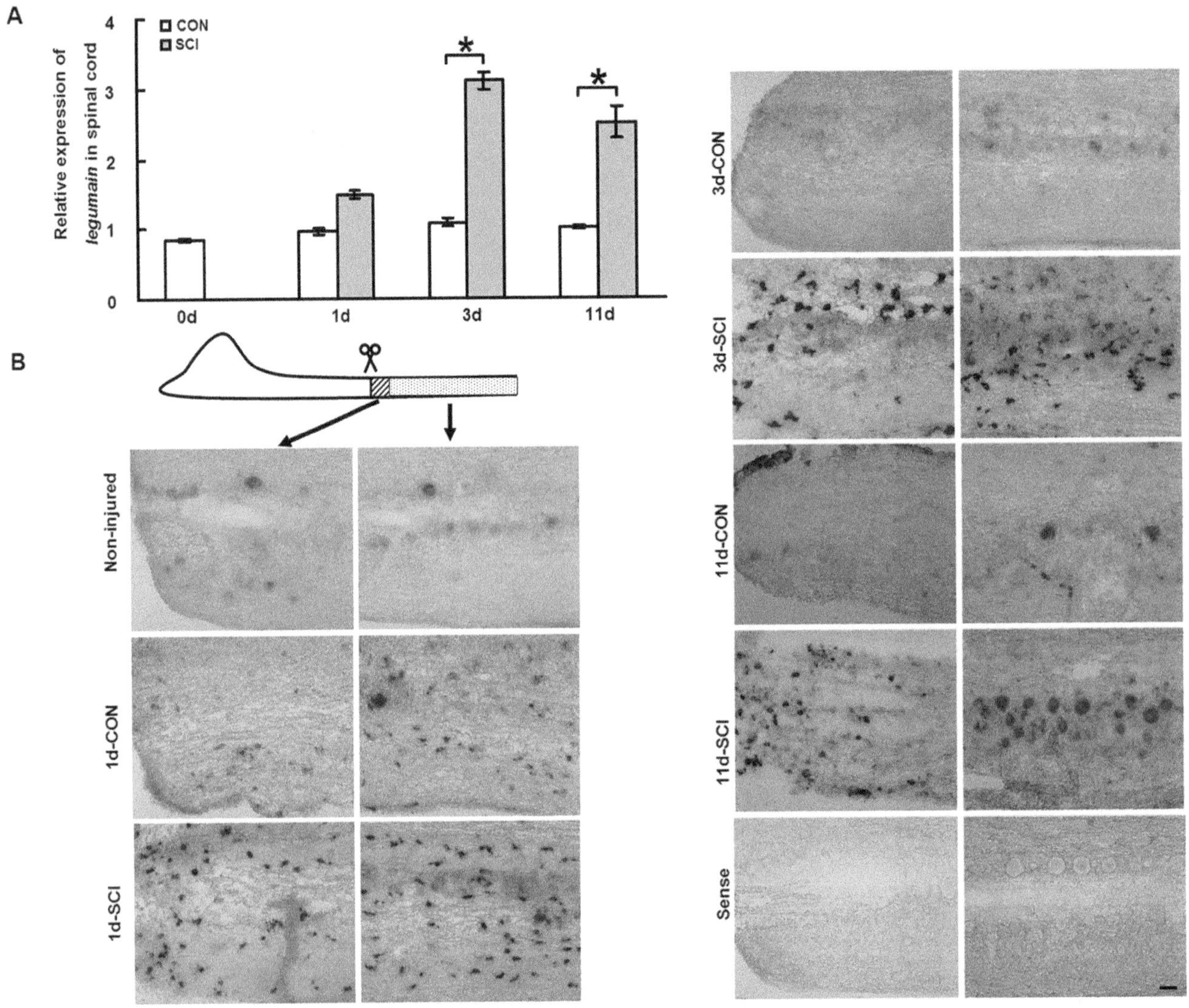

Figure 3. *Legumain* mRNA expression is upregulated in the caudal spinal cord after SCI. (A) Quantitative real-time PCR (qPCR) shows that *legumain* mRNA expression increases from 3 days post-injury and remains upregulated at 11 days after SCI. (B) *In situ* hybridization for *legumain* mRNA in the caudal spinal cord shows different expression patterns in the lesion site (area with stripes) and the caudal part of spinal cord (area with dots). In the non-injured spinal cord, *legumain* mRNA is only observed in neurons. In the lesion site, *legumain* mRNA is observed in many small cells at all time points tested after SCI. In the spinal cord caudal to the lesion site, *legumain* mRNA is detectable in small cells in both the sham-injured and SCI groups at 1 day, with a stronger signal for *legumain* mRNA after SCI compared to the sham injury group. At 3 days, while the signal for *legumain* mRNA in small cells is not detectable anymore in the sham-injured group, strong positive signal for *legumain* mRNA expression is observed in small cells in the SCI group. At 11 days, more positive neurons are seen after SCI compared to the sham-injury group. No signal is detectable with the sense probe. Rostral is left and caudal is right. A, $n=3$ experiments; B, $n=4$ fish for each group. * $P<0.05$, two-way ANOVA with Tukey's *post hoc* test; mean values ±SEM are shown. Scale bar, 50 μm.

legumain under these conditions. Interestingly, at 11 days after SCI, *legumain* in the small cells in the spinal cord caudal to the lesion site was no longer detectable, while more neurons showed upregulation of *legumain* expression after SCI when compared to the sham-injured control group (Fig. 3B, 11d-CON, 100±5.25%; 11d-SCI, 261.44±15.26% (normalized to 11d-CON), $n=3$ fish, two-tailed *t*-test, $P=0.0006$).

The combined observations indicate that upregulation of *legumain* expression in the caudal spinal cord is due to its expression by small cells in the lesion site at all time points tested. At 1 day and 3 days after SCI, upregulation of *legumain* is also due to increased expression by small cells in the spinal cord caudal to the lesion site. At 11 days after SCI, neurons contribute to this upregulation.

Identification of legumain positive cells in the spinal cord

Cells expressing legumain in the spinal cord caudal to the lesion site were identified by immunohistochemistry using NeuN as a marker for neurons and GFAP for astrocytes. Macrophages/microglia were identified by antibody 4C4 [34–35]. Since highest expression of *legumain* by small cells was observed 3 days after SCI (Fig. 3B), double immunostaining of GFAP and 4C4 with Legumain was performed in sections taken from spinal cord caudal to the lesion site 3 days after SCI. Similarly, double immunostaining of NeuN with Legumain was performed using sections from fish 11 days after SCI, showing colocalization of NeuN with Legumain (Fig. 4 I–L). No colocalization GFAP and Legumain was observed (Fig. 4 A–D). In the non-injured spinal cord, only very few cells were positive for 4C4, which are negative for Legumain. Three days after SCI, almost all 4C4 positive cells expressed Legumain in the spinal cord caudal to the lesion site (Fig. 4 E–H). In the lesion site, Legumain expressing cells were also positive for 4C4 (data not shown). Interestingly, at 11 days after SCI, 4C4 immunopositive macrophages/microglia did not express detectable levels of Legumain (data not shown), demonstrating down-regulated expression of legumain in macrophages/microglia to basal levels as seen in the non-injured spinal cord. These observations suggest that expression of legumain in macrophages/ microglia is limited to their early activation stages.

Legumain is essential for spinal cord regeneration in adult zebrafish

As legumain expression is upregulated after SCI, we used anti-sense morpholinos (MOs) to knockdown expression of Legumain to investigate whether this molecule is essential in spinal cord regeneration. Two different MOs used here were labeled with fluorescein, allowing identification of the cells that had taken up the MOs. To validate the knockdown of Legumain at the protein level, immunohistochemistry was performed on brainstem sections from animals treated with standard control and legumain MOs 11 days after SCI. As shown in Figs. 1, 2 and 5, expression of Legumain in NMLF neurons was strongly increased after SCI. Application of *legumain* MO1 or MO2 (Fig. 5 A, B) dramatically reduced the numbers of Legumain protein expressing neurons in the NMLF compared to standard control MO treatment (Fig. 5 A, B). In the *legumain* anti-sense MO treated groups, neurons positive for fluorescein were not positive for Legumain by immunohistochemistry, while in the control MO treated group, neurons positive for MO also were positive for Legumain.

The locomotor recovery after complete spinal cord transection in adult zebrafish is measured by their free swimming ability at 6 weeks after SCI. The ability of injured fish to swim reaches maximal levels at 6 weeks after SCI with no additional improvement 10 weeks after SCI [19]. Locomotor recovery was quantified in terms of total distance moved by undisturbed fish during 5 min at 6 weeks after SCI. Fish treated with *legumain* MO1 or MO2 showed impaired recovery compared to fish treated with standard control MO: the total distances moved by fish treated with *legumain* MO1 (Fig. 5C) or *legumain* MO2 (Fig. 5C) were highly reduced relative to standard control MO treated fish, indicating that legumain contributes to functional recovery.

To investigate the effect of *legumain* MOs on axonal regrowth after SCI, retrograde tracing of brainstem neurons was performed

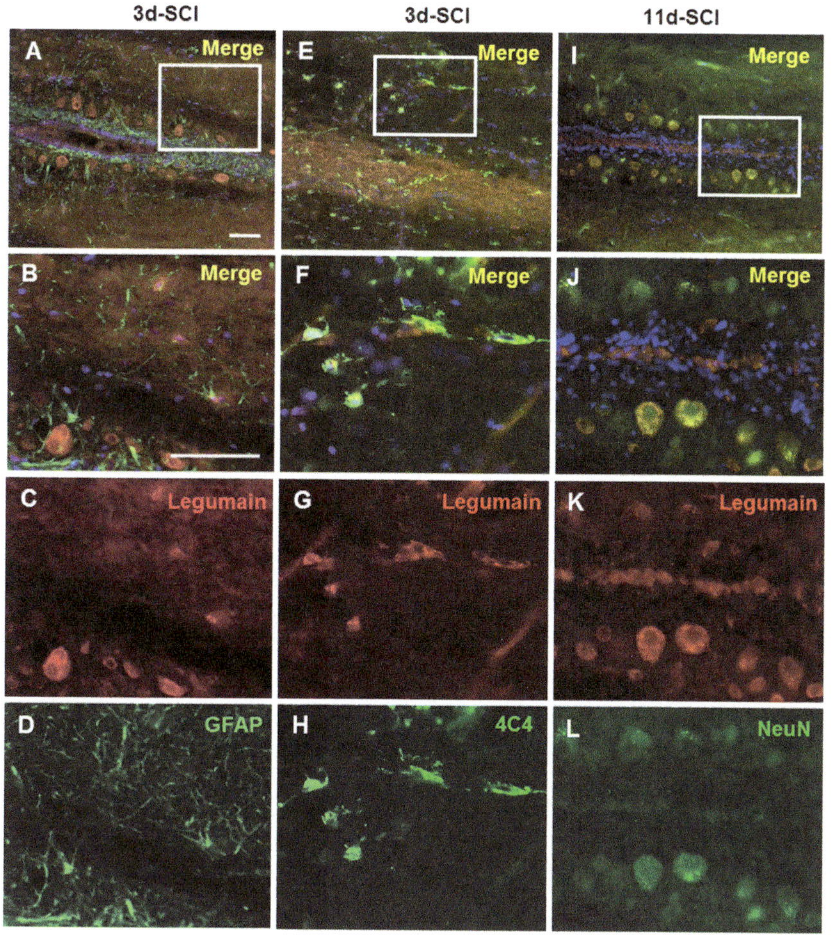

Figure 4. Neurons and macrophages/microglia express Legumain in the caudal spinal cord after SCI. Spinal cord sections from fish 3 days after SCI were used for double staining of Legumain and GFAP (A–D) or 4C4 (E–H). Spinal cord sections from fish 11 days after SCI were used for double staining of Legumain and NeuN (I–L). B, F, and J are the magnifications of A, E and I, respectively. No co-localization of Legumain and GFAP is observed (A–D). Double immunostaining of Legumain with 4C4 antibody identifies the positive small cells as macrophages/microglia (E–H). Double staining with NeuN shows that neurons express Legumain at 11 days after SCI (I–L). $n=3$ experiments. Scale bar, 50 μm.

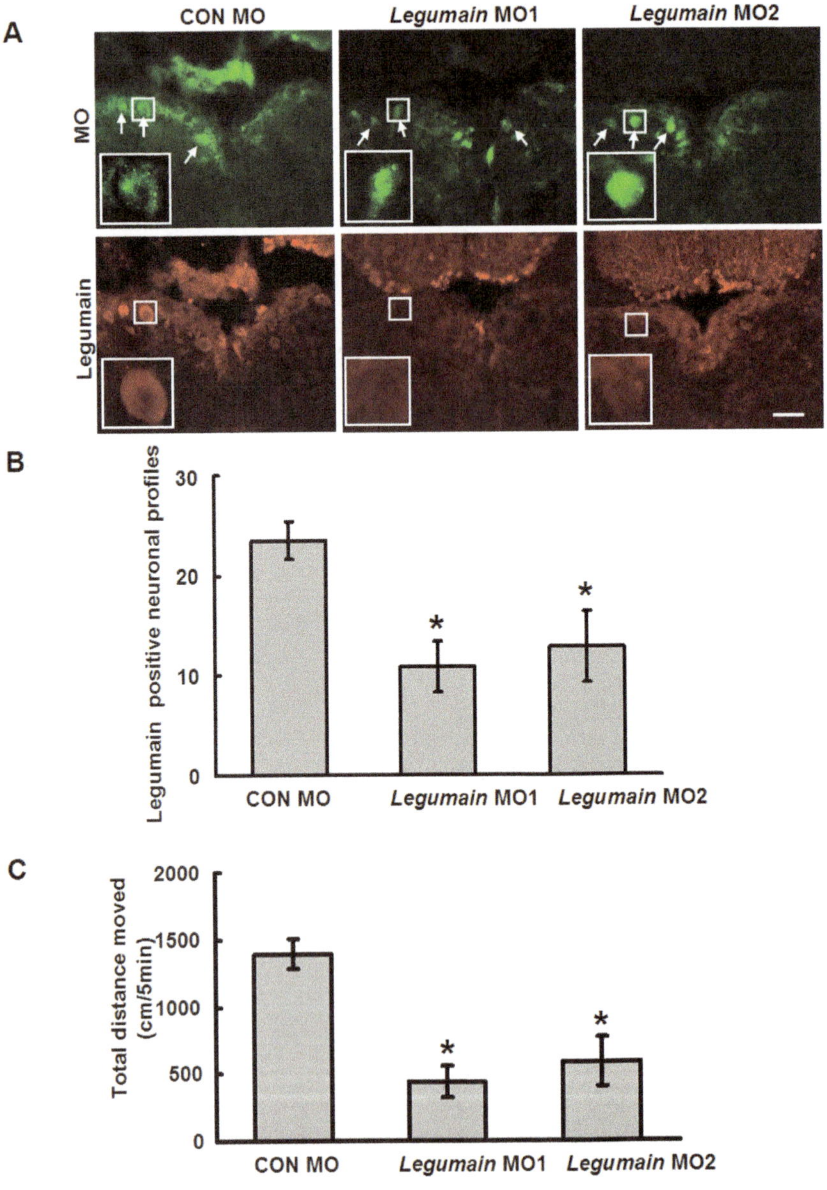

Figure 5. *Legumain* MO treatment inhibits locomotor recovery after SCI. (A, B) *Legumain* MO1 and MO2 knockdown Legumain protein expression as tested at 11 days after SCI. *Legumain* MO1 and *legumain* MO2 reduce the numbers of Legumain expressing neurons. Magnifications of the squared area are shown. (C) Total distance moved by fish treated with standard control (CON) MO, *legumain* MO1, or *legumain* MO2 was measured at 6 weeks after MO treatment. *Legumain* MO1 ($n = 14$ fish) or *legumain* MO2 ($n = 11$ fish) treatments reduce the total distance moved when compared with CON MO treatment ($n = 11$ fish). Dorsal is up. A, $n = 3$ experiments. * $P < 0.05$, one-way ANOVA with Tukey's *post hoc* test; mean values ±SEM are shown. Scale bar, 50 μm.

after analysis of locomotor recovery of the fish. The tracer, biocytin, was applied 3.5 mm caudal to the first lesion site. Fish treated with *legumain* anti-sense MOs showed reduced numbers of biocytin labeled neurons compared to control MO treated fish. The numbers of retrogradely labeled neurons were reduced in *legumain* anti-sense MO1 or MO2 treated fish in comparison to control MO treated fish in the NMLF or the IMRF (Fig. 6A, B). Since the *legumain* MOs were tagged with fluorescein, we were able to detect their presence 6 weeks after application as reported [2,19]. As the standard control MO does not affect cell viability [19], we compared the numbers of fluorescein-positive cell profiles from *legumain* MO1 or MO2-treated fish with those from control MO-treated fish. No difference was found in the numbers of fluorescein-positive cells in the NMLF between control and experimental animals (data not shown), indicating that neurons are not affected in their survival by MO treatment. Altogether, observations showed reduced locomotor recovery and reduced numbers of retrogradely labeled NMLF neurons in animals treated with *legumain* MOs, indicating that legumain contributes to locomotor recovery and axonal regrowth after SCI in adult zebrafish.

Discussion

In this study, we have identified legumain as an essential component for successful spinal cord regeneration after complete

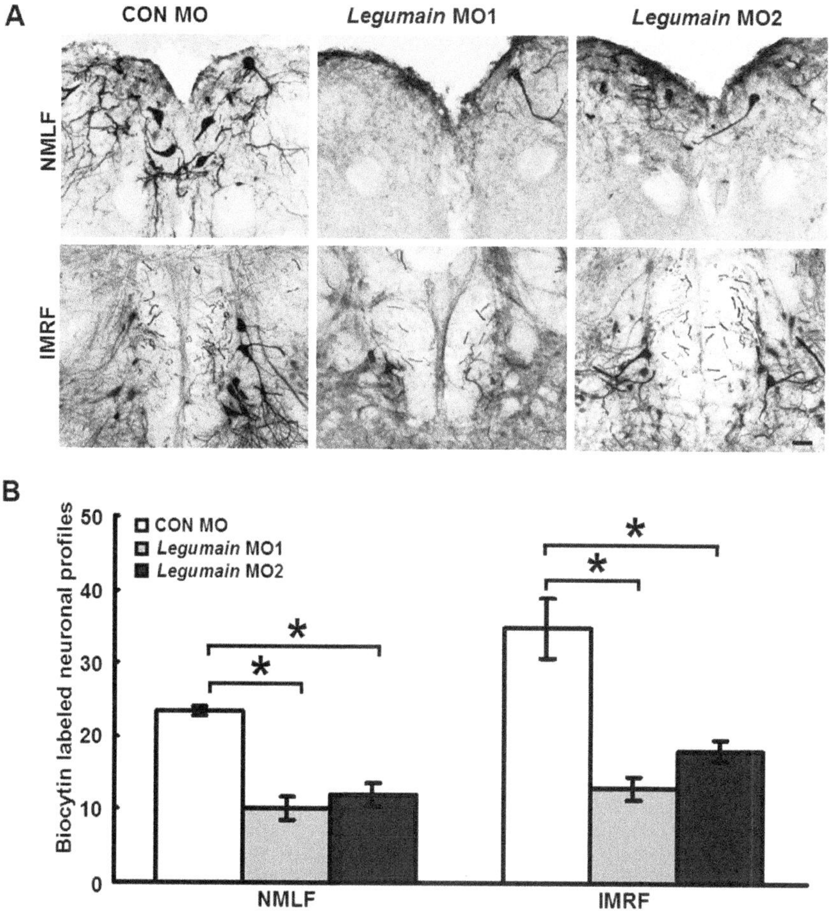

Figure 6. *Legumain* MOs inhibit axonal regrowth after SCI. (A) Representative images of neurons retrogradely labeled in the NMLF and IMRF 6 weeks after SCI. (B) Quantification of biocytin-labeled neuronal profiles in fish that had received *legumain* MO1 ($n = 7$ fish), *legumain* MO2 ($n = 6$ fish) or CON MO ($n = 6$ fish). *Legumain* MO1 and MO2 treatments reduce the numbers of biocytin-labeled neuronal profiles in the NMLF and IMRF when compared with CON MO treatment. Dorsal is up. * $P < 0.05$, one-way ANOVA with Tukey's *post hoc* test; mean values ±SEM are shown. Scale bar, 50 μm.

spinal cord transection in adult zebrafish. We found that legumain is one of the upregulated genes in the NMLF during axon regeneration by microarray analysis, *in situ* hybridization and immunohistochemistry. Moreover, levels of *legumain* mRNA are also increased in the caudal part spinal cord, which provides a permissive environment for regeneration. This upregulation of legumain expression has a biological function, since knockdown of Legumain expression strongly impaired locomotor recovery and axonal regrowth of brainstem neurons.

Microarray analysis had shown that there is no change of *legumain* mRNA expression during the early injury response period, i.e. 4 and 12 hours, suggesting that legumain is not involved in early responses after injury in neurons capable of axonal regeneration. At 3 days after SCI, upregulation of *legumain* expression becomes detectable and is very prominent at 11 days after SCI (Fig. 7), a time point of active axonal regrowth. Similar to our present results, upregulation of legumain expression occurs also at later phases after injury in retinal ganglion cells [36], optic nerve [37] and heart [38], suggesting that different organs use similar molecular mechanisms in regeneration. Similarly, upregulation of legumain is observed not only in the NMLF neurons, but also the IMRF neurons, indicating similar molecular mechanisms in neurons capable of axonal regrowth. Mauthner cells with no or limited capacity for regeneration, do not express *legumain* neither in sham-injured nor spinal cord injured fish at any time point after SCI, suggesting that upregulation of legumain expression is specifically associated with neurons capable of axonal regrowth.

In addition to the upregulation of *legumain* in brainstem neurons capable of axonal regeneration after SCI, cells in the spinal cord caudal to the lesion site also express higher levels of *legumain* after injury at all time points tested, with increased *legumain* expression reaching the highest level at 3 days after SCI. At 1 day and 3 days after SCI (Fig. 7), *legumain* expression is distinctly upregulated in macrophages/microglia, not only in the lesion site, but also caudal to the lesion site. Interestingly, however, *legumain* expression in macrophages/microglia is no more detectable at 11 days after SCI when neurons in spinal cord upregulate *legumain* expression (Fig. 7). Surprisingly, macrophages/microglia cells also express *legumain* in 1 day sham-injured control fish, in contrast to absence of *legumain* expression in these cells in non-injured fish. Of note, *legumain* expression in macrophages/microglia in sham-injured spinal cord is no more detectable at 3 days (Fig. 7), which differs from conditions of SCI under which *legumain* expression is upregulated at this time point. Insights into the molecular mechanisms underlying the transient expression after sham-injury are difficult to explain at present, but it is conceivable that deafferentation of muscle innervation induced by cutting muscles at the thoracic level could activate macrophages/microglia. It should

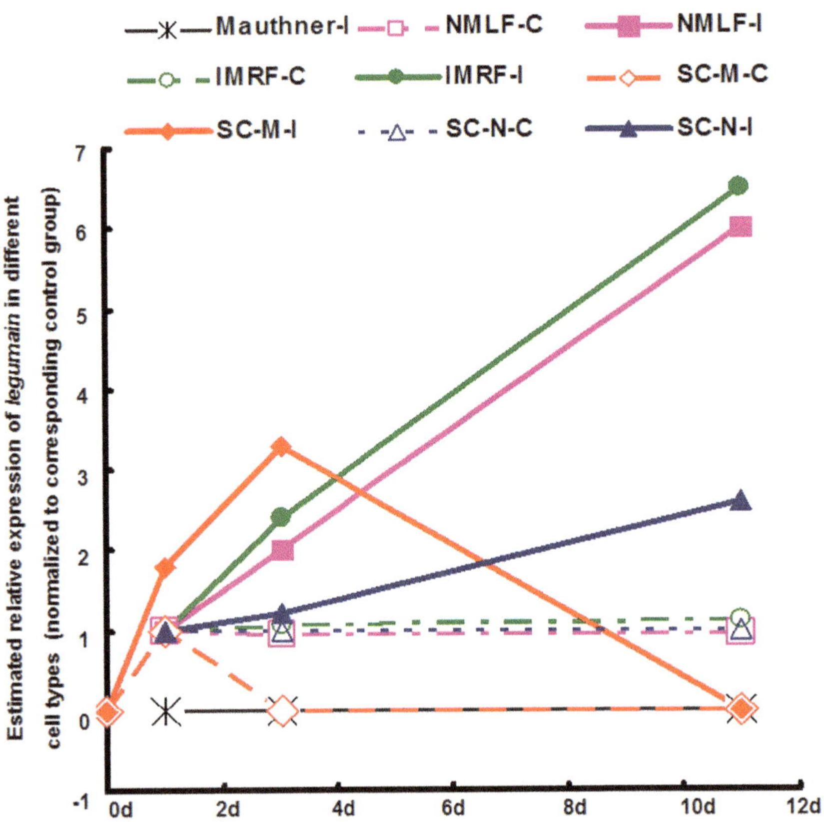

Figure 7. Summary scheme of *legumain* expression patterns in distinct cell types in brain and spinal cord after SCI. No signal for *legumain* expression was set as 0. When signal for *legumain* is detected in sham-injured control at 1 day post-injury, the value for *legumain* expression in 1 day sham-injured control is set as 1 and the relative expression in all other groups is normalized to the 1 day sham-injured control. The expression of *legumain* in brainstem neurons (NMLF-I, IMRF-I) is increased sharply after 1 day post-SCI. *Legumain* in spinal cord neurons (SC-N-I) is increased only at 11 days post-SCI. In the sham-injured control group, *legumain* expression in macrophages/microglia in the caudal spinal cord (SC-M-C) is detectable at 1 day and no more detectable thereafter. In the SCI group (SC-M-I), *legumain* expression in macrophages/microglia is increased 1 day, reaches a peak at 3 days and disappears 11 days after SCI. Abbreviations: Mauthner-I, Mauthner neurons of the SCI group; NMLF-C, NMLF neurons of the sham-injured control group; NMLF-I, NMLF neurons of the SCI group; IMRF-C, IMRF neurons of the sham-injured control group; IMRF-I, IMRF neurons of the SCI group; SC-M-C, macrophages/microglia in the caudal spinal cord of the sham-injured group; SC-M-I, macrophages/microglia in caudal spinal cord of the SCI group; SC-N-C, neurons in caudal spinal cord of the sham-injured group; SC-N-I, neurons in caudal spinal cord of the SCI group.

be emphasized that this transient *legumain* expression after sham-injury is weak in comparison to the reaction after SCI, but shows the sensitivity of macrophages/microglia to relatively mild interventions with physiological homeostasis. Similarly, legumain is detectable in mammalian macrophages [39–43] where its lysosomal proteolytic activity contributes to protein degradation and antigen presentation. However, the detailed molecular mechanisms of legumain's functions in macrophages/microglia have remained unclear. To the best of our knowledge, our study is the first to show that legumain expression is limited to a specifically transient stage of macrophages/microglia activation after tissue injury. Thus, legumain may become a useful early activation marker for macrophages/microglia.

The expression of legumain in macrophages/microglia raises the question as to the involvement of the immune system in zebrafish regeneration. In a recent study, acute inflammation initiates the regenerative response and is required for successful regeneration in the acutely injured adult zebrafish brain [44]. Similarly, application of anti-inflammatory glucocorticoid significantly reduces heart regenerative capacities in adult zebrafish [45]. Expression of legumain in macrophages/microglia in the early responses to injury in the spinal cord suggests that legumain expression might be supportive to recovery from trauma in zebrafish. Similarly, we found increased legumain expression at the lesion site of the mouse spinal cord at 7 days after SCI and this increase is attributable to accumulation of macrophages/microglia (unpublished observation). However, we did not observe upregulation of legumain in spinal motor neurons as we did in the zebrafish. In future experiments, we will test if increased expression of legumain in spinal cord and projection neurons can positively affect axon outgrowth after SCI in mammals.

After its discovery as a robust acidic cysteine endopeptidase, a considerable number of target proteins for legumain were described, such as extracellular matrix (ECM) component fibronectin [12]. The expression and functions of legumain in solid tumors has also been explored. In contrast to its low expression level in most normal tissues [9,46], legumain is highly expressed in many solid tumors, being related to a more invasive and metastatic phenotype [9,16–17,47]. Tumor invasion and metastasis is a complex process involving interactions between the invasive cells and the ECM, where proteases are essential for tumor cell-mediated ECM proteolysis. Notably, legumain is present extracellularly in the tumor microenviroment and associated with matrix as well as cell surfaces [9,11,48]. The association of secreted legumain with the extracellular matrix has been repeatedly described [10–13,16,49], an observation which has instigated the design legumain-activated anti-cancer prodrugs [13]. Furthermore, legumain is able to activate the secreted inactive proenzyme of matrix metalloproteinase-2 [9,50], the role of which in tumor cell-mediated ECM proteolysis and metastasis has been well established [51]. Similar to mechanisms in tumor metastasis, growth cones of regenerating axons degrade ECM molecules for motility and neurite extension, pointing to share similar mechanisms in proteolysis [52]. The extracellular activity of legumain is indicated in our study, where we could show that legumain is secreted by legumain positive cell types, such as microglia/macrophages and neurons (Figure S2). It is also possible that the upregulation of legumain in the caudal spinal cord after SCI may play a role in remodeling the extracellular environment to facilitate axon regeneration into the caudal spinal cord. It is noteworthy in this context that legumain is optimally active under acidic conditions, which are acutely generated in the spinal cord after injury and which are present in the microenvironment of tumors. Unfortunately, the investigation of the mechanisms underlying the functions of legumain with different cell types *in vitro* is hampered by the fact that cultured cells cannot be maintained under acidic conditions for time periods necessary for functional studies, thereby preventing the establishment of conditions that mirror those *in vivo* after injury.

It is noteworthy that some functions of legumain do not require its enzyme activity. The expression of legumain in the nucleus is regulated by nuclear calcium concentration and nuclear legumain is involved in cell proliferation, independent on its enzyme activity [7]. Also legumain's presence in human bone marrow is reported to inhibit osteoclast formation and bone resorption without its enzymatic activity [10]. Moreover, identification of legumain as a carboxypeptidase may allow novel insights into the functions of legumain under different physiological conditions [18]. In future experiments, we plan to examine the mechanism through which legumain appears to enhance recovery from CNS injury in zebrafish. Discovery of other target proteins for legumain and further biochemical studies may be helpful in elucidating mechanistic features of legumain function to develop potential therapies to promote CNS repair in mammals.

Supporting Information

Figure S1 Determination of the ability of legumain antibody to specifically detect Legumain in zebrafish as assayed by Western blot analysis. N2a cells was used as positive control (lane 1) and zebrafish spinal cord was used for this analysis (lane 3). Protein marker was loaded in lane 2. The antibody detects two major bands at 50 kDa and 37 kDa with N2a cells, the inactive proenzyme form and active form of mouse legumain, respectively. A band with the same size at 50 kDa is detected with zebrafish spinal cord as for N2a cells. n = 3 experiments.

Figure S2 Assays for detecting secretion of Legumain by different cell types *in vitro*. The secreted Legumain is mainly presented by the inactive proenzyme form at 50 kDa (the bands with arrows) in Western blot analysis. (A) Cultured macrophages secrete Legumain into the culture medium (lane 2) compared to non-cultured fresh control medium (lane 1). (B) N2a neuroblastoma cells (lane 2) secrete Legumain into the culture medium compared to non-cultured control medium (lane 1). (C) Primary cultured E18 embryonic hippocampal neurons secrete Legumain into the medium as tested by ELISA compared to non-cultured control medium. * $P<0.05$, two-tailed *t*-test; mean values ±SEM are shown. n = 3 experiments.

Acknowledgments

We are grateful to Alexandra Lepier for the kind gift of 4C4 antibody and Nakul Shah for careful reading the manuscript. We also thank Brian Siwek for his diligent care of the fish. Melitta Schachner is New Jersey Professor of Spinal Cord Research and a consultant at the Center for Neuroscience of the Li Kashing Shantou University Medical College, China.

Author Contributions

Conceived and designed the experiments: LM MS. Performed the experiments: LM HPK. Analyzed the data: LM YQS MS. Wrote the paper: LM MS.

References

1. Becker CG, Becker T (2008) Adult zebrafish as a model for successful central nervous system regeneration. Restor Neurol Neurosci 26: 71–80.
2. Ma L, Yu YM, Guo Y, Hart RP, Schachner M (2012) Cysteine- and glycine-rich protein 1a is involved in spinal cord regeneration in adult zebrafish. Eur J Neurosci 35: 353–365.
3. Van Hove I, Lemmens K, Van de Velde S, Verslegers M, Moons L (2012) Matrix metalloproteinase-3 in the central nervous system: a look on the bright side. J Neurochem 123: 203–216.
4. Zhang H, Chang M, Hansen CN, Basso DM, Noble-Haeusslein LJ (2011) Role of matrix metalloproteinases and therapeutic benefits of their inhibition in spinal cord injury. Neurotherapeutics 8: 206–220.
5. Chen JM, Dando PM, Rawlings ND, Brown MA, Young NE, et al. (1997) Cloning, isolation, and characterization of mammalian legumain, an asparaginyl endopeptidase. J Biol Chem 272: 8090–8098.
6. Chen JM, Dando PM, Stevens RA, Fortunato M, Barrett AJ (1998) Cloning and expression of mouse legumain, a lysosomal endopeptidase. Biochem J 335 (Pt 1): 111–117.
7. Andrade V, Guerra M, Jardim C, Melo F, Silva W, et al. (2011) Nucleoplasmic calcium regulates cell proliferation through legumain. J Hepatol 55: 626–635.
8. Haugen MH, Johansen HT, Pettersen SJ, Solberg R, Brix K, et al. (2013) Nuclear legumain activity in colorectal cancer. PLoS One 8: e52980.
9. Liu C, Sun C, Huang H, Janda K, Edgington T (2003) Overexpression of legumain in tumors is significant for invasion/metastasis and a candidate enzymatic target for prodrug therapy. Cancer Res 63: 2957–2964.
10. Choi SJ, Reddy SV, Devlin RD, Menaa C, Chung H, et al. (1999) Identification of human asparaginyl endopeptidase (legumain) as an inhibitor of osteoclast formation and bone resorption. J Biol Chem 274: 27747–27753.
11. Liu Y, Bajjuri KM, Liu C, Sinha SC (2012) Targeting cell surface alpha(v)beta(3) integrin increases therapeutic efficacies of a legumain protease-activated auristatin prodrug. Mol Pharm 9: 168–175.
12. Morita Y, Araki H, Sugimoto T, Takeuchi K, Yamane T, et al. (2007) Legumain/asparaginyl endopeptidase controls extracellular matrix remodeling through the degradation of fibronectin in mouse renal proximal tubular cells. FEBS Lett 581: 1417–1424.
13. Wu W, Luo Y, Sun C, Liu Y, Kuo P, et al. (2006) Targeting cell-impermeable prodrug activation to tumor microenvironment eradicates multiple drug-resistant neoplasms. Cancer Res 66: 970–980.
14. Manoury B, Hewitt EW, Morrice N, Dando PM, Barrett AJ, et al. (1998) An asparaginyl endopeptidase processes a microbial antigen for class II MHC presentation. Nature 396: 695–699.
15. Shirahama-Noda K, Yamamoto A, Sugihara K, Hashimoto N, Asano M, et al. (2003) Biosynthetic processing of cathepsins and lysosomal degradation are abolished in asparaginyl endopeptidase-deficient mice. J Biol Chem 278: 33194–33199.
16. Briggs JJ, Haugen MH, Johansen HT, Riker AI, Abrahamson M, et al. (2010) Cystatin E/M suppresses legumain activity and invasion of human melanoma. BMC Cancer 10: 17.
17. Ohno Y, Nakashima J, Izumi M, Ohori M, Hashimoto T, et al. (2013) Association of legumain expression pattern with prostate cancer invasiveness and aggressiveness. World J Urol 31: 359–364.
18. Dall E, Brandstetter H (2013) Mechanistic and structural studies on legumain explain its zymogenicity, distinct activation pathways, and regulation. Proc Natl Acad Sci U S A 110: 10940–10945.

19. Becker CG, Lieberoth BC, Morellini F, Feldner J, Becker T, et al. (2004) L1.1 is involved in spinal cord regeneration in adult zebrafish. J Neurosci 24: 7837–7842.
20. Becker T, Wullimann MF, Becker CG, Bernhardt RR, Schachner M (1997) Axonal regrowth after spinal cord transection in adult zebrafish. J Comp Neurol 377: 577–595.
21. Guo Y, Ma L, Cristofanilli M, Hart RP, Hao A, et al. (2011) Transcription factor Sox11b is involved in spinal cord regeneration in adult zebrafish. Neuroscience 172: 329–341.
22. Yu YM, Cristofanilli M, Valiveti A, Ma L, Yoo M, et al. (2011) The extracellular matrix glycoprotein tenascin-C promotes locomotor recovery after spinal cord injury in adult zebrafish. Neuroscience 183: 238–250.
23. Yu YM, Gibbs KM, Davila J, Campbell N, Sung S, et al. (2011) MicroRNA miR-133b is essential for functional recovery after spinal cord injury in adult zebrafish. Eur J Neurosci 33: 1587–1597.
24. Goff LA, Bowers J, Schwalm J, Howerton K, Getts RC, et al. (2004) Evaluation of sense-strand mRNA amplification by comparative quantitative PCR. BMC Genomics 5: 76.
25. Becker T, Bernhardt RR, Reinhard E, Wullimann MF, Tongiorgi E, et al. (1998) Readiness of zebrafish brain neurons to regenerate a spinal axon correlates with differential expression of specific cell recognition molecules. J Neurosci 18: 5789–5803.
26. Lieberoth BC, Becker CG, Becker T (2003) Double labeling of neurons by retrograde axonal tracing and non-radioactive in situ hybridization in the CNS of adult zebrafish. Methods Cell Sci 25: 65–70.
27. Wullimann MF, B Rupp, and H Reichert (1996) Neuroanatomy of the Zebrafish Brain: A Topological Atlas. Basel: Birkhauser
28. Ma L, Yin M, Wu X, Wu C, Yang S, et al. (2006) Expression of trophinin and bystin identifies distinct cell types in the germinal zones of adult rat brain. Eur J Neurosci 23: 2265–2276.
29. Lin JF, Pan HC, Ma LP, Shen YQ, Schachner M (2012) The cell neural adhesion molecule contactin-2 (TAG-1) is beneficial for functional recovery after spinal cord injury in adult zebrafish. PLoS One 7: e52376.
30. Pan HC, Lin JF, Ma LP, Shen YQ, Schachner M (2013) Major vault protein promotes locomotor recovery and regeneration after spinal cord injury in adult zebrafish. Eur J Neurosci 37: 203–211.
31. Yu Y, Schachner M (2013) Syntenin-a promotes spinal cord regeneration following injury in adult zebrafish. Eur J Neurosci 38: 2280–2289.
32. Dias TB, Yang YJ, Ogai K, Becker T, Becker CG (2012) Notch signaling controls generation of motor neurons in the lesioned spinal cord of adult zebrafish. J Neurosci 32: 3245–3252.
33. Reimer MM, Kuscha V, Wyatt C, Sorensen I, Frank RE, et al. (2009) Sonic hedgehog is a polarized signal for motor neuron regeneration in adult zebrafish. J Neurosci 29: 15073–15082.
34. Baumgart EV, Barbosa JS, Bally-Cuif L, Gotz M, Ninkovic J (2012) Stab wound injury of the zebrafish telencephalon: a model for comparative analysis of reactive gliosis. Glia 60: 343–357.
35. Becker T, Becker CG (2001) Regenerating descending axons preferentially reroute to the gray matter in the presence of a general macrophage/microglial reaction caudal to a spinal transection in adult zebrafish. J Comp Neurol 433: 131–147.
36. Veldman MB, Bemben MA, Thompson RC, Goldman D (2007) Gene expression analysis of zebrafish retinal ganglion cells during optic nerve regeneration identifies KLF6a and KLF7a as important regulators of axon regeneration. Dev Biol 312: 596–612.
37. McCurley AT, Callard GV (2010) Time Course Analysis of Gene Expression Patterns in Zebrafish Eye During Optic Nerve Regeneration. J Exp Neurosci 2010: 17–33.
38. Lien CL, Schebesta M, Makino S, Weber GJ, Keating MT (2006) Gene expression analysis of zebrafish heart regeneration. PLoS Biol 4: e260.
39. Edgington LE, Verdoes M, Ortega A, Withana NP, Lee J, et al. (2013) Functional imaging of legumain in cancer using a new quenched activity-based probe. J Am Chem Soc 135: 174–182.
40. Hashimoto S, Suzuki T, Dong HY, Yamazaki N, Matsushima K (1999) Serial analysis of gene expression in human monocytes and macrophages. Blood 94: 837–844.
41. Lecaille F, Muno D, Kominami E, Ishidoh K (2004) Proteinases participating in the processing and activation of prolegumain in primary cultured rat macrophages. Biol Chem 385: 511–516.
42. Lin Y, Wei C, Liu Y, Qiu Y, Liu C, et al. (2013) Selective ablation of tumor-associated macrophages suppresses metastasis and angiogenesis. Cancer Sci 104: 1217–1225.
43. Luo Y, Zhou H, Krueger J, Kaplan C, Lee SH, et al. (2006) Targeting tumor-associated macrophages as a novel strategy against breast cancer. J Clin Invest 116: 2132–2141.
44. Kyritsis N, Kizil C, Zocher S, Kroehne V, Kaslin J, et al. (2012) Acute inflammation initiates the regenerative response in the adult zebrafish brain. Science 338: 1353–1356.
45. Huang WC, Yang CC, Chen IH, Liu YM, Chang SJ, et al. (2013) Treatment of Glucocorticoids Inhibited Early Immune Responses and Impaired Cardiac Repair in Adult Zebrafish. PLoS One 8: e66613.
46. Yamane T, Takeuchi K, Yamamoto Y, Li YH, Fujiwara M, et al. (2002) Legumain from bovine kidney: its purification, molecular cloning, immunohistochemical localization and degradation of annexin II and vitamin D-binding protein. Biochim Biophys Acta 1596: 108–120.
47. Wang L, Chen S, Zhang M, Li N, Chen Y, et al. (2012) Legumain: a biomarker for diagnosis and prognosis of human ovarian cancer. J Cell Biochem 113: 2679–2686.
48. Wu B, Yin J, Texier C, Roussel M, Tan KS (2010) Blastocystis legumain is localized on the cell surface, and specific inhibition of its activity implicates a pro-survival role for the enzyme. J Biol Chem 285: 1790–1798.
49. Smith R, Johansen HT, Nilsen H, Haugen MH, Pettersen SJ, et al. (2012) Intra- and extracellular regulation of activity and processing of legumain by cystatin E/M. Biochimie 94: 2590–2599.
50. Chen JM, Fortunato M, Stevens RA, Barrett AJ (2001) Activation of progelatinase A by mammalian legumain, a recently discovered cysteine proteinase. Biol Chem 382: 777–783.
51. Deryugina EI, Quigley JP (2006) Matrix metalloproteinases and tumor metastasis. Cancer Metastasis Rev 25: 9–34.
52. Zuo J, Ferguson TA, Hernandez YJ, Stetler-Stevenson WG, Muir D (1998) Neuronal matrix metalloproteinase-2 degrades and inactivates a neurite-inhibiting chondroitin sulfate proteoglycan. J Neurosci 18: 5203–5211.

10

Passive Exercise of the Hind Limbs after Complete Thoracic Transection of the Spinal Cord Promotes Cortical Reorganization

Alessandro Graziano[2*¶], Guglielmo Foffani[1,4¶], Eric B. Knudsen[1], Jed Shumsky[3], Karen A. Moxon[1,3]

1 School of Biomedical Engineering, Science and Health Systems, Drexel University, Philadelphia, Pennsylvania, United States of America, **2** Department of Physiology and Pharmacology, Drexel University College of Medicine, Philadelphia, Pennsylvania, United States of America, **3** Department of Neurobiology and Anatomy, Drexel University College of Medicine, Philadelphia, Pennsylvania, United States of America, **4** Hospital Nacional de Parapléjicos, Servicio de Salud de Castilla-La Mancha, Toledo, Spain

Abstract

Physical exercise promotes neural plasticity in the brain of healthy subjects and modulates pathophysiological neural plasticity after sensorimotor loss, but the mechanisms of this action are not fully understood. After spinal cord injury, cortical reorganization can be maximized by exercising the non-affected body or the residual functions of the affected body. However, exercise per se also produces systemic changes – such as increased cardiovascular fitness, improved circulation and neuroendocrine changes – that have a great impact on brain function and plasticity. It is therefore possible that passive exercise therapies typically applied below the level of the lesion in patients with spinal cord injury could put the brain in a more plastic state and promote cortical reorganization. To directly test this hypothesis, we applied passive hindlimb bike exercise after complete thoracic transection of the spinal cord in adult rats. Using western blot analysis, we found that the level of proteins associated with plasticity – specifically ADCY1 and BDNF – increased in the somatosensory cortex of transected animals that received passive bike exercise compared to transected animals that received sham exercise. Using electrophysiological techniques, we then verified that neurons in the deafferented hindlimb cortex increased their responsiveness to tactile stimuli delivered to the forelimb in transected animals that received passive bike exercise compared to transected animals that received sham exercise. Passive exercise below the level of the lesion, therefore, promotes cortical reorganization after spinal cord injury, uncovering a brain-body interaction that does not rely on intact sensorimotor pathways connecting the exercised body parts and the brain.

Editor: Colin Combs, University of North Dakota, United States of America

Funding: This work was supported by grant 36206 from the Neilsen Foundation and grants P01 NS 055976 and R01 NS05741 from the National Institutes of Health. The funders had no role in study design, data collection and analysis, decision to publish, or preparation of the manuscript.

Competing Interests: The authors have declared that no competing interests exist.

* E-mail: Alessandro.Graziano@DrexelMed.edu

¶ These authors contributed equally to this work.

Introduction

Limb amputation, damage to peripheral nerves and spinal cord injury can alter the somatotopic organization of the primary somatosensory cortex [1,2,3,4,5,6]. Cortical reorganization subserves functional recovery [7,8,9,10,11,12] but excessive reorganization can have pathological consequences, such as phantom limb sensations [13,14] and neuropathic pain [15,16,17,18]. It is therefore important to fully understand the mechanisms of cortical reorganization and to develop optimal strategies to modulate it after deafferentation [19].

Cortical reorganization after somatosensory deafferentation can lead to the enlargement of cortical representations of intact body areas into cortical representations of deafferented body areas. A conceptually similar cortical enlargement is induced by increasing the activity of a cortical area through enhanced sensory experience [20]. A natural strategy to maximize cortical reorganization after somatosensory deafferentation is therefore to increase the activity of the intact cortex by exercising the non-affected body or the residual functions of the affected body, as investigated in previous works in rat models [9,21,22] and in patients with spinal cord injury [23,24,25,26]. An alternative strategy would be to put the overall cortex in a more plastic state, e.g. using systemic drugs or other manipulations that generically promote cortical plasticity [27,28,29].

A possible intriguing way to generically promote cortical plasticity is indirectly suggested by exercise therapies employed after spinal cord injury, which are often applied to the *affected* body in order to improve functions below the level of the lesion [30]. For example, passive exercise of the lower limbs after spinal cord injury has been shown to reduce spasticity [31,32,33,34], reduce the rate of bone density loss [35,36] and reduce lower limb blood pooling [37]. Interestingly, passive exercise also produces the systemic effects that are typical of exercise per se, such as increases in cardiovascular fitness [38], improved circulation [39] and neuroendocrine changes [40]. These systemic effects of exercise are known to have a great impact on brain function [41], as they contribute to stimulate neurogenesis and to increase the levels of growth factors such as BDNF, thereby promoting brain plasticity

[42,43,44,45]. Even though at first glance it might appear counter-intuitive, it is reasonable to suggest that exercise below the level of the lesion after complete spinal cord injury might promote cortical reorganization.

In order to directly test this hypothesis, we applied passive hindlimb bike exercise after complete thoracic transection of the spinal cord in adult rats. The rationale for employing the thoracic transection rat model of spinal cord injury is that it has been shown to produce cortical reorganization associated with alterations of BDNF regulation in the brain [46,47]. The rationale for employing passive hindlimb bike exercise is three-fold: (*1*) it is well established in rat models of spinal cord injury [48], (*2*) it has direct translational relevance for spinal cord injury patients, and (*3*) it specifically confines the exercise below the level of the lesion. We first investigated whether passive hindlimb bike training after thoracic transection of the spinal cord affected the expression in the somatosensory cortex of proteins associated with plasticity (Fig. 1A). We then verified that these changes in markers of cortical plasticity were associated with increased neurophysiological reorganization of the deafferented hindlimb cortex (Fig. 1B).

Results

Hindlimb Bike Exercise after Thoracic Transection of the Spinal Cord Induces Changes in the Levels of Proteins Associated with Plasticity in the Somatosensory Cortex

We performed western blot analysis to assess the levels of plasticity-related proteins in the somatosensory cortex of 32 rats, divided in 5 groups (Fig. 1A): one group of normal animals (n = 6); two groups of 'bike-exercise' transected animals, which received either 1 week (n = 8) or 8 weeks (n = 5) of hindlimb bike exercise after complete thoracic (T9/T10) transection of the spinal cord; two groups of 'sham-exercise' transected animals, which received either 1 week (n = 7) or 8 weeks (n = 6) of sham bike exercise after the spinal cord transection. Passive hindlimb bike exercise or sham bike exercise started the week after the spinal transection (two 30-min sessions per day on Monday, Wednesday and Friday) and animals were sacrificed within one hour after the last session. This exercise protocol is based on previous work showing that at least 1 week of hindlimb bike exercise after spinal cord injury is necessary to induce significant plastic changes in the spinal cord below the level of the lesion (Keeler et al., 2009). We focused on the following 6 proteins known to be involved in neuronal plasticity in the brain: ADCY1, BDNF and its receptor trkB, GAP43, LINGO-1 and p35 [49,50,51,52,53,54,55,56,57,58,59,60,61,62]. Data

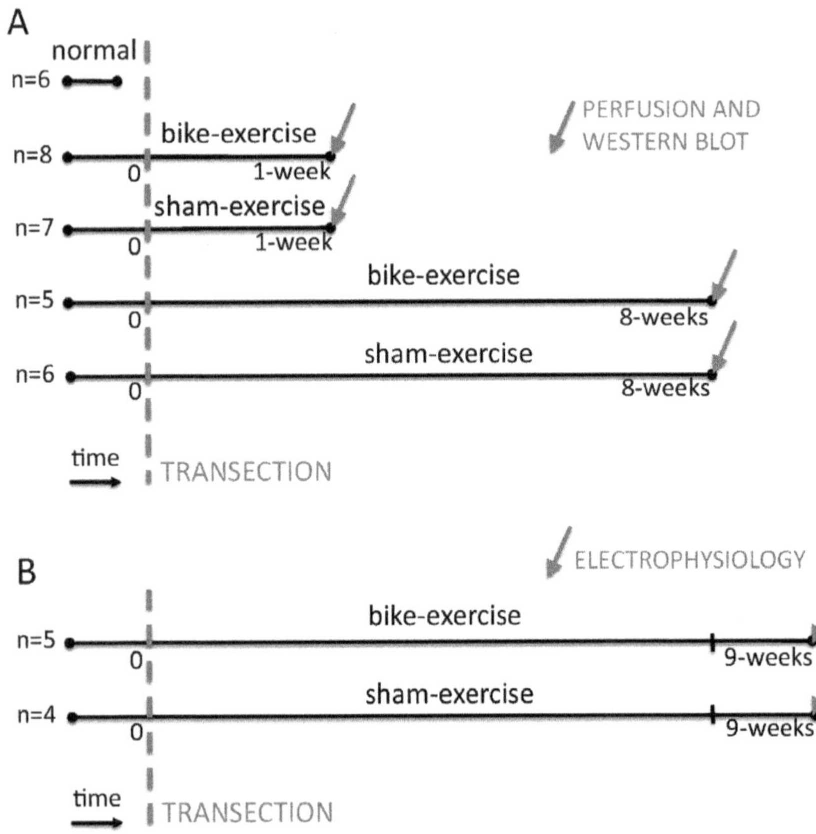

Figure 1. Experimental protocol. (**A**) In 32 rats western blot analysis was performed to assess the levels of plasticity-related proteins in the somatosensory cortex: one group of normal animals (n = 6); two groups of 'bike-exercise' transected animals, which received either 1 week (n = 8) or 8 weeks (n = 5) of hindlimb bike exercise after complete thoracic (T9/T10) transection of the spinal cord; two groups of 'sham-exercise' transected animals, which received either 1 week (n = 7) or 8 weeks (n = 6) of sham bike exercise after the spinal cord transection. (**B**) In 9 additional rats, an electrophysiological study was performed to assess the functional reorganization of the deafferented somatosensory cortex: one group of 'bike-exercise' transected animals (n = 5) and one group of 'sham-exercise' transected animals (n = 4). Both groups received real or sham passive hindlimb bike exercise for 8 weeks after transection, and the electrophysiological study was performed one week after the last bike session (i.e. 9 weeks after the spinal transection).

from 'bike-exercise' and 'sham-exercise' animals were expressed as percentage of normal animals (as in [46]).

It has been previously shown that complete transection of the spinal cord changes the transcriptional activities of several genes related to plasticity in the primary somatosensory cortex, including BDNF, the Nogo receptor and its co-receptor LINGO-1, as assessed by *in situ* hybridization [46]. In order to corroborate the sensitivity of our experimental approach to detect changes in cortical plasticity after spinal cord transection, we first compared 'sham-exercise' transected animals to normal animals (Fig. 2A). Spinal transection affected the levels of most of the proteins of interest (two-way ANOVA, time from lesion: $F = 3.6$, $p = 0.0514$; interaction time from lesion × protein: $F = 12.1$, $p<0.0001$; follow-up one-way ANOVAs, ADCY1: $F = 27.4$, $p<0.0001$; BDNF: $F = 5.9$, $p = 0.0120$; trkB: $F = 0.93$, $p = 0.41$; GAP43: $F = 19.5$, $p<0.0001$; LINGO-1: $F = 3.6$, $p = 0.0524$; p35: $F = 11.2$, $p = 0.0009$). Specifically, 1 week after spinal transection there was only a marginal increase in the level of ADCY1 (post-hoc: $p = 0.0505$) and BDNF ($p = 0.0780$), but 8 weeks after spinal transection all proteins but trkB were altered compared to 1 week: ADCY1, BDNF and p35 were decreased ($p<0.0001$, $p = 0.0035$, $p = 0.0007$), whereas GAP43 and LINGO-1 were increased ($p<0.0001$, $p = 0.0279$). ADCY1, GAP43, LINGO-1 and p35 were also significantly different 8 weeks after spinal transection compared to normal animals ($p = 0.0001$, $p<0.0001$, $p = 0.0410$, $p = 0.0010$). These data show that spinal cord injury per se affects the levels of plasticity-related proteins in the rat primary somatosensory cortex.

We then investigated the effect of passive hindlimb bike exercise after spinal transection by jointly analyzing the data from 'bike-exercise' and 'sham-exercise' animals (Fig. 2B). Passive hindlimb bike exercise after spinal transection increased the levels of plasticity-related proteins in the somatosensory cortex of our animals (three-way ANOVA, exercise: $F = 8.7$, $p = 0.0076$). This increase tended to be stronger in animals that received 8 weeks compared to 1 week of bike exercise after spinal cord transection (interaction exercise × weeks: $F = 3.2$, $p = 0.0868$), and was highly protein-dependent (interaction exercise × protein: $F = 5.1$, $p = 0.0003$). More specifically, the proteins that appeared more sensitive to hindlimb bike exercise were ADCY1 (follow-up two-way ANOVA, exercise: $F = 10.7$, $p = 0.0034$) and BDNF ($F = 7.2$, $p = 0.0141$). These results show that exercise below the lesion induces changes in the levels of proteins associated with plasticity in the somatosensory cortex after complete spinal cord injury.

Hindlimb Bike Exercise after Thoracic Transection of the Spinal Cord Enhances the Neurophysiological Reorganization of the Deafferented Hindlimb Cortex

In order to verify the functional relevance of the above changes in proteins associated with cortical plasticity, we directly assessed whether passive hindlimb bike exercise after spinal cord transection affected the neurophysiological reorganization of the deafferented hindlimb cortex. To this end, we studied two additional groups of 'bike-exercise' transected animals ($n = 5$) and 'sham-exercise' transected animals ($n = 4$) (Fig. 1B). These new groups received passive hindlimb real or sham bike exercise for 8 weeks after transection. One week after the last bike session (i.e. 9 weeks after the spinal transection), animals were anesthetized to perform an acute, single-neuron mapping study in the deafferented hindlimb cortex. Similar to our previous study [9], high-impedance single tungsten microelectrodes were inserted into the hindlimb primary somatosensory cortex with multiple penetrations (4–6 per animal), and single neurons from the supragranular (bike: $n = 142$; sham: $n = 64$) granular (bike: $n = 95$; sham: $n = 65$) and infragranular (bike: $n = 253$; sham: $n = 121$) layers were isolated and identified as either responsive or not responsive to cutaneous stimulation of the forelimbs (Fig. 3A, Table 1).

In sham-exercise transected animals, the percentage of cells stereotaxically located in the deafferented hindlimb cortex that responded to stimulation of the intact forelimb was extremely low: 1.3% considering all cells ($n = 233$), 0% in the supragranular layers, 3.2% in the granular layers, and <1% in the infragranular layers. In bike-exercise transected animals, the percentage of cells stereotaxically located in the deafferented hindlimb cortex that responded to stimulation of the intact forelimb dramatically increased at all cortical layers: 11.6% considering all cells ($n = 490$, two-proportion test: $p<0.0001$), 14.8% in the supragranular layers ($p = 0.0019$), 20% in the granular layers ($p = 0.0030$) and 10.7% in the infragranular layers ($p = 0.0014$). Essentially the same results were obtained with a two-way ANOVA, considering each track as an independent sample (Fig. 3B). The data for each individual animal are given in Table 1. The completeness of the spinal cord transection was histologically verified in all animals at the end of the study (Fig. 3C). There were no differences (t-test, $p = 0.53$) in the rostrocaudal extent of the lesion between animals that received bike exercise (6.2±0.6 mm) and animals that received sham exercise (6.0±0.4 mm) after the spinal transection.

These results represent the electrophysiological counterpart to the exercise-induced protein regulation reported in the previous section and overall show that exercise below the level of the lesion promotes cortical reorganization after complete spinal cord injury.

Discussion

We previously showed that exercise (treadmill) above the level of the lesion promotes cortical reorganization in adult rats spinalized as neonates [9,22]. The main result of the present work is that passive exercise *below* the level of the lesion promotes cortical reorganization in adult rats spinalized as adults. Specifically, we show that passive hindlimb bike exercise after thoracic transection of the spinal cord induces changes in the levels of proteins associated with plasticity in the sensorimotor cortex and enhances the neurophysiological reorganization of the deafferented hindlimb cortex.

Hindlimb Bike Exercise after Thoracic Transection of the Spinal Cord Induces Changes in the Levels of Proteins Associated with Plasticity in the Sensorimotor Cortex

Spinal cord transection alone ('sham-exercise' transected animals compared to normal animals) had a profound impact on the levels of plasticity-related proteins in the somatosensory cortex. On the one hand, ADCY1 and BDNF tended to increase 1 week after spinal transection and significantly decreased 8 weeks after spinal transection – even below normal levels for ADCY1, together with p35. On the other hand, GAP43 and LINGO-1 increased 8 weeks after the spinal transection.

BDNF is critical for neuronal growth and differentiation (Huang and Reichardt, 2001) and for the establishment of long-term synaptic plasticity [55,56], whereas LINGO-1 promotes neuronal survival and branching [54,58] but negatively regulates central myelination and axonal sprouting after spinal cord injury [52,53]. These two proteins have been previously implicated in brain reorganization after spinal cord injury, with complex temporal patterns of up-regulation and down-regulation [46,47,63,64]. In the only previous study specifically investigating the neocortex, Endo et al. [46] used in situ hybridization to quantify changes in the levels of BDNF and LINGO-1 mRNAs after spinal cord

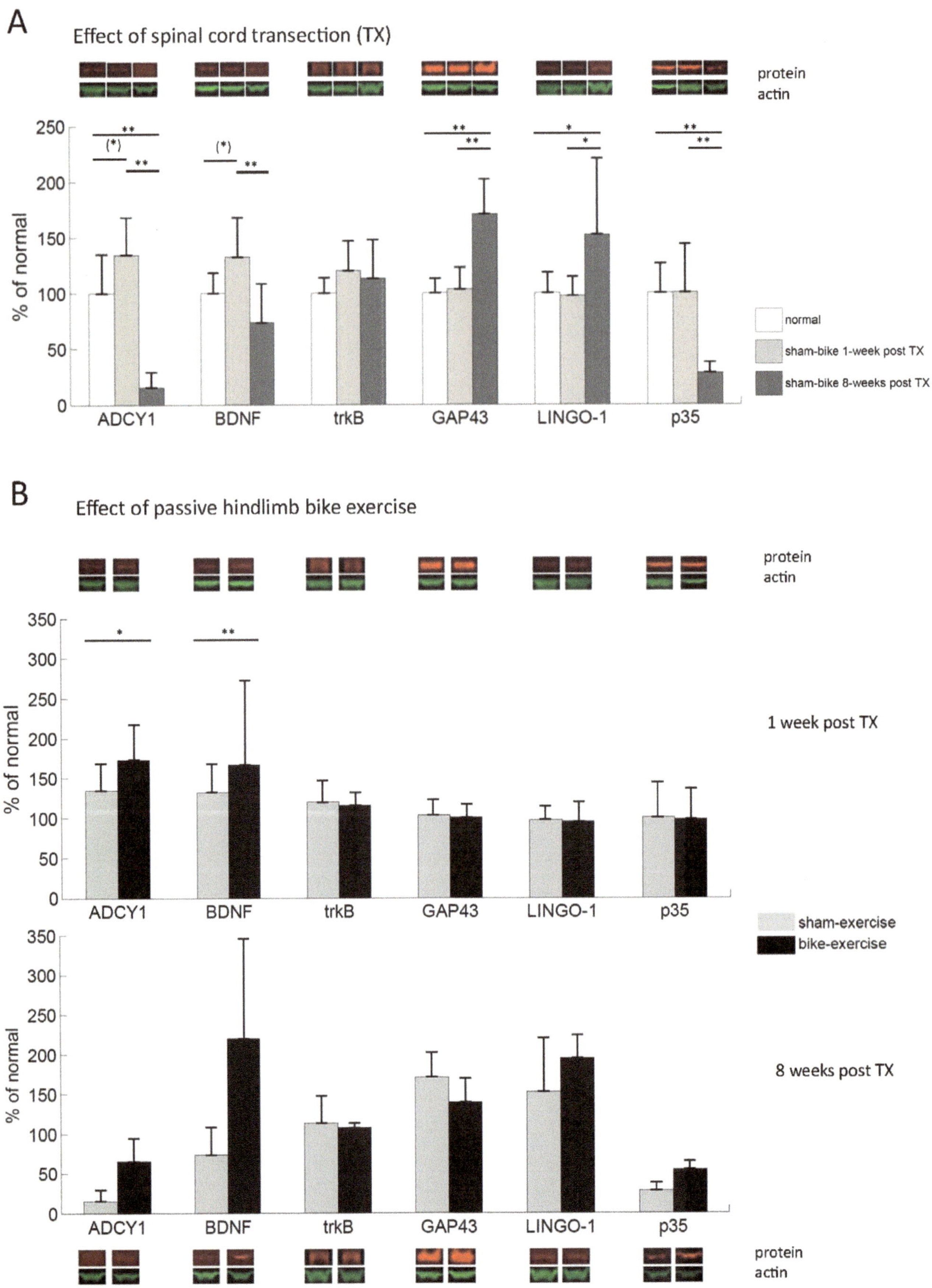
A
Effect of spinal cord transection (TX)
protein
actin
250
200
150
100
50
0
% of normal
**
(*)
**
*
ADCY1
BDNF
trkB
GAP43
LINGO-1
p35
normal
sham-bike 1-week post TX
sham-bike 8-weeks post TX
B
Effect of passive hindlimb bike exercise
350
300
1 week post TX
8 weeks post TX
sham-exercise
bike-exercise

Figure 2. Changes in the levels of proteins associated with plasticity in the somatosensory cortex. (**A**) Effect of spinal cord transection alone ('sham-exercise' transected animals compared to normal animals). (**B**) Effect of passive hindlimb exercise. Representative western blot bands are shown for each case. Error bars indicate standard deviations. (*) = p<0.1, * = p<0.05, ** = p<0.01.

transection, reporting changes in gene expression that only in part match the changes in protein levels we observed.

After spinal cord transection in the absence of passive exercise, LINGO-1 mRNA was reduced in the deafferented hindlimb cortex and the adjacent forelimb cortex [46], while in our study protein levels are unchanged 1 week after transection and are even increased 8 weeks after transection. Endo et al. measured mRNA levels in discrete cortical sub-regions and the observed changes involved only a subset of these regions. Because we extracted total protein from the whole sensorimotor cortex, it is possible that changes affecting only part of it where diluted and hence not detectable. A more intriguing possibility, however, is that post-transcriptional and posttranslational modifications are responsible for the uncoupling of LINGO-1 mRNA and protein levels. One important mechanism is represented by micro-RNAs (miRNA), which affect protein translation by binding to their target mRNA and effectively controlling protein levels (see for example [65]). Moreover, LINGO-1 proteins form very stable membrane-bound homotetramers that act as a scaffold with multiple sites available for protein-protein interactions [66]. It is therefore likely that

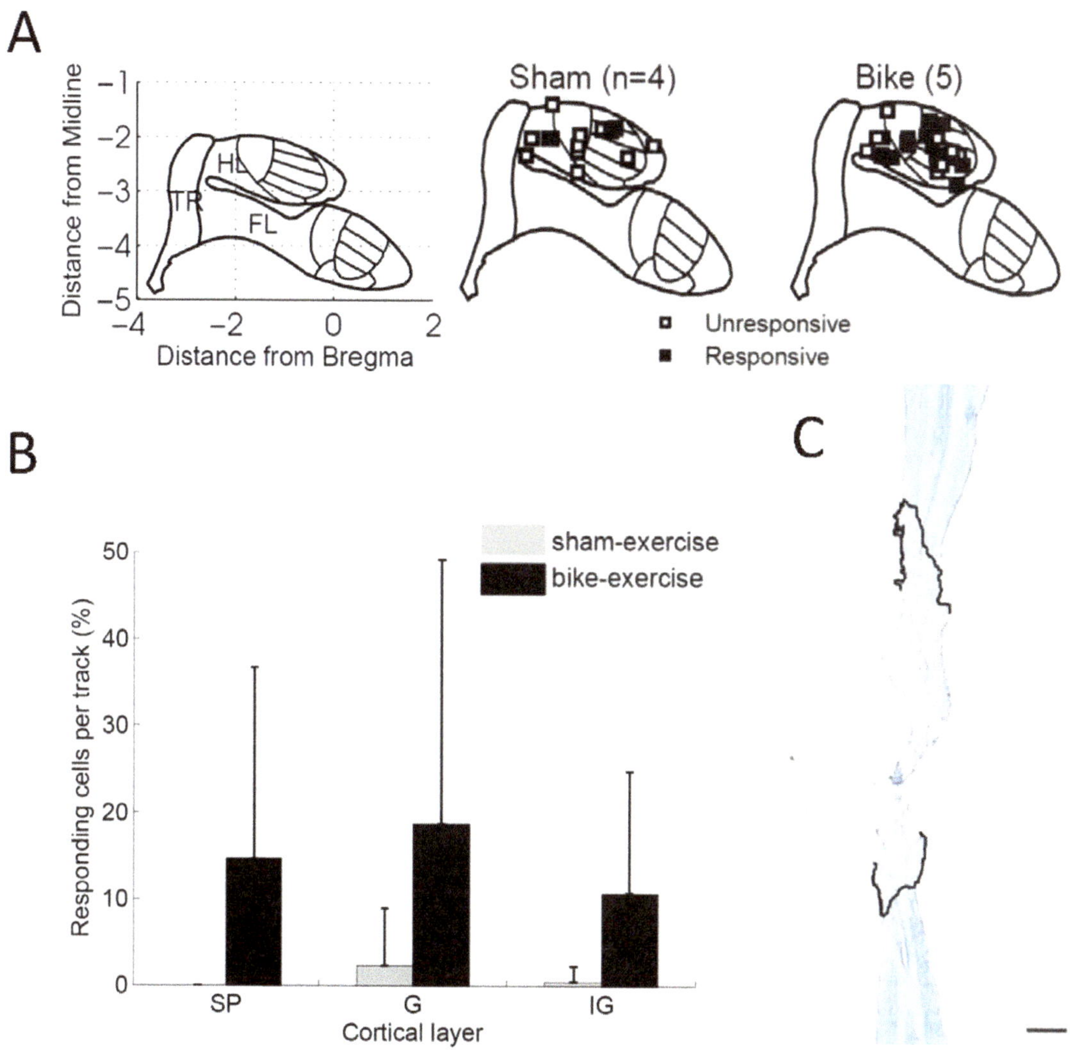

Figure 3. Neurophysiological reorganization of the somatosensory cortex. (A) Cartoon of the hindlimb (HL), forelimb (FL) and trunk (TR) areas in the primary somatosensory cortex in stereotaxic coordinates (left), and visual representation of responsive (filled squares) and unresponsive (empty squares) tracks in the electrophysiological study for sham-exercise transected animals (center) and bike-exercise transected animals (right). (**B**) Percentage of responding cells per track in sham exercise transected animals and bike-exercise transected animals, separated by cortical layer. supragranular (SP), granular (G) and infragranular (IG). In bike-exercise transected animals, the percentage of cells stereotaxically located in the deafferented hindlimb cortex that responded to stimulation of the intact forelimb dramatically increased (two-way mixed ANOVA, exercise: $F = 7.54$, $p = 0.0091$) at all cortical layers (interaction exercise × cortical layer: $F = 0.88$, $p = 0.42$). Error bars indicate standard deviations. (**C**) Nissl/myelin staining of the spinal cord of a representative animal that received bike exercise after spinal cord transection. No cell bodies or axons were observed in the transection site (marked by the black lines). The extent of this representative injury was comparable with the other injuries. Scale bar: 1.0 mm.

Table 1. Electrophysiological data.

	Responsive tracks per animal				Responsive cells per animal			
	SG	G	IG	TOT	SG	G	IG	TOT
SHAM 1	0 of 4	0 of 4	0 of 4	0 of 4	0 of 13	0 of 20	0 of 30	0 of 63
SHAM 2	0 of 5	0 of 5	0 of 5	0 of 5	0 of 14	0 of 18	0 of 18	0 of 50
SHAM 3	0 of 4	0 of 4	0 of 4	0 of 4	0 of 16	0 of 7	0 of 28	0 of 51
SHAM 4	0 of 4	2 of 4	1 of 4	2 of 4	0 of 17	2 of 17	1 of 35	3 of 69
TOT	**0 of 17**	**2 of 17**	**1 of 17**	**2 of 17**	**0 of 60**	**2 of 62**	**1 of 111**	**3 of 233**
BIKE 1	6 of 6	6 of 6	5 of 6	6 of 6	13 of 54	10 of 30	12 of 54	35 of 138
BIKE 2	1 of 5	1 of 5	2 of 5	3 of 5	1 of 22	1 of 18	3 of 55	5 of 95
BIKE 3	1 of 4	1 of 4	4 of 4	4 of 4	1 of 12	1 of 7	4 of 56	6 of 75
BIKE 4	2 of 5	2 of 5	2 of 5	2 of 5	6 of 30	7 of 22	8 of 48	21 of 100
BIKE 5	0 of 4	0 of 4	0 of 4	0 of 4	0 of 24	0 of 18	0 of 40	0 of 82
TOT	**10 of 24**	**10 of 24**	**13 of 24**	**15 of 24**	**21 of 142**	**19 of 95**	**27 of 253**	**57 of 490**

SG = supragranular, G = granular, IG = infragranular.

numerous post-translational modifications may affect its subcellular targeting, processing and degradation rate, hence affecting the net protein level, at least in part independent of its mRNA levels. Since ours is the first study to address changes in cortical LINGO-1 protein levels after spinal cord transection, such possibilities cannot be ruled out and suggest interesting new lines of investigation on the mechanisms of cortical reorganization after spinal cord injury and new therapeutic options.

Similar considerations hold for the difference between mRNA and protein levels of BDNF. Endo et al. [46] showed long-lasting up-regulation of BDNF mRNA levels in transected rats; on the contrary, 8 weeks after transection we observed increased BDNF levels only in transected animals under bike exercise regimen, while in non-exercising transected animals BDNF levels were actually decreased. Again, it is possible that post-transcriptional and post-translational mechanisms uncoupled the regulation of protein levels from mRNA levels, causing the discrepancy between the two studies. Our study further shows that other proteins known to be associated with different aspects of morphological and functional plasticity are regulated after spinal cord transection. These include ADCY1, which is involved in long-term synaptic plasticity, learning and memory [51]; GAP43, which is critical for the normal establishment of ordered topography in the developing barrel cortex [67,68] and mediates functional recovery after lesions in the adult central nervous system [21,57,60]; p35, which is regulated in neurodegeneration [61], has an important neuroprotective role in vivo [49] and contributes to different forms of synaptic plasticity [62]. A complex network of proteins is therefore involved in cortical reorganization after spinal cord injury.

Passive hindlimb bike exercise consistently modulated only the levels of two of the above proteins (increasing them): BDNF and ADCY1. On the one hand, exercise has been associated with increased brain levels of BDNF in several previous studies [45,69,70,71]. Our data suggest that exercise-dependent modulation of BDNF levels in the brain is not necessarily mediated by the sensorimotor system, but could also be mediated by cardiovascular and/or neuroendocrine mechanisms [41]. On the other hand, the involvement of ADCY1 is intriguing because of the critical role of this protein in multiple forms of plasticity, including the formation of cortical barrels [72,73,74], experience-dependent strengthening of whisker thalamic relay synapses [51] and the refinement of retinal projection maps [75,76] during development. It therefore seems possible that molecular mechanisms mediating cortical plasticity during development might be reactivated in adulthood after a massive injury such as spinal cord injury. The demonstration that cortical ADCY1 has a causal role in central sensitization and behavioral allodynia after peripheral nerve injury [77] and, more recently, that it affects behavioral sensitization by controlling PKMz levels independently of transcription [78] has important clinical implications, as its regulation may represent the mechanism underlying the emergence and maintenance of pain after spinal cord injury. Our data indicate that passive exercise, even in absence of sensorimotor spinal connections, can modulate these molecular mechanisms and suggest possible novel targets to selectively control central pain after spinal cord injury.

Hindlimb Bike Exercise after Thoracic Transection of the Spinal Cord Enhances the Neurophysiological Reorganization of the Deafferented Hindlimb Cortex

The altered levels of plasticity-related proteins were not sufficient – without passive bike exercise – to induce a detectable electrophysiological reorganization: in 'sham-exercise' transected animals, the probability of neurons in the deafferented hindpaw cortex to respond to forepaw/forelimb tactile stimulation 8 weeks after spinal transection was extremely low, as expected from normal animals under deep anesthesia [9]. This observation is consistent with the absence of cortical reorganization reported by Jain et al. (1995) based on the responses to tactile stimuli after dorsal columns section [79], and is not in contradiction with the reorganization observed with functional magnetic resonance imaging (fMRI), based on the responses to high-intensity electrical stimuli after complete transection of the spinal cord [46,80]. In fact, a similar dependence on stimulus-intensity is observed immediately after spinal cord injury [81], when the responses to low-intensity electrical stimuli are not sufficiently consistent to uncover cortical reorganization, but cortical reorganization is revealed by high-intensity stimuli. The dependence of long-term cortical reorganization after spinal cord injury on stimulus-intensity, possibly due to differences between dorsal columns inputs and spinothalamic inputs [82], is beyond the scope of the present study and will deserve further investigation.

The data presented here show that passive bike training after spinal cord transection is indeed sufficient to increase the neural responsiveness of the deafferented hindpaw cortex to tactile stimuli delivered to the forepaw/forelimb under deep anesthesia. This increase in responsiveness was observed at all cortical layers – differently from our previous experiments with forelimb training in neonatally spinalized rats, in which we did not observe changes in the granular layer [9]. Interestingly, a similar increase in responsiveness of the hindpaw cortex to tactile stimuli delivered to the forepaw/forelimb can be obtained by decreasing the depth of anesthesia [83]. This suggests that the exercise-dependent increase of neural responsiveness might be mediated not only by axonal sprouting [84,85,86], but also by the alteration of the dynamic equilibrium of dendritic spines and axonal boutons between interneurons and pyramidal neurons [10,87], possibly as a compensatory process to maintain the delicate cortical balance between excitation and inhibition [88], or even by the alteration of more subtle intrinsic properties of cortical neurons. Combining our electrophysiological and molecular observations, even though we did not show a causal link, it is tempting to suggest that BDNF and ADCY1 could be particularly critical for the reorganization of the cortical architecture dedicated to the processing of dorsal column inputs. Nonetheless, because the neurophysiological reorganization we observed in the deafferented hindlimb cortex was not layer-specific, we cannot exclude a subcortical contribution to the cortical reorganization [12,89,90,91,92,93]. We speculatively propose that the cardiovascular and neuroendocrine systemic effects produced by passive exercise can boost or simply accelerate the cascade of plasticity-related events that are already occurring in the massively deafferented somatosensory cortex after spinal cord injury.

Independently of the exact mechanism, our data show that passive exercise of the lower limbs after complete transection of the spinal cord is indeed sufficient to promote cortical reorganization.

Conclusions

We showed that passive exercise below the level the lesion in rats both alters plasticity-related proteins in the sensorimotor cortex and promotes an electrophysiologically measurable re-organization in the deafferented hindlimb cortex after complete spinal cord injury. These results support the important role of physical exercise for learning and plasticity, suggest that exercise should be considered – among its other effects – as a re-habilitation strategy that generically promotes cortical plasticity, and uncover a brain-body interaction that does not rely on intact sensorimotor pathways connecting the exercised body parts and the brain.

Materials and Methods

A total of 41 adult Sprague-Dawley were used in this study. The different experimental groups are indicated in Figure 1. In 32 animals we used western blot analysis to assess whether passive hindlimb bike training after thoracic transection of the spinal cord affected the expression in the somatosensory cortex of proteins associated with plasticity (Fig. 1A). In 9 additional animals we performed single-neuron mapping in the deafferented somatosensory cortex at the end of the study to electrophysiologically verify the presence of exercise-dependent cortical reorganization (Fig. 1B). All procedures were performed under the guidelines of the National Institutes of Health, and approved by the Institutional Animal Care and Use Committee of Drexel University.

Spinal Cord Transection

Animals received a complete thoracic transection of the spinal cord with procedures that are similar to our previous studies [81,94]. Briefly, adult female Sprague-Dawley (Charles River) rats were anesthetized with isoflurane (2–3% with oxygen) and the spinal cord was exposed by laminectomy at the T8/T9 level. The cord was transected with iridectomy scissors followed by aspiration of tissue within the cavity. A collagen matrix, Vitrogen, was injected into the site of the transection to fill the cavity. The muscle and skin were sutured in layers with 5-0 silk. Animals were then warmed, and when they became active, returned to their home cages. Bladders were manually expressed until the animals were able to void on their own. Animals were housed under a 12 h light/dark cycle (lights on at 07:00) with free access to food and water.

Passive Hindlimb Bike Exercise

As in previous studies, hindlimb bike exercise consisted of two 30-minute sessions with a 10-minute break, 3 days per week (M, W and F) [48]. This exercise regimen involved suspending the rats on a sling with the hindlimbs hanging down and the hind feet strapped onto the pedals of a bicycle-type device that was driven by a motorized belt. The exercise consisted of a pedaling motion that flexed one limb while extending the other without over-stretching the limbs. Cycling speed was 0.5 Hz. This was, therefore, a passive exercise of the hindlimbs only. Animals did not watch the exercised hindlimbs. Sham exercise consisted of placing the animals on the bike for 70 minutes, 3 days per week, but without moving the pedals.

Western Blot Analysis

Immediately following their last exercise session, animals were anesthetized with isoflurane and then decapitated. The brain and spinal cord were immediately removed, sliced on ice into 2 mm thick coronal slices and flash-frozen on dry ice. We focused on the sensorimotor cortex. Each tissue sample was placed into a FastPrep 120 tube (MP Biomedicals, Irvine, CA) in cold homogenization buffer and homogenized with FastPrep 120 for 40 sec, centrifuged at 1000 g for 10 min, transferred into 1.5 ml microfuge tubes and centrifuged at 20,000 g for 15 min. Protein concentration was assessed by using BioRad DC protein assay method (BioRad, Hercules, CA). Homogenates were fast frozen on dry ice and stored at −80°C until further processing. Proteins were run on pre-cast 26 well SDS gels (BioRad) either 10% or 4–15% gradient, depending upon expected protein molecular weight. Protein standards (Biorad) were used to determine protein size. For each antibody an initial amount of 30 μg total protein/well was loaded at four different dilutions (1:1, 1:2, 1:5, 1:10). Once the optimal dilution was identified, it was held constant across all samples. Gelled proteins were transferred to 0.2 μ nitrocellulose membrane using I Blot system (Invitrogen). After transfer the membrane was incubated for 1 hr at room temperature in Li Cor western block (Li Cor, Lincoln NE) solution and then overnight at 4°C in primary antibody solution (Li Cor Block +0.1% Tween) with one of the following primary antibodies: adenylate cyclase isoform 1 (ADCY1; Bioworlde BS2391), brain derived neurotrophic factor (BDNF; Santa Cruz SC-20981), tyrosine kinase B (trkB; Millipore 07–225), 43 kD growth associated protein (GAP43; Epitomics 2259-1), leucine-rich repeat and Ig domain-containing Nogo receptor-interacting protein (LINGO-1; Santa Cruz SC-134597), Cyclin-dependent kinase 5 activator 1 (p35; Bioworlde BS2065).

Antibody anti Beta-actin (Sigma A5441) was added to the incubation solution for endogenous control. After incubation in primary antibodies the blots were rinsed 3×10 min in PBS +0.1% Tween and incubated 1 hr and RT in block solution containing the following secondary antibodies developed in goat: anti-rabbit IgG IRDye700DX-conjugated, cat #611-130-122 and anti-mouse IgG IRDye800DX-conjugated, cat #610-132-121 (Rockland, Gilbertsville, PA) and HRP conjugated streptactin (BioRad 161-0382), then washed 3×10 min in PBS+Tween and rinsed in PBS. Processed membranes were exposed on Li-Cor Odyssey infrared imager at both 700 and 800 nm wavelengths for appropriate exposure times. All protein level values were obtained on the gel image by subtracting the background intensity from the signal for the protein of interest. The same procedure was performed for the control protein (Beta-actin) and each blot was normalized to its corresponding actin value. For statistical and illustration purposes, all western blot data for each animal and each protein were divided by the average value of the corresponding protein in the normal animals group and expressed as percentage. Note that in this way the average value for normal animals is 100% but the variability between animals (see error bars) is maintained.

Electrophysiology

Acute single-neuron mapping of the deafferented hindpaw cortex was performed at the end of the study with similar techniques as in our previous study [9]. Rats were anesthetized by intraperitoneal injection of urethane anesthesia (1.3 g/Kg) and placed in a stereotaxic frame. Craniotomies were performed over either the right or left cortex to expose the hindlimb representations in the primary somatosensory cortex. The stereotaxic coordinates for hindlimb craniotomy were from 0 to 3 mm posterior to bregma and from 2 to 3 mm lateral [95]. Electrode penetrations were defined using the stereotaxic coordinates for the hindlimb somatosensory cortex [96,97]. For all animals, the anesthesia level was maintained at Stage III-4 [98].

A high impedance (10 MΩ) tungsten microelectrode (FHC, Inc, Bowdoin, ME) was mounted on a stereotaxic electrode manipulator. A ground wire was inserted into the brain adjacent to the craniotomies. The microelectrode was then moved to the anterior-posterior and medial-lateral coordinates that defined a predetermined location above the hindlimb somatosensory cortex, and lowered, perpendicular to the surface of the brain, to penetrate the dura and pia. The microelectrode was then slowly inserted into the brain.

The signals from the microelectrode were continuously monitored on the oscilloscope and audio speakers as the electrode was lowered. When a neuron was encountered, the dorsal/ventral coordinates of the cell were noted. Two experimenters then determined whether the identified cell responded to sensory stimulation. The first experimenter, with knowledge of the electrode placement, used wooden probes to touch the hair/skin on the forelimb and shoulder. The second experimenter, blind to the position of the electrode and treatment group of the animal, determined if the cell responded to the stimulus, predominately by listening for a change in firing rate. If the cell did not modulate its firing rate in response to the stimulation, the cell was noted as negative. If the cell did modulate its firing rate, the cell was noted as positive. If the cell was noted as positive, then the receptive field of the cell was identified by tapping locations on the body rostral to the level of the injury. Stimulation of any body surface that modulated the cell's firing rate was considered part of the cell's receptive field. To ensure that tapping forces between animals and across sites were uniform, the responses elicited by the wooden probe were periodically compared to responses elicited by von Frey filaments to calibrate the stimulus applied by the wooden probe. The stimulation consisted of pressing a filament gently against the skin, perpendicular to its surface until the filament bent 90 degrees. This procedure was done 5 times for each filament and skin site, to ensure reproducibility of the results. The filament necessary to elicit a response similar to the wooden probe was noted and compared across animals and locations. The filaments required to produce an equivalent response ranged from 4.31 (bending force of 2 g) to 4.93 (bending force of 8 g) across animals and animal groups. There were no identifiable differences in the distribution of filaments used between the groups.

After a cell was characterized, the microelectrode was moved at least 50 microns deeper (with respect to the cortical surface) before another cell could be identified in the same penetration to ensure a new cell was encountered. For every cell identified, the stereotaxic coordinates of the microelectrode position were identified allowing us to evaluate neuronal responsiveness for each layer of the cortex. To minimize tissue damage and its possible effects on cell responsiveness during later penetrations, no more than 6 penetrations were performed per animal.

Perfusion and Histological Processing of the Brain and Spinal Cord

At the end of the mapping sessions, the rats were perfused transcardially with buffered saline, followed by buffered 2% paraformaldehyde, and then by buffered 2% paraformaldehyde containing 10% sucrose. The cortex was removed and flattened between two glass slides. The tissue was cryoprotected in 30% sucrose and sectioned (70 microns parallel to the pial surface) frozen on a sliding microtome. Series of these sections from the cortex were stained for cytochrome oxidase (CO) activity [99]. Spinal cords were removed and placed in phosphate buffer containing 30% sucrose for 72 h. Specimens were frozen in OCT and sectioned on a freezing microtome at 20 μm. The transection segments of the spinal cords were sectioned parasagitally, and alternate sections were Nissl-myelin stained. The resulting sections were examined under a microscope to confirm completeness of the transection.

Statistical Analyses

To assess the effects of spinal cord transection alone on plasticity-related proteins in the sensorimotor cortex, we compared 'sham-exercise' transected animals to normal animals by entering the data into a two-way independent-measures analysis of variance (ANOVA). The factors were 'protein' (ADCY1, BDNF, trkB, GAP43, LINGO-1 and p35), and 'time from lesion' (normal, 1 week after transection, 8 weeks after transection). In case of significant interaction, we performed follow-up one-way ANOVAs on individual proteins, followed by Fisher's post-hoc test (as in Endo et al., 2007).

To assess the effects of passive hindlimb bike exercise after spinal transection on plasticity-related proteins in the sensorimotor cortex, the data from 'bike-exercise' and 'sham-exercise' animals were entered into a three-way independent-measures analysis of variance (ANOVA). The factors were 'exercise' (bike or sham), 'protein' (ADCY1, BDNF, trkB, GAP43, LINGO-1 and p35) and 'weeks' (1 or 8 weeks). In case of significant interactions, we performed follow-up two-way ANOVAs on individual proteins.

To assess the effects of passive hindlimb bike exercise after spinal transection on the electrophysiological reorganization of the deafferented cortex, we performed two types of analyses. First, the percentage of cells stereotaxically located in the deafferented hindlimb cortex that responded to stimulation of the intact forelimb were compared between bike animals and sham animals using two-proportion tests, separately for all cells and for each cortical layer. Second, the percentage of cells *per track* stereotaxically located in the deafferented hindlimb cortex that responded to stimulation of the intact forelimb were entered into a two-way mixed ANOVA, considering each track as an independent sample. The factors were exercise (bike or sham, independent measures) and cortical layer (supragranular, granular, infragranular, repeated measures).

Results were considered significant at $p<0.05$.

Acknowledgments

We thank Dr. Elizabeth Dugan for assistance with the transection surgery, animal care and bicycle therapy, Jennifer Garcia for performing the spinal surgeries, managing the therapy protocols and caring for the animals, and Kamal Laroiya for technical assistance in tissue collecting and processing. We would also like to thank Dr. Tim Himes and Theresa Connors and the Spinal Cord Research Center at Drexel University for assistance with the therapy protocols, animal care, transection surgery and histological analysis and Dr. Robert Flint, Patrick Ganzer and Matt Cozon for their assistance during the electrophysiological recordings.

Author Contributions

Conceived and designed the experiments: KAM JS AG. Performed the experiments: KAM JS AG EBK. Analyzed the data: KAM AG GF. Contributed reagents/materials/analysis tools: KAM AG JS. Wrote the paper: KAM AG GF.

References

1. Wall PD, Egger MD (1971) Formation of new connexions in adult rat brains after partial deafferentation. Nature 232: 542–545.
2. Calford MB, Tweedale R (1988) Immediate and chronic changes in responses of somatosensory cortex in adult flying-fox after digit amputation. Nature 332: 446–448.
3. Pons TP, Garraghty PE, Ommaya AK, Kaas JH, Taub E, et al. (1991) Massive cortical reorganization after sensory deafferentation in adult macaques. Science 252: 1857–1860.
4. Jain N, Catania KC, Kaas JH (1997) Deactivation and reactivation of somatosensory cortex after dorsal spinal cord injury. Nature 386: 495–498.
5. Florence SL, Taub HB, Kaas JH (1998) Large-scale sprouting of cortical connections after peripheral injury in adult macaque monkeys. Science 282: 1117–1121.
6. Kaas JH (2000) The reorganization of somatosensory and motor cortex after peripheral nerve or spinal cord injury in primates. Prog Brain Res 128: 173–179.
7. Green JB, Sora E, Bialy Y, Ricamato A, Thatcher RW (1998) Cortical sensorimotor reorganization after spinal cord injury: an electroencephalographic study. Neurology 50: 1115–1121.
8. Nishimura Y, Onoe H, Morichika Y, Perfiliev S, Tsukada H, et al. (2007) Time-dependent central compensatory mechanisms of finger dexterity after spinal cord injury. Science 318: 1150–1155.
9. Kao T, Shumsky JS, Murray M, Moxon KA (2009) Exercise induces cortical plasticity after neonatal spinal cord injury in the rat. J Neurosci 29: 7549–7557.
10. Ghosh A, Peduzzi S, Snyder M, Schneider R, Starkey M, et al. (2011) Heterogeneous spine loss in layer 5 cortical neurons after spinal cord injury. Cereb Cortex 22: 1309–1317.
11. Ghosh A, Sydekum E, Haiss F, Peduzzi S, Zorner B, et al. (2009) Functional and anatomical reorganization of the sensory-motor cortex after incomplete spinal cord injury in adult rats. J Neurosci 29: 12210–12219.
12. Bowes C, Massey JM, Burish M, Cerkevich CM, Kaas JH (2012) Chondroitinase ABC promotes selective reactivation of somatosensory cortex in squirrel monkeys after a cervical dorsal column lesion. Proc Natl Acad Sci U S A 109: 2595–2600.
13. Moore CI, Stern CE, Dunbar C, Kostyk SK, Gehi A, et al. (2000) Referred phantom sensations and cortical reorganization after spinal cord injury in humans. Proc Natl Acad Sci U S A 97: 14703–14708.
14. Simoes EL, Bramati I, Rodrigues E, Franzoi A, Moll J, et al. (2012) Functional expansion of sensorimotor representation and structural reorganization of callosal connections in lower limb amputees. J Neurosci 32: 3211–3220.
15. Flor H, Elbert T, Knecht S, Wienbruch C, Pantev C, et al. (1995) Phantom-limb pain as a perceptual correlate of cortical reorganization following arm amputation. Nature 375: 482–484.
16. Lotze M, Grodd W, Birbaumer N, Erb M, Huse E, et al. (1999) Does use of a myoelectric prosthesis prevent cortical reorganization and phantom limb pain? Nat Neurosci 2: 501–502.
17. Klit H, Finnerup NB, Jensen TS (2009) Central post-stroke pain: clinical characteristics, pathophysiology, and management. Lancet Neurol 8: 857–868.
18. Wrigley PJ, Press SR, Gustin SM, Macefield VG, Gandevia SC, et al. (2009) Neuropathic pain and primary somatosensory cortex reorganization following spinal cord injury. Pain 141: 52–59.
19. Engineer ND, Riley JR, Seale JD, Vrana WA, Shetake JA, et al. (2011) Reversing pathological neural activity using targeted plasticity. Nature 470: 101–104.
20. Feldman DE, Brecht M (2005) Map plasticity in somatosensory cortex. Science 310: 810–815.
21. Girgis J, Merrett D, Kirkland S, Metz GA, Verge V, et al. (2007) Reaching training in rats with spinal cord injury promotes plasticity and task specific recovery. Brain 130: 2993–3003.
22. Kao T, Shumsky JS, Knudsen EB, Murray M, Moxon KA (2011) Functional role of exercise-induced cortical organization of sensorimotor cortex after spinal transection. J Neurophysiol 106: 2662–2674.
23. Thomas SL, Gorassini MA (2005) Increases in corticospinal tract function by treadmill training after incomplete spinal cord injury. J Neurophysiol 94: 2844–2855.
24. Winchester P, McColl R, Querry R, Foreman N, Mosby J, et al. (2005) Changes in supraspinal activation patterns following robotic locomotor therapy in motor-incomplete spinal cord injury. Neurorehabil Neural Repair 19: 313–324.
25. Hoffman LR, Field-Fote EC (2007) Cortical reorganization following bimanual training and somatosensory stimulation in cervical spinal cord injury: a case report. Phys Ther 87: 208–223.
26. Knikou M (2012) Plasticity of corticospinal neural control after locomotor training in human spinal cord injury. Neural Plast 2012: 254948.
27. Juliano SL, Ma W, Eslin D (1991) Cholinergic depletion prevents expansion of topographic maps in somatosensory cortex. Proc Natl Acad Sci U S A 88: 780–784.
28. Kilgard MP, Merzenich MM (1998) Cortical map reorganization enabled by nucleus basalis activity. Science 279: 1714–1718.
29. Conner JM, Chiba AA, Tuszynski MH (2005) The basal forebrain cholinergic system is essential for cortical plasticity and functional recovery following brain injury. Neuron 46: 173–179.
30. Hutchinson KJ, Gomez-Pinilla F, Crowe MJ, Ying Z, Basso DM (2004) Three exercise paradigms differentially improve sensory recovery after spinal cord contusion in rats. Brain 127: 1403–1414.
31. De Mello MT, Esteves AM, Tufik S (2004) Comparison between dopaminergic agents and physical exercise as treatment for periodic limb movements in patients with spinal cord injury. Spinal Cord 42: 218–221.
32. Kiser TS, Reese NB, Maresh T, Hearn S, Yates C, et al. (2005) Use of a motorized bicycle exercise trainer to normalize frequency-dependent habituation of the H-reflex in spinal cord injury. J Spinal Cord Med 28: 241–245.
33. Phadke CP, Flynn SM, Thompson FJ, Behrman AL, Trimble MH, et al. (2009) Comparison of single bout effects of bicycle training versus locomotor training on paired reflex depression of the soleus H-reflex after motor incomplete spinal cord injury. Arch Phys Med Rehabil 90: 1218–1228.
34. Rayegani SM, Shojaee H, Sedighipour L, Soroush MR, Baghbani M, et al. (2011) The effect of electrical passive cycling on spasticity in war veterans with spinal cord injury. Front Neurol 2: 39.
35. Hangartner TN, Rodgers MM, Glaser RM, Barre PS (1994) Tibial bone density loss in spinal cord injured patients: effects of FES exercise. J Rehabil Res Dev 31: 50–61.
36. Lauer RT, Smith BT, Mulcahey MJ, Betz RR, Johnston TE (2011) Effects of cycling and/or electrical stimulation on bone mineral density in children with spinal cord injury. Spinal Cord 49: 917–923.
37. Phillips WT, Kiratli BJ, Sarkarati M, Weraarchakul G, Myers J, et al. (1998) Effect of spinal cord injury on the heart and cardiovascular fitness. Curr Probl Cardiol 23: 641–716.
38. Phillips AA, Cote AT, Warburton DE (2011) A systematic review of exercise as a therapeutic intervention to improve arterial function in persons living with spinal cord injury. Spinal Cord 49: 702–714.
39. Faghri PD, Van Meerdervort HF, Glaser RM, Figoni SF (1997) Electrical stimulation-induced contraction to reduce blood stasis during arthroplasty. IEEE Trans Rehabil Eng 5: 62–69.
40. Twist DJ, Culpepper-Morgan JA, Ragnarsson KT, Petrillo CR, Kreek MJ (1992) Neuroendocrine changes during functional electrical stimulation. Am J Phys Med Rehabil 71: 156–163.
41. Seifert T, Secher NH (2011) Sympathetic influence on cerebral blood flow and metabolism during exercise in humans. Prog Neurobiol 95: 406–426.
42. van Praag H, Christie BR, Sejnowski TJ, Gage FH (1999) Running enhances neurogenesis, learning, and long-term potentiation in mice. Proc Natl Acad Sci U S A 96: 13427–13431.
43. van Praag H, Kempermann G, Gage FH (1999) Running increases cell proliferation and neurogenesis in the adult mouse dentate gyrus. Nat Neurosci 2: 266–270.

44. Ang ET, Gomez-Pinilla F (2007) Potential therapeutic effects of exercise to the brain. Curr Med Chem 14: 2564–2571.
45. Cotman CW, Berchtold NC, Christie LA (2007) Exercise builds brain health: key roles of growth factor cascades and inflammation. Trends Neurosci 30: 464–472.
46. Endo T, Spenger C, Tominaga T, Brene S, Olson L (2007) Cortical sensory map rearrangement after spinal cord injury: fMRI responses linked to Nogo signalling. Brain 130: 2951–2961.
47. Gomez-Pinilla F, Ying Z, Zhuang Y (2012) Brain and spinal cord interaction: protective effects of exercise prior to spinal cord injury. PLoS One 7: e32298.
48. Skinner RD, Houle JD, Reese NB, Berry CL, Garcia-Rill E (1996) Effects of exercise and fetal spinal cord implants on the H-reflex in chronically spinalized adult rats. Brain Res 729: 127–131.
49. Viswanath V, Wu Z, Fonck C, Wei Q, Boonplueang R, et al. (2000) Transgenic mice neuronally expressing baculoviral p35 are resistant to diverse types of induced apoptosis, including seizure-associated neurodegeneration. Proc Natl Acad Sci U S A 97: 2270–2275.
50. Huang EJ, Reichardt LF (2001) Neurotrophins: roles in neuronal development and function. Annu Rev Neurosci 24: 677–736.
51. Wang H, Ferguson GD, Pineda VV, Cundiff PE, Storm DR (2004) Overexpression of type-1 adenylyl cyclase in mouse forebrain enhances recognition memory and LTP. Nat Neurosci 7: 635–642.
52. Mi S, Miller RH, Lee X, Scott ML, Shulag-Morskaya S, et al. (2005) LINGO-1 negatively regulates myelination by oligodendrocytes. Nat Neurosci 8: 745–751.
53. Ji B, Li M, Wu WT, Yick LW, Lee X, et al. (2006) LINGO-1 antagonist promotes functional recovery and axonal sprouting after spinal cord injury. Mol Cell Neurosci 33: 311–320.
54. Inoue H, Lin L, Lee X, Shao Z, Mendes S, et al. (2007) Inhibition of the leucine-rich repeat protein LINGO-1 enhances survival, structure, and function of dopaminergic neurons in Parkinson's disease models. Proc Natl Acad Sci U S A 104: 14430–14435.
55. Bekinschtein P, Cammarota M, Igaz LM, Bevilaqua LR, Izquierdo I, et al. (2007) Persistence of long-term memory storage requires a late protein synthesis-and BDNF- dependent phase in the hippocampus. Neuron 53: 261–277.
56. Bekinschtein P, Cammarota M, Katche C, Slipczuk L, Rossato JI, et al. (2008) BDNF is essential to promote persistence of long-term memory storage. Proc Natl Acad Sci U S A 105: 2711–2716.
57. Mendonca HR, Araujo SE, Gomes AL, Sholl-Franco A, da Cunha Faria Melibeu A, et al. (2010) Expression of GAP-43 during development and after monocular enucleation in the rat superior colliculus. Neurosci Lett 477: 23–27.
58. Petrinovic MM, Duncan CS, Bourikas D, Weinman O, Montani L, et al. (2010) Neuronal Nogo-A regulates neurite fasciculation, branching and extension in the developing nervous system. Development 137: 2539–2550.
59. Mizutani K, Sonoda S, Yamada K, Beppu H, Shimpo K (2011) Alteration of protein expression profile following voluntary exercise in the perilesional cortex of rats with focal cerebral infarction. Brain Res 1416: 61–68.
60. Wei HF, Zeng BF, Chen YF, Chen L, Gu YD (2011) BDNF and GAP43 contribute to dynamic transhemispheric functional reorganization in rat brain after contralateral C7 root transfer following brachial plexus avulsion injuries. Neurosci Lett 500: 187–191.
61. Lopes JP, Agostinho P (2011) Cdk5: multitasking between physiological and pathological conditions. Prog Neurobiol 94: 49–63.
62. Su SC, Tsai LH (2011) Cyclin-dependent kinases in brain development and disease. Annu Rev Cell Dev Biol 27: 465–491.
63. Fumagalli F, Madaschi L, Caffino L, Marfia G, Di Giulio AM, et al. (2009) Acute spinal cord injury reduces brain derived neurotrohic factor expression in rat hippocampus. Neuroscience 159: 936–939.
64. Felix MS, Popa N, Djelloul M, Boucraut J, Gauthier P, et al. (2012) Alteration of forebrain neurogenesis after cervical spinal cord injury in the adult rat. Front Neurosci 6: 45.
65. Zhu HC, Wang LM, Wang M, Song B, Tan S, et al. (2012) MicroRNA-195 downregulates Alzheimer's disease amyloid-beta production by targeting BACE1. Brain Res Bull.
66. Mosyak L, Wood A, Dwyer B, Buddha M, Johnson M, et al. (2006) The structure of the Lingo-1 ectodomain, a module implicated in central nervous system repair inhibition. J Biol Chem 281: 36378–36390.
67. Erzurumlu RS, Jhaveri S, Benowitz LI (1990) Transient patterns of GAP-43 expression during the formation of barrels in the rat somatosensory cortex. J Comp Neurol 292: 443–456.
68. Maier DL, Mani S, Donovan SL, Soppet D, Tessarollo L, et al. (1999) Disrupted cortical map and absence of cortical barrels in growth-associated protein (GAP)-43 knockout mice. Proc Natl Acad Sci U S A 96: 9397–9402.
69. Gomez-Pinilla F, Ying Z, Roy RR, Molteni R, Edgerton VR (2002) Voluntary exercise induces a BDNF-mediated mechanism that promotes neuroplasticity. J Neurophysiol 88: 2187–2195.
70. Griesbach GS, Hovda DA, Molteni R, Wu A, Gomez-Pinilla F (2004) Voluntary exercise following traumatic brain injury: brain-derived neurotrophic factor upregulation and recovery of function. Neuroscience 125: 129–139.
71. Vaynman S, Gomez-Pinilla F (2005) License to run: exercise impacts functional plasticity in the intact and injured central nervous system by using neurotrophins. Neurorehabil Neural Repair 19: 283–295.
72. Welker E, Armstrong-James M, Bronchti G, Ourednik W, Gheorghita-Baechler F, et al. (1996) Altered sensory processing in the somatosensory cortex of the mouse mutant barrelless. Science 271: 1864–1867.
73. Abdel-Majid RM, Leong WL, Schalkwyk LC, Smallman DS, Wong ST, et al. (1998) Loss of adenylyl cyclase I activity disrupts patterning of mouse somatosensory cortex. Nat Genet 19: 289–291.
74. Lu HC, She WC, Plas DT, Neumann PE, Janz R, et al. (2003) Adenylyl cyclase I regulates AMPA receptor trafficking during mouse cortical 'barrel' map development. Nat Neurosci 6: 939–947.
75. Ravary A, Muzerelle A, Herve D, Pascoli V, Ba-Charvet KN, et al. (2003) Adenylate cyclase 1 as a key actor in the refinement of retinal projection maps. J Neurosci 23: 2228–2238.
76. Nicol X, Muzerelle A, Rio JP, Metin C, Gaspar P (2006) Requirement of adenylate cyclase 1 for the ephrin-A5-dependent retraction of exuberant retinal axons. J Neurosci 26: 862–872.
77. Wei F, Qiu CS, Kim SJ, Muglia L, Maas JW, et al. (2002) Genetic elimination of behavioral sensitization in mice lacking calmodulin-stimulated adenylyl cyclases. Neuron 36: 713–726.
78. Li XY, Ko HG, Chen T, Descalzi G, Koga K, et al. (2010) Alleviating neuropathic pain hypersensitivity by inhibiting PKMzeta in the anterior cingulate cortex. Science 330: 1400–1404.
79. Jain N, Florence SL, Kaas JH (1995) Limits on plasticity in somatosensory cortex of adult rats: hindlimb cortex is not reactivated after dorsal column section. J Neurophysiol 73: 1537–1546.
80. Ghosh A, Haiss F, Sydekum E, Schneider R, Gullo M, et al. (2010) Rewiring of hindlimb corticospinal neurons after spinal cord injury. Nat Neurosci 13: 97–104.
81. Aguilar J, Humanes-Valera D, Alonso-Calvino E, Yague JG, Moxon KA, et al. (2010) Spinal cord injury immediately changes the state of the brain. J Neurosci 30: 7528–7537.
82. Yague JG, Foffani G, Aguilar J (2011) Cortical hyperexcitability in response to preserved spinothalamic inputs immediately after spinal cord hemisection. Exp Neurol 227: 252–263.
83. Moxon KA, Hale LL, Aguilar J, Foffani G (2008) Responses of infragranular neurons in the rat primary somatosensory cortex to forepaw and hindpaw tactile stimuli. Neuroscience 156: 1083–1092.
84. Darian-Smith C, Gilbert CD (1994) Axonal sprouting accompanies functional reorganization in adult cat striate cortex. Nature 368: 737–740.
85. Yamahachi H, Marik SA, McManus JN, Denk W, Gilbert CD (2009) Rapid axonal sprouting and pruning accompany functional reorganization in primary visual cortex. Neuron 64: 719–729.
86. Marik SA, Yamahachi H, McManus JN, Szabo G, Gilbert CD (2010) Axonal dynamics of excitatory and inhibitory neurons in somatosensory cortex. PLoS Biol 8: e1000395.
87. Keck T, Scheuss V, Jacobsen RI, Wierenga CJ, Eysel UT, et al. (2011) Loss of sensory input causes rapid structural changes of inhibitory neurons in adult mouse visual cortex. Neuron 71: 869–882.
88. House DR, Elstrott J, Koh E, Chung J, Feldman DE (2011) Parallel regulation of feedforward inhibition and excitation during whisker map plasticity. Neuron 72: 819–831.
89. Faggin BM, Nguyen KT, Nicolelis MA (1997) Immediate and simultaneous sensory reorganization at cortical and subcortical levels of the somatosensory system. Proc Natl Acad Sci U S A 94: 9428–9433.
90. Jones EG, Pons TP (1998) Thalamic and brainstem contributions to large-scale plasticity of primate somatosensory cortex. Science 282: 1121–1125.
91. Jones EG (2000) Cortical and subcortical contributions to activity-dependent plasticity in primate somatosensory cortex. Annu Rev Neurosci 23: 1–37.
92. Jain N, Qi HX, Collins CE, Kaas JH (2008) Large-scale reorganization in the somatosensory cortex and thalamus after sensory loss in macaque monkeys. J Neurosci 28: 11042–11060.
93. Graziano A, Jones EG (2009) Early withdrawal of axons from higher centers in response to peripheral somatosensory denervation. J Neurosci 29: 3738–3748.
94. Nothias JM, Mitsui T, Shumsky JS, Fischer I, Antonacci MD, et al. (2005) Combined effects of neurotrophin secreting transplants, exercise, and serotonergic drug challenge improve function in spinal rats. Neurorehabil Neural Repair 19: 296–312.
95. Paxinos G, Watson C (1986) The rat brain in stereotaxic coordinates. Sydney; Orlando: Academic Press. xxvi, [237] p. p.
96. Chapin JK, Lin CS (1984) Mapping the body representation in the SI cortex of anesthetized and awake rats. J Comp Neurol 229: 199–213.
97. Leergaard TB, Alloway KD, Pham TA, Bolstad I, Hoffer ZS, et al. (2004) Three-dimensional topography of corticopontine projections from rat sensorimotor cortex: comparisons with corticostriatal projections reveal diverse integrative organization. J Comp Neurol 478: 306–322.
98. Friedberg MH, Lee SM, Ebner FF (1999) Modulation of receptive field properties of thalamic somatosensory neurons by the depth of anesthesia. J Neurophysiol 81: 2243–2252.
99. Wong-Riley M (1979) Changes in the visual system of monocularly sutured or enucleated cats demonstrable with cytochrome oxidase histochemistry. Brain Res 171: 11–28.

11

NK1 Receptor Blockade Is Ineffective in Improving Outcome following a Balloon Compression Model of Spinal Cord Injury

Anna Victoria Leonard[1]*, Emma Thornton[1], Robert Vink[2]

1 School of Medical Sciences, University of Adelaide, Adelaide, South Australia, Australia, 2 Division of Health Sciences, University of South Australia, Adelaide, South Australia, Australia

Abstract

The neuropeptide substance P (SP) is a well-known mediator of neurogenic inflammation following a variety of CNS disorders. Indeed, inhibition of SP through antagonism of its receptor, the tachykinin NK1 receptor, has been shown to be beneficial following both traumatic brain injury and stroke. Such studies demonstrated that administration of an NK1 receptor antagonist reduced blood-brain-barrier permeability, edema development and improved functional outcome. Furthermore, our recent studies have demonstrated a potential role for SP in mediating neurogenic inflammation following traumatic spinal cord injury (SCI). Accordingly, the present study investigates whether inhibition of SP may similarly play a neuroprotective role following traumatic SCI. A closed balloon compression injury was induced at T10 in New Zealand White rabbits. At 30 minutes post-injury an NK1 receptor antagonist was administered intravenously. Animals were thereafter assessed for blood spinal cord barrier (BSCB) permeability, spinal water content (edema), intrathecal pressure (ITP), and histological and functional outcome from 5 hours to 2 weeks post-SCI. Administration of an NK1 receptor antagonist was not effective in reducing BSCB permeability, edema, ITP, or functional deficits following SCI. We conclude that SP mediated neurogenic inflammation does not seem to play a major role in BSCB disruption, edema development and consequential tissue damage seen in acute traumatic SCI. Rather it is likely that the severe primary insult and subsequent hemorrhage may be the key contributing factors to ongoing SCI injury.

Editor: Pranela Rameshwar, Rutgers - New Jersey Medical School, United States of America

Funding: The study was funded by the Neil Sachse Foundation (http://www.nsf.org.au/) and the University of Adelaide. AVL is the Neil Sachse Foundation Fellow. The funders had no role in study design, data collection and analysis, decision to publish, or preparation of the manuscript.

Competing Interests: The authors have declared that no competing interests exist.

* E-mail: anna.leonard@adelaide.edu.au

Introduction

Spinal cord injury (SCI) remains a major cause of disability within society, frequently affecting individuals in the prime of their life. To date, therapies have very limited efficacy in attenuating any resultant functional deficits, and accordingly, novel therapeutic approaches are urgently required. SCI is characterized by both primary and secondary injury mechanisms. While the primary injury is clearly irreversible, secondary injury mechanisms are considered reversible and are thus targeted for potential therapeutic interventions. Edema is one of the major secondary injury mechanisms in CNS injury, being considered to significantly contribute to further potentiation of injury development and tissue damage. The development of edema following SCI has been well characterized both within the injury epicentre [1,2,3,4,5,6] and in the adjacent segments where a delayed rostrocaudal spread of edema has been demonstrated with time [7,8]. Such edema may be both vasogenic and cytotoxic in nature, however it has been hypothesized that the initial edema is predominantly vasogenic in nature given that blood-spinal cord-barrier (BSCB) disruption is also present [1,2,9,10,11]. Importantly, increased edema following injury may lead to raised intrathecal pressure (ITP) [12], which in turn can result in greater tissue damage, and ultimately profound functional deficits.

Neurogenic inflammation has recently been shown to play an important role in the development of edema following a range of CNS injuries [13,14,15,16,17,18,19,20]. Neurogenic inflammation is a response of perivascular, unmyelinated afferent nerve fibres to injury or infection and is typically characterized by vasodilation, protein extravasation and edema [13,14,21]. The vascular response is facilitated by the release of neuropeptides such as substance P (SP) and calcitonin gene related peptide (CGRP). SP is known to preferentially bind to the tachykinin NK1 receptor, activation of which results in increased barrier permeability and edema development [14]. Increased SP immunoreactivity has been associated with increased blood brain barrier (BBB) permeability and edema development following both TBI [13,17] and stroke [16], whilst antagonism of the NK1 receptor has been shown to reduce BBB permeability and edema, as well as improve functional outcome [13,17,22]. Furthermore, our recent investigation following SCI has demonstrated that SP stores are reduced following injury, indicative of SP release, whilst NK1 receptor immunoreactivity increased [20]. Such results implicate a role for SP as a mediator of neurogenic inflammation following

SCI. However, whether inhibition of SP may similarly produce a neuroprotective effect following SCI has not yet been investigated.

Accordingly, the current study investigates the effect of administration an NK1 receptor antagonist following a balloon compression model of SCI. Specifically, this paper will assess SP immunoreactivity, BSCB permeability, edema, ITP, histological outcome, and functional outcome from 5 hours to 2 weeks post-SCI. We have utilized the balloon compression model of SCI due to its closed nature, thus facilitating development of increased ITP, and its replication of key primary injury mechanisms in clinical SCI as previously reported [20,23,24,25].

Materials and Methods

All experimental protocols were conducted according to the guidelines established by the National Health and Medical Research Council and were approved by the animal ethics committees of the University of Adelaide (M-2010-140) and the Institute of Medical and Veterinary Sciences (98/10), Adelaide, South Australia.

2.1. Balloon compression model of SCI

New Zealand white rabbits (n = 88) were subject to a balloon compression spinal cord injury as previously described [26,27]. Briefly, during the 12-hour day cycle, animals were removed from their home cages and anesthetized via a subcutaneous injection of Ketamine (2.5 mg/kg) and Domitor (0.25 mg/kg) mixture. Once a surgical level of anesthesia was achieved, the animal was placed onto a thermostatically controlled heating pad in the prone position. Initially, the dorsal surface of the animal's back was shaved and a midline incision of approximately 10 cm in length was made along the spinous processors (approximately T11 – L2). Paraspinal muscles were retracted and a laminectomy performed. A balloon catheter (ApexTM MonorailTM 4 mm×8 mm, Boston Scientific) was then advanced approximately 4 cm to T10 and rapidly inflated using an inflation device (Boston Scientific) to 8 atm of pressure. The balloon remained inflated for a 5-minute period before being deflated and removed. The muscular wound was sutured closed followed by closure of the skin with surgical clips. An additional group of animals were subject to all surgical procedures except inflation of the balloon catheter (sham; surgery controls).

2.2. n-acetyl L-tryptophan (NAT)

Animals were randomly assigned to receive the NK1 receptor antagonist, n-acetyl tryptophan (NAT), or equal volume vehicle (0.9% saline). NAT was administered intravenously at 30 minutes post-SCI at 2.5 mg/kg, with this optimal dose of NAT having been previously determined in studies conducted in our laboratory [28]. For studies with survival times greater than 24 hours, 2 additional i.v. doses were administered daily on day 1 and 2 post-SCI.

2.3. BSCB permeability

The Evan's Blue (EB) dye extravasation method, as previously described [14], was used to assess BSCB permeability at 5 hours (vehicle, n = 5; NAT, n = 6) post-SCI (or sham, n = 5). Briefly, 30 minutes prior to perfusion, EB was injected intravenously. The animals were then saline perfused and the spinal cord dissected and 10 mm segments cut. Each segment was homogenized and the absorbance of the supernatant was measured at 610 nm using a spectrophotometer. The level of extravasated EB within each tissue sample was then determined using a previously obtained EB standard curve, and was expressed as ug/mg of spinal cord tissue.

2.4. Edema measurement

Animals were assessed for edema at 3 days post-SCI (NAT and vehicle; n = 4/group) or sham (n = 5) using the wet weight/dry weight method as previously described [14]. Briefly, animals were administered a lethal injection of pentobarbital and the spinal cord rapidly removed. The spinal cord was cut into 10 mm segments and the wet weight was obtained. Spinal cord segments were then oven dried at 100°C for 48 hours before the dry weight was measured. The percentage of tissue water content was then calculated using the equation: % Water Content = ((Wet Weight – Dry Weight)/Wet weight) X 100

2.5. Intrathecal pressure measurement

Animals (vehicle, n = 6; NAT, n = 5; sham, n = 5) underwent a tracheotomy and the right and left femoral artery were dissected. The right femoral artery was cannulated and connected to a syringe pump containing saline, which was administered at 2 ml/h except when taking a blood sample for blood gas analysis. A Codman MICROSENSOR ICP probe was inserted into the left artery to monitor blood pressure. Following balloon compression, a Codman MICROSENSOR ICP probe was introduced into the intrathecal space and extended to the injury epicentre. The Codman probes were connected to an 8 channel Powerlab system (AD instruments) and the output was viewed live and recorded with Labchart (AD instruments). Intrathecal pressure was monitored for a 5 hour period. Blood pressure and blood gases were monitored to ensure physiological parameters were maintained.

2.6. Functional outcome

Animals were randomly assigned to sham, vehicle or NAT treated groups (n = 6 per group) and were assessed on days 3, 7, 10 and 14 post-SCI for both sensory and motor outcome. A modified Tarlov Score [23] was used to assess motor function of the hindlimbs. The criteria were as follows: 0 = No movement; 1 = minor movement of the hind limb joints; 2 = major movement of the hind limb joints; 3 = able to stand properly but unable to hop; 4 = able to hop, but not properly; 5 = normal movement. Animals were scored following a recorded 5-minute monitoring period. In addition, a forelimb to hindlimb ratio was calculated by recording the number of hindlimb movements per the first 20 forward moving forelimb steps. This ratio was then converted into a percentage.

The sensory outcome test involved applying the tip end of Dumont #4 fine forceps to the shaved plantar surface of animal's hind paw and assessing the withdrawal time. Animals were placed into an enclosed plastic box with a wire bottom with food provided as a distraction. The fine forceps were then applied to each hind paw 10 times with a 30 second interval between each application. The withdrawal response of the animals to the stimulus was graded as either; 0 = no response, 1 = weak response (slight movement of one joint of the hindlimb), 2 = moderate response (extensive movement of 2 or more joints of the hindlimb), or 3 = normal response. A sensory score out of 30 was given to each hind paw.

2.7. Histological outcome

Animals were randomly assigned to sham (n = 11), vehicle (n = 23) and NAT treated groups (n = 21) and were assessed for histological outcome using immunohistochemical techniques. Briefly animals were perfuse fixed with 10% formalin at 5 hours, 24 hours, 3 days, or 2 weeks post-SCI. Spinal cord tissue was then processed, embedded in paraffin and 5 μm cross sections were cut for assessment of morphological features (H&E stain), SP (Santa

Cruz Sc-9758; 1:2000, EDTA retrieval), NK1 receptor (Advanced Targeting Systems #AB-N33AP; 1:4000, Citrate retrieval), Albumin (Cappel #0113-0341; 1:20,000), microglia (Griffonia simplicifolia – Sigma L2140; 1:200), and AQP4 (Abcam Ab9512; 1:200, Citrate retrieval).

All sections underwent a similar immunohistochemical procedure, with all antibodies incubated at room temperature and PBS washes applied between each antibody. Briefly, sections were dewaxed, dehydrated and placed in methanol with 30% hydrogen peroxide. Specified microwave antigen retrieval was performed as required and sections incubated for 45 min in 3% normal horse serum. Primary antibody was added overnight before specific biotinylated secondary antibody (Vector,1:250) was added for 30 minutes. Tertiary streptavidin peroxidase conjugate (SPC; Pierce, 1:1000) was added for 1 hour and the immunocomplex visualised using 3,3′diaminobenzidine (DAB; Sigma) as a chromogen in the peroxidase reaction.

All sections were scanned at high resolution using the Hamamatsu Nanozoomer. Slides were viewed using the associated proprietary viewing software (NDP.view v1.1.27, Hamamatsu). Qualitative assessments were made by a blinded assessor using a ranking system (0 = no staining to 10 = extensive dark staining). Alternatively, whole sections were exported and assessed using our previously published color deconvolution method [29].

2.8. Statistical Analysis

All statistical tests were undertaken using GraphPad PRISM®. Evan's Blue extravasation, edema, ITP, Plantar prick test, and color deconvolution were analyzed using a two-way analysis of variance (ANOVA) followed by Bonferroni post-tests, with data expressed as mean ± standard error of the mean (SEM). Immunohistochemistry ranking and modified Tarlov score were analyzed using the Kruskal Wallis ANOVA followed by Dunn's multiple comparisons test. This data was expressed as the median and interquartile range (immunohistochemical ranking) or as the median and individual data points (Tarlov score).

Results

3.1. BSCB Permeability– Evan's Blue extravasation

Sham animals demonstrated minimal EB extravasation with an average of 6.93±1.25 μg EB/g tissue measured along all segments of the spinal cord (Figure 1A). After injury, a significant ($p<0.001$) increase in EB extravasation to 15.43±3.04 μg EB/g tissue was observed in vehicle treated animals within the injury epicentre at 5 hours post-SCI, with adjacent segments recording similar values to sham. NAT treated animals had similar EB extravasation to vehicles within the injury epicentre ($p<0.001$), however recorded significantly greater EB values ($0.01<p<0.05$) in the immediate adjacent segments when compared to shams. No significant differences were seen between vehicle and NAT treated groups.

3.2. Edema measurement

The spinal cord tissue water content of sham animals was 65.55±2.08% (Figure 1B). By 3 days post-SCI in vehicle treated animals, spinal cord water content had significantly increased ($p<0.001$) to 77.47±1.00% in the injury epicentre and to 68.82±1.39% and 70.4±1.56% within the immediate rostral ($p<0.05$) and caudal ($p<0.001$) segments, respectively. NAT treated animals had a similar edema profile to vehicle treated animals at this time, although a greater increase was apparent within the most distal caudal segment of the spinal cord, which was significant compared to sham ($p<0.05$).

3.3. Intrathecal pressure measurement

The intrathecal pressure of sham animals was 0.65±1.61 mmHg at the beginning of the recording period then stabilized and reached 3.75±1.26 mmHg by the end of monitoring (Figure 1C). An immediate significant increase in ITP was observed following injury with vehicle treated animals recording 5.31±3.98 mmHg ($p<0.001$) at 30 min post-SCI. ITP continued to gradually rise, reaching a maximal ITP of 7.36±0.79 mmHg by the end of 5 hour monitoring period ($p<0.001$). A similar significant increase in ITP was observed at the beginning of the monitoring period within the NAT treated group, with a recorded ITP measurement of 6.82±1.48 mmHg ($p<0.001$). Thereafter, a gradual increase in ITP was observed in the NAT treated group reaching a maximal recording of 9.42±1.34 mmHg at the end of the monitoring period ($p<0.001$). Whilst the NAT treated animals appear to trend slightly higher, no significant difference was observed between treatment groups over time.

3.4. Functional outcome

3.4.1. Motor function - Modified Tarlov Scale. Sham animals demonstrated normal motor function on all assessment days and ranked 5 (Figure 2A). Following injury, vehicle treated animals demonstrated a significant decrease in hindlimb motor function with severe paralysis observed on days 3 and 6 post-SCI. By day 10 and 14, vehicle treated animals ranked 1 and had regained some motor function. In contrast, NAT treated animals had recovered some minor hindlimb joint movement on day 6 post-SCI and accordingly had a significant improvement when compared to vehicle treated animals ($p<0.05$). However, from day 10 onwards, vehicle and NAT treated animals both had only minor motor function as assessed by the Tarlov score.

3.4.2. Motor function - hindlimb to forelimb ratio. The frequency of the hind limb movement was recorded as the number of hindlimb movements per 20 forelimb steps (Figure 2B). Sham animals demonstrated normal movement with every forelimb step followed by a hindlimb step, resulting in a 100% normal hindlimb movement. Vehicle treated injured animals showed no hind limb movement on day 3 and subsequently recorded 0% for the frequency of hind limb movement. Thereafter, a gradual increase in the frequency of hindlimb movement was observed, reaching 20±15.17% by day 14 post-SCI. As in the Tarlov score, NAT treated animals demonstrated earlier increases in the frequency of hindlimb movement with 10.83±12.81% recorded on day 6 post-SCI, and had a higher maximal frequency of movement of 25.83±18.82% observed on day 14 post-SCI. However, the improvement in hindlimb motor function produced by NAT treatment was only slight and was not significant.

3.4.3. Sensory function – prick test. Sham animals demonstrated normal sensory function over the 14 day assessment period, with only a slight deficit observed on day 3 in the left hindlimb. Such results suggest that the surgical procedure did not affect sensory function (Figure 2C and 2D). Vehicle treated animals demonstrated a significant decrease on day 3 post-SCI to 11.75±4.57 and 13.00±6.38 for the left and right hindlimbs, respectively ($p<0.001$). Some spontaneous improvement was observed over the assessment period and by day 14 the pain withdrawal score was 17.00±4.96 and 16.50±4.43 for the left and right hindlimbs, respectively ($p<0.001$). NAT animals similarly demonstrated a significant decrease in sensory function following injury, obtaining a pain withdrawal score of 13.00±2.98 and 10.00±4.99 for the left and right hindlimbs, respectively, on day 3 post-SCI ($P<0.001$). Similarly to vehicle treated animals, NAT treated animals recorded a slight spontaneous improvement in sensory function in both hindlimbs during the assessment period

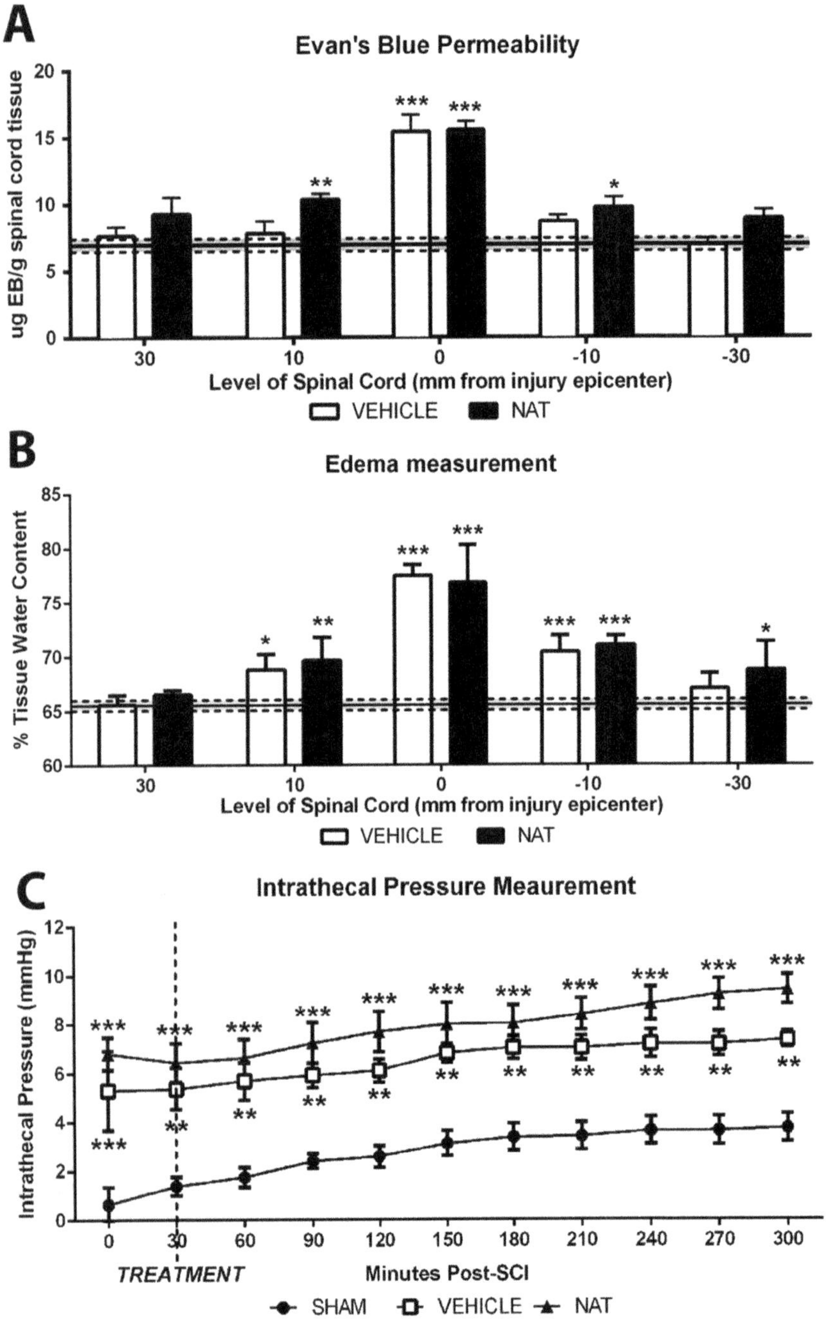

Figure 1. The effect of NAT administration on barrier permeability at 5 hours post-SCI was determined by the extent of EB extravasation (A). The percentage of spinal cord tissue water content was measured to determine the extent of edema development at 3 days post-SCI (B). The effect of NAT administration on ITP was measured for a 5 hour monitoring period (C). Sham levels indicated by the dashed line in (A) & (B). *denotes $p<0.05$, ** denotes $p<0.01$, *** denotes $p<0.001$ compared to sham.

recording a pain withdrawal score on day 14 post-SCI of 18±6.24 and 17.5±1.71 in the left and right hindlimbs respectively.

3.5. Histological outcome

3.5.1. Morphological features – H&E staining. Sham animals had normal tissue morphology and architecture (Figure 3). SCI resulted in focal areas of severe hemorrhage within the injury epicentre, predominantly within the grey matter, and substantial tissue disruption at 5 hours. The hemorrhage continued to spread and was diffusively located through the injury epicentre by 24 hours. Localized hemorrhage was also observed predominantly within the dorsal aspect of the white matter in the adjacent segments at this time. By 3 days post-SCI, moderate diffuse hemorrhage was observed within the injury epicentre, whilst minor hemorrhage was still apparent within the adjacent segments. Additionally by this time, loss of tissue morphology and architecture are clearly evident in the injury epicentre. By 2 weeks post-SCI extensive tissue loss was evident within the injury

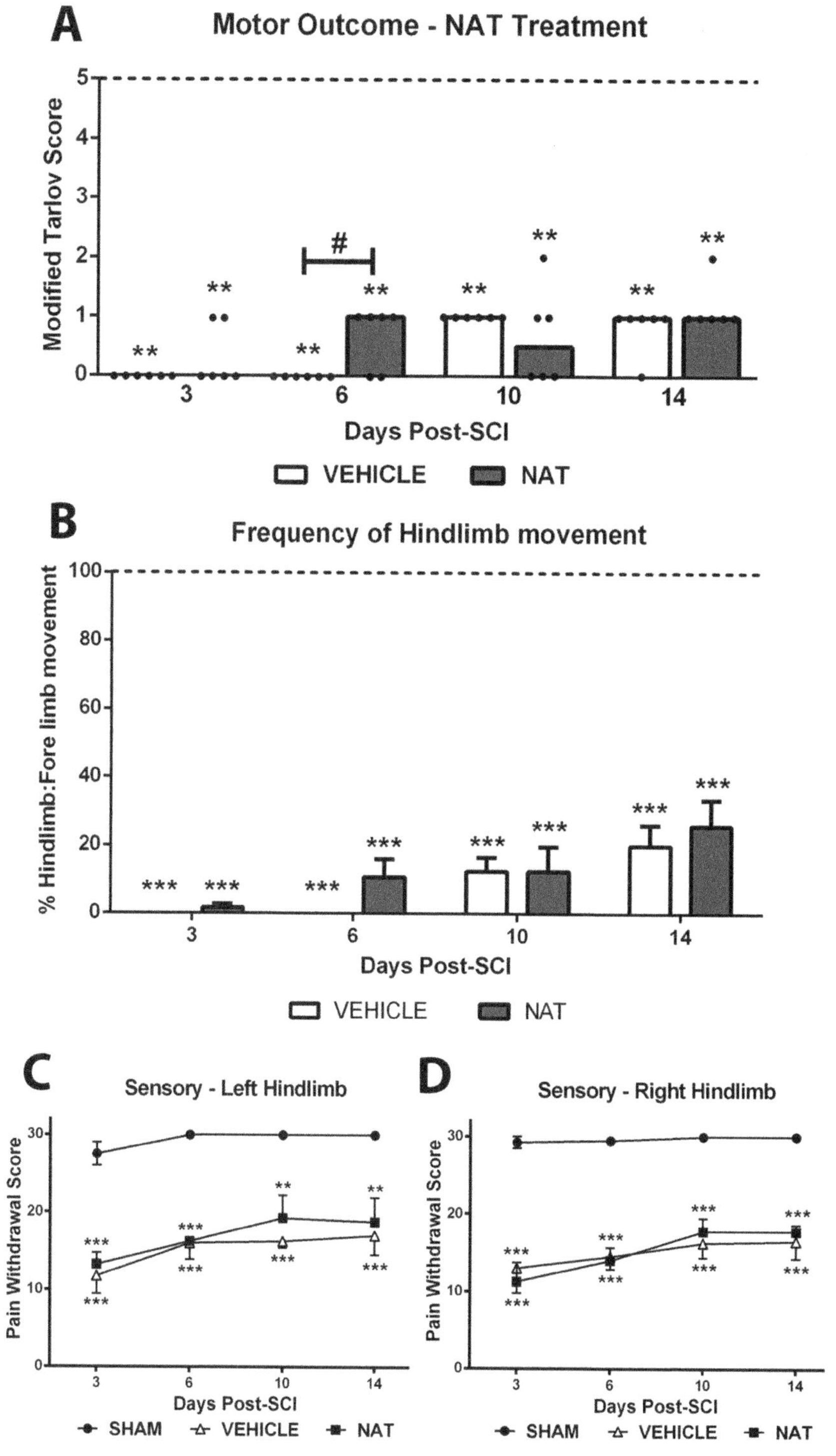

Figure 2. The effect of NAT administration on motor and sensory function following SCI. A modified Tarlov score was used to assess crude motor function (A), data is expressed as the median with individual data points plotted. Whilst a significant improvement was observed at 6 days post-SCI following NAT administration, this improvement was not significantly different to vehicle on days 10 and 14 post-injury. The frequency of hindlimb movement gradually increased in both treatment groups over time (B). Whilst NAT treated animals demonstrated earlier increases in movement frequency, no significant difference was observed between groups. A similar significant decrease in sensory function was observed in both the left (C) and right (D) hindlimbs of both treatment groups. ** denotes $p<0.01$, *** denotes $p<0.001$ when compared to sham. # denotes $p<0.05$ compared to vehicle.

epicentre with minimal white matter sparing and minor hemorrhage. The adjacent segments also demonstrated loss of tissue centred within the grey matter and radiating outwards. No differences in morphological features were observed between treatment groups at any time point post-SCI.

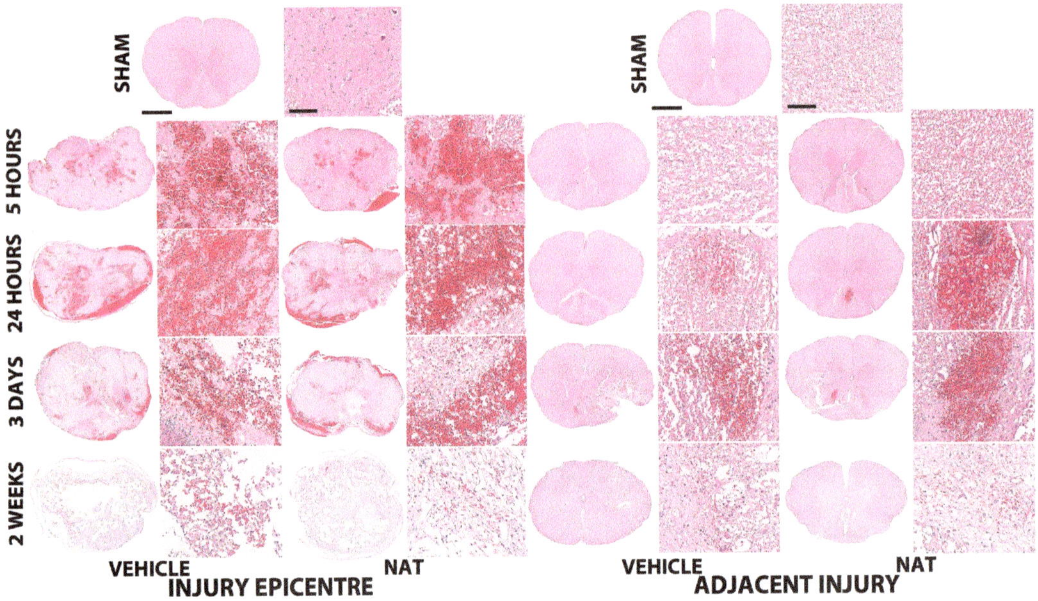

Figure 3. H&E staining demonstrates the morphological changes within the injury epicentre from 5 hours to 2 weeks post-SCI. Hemorrhage was predominant within 24 hours post-SCI, with marked tissue loss observed by 2 weeks post-SCI. No differences were observed between vehicle and NAT treatment groups. Cross section scale bar = 1 mm, high magnification scale bar = 100 μm.

3.5.2. Substance P immunoreactivity - Dorsal Horn region. Sham animals demonstrated a moderate level of SP immunoreactivity (median = 6) within the grey matter with particular predominance in lamina I and II of the dorsal horn (Figure 4). Within the injury epicentre, there was a significant decrease in SP immunoreactivity in both treatment groups when compared to sham ($p<0.001$), with further decreases in both groups at 24 hours (vehicle = 0 $p<0.001$; NAT = 1 $p<0.01$) and 3 days post-SCI ($p<0.001$ for both groups). By 2 weeks, the injury epicentre in both groups was completely devoid of SP immunoreactivity ($p<0.001$). The loss in SP immunoreactivity within the adjacent sections was not as pronounced as in the injury epicentre until day 3 in the 10 mm caudal section (median = 2; $p<0.001$) and 2 weeks in the 10 mm rostral section (median = 2). Interestingly at day 3 within the 10 mm caudal section, NAT treated animals had greater SP expression, with a median ranking of 4. Similarly, in the rostral section at 2 weeks, NAT treated animals recorded a higher median ranking of 4 suggesting NAT treatment resulted in greater SP immunoreactivity.

3.5.3. Substance P immunoreactivity - Perivascular region. The perivascular region was assessed within the grey matter of the spinal cord (Figure 5). The injury epicentre could not be examined because of severe tissue disruption. Sham animals demonstrated moderate SP immunoreactivity surrounding the vasculature with a median of 6. At 5 hours post-SCI a slight decrease was observed within both adjacent segments in both treatment groups, with this trend remaining at 24 hours post-SCI. Interestingly in both adjacent segments, by 3 days post-SCI the NAT treated group had returned to sham levels, recording a median ranking of 6. By 2 weeks post-SCI, both treatment groups demonstrated comparable immunoreactivity to sham levels in the rostral segment, though remained below sham levels within the caudal segment. No significant differences were detected between treatment groups at any time post-SCI.

3.5.4. NK1 immunoreactivity - Grey Matter. Sham sections demonstrated diffuse immunoreactivity within the grey matter with greater intensity observed within the dorsal horn resulting in a median ranking of 7 (Figure 6). At 5 and 24 hours post-SCI within the injury epicentre, a significant increase in NK1 receptor immunoreactivity to a median ranking to 9 was observed within the injury epicentre in both treatment groups (vehicle = $p<0.01$, NAT = $p<0.05$–0.01). Such immunoreactivity remained elevated in both treatment groups on day 3 post-SCI. By 24 hours post-SCI, the adjacent segments also demonstrated a slight increase in NK1 expression centrally within the grey matter in both groups. However by day 3, a slight reduction in NK1 immunoreactivity within these segments was observed in both groups (median = 5). By 2 weeks post-SCI, the loss of tissue made it difficult to assess NK1 immunoreactivity in the injury epicentre, whereas NK1 immunoreactivity had further decreased in the adjacent segments of both groups, recording a median ranking of 4 (rostral = $p<0.05$, caudal $p<0.001$).

3.5.5. NK1 immunoreactivity – Perivascular. Sham sections demonstrated faint NK1 receptor immunoreactivity surrounding the vasculature with a median ranking of 4 (Figure 7). Due to severe tissue disruption, NK1 immunoreactivity was not assessed within the injury epicentre. A slight increase in NK1 immunoreactivity was observed within the adjacent segments of both treatment groups at 5 hours post-SCI. Further increases were observed at 24 hours post-SCI within the caudal segment recording a median ranking of 7 for both treatment groups, whilst the rostral segment was only slightly increased to a median ranking of 6. By day 3, NAT treated caudal segments remained at a median of 7, whereas vehicle treated animals had slightly reduced further to 6, although this was still increased compared to shams. Similarly, within the rostral segment NAT treatment resulted in slightly greater immunoreactivity compared to both vehicle and sham, whereas vehicle treated animals had comparable NK1 immunoreactivity to shams. Vehicle treated animals remained at sham levels at 2 weeks post-SCI in both sections, whilst NAT treatment still recorded above sham levels (rostral median = 5; caudal median 6).

3.5.6. Albumin immunoreactivity. Albumin immunoreactivity was assessed to quantify the effect of NAT administration on

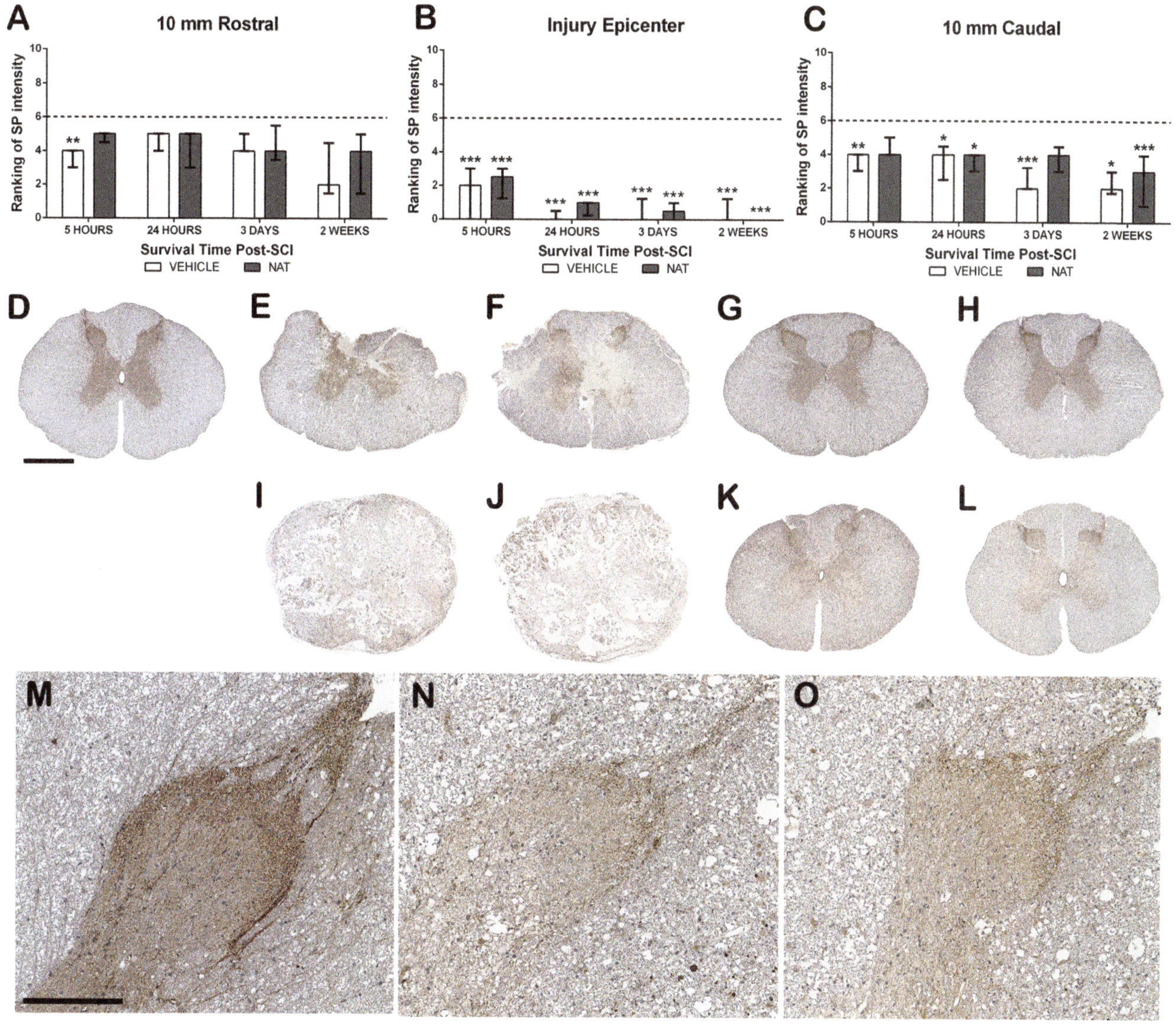

Figure 4. Assessment of the effect of NAT treatment on SP immunoreactivity within the dorsal horn region following SCI. Ranking of SP immunoreactivity within the injury epicentre (B) and at 10 mm rostral (A) and 10 mm caudal (C). Sham sections demonstrated moderate SP immunoreactivity (D). At 5 hours post-SCI reduced immunoreactivity was observed in both vehicle and NAT treatment groups within the injury epicentre (E = Vehicle, F = NAT), whilst a slight reduction was apparent within the adjacent segments (G = Vehicle, H = NAT). However, a significant loss was observed by 2 weeks post-SCI within the injury epicentre (I = Vehicle, J = NAT) and within the adjacent segments (K = Vehicle, L = NAT). Higher magnification images clearly demonstrate this difference (M = sham, N = 2 week Vehicle adjacent, O = 2 week NAT adjacent). Low magnification scale bar = 1 mm, High magnification scale bar = 200 μm. Dashed line (A–C) represents sham median.

the extent of BSCB permeability following SCI (Figure 8). Sham sections of spinal cord demonstrated minimal albumin immunoreactivity with a DABwt% of 4.7±0.42, indicating that sham surgery did not disrupt the BSCB. Following injury, a significant increase in albumin immunoreactivity was observed within the injury epicentre and became maximal at 24 hours post-SCI reaching 24.64±2.77 DABwt% ($p<0.001$). Albumin immunoreactivity then decreased over time, although was still significantly greater than shams at 2 weeks ($p<0.001$). The NAT treated animals had a similar expression of albumin to vehicle treated animals in the injury epicentre, although they recorded significantly greater albumin than vehicle treated animals at day 3 ($p<0.05$). However by 2 weeks, they had decreased below vehicle treated animals but were still had significantly greater albumin than sham ($p<0.05$). Similarly, the adjacent segments demonstrated maximal increases at 24 hours post-SCI for both treatment groups ($p<0.001$), with a decrease over time so that by 2 weeks both groups had returned to sham levels. Moreover, NAT treated animals were comparable to vehicles at all assessment times in the adjacent segments.

3.5.7. Microglial immunoreactivity (ISOB4) - White Matter. Sham sections demonstrated low numbers of resting microglia with long fine processes. After injury, small numbers of microglia were observed within the injury epicentre of both treatment groups (Figure 9A). At 24 hours post-SCI many cells with a small round phenotype suggestive of phagocytic activity can be seen. Furthermore, increased numbers of immunoreactive cells can also be seen within the adjacent segments at this time. At 3 days post-SCI, tissue loss is apparent and further increases in immunoreactive cells are seen within the injury epicentre in both

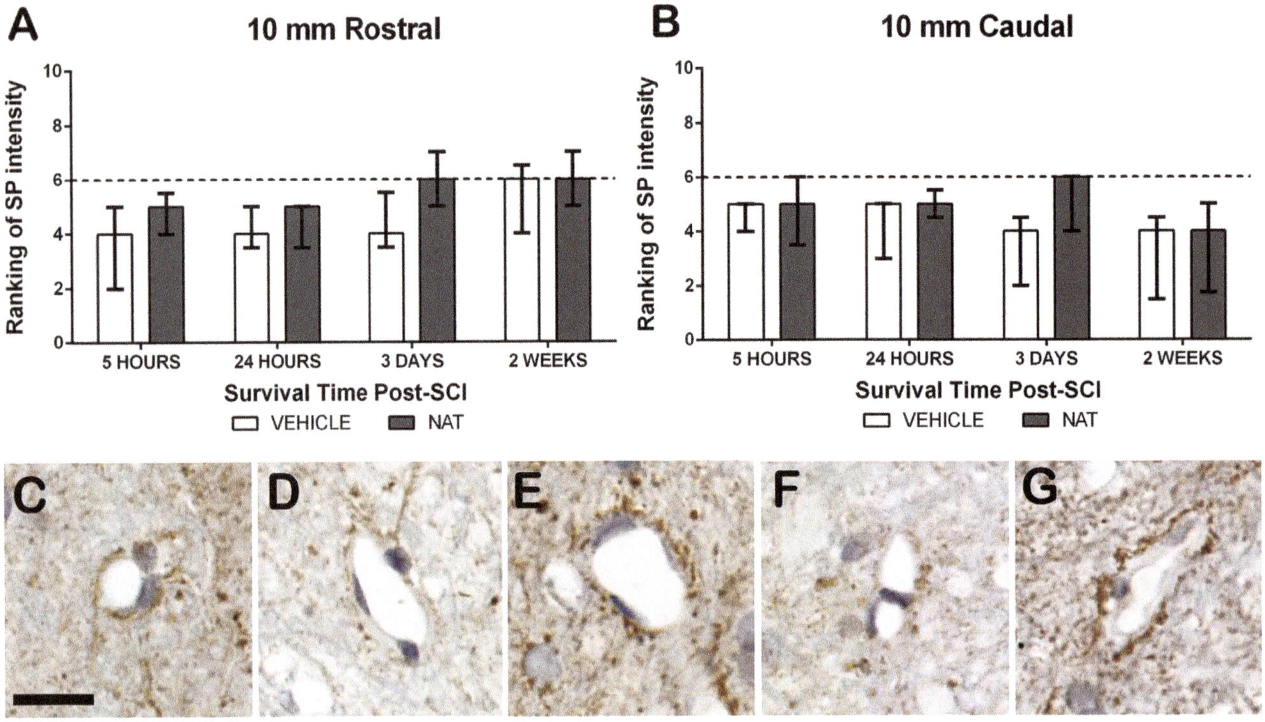

Figure 5. Assessment of the effect of NAT treatment on SP immunoreactivity within the perivascular region following SCI. Ranking of SP immunoreactivity at 10 mm rostral (A) and 10 mm caudal (B) to the injury epicentre. Sham sections demonstrated moderate SP immunoreactivity (C). At both 5 and 24 hours post-SCI a slight decrease was observed within both segments of vehicle and NAT treatment groups. However at 3 days post-SCI NAT treated sections at both 10 mm rostral (E) and caudal (G) demonstrated a return to sham levels whilst vehicle treated remained reduced (D = 10 mm rostral; F = 10 mm caudal). *denotes $p<0.05$, **denotes $p<0.01$, ***denotes $p<0.001$, sham median ranking indicated by the dashed line. Scale bar = 25 μm.

treatment groups. By 2 weeks post-SCI greater tissue loss is apparent and florid microglia are present within the white matter, becoming amoeboid in shape by 2 weeks post-SCI. At this time, the adjacent segments of spinal cord also demonstrate increased microglia immunoreacitivty, with many amoeboid cells apparent within the white matter of both treatment groups. No differences in microglia immunoreactivity were observed between vehicle and NAT treated animals.

3.5.8. Microglial immunoreactivity (ISOB4) - Grey Matter. Sham sections again demonstrate low numbers of resting microglia with fine long processes (Figure 9B). At 5 hours post-SCI, hemorrhage is visible in addition to small round immunoreactive cells, suggestive of phagocytic activity, present within the injury epicentre of both treatment groups. At 24 hours post-SCI florid microglia can be seen within the injury epicentre whilst the adjacent segments also demonstrate increased microglia particularly surrounding the blood vessels within both treatment groups. At 3 days post-SCI greater tissue loss was observed within the injury epicentre with many immunoreactive cells still present, and becoming larger in size. The adjacent segments demonstrated numerous activated microglia that appear ramified in nature. By 2 weeks post-SCI increased tissue loss was observed within the injury epicentre with larger phagocytic cells apparent within both vehicle and NAT treated sections. The adjacent segments similarly demonstrate florid microglial activity with many observed as fully ramified and amoeboid in appearance, representing phagocytic activity. No differences in microglial immunoreactivity between vehicle and NAT treated groups were observed.

3.5.9. AQP4 immunoreactivity - Perivascular region. Sham sections of spinal cord demonstrated faint AQP4 immunoreactivity surrounding the vasculature within the grey matter, assessed as a median ranking of 3 (Figure 10). Due to severe tissue disruption the injury epicentre was not assessed. Following injury increased AQP4 immunoreactivity was observed by 5 hours and reached a median ranking of 6 by 24 hours post-SCI. A slight decrease was observed at 3 days post-SCI in the caudal section, whereas the rostral section still ranked 6. A further decrease to below sham levels was apparent by 2 weeks (rostral = 2; caudal = 1). NAT treatment had a similar pattern of immunoreactivity to vehicle treated animals in the rostral section, apart from on day 3 when they ranked slightly less (median = 4). Within the caudal section, NAT treated animals recorded slightly higher than vehicles at 5 hours, but then decreased over time so that they were less than vehicles at 24 hours but similar at 3 days and 2 weeks.

3.5.10. AQP4 immunoreactivity - Central Canal region. Sham sections of spinal cord demonstrated faint AQP4 immunoreactivity in the ependymal cells of the central canal with a median ranking of 3 (Figure 10). The injury epicentre was too disrupted to accurately assess AQP4 immunoreactivity. Following injury an increase was observed in the rostral section by 5 hours (median = 4.5) with a slightly further rise to 5 at 24 hours and 3 days before returning to sham levels at 2 weeks. In contrast, NAT treated animals had maximal AQP4 immunoreactivity in this section by 5 hours (median = 5), which remained until day 3 when a reduced ranking of 4 was recorded. A further decrease was seen at 2 weeks, although they were still just above shams (median 3.5). Within the caudal section, AQP4 was not increased until 24 hours when a median ranking of 6 was recorded in the vehicle treated animals. AQP4 then declined over time to be near to sham

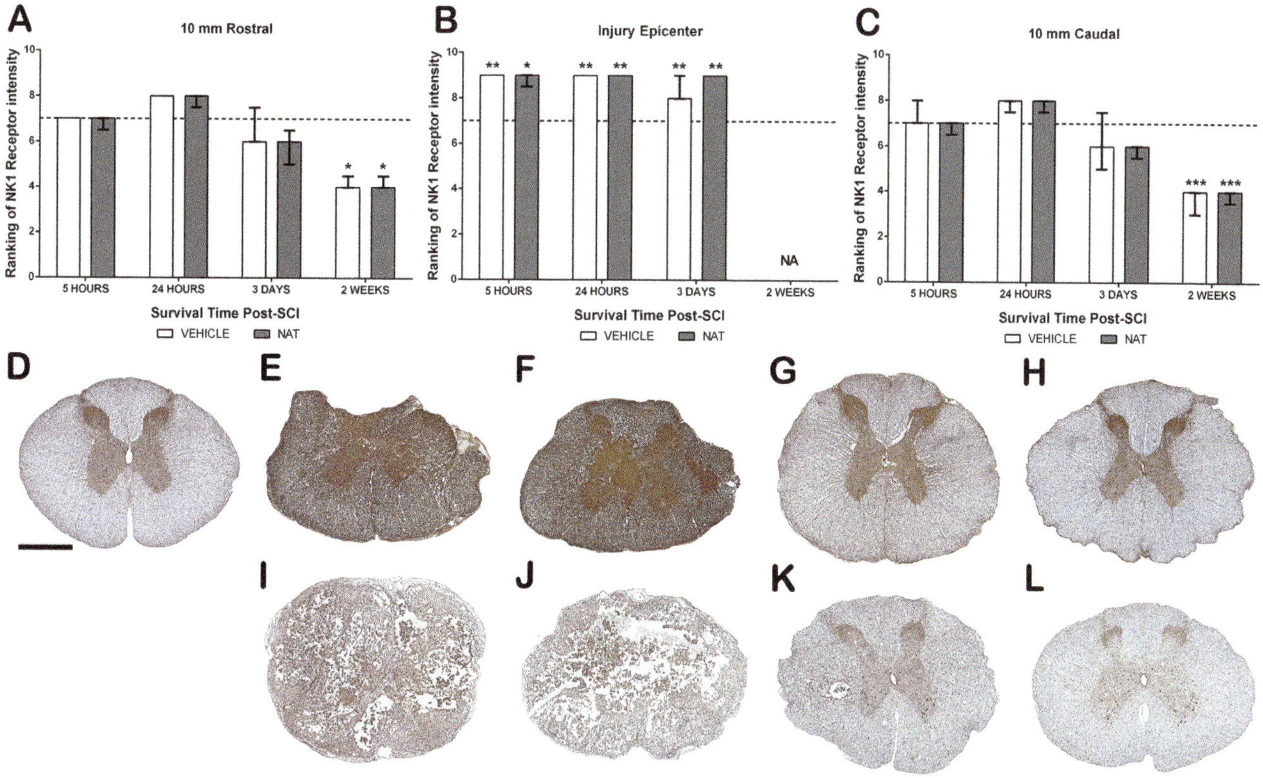

Figure 6. The effect of NAT administration on NK1 receptor immunoreactivity within the grey matter following SCI. Ranking of NK1 receptor immunoreactivity at 10 mm rostral (A), within the injury epicentre (B) and at 10 mm caudal (C). At 24 hours post-SCI a significant increase was observed within the injury epicentre (E= vehicle and F=NAT), whilst adjacent segments demonstrated a slight increase (G= vehicle and H=NAT). By 2 weeks post-SCI tissue loss was too great to assess NK1 immunoreactivity within the injury epicentre (I-vehicle, J-NAT) although adjacent segments had reduced immunoreactivity (K-vehicle, L-NAT). No differences were observed between treatment groups at any time point. *denotes $p<0.05$, **denotes $p<0.01$, ***denotes $p<0.001$, sham median ranking indicated by the dashed line (A,B & C). Scale bar =1 mm.

levels by 2 weeks. In contrast, NAT treatment resulted in a increase in AQP4 by 5 hours recording a median ranking of 5, however then declined to 4 at 24 hours and had returned to sham levels by day 3. No significant differences were observed between treatment groups at any assessment time.

Discussion

The present study has demonstrated that administration of the NK1 receptor antagonist, NAT, does not reduce BSCB permeability, edema, ITP or significantly improve neurological function following SCI. These results suggest that SP mediated neurogenic inflammation does not play a major role in the acute development of such injury processes following traumatic SCI. However, a release of SP was observed, demonstrated by reduced SP immunoreactivity, whilst perivascular NK1 receptor immunoreactivity initially increased before decreasing, which is suggestive of NK1 receptor activation and internalisation. This reflects manifestation of SP mediated neurogenic inflammation, albeit that neurogenic inflammation may not be the predominant driver of these injury processes in the acute phase of SCI.

Although only a bolus dose of NAT was administered on the day of surgery, and for two consecutive days for survival times of 3 days or more, such dosage regimes have previously been used in acute CNS injury with highly beneficial outcomes [13,17,22]. Indeed administration of an NK1 receptor antagonist at 30 minutes post-TBI reduced barrier permeability, edema and improved functional outcome, demonstrating that inhibition of SP effects was possible despite a 30 minute delay post-injury [13,17]. It is unlikely that a shorter timeframe for pharmacological intervention would be clinically relevant. Furthermore, whilst NAT is not barrier permeable, our results demonstrate that the BSCB was disrupted for at least 5 hours post-SCI. Given the severe extent of hemorrhage and destruction of vasculature observed at the site of impact, intravenous administration may have not provided sufficient delivery of NAT. Nonetheless, some differences between vehicle and NAT treated groups were observed in the current study beyond the injury site, indicating that NAT administration was likely successfully delivered centrally. A more direct route of administration, such as an injection into the intrathecal space may provide a more efficient method of administration for future investigations. Given the highly preserved nature of NK1 receptors across different vertebrate species [30], it is unlikely that any lack of effectiveness of NAT treatment was due to low affinity for the rabbit NK1 receptor.

Whilst two isoforms of the NK1 receptor exist, a long complete isoform and a truncated isoform, the binding site of the antagonist is identical in both, and thus the NK1 receptor antagonist used in the current study would be equally effective on both isoforms. However, the long NK1 isoform is known to predominate within the CNS whilst the truncated isoform is most represented within peripheral tissue [31]. Additionally, consideration must be given to related tachykinin receptors, the NK2 receptor and NK3 receptor. Our results do not exclude the possibility that the NK2 or NK3 receptors might play an important role and that inhibition of these receptors may be beneficial to outcome after SCI. However, SP

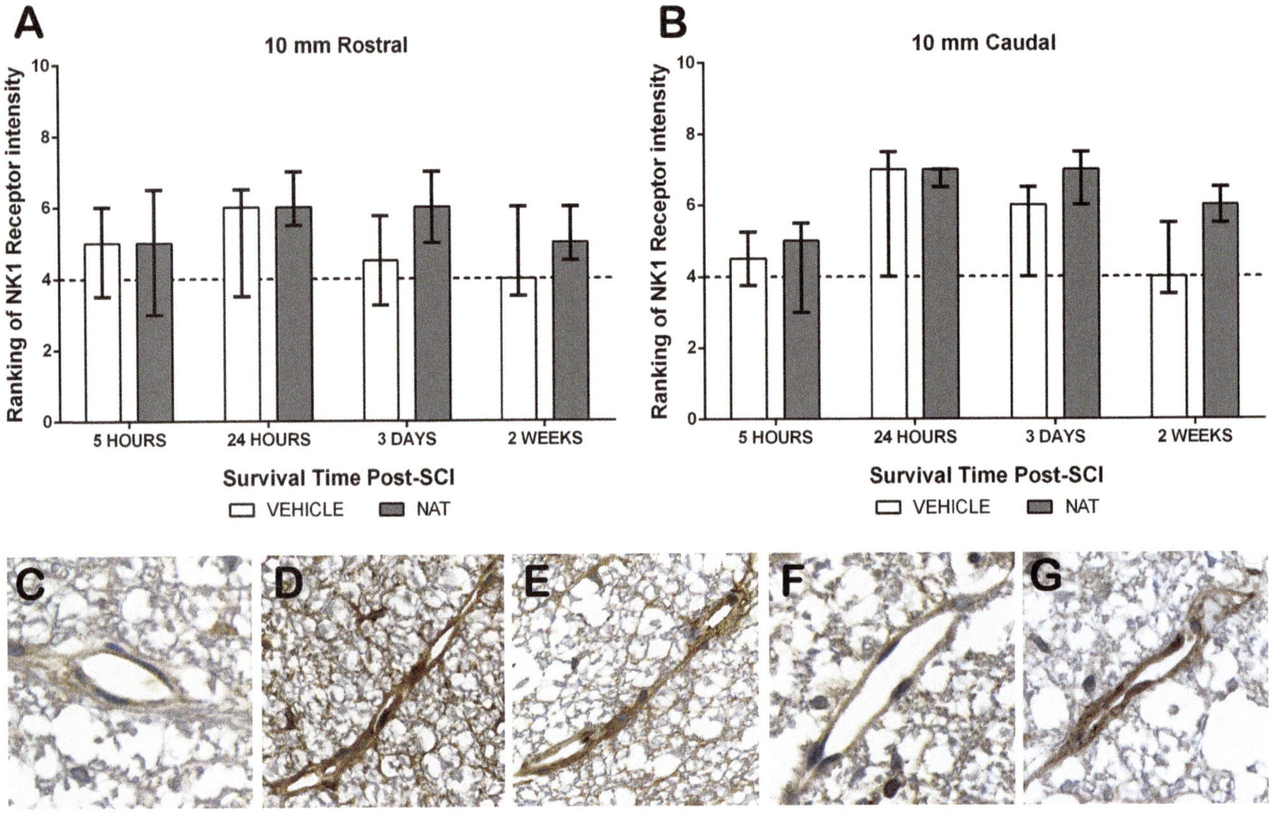

Figure 7. The effect of NAT administration on NK1 receptor immunoreactivity within the perivascular region following SCI. NK1 receptor immunoreactivity ranking at 10 mm rostral (A) and caudal (B). Sham sections demonstrated faint immunoreactivity surrounding the vasculature (C). Notably, at 24 hours post-SCI a marked increase was observed in both vehicle (D) and NAT (E) treatment groups. By 2 weeks post-SCI at 10 mm caudal vehicle treated (F) returned to sham levels, whilst NAT treated remained elevated (G). Median sham ranking indicated by the dashed line (A&B).

binds preferentially to the NK1 receptor [32], and it is only activation of this receptor that is thought to result in the initiation of neurogenic inflammation. Indeed, It has been demonstrated that the NK2 and NK3 receptors have no direct role in plasma protein extravasation within the CNS [33].

After receiving 3 consecutive daily doses of NAT or saline, NAT treated animals demonstrated a trend for greater perivascular and dorsal horn SP immunoreactivity than vehicle treated animals. Such increases in SP may be explained by the presence of an NK1 autoreceptor, which is thought to regulate SP release through a negative feedback loop [34,35]. In the current study, blockade of the NK1 autoreceptor due to NAT administration would prevent SP from exerting negative feedback on its own synthesis and release, resulting in greater expression of SP. However, the comparative increase in SP would not have been functional, as blockade of the NK1 receptor with NAT prevents SP from binding and mediating downstream effects.

Interestingly, at 3 days post-injury NAT treatment resulted in significantly higher BSCB permeability compared to vehicle as assessed by albumin. This finding paradoxically implies that inhibition of the NK1 receptor resulted in greater BSCB permeability. Such results are in contrast to previous studies where NAT treatment resulted in reduced BSCB permeability following TBI and stroke [13,22]. These findings imply that despite similar secondary injury processes arising following SCI, the role of SP may be vastly different in SCI than its role in other acute CNS injuries. One important difference may be the extent of primary mechanical damage, resulting in severe hemorrhage. Previous studies within our group have demonstrated that in severe subarachnoid hemorrhage, NAT administration worsened outcome [36]. These combined results suggest that in models of severe hemorrhage, the primary induced tissue and vasculature damage may dominate over SP mediated neurogenic inflammation in the development of BSCB permeability. Furthermore, as the current study provided evidence that NAT treatment worsened BSCB permeability, SP may actually play a protective role in such severe hemorrhage models. Indeed, a recent study demonstrated that SP treatment promoted a more anti-inflammatory environment following SCI by inducing interlukin-10 and M2 macrophages whilst suppressing nitric oxide synthase and tumour necrosis factor-α [37]. Our own results demonstrate an increase in microglial activity following SCI, though predominantly phagocytic in nature, with no differences between treatment groups. In addition, intrathecal administration of a SP antagonist has been shown to cause a marked decrease in spinal cord blood flow (SCBF) [38] and likely contributed to further damage and BSCB permeability by promoting an ischemic environment. These findings together with the current study suggest that SP may be beneficial following acute SCI.

Regardless of the role of SP following SCI, edema remains a serious complication leading to raised ITP [39,40], reduced SCBF [9,40] and myelin damage [1]. Indeed, numerous studies have shown that the extent of edema corresponds to the degree of functional deficits observed following injury [41,42,43,44,45]. The

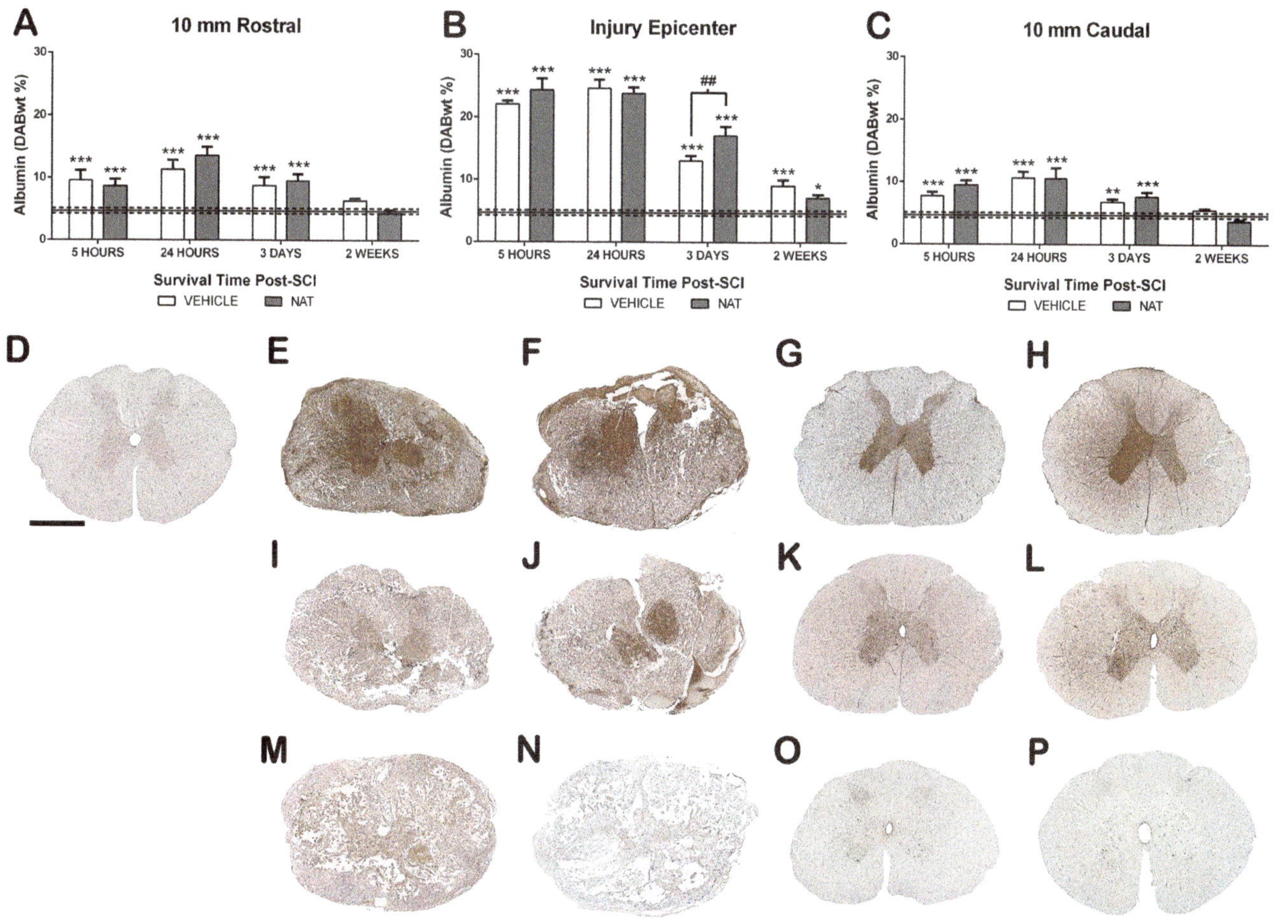

Figure 8. The effect of NAT treatment on albumin immunoreactivity following SCI. Albumin immunoreactivity at 10 mm rostral (A), within the injury epicentre (B) and at 10 mm caudal (C). Sham sections (D) demonstrated minimal immunoreactivity. Immunoreactivity was significantly increased at both 5 and 24 hours post-SCI. Representative images at 24 hours are shown within the injury epicentre (E-vehicle, F-NAT) and adjacent segment (G-vehicle, H-NAT). By 3 days post-SCI albumin immunoreactivity began to reduce within the injury epicentre (I-vehicle, J-NAT) and adjacent segment (K-vehicle, L-NAT), though NAT treatment resulted in significantly greater albumin immunoreactivity when compared to vehicle. Albumin immunoreactivity reduced further by 2 weeks post-SCI within the injury epicentre (M-vehicle, N-NAT), returning to sham levels within the adjacent segments (O-vehicle, P-NAT). *denotes $p<0.05$, **denotes $p<0.01$, ***denotes $p<0.001$ when compared to sham. Mean sham values indicated by the dashed line. Scale bar = 1 mm.

present study demonstrated increased edema associated with raised ITP following injury, which was maximal at 3 days post-SCI. Furthermore, at this time it was apparent that the adjacent segments, uninjured by the balloon compression, also demonstrated significant increases in edema. Therefore, substantial rostrocaudal spread of edema had occurred following the balloon compression model by 3 days post-SCI. However, albumin immunoreactivity, a marker of BSCB permeability, was maximal at 24 hours post-SCI with a reduction observed at 3 days post-SCI within the adjacent segments. Therefore, significant disparity exists between BSCB permeability and edema formation, indicating that the rostrocaudal spread of edema was not due to BSCB disruption and thus not vasogenic in nature. These results further suggest that neurogenic inflammation is not primarily responsible for the developed edema and may account for the ineffectiveness of NAT administration to reduce edema.

It is possible that the spread of edema may be a compensatory mechanism to reduce the edema present within the injury epicentre. Alternatively, the BSCB may in fact still remain permeable to smaller molecules than albumin. Previous studies have employed alternative smaller tracers of extravasation such as hydrazide [46], horseradish peroxidase [10,47,48], protein luciferase [49], and iodine [4,50] and found greater extension of BSCB permeability. Alternatively, such increases in edema may be due to an ultrafiltration mechanism rather than extravasation as previously described by Nemecek and colleagues [7]. Such ultrafiltration may be aided by reduced blood flow and severe hemorrhage. As NAT treatment has no ability to reduce hemorhage and SP antagonists can markedly reduce SCBF [38], the greater edema within the adjacent segments of NAT treated animals may be due to increased ultrafiltration. Alternatively, in the absence of BSCB disruption, the increased edema may be facilitated by AQP4 water channels.

Indeed, within the current study, AQP4 immunoreactivity was increased following injury at similar times to maximal edema. Although such an increase implies that AQP4 may facilitate edema development, NAT administration resulted in a slight increase in edema and a concurrent reduction in AQP4 immunoreactivity. Therefore, injury induced increases in AQP4 may actually be a compensatory mechanism to assist in fluid clearance. These changes in AQP4 and edema formation contrast to that in TBI, where injury reduced AQP4 expression and NAT

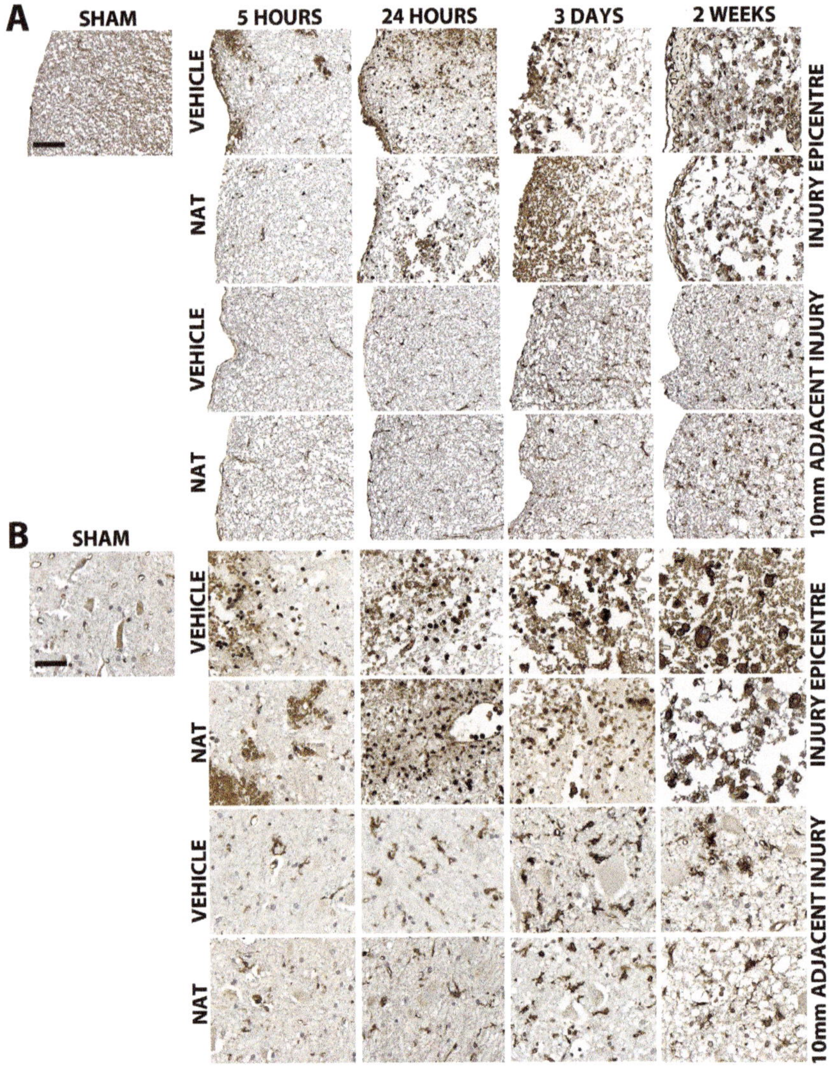

Figure 9. The effect of NAT administration on microglial immunoreactivity following SCI within the white matter (A) and grey matter (B). Sham sections demonstrate minimal microglial immunoreactivity in both the white and grey matter. Within the white matter microglia immunoreactivity is maximal by 2 weeks post-SCI within the injury epicentre and adjacent segment for both treatment groups. Within the grey matter, many small round microglia can be seen within the injury epicentre, increasing in size by 2 weeks post-SCI. Within the adjacent segment of the grey matter many ramified microglia can be seen by 3 days post-SCI and becoming amoeboid in shape by 2 week post-SCI. No differences between treatment groups were observed. Scale bar (A) = 200 µm, (B) = 50 µm.

treatment restored AQP4 levels, whilst reducing edema [28]. These opposing effects of NAT treatment in TBI and SCI further illustrate the differences in their injury mechanisms. Moreover, these results demonstrate that the relationship between SP and AQP4 warrants further investigation. Taken together, these results demonstrate that AQP4 may play an essential role in the elimination of excess fluid. Indeed, previous investigations have similarly demonstrated that AQP4 plays an integral role in facilitating water clearance following SCI [2,51,52]. However, to date, almost all studies of AQP4 following SCI have assessed its function through altered expression [2,51], or employed AQP4-null mice [12,52]. As such, further investigation to fully elucidate the role of AQP4 following SCI is required. Ideally, this could be through the pharmacological modulation of the AQP4 water channels, which may then be utilized as a novel therapeutic intervention.

Conclusions

The current study has demonstrated that despite a release of SP and therefore induction of SP mediated neurogenic inflammation, the severe primary damage that results in destruction of vasculature and hemorrhage may play a greater role in BSCB disruption, subsequent edema development and associated tissue damage and functional deficits following traumatic SCI. Thus, administration of the NK1 receptor antagonist, NAT, did not reduce BSCB permeability, edema, ITP, or improve neurological function following SCI. In contrast, SP may actually play a beneficial role in reducing this ongoing damage associated with traumatic SCI.

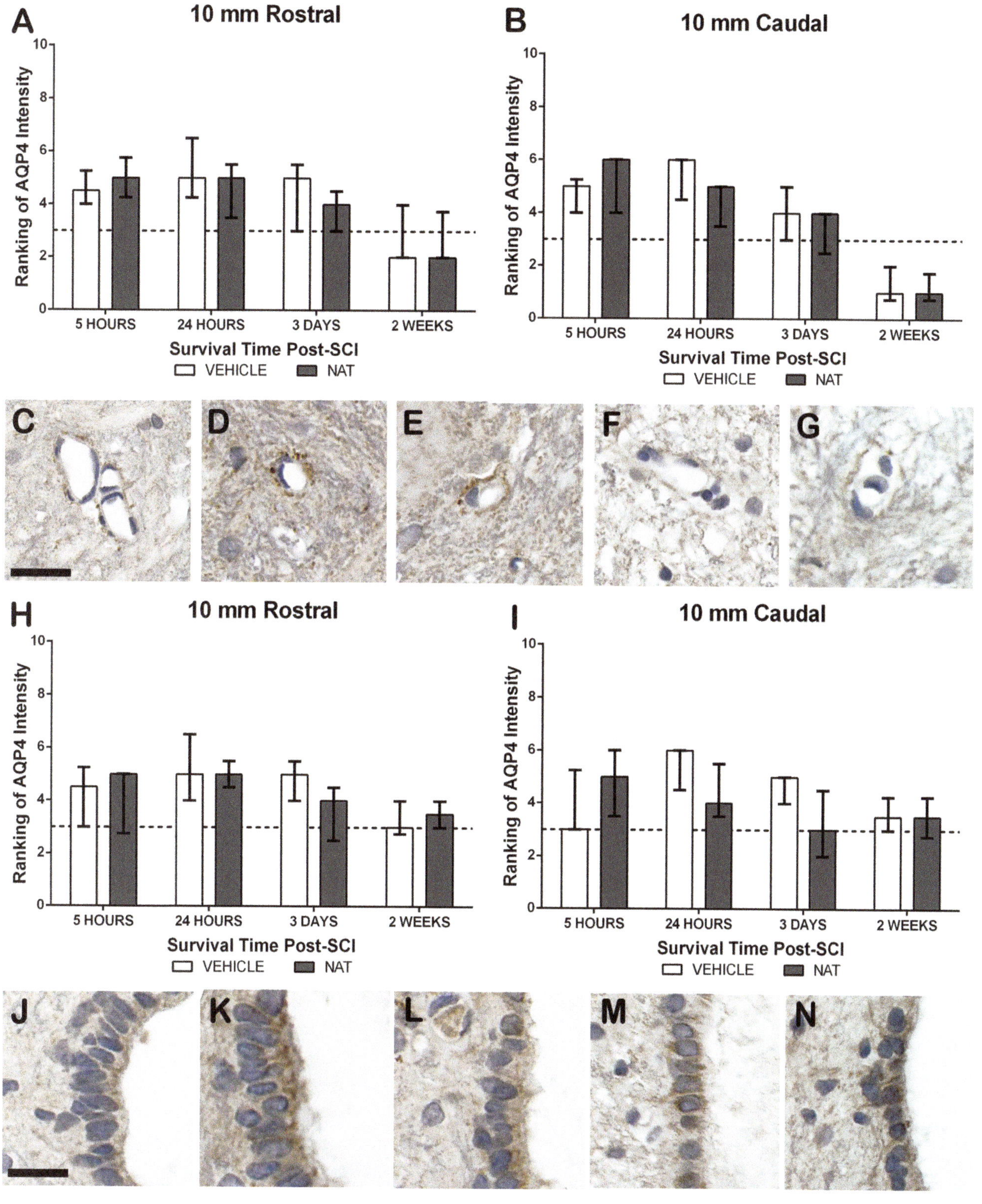

Figure 10. The effect of NAT administration on perivascular and ependymal AQP4 immunoreactivity following SCI. Ranking of perivascular AQP4 immunoreactivity at 10 mm rostral (A) and 10 mm caudal (B). Sham sections demonstrated faint immunoreactivity surrounding the vessels (C). Increased immunoreactivity can be seen at 24 hours following both vehicle (D) and NAT (E) treatment. Reduced immunoreacticity below sham levels was observed at 2 weeks (H-vehicle, I-NAT). Dashed line indicated mean sham values. Ranking of ependymal AQP4 immunoreactivity at 10 mm rostral (H) and 10 mm caudal (I). Sham sections demonstrated faint immunoreactivity within the ependymal cells of the central canal (J). At 24 hours post-SCI increases were apparent, with greater increases in the caudal segments of vehicle treated sections (K) than NAT treated (L). By 2 weeks post-SCI both treatment groups demonstrated comparable AQP4 immunoreactivity to sham levels (M-vehicle, N-NAT). Scale bars = 25 μm.

Author Contributions

Conceived and designed the experiments: AVL ET RV. Performed the experiments: AVL. Analyzed the data: AVL ET RV. Contributed to the writing of the manuscript: AVL ET RV.

References

1. Sharma HS (2005) Pathophysiology of blood-spinal cord barrier in traumatic injury and repair. Curr Pharm Des 11: 1353–1389.
2. Nesic O, Lee J, Ye Z, Unabia GC, Rafati D, et al. (2006) Acute and chronic changes in aquaporin 4 expression after spinal cord injury. Neuroscience 143: 779–792.
3. Sharma HS, Winkler T, Stalberg E, Olsson Y, Dey PK (1991) Evaluation of traumatic spinal cord edema using evoked potentials recorded from the spinal epidural space. An experimental study in the rat. J Neurol Sci 102: 150–162.
4. Sharma HS, Olsson Y, Nyberg F, Dey PK (1993) Prostaglandins modulate alterations of microvascular permeability, blood flow, edema and serotonin levels following spinal cord injury: an experimental study in the rat. Neuroscience 57: 443–449.
5. Winkler T, Sharma HS, Stalberg E, Olsson Y, Nyberg F (1994) Opioid receptors influence spinal cord electrical activity and edema formation following spinal cord injury: experimental observations using naloxone in the rat. Neurosci Res 21: 91–101.
6. Ates O, Cayli SR, Gurses I, Turkoz Y, Tarim O, et al. (2007) Comparative neuroprotective effect of sodium channel blockers after experimental spinal cord injury. J Clin Neurosci 14: 658–665.
7. Nemecek S, Petr R, Suba P, Rozsival V, Melka O (1977) Longitudinal extension of oedema in experimental spinal cord injury–evidence for two types of post-traumatic oedema. Acta Neurochir (Wien) 37: 7–16.
8. Demediuk P, Lemke M, Faden AI (1990) Spinal cord edema and changes in tissue content of Na+, K+, and Mg2+ after impact trauma in rats. Adv Neurol 52: 225–232.
9. Wang R, Ehara K, Tamaki N (1993) Spinal cord edema following freezing injury in the rat: relationship between tissue water content and spinal cord blood flow. Surg Neurol 39: 348–354.
10. Noble LJ, Wrathall JR (1989) Distribution and time course of protein extravasation in the rat spinal cord after contusive injury. Brain Res 482: 57–66.
11. Goodman JH, Bingham WG Jr, Hunt WE (1976) Ultrastructural blood-brain barrier alterations and edema formation in acute spinal cord trauma. J Neurosurg 44: 418–424.
12. Saadoun S, Bell BA, Verkman AS, Papadopoulos MC (2008) Greatly improved neurological outcome after spinal cord compression injury in AQP4-deficient mice. Brain 131: 1087–1098.
13. Donkin JJ, Nimmo AJ, Cernak I, Blumbergs PC, Vink R (2009) Substance P is associated with the development of brain edema and functional deficits after traumatic brain injury. J Cereb Blood Flow Metab.
14. Vink R, Young A, Bennett CJ, Hu X, Connor CO, et al. (2003) Neuropeptide release influences brain edema formation after diffuse traumatic brain injury. Acta Neurochir Suppl 86: 257–260.
15. Nimmo AJ, Cernak I, Heath DL, Hu X, Bennett CJ, et al. (2004) Neurogenic inflammation is associated with development of edema and functional deficits following traumatic brain injury in rats. Neuropeptides 38: 40–47.
16. Turner RJ, Blumbergs PC, Sims NR, Helps SC, Rodgers KM, et al. (2006) Increased substance P immunoreactivity and edema formation following reversible ischemic stroke. Acta Neurochir Suppl 96: 263–266.
17. Corrigan F, Leonard A, Ghabriel M, Van Den Heuvel C, Vink R (2012) A substance P antagonist improves outcome in female Sprague Dawley rats following diffuse traumatic brain injury. CNS Neurosci Ther 18: 513–515.
18. Harford-Wright E, Thornton E, Vink R (2010) Angiotensin-converting enzyme (ACE) inhibitors exacerbate histological damage and motor deficits after experimental traumatic brain injury. Neurosci Lett 481: 26–29.
19. Thornton E, Vink R (2012) Treatment with a substance P receptor antagonist is neuroprotective in the intrastriatal 6-hydroxydopamine model of early Parkinson's disease. PLoS One 7: e34138.
20. Leonard AV, Thornton E, Vink R (2013) Substance P as a mediator of neurogenic inflammation following balloon compression induced spinal cord injury. J Neurotrauma.
21. Thornton E, Ziebell JM, Leonard AV, Vink R (2010) Kinin receptor antagonists as potential neuroprotective agents in central nervous system injury. Molecules 15: 6598–6618.
22. Turner RJ, Helps SC, Thornton E, Vink R (2011) A substance P antagonist improves outcome when administered 4 h after onset of ischaemic stroke. Brain Res 1393: 84–90.
23. Tarlov IM, Klinger H (1954) Spinal cord compression studies. II. Time limits for recovery after acute compression in dogs. AMA Arch Neurol Psychiatry 71: 271–290.
24. Tarlov IM, Klinger H, Vitale S (1953) Spinal cord compression studies. I. Experimental techniques to produce acute and gradual compression. AMA Arch Neurol Psychiatry 70: 813–819.
25. Fukuda S, Nakamura T, Kishigami Y, Endo K, Azuma T, et al. (2005) New canine spinal cord injury model free from laminectomy. Brain Res Brain Res Protoc 14: 171–180.
26. Martin D, Schoenen J, Delree P, Gilson V, Rogister B, et al. (1992) Experimental acute traumatic injury of the adult rat spinal cord by a subdural inflatable balloon: methodology, behavioral analysis, and histopathology. J Neurosci Res 32: 539–550.
27. Vanicky I, Urdzikova L, Saganova K, Cizkova D, Galik J (2001) A simple and reproducible model of spinal cord injury induced by epidural balloon inflation in the rat. J Neurotrauma 18: 1399–1407.
28. Donkin J (2006) The effects of the neuropeptide Substance P on outcome following experimental brain injury in rats. Adelaide: University of Adelaide.
29. Helps SC, Thornton E, Kleinig TJ, Manavis J, Vink R (2012) Automatic nonsubjective estimation of antigen content visualized by immunohistochemistry using color deconvolution. Appl Immunohistochem Mol Morphol 20: 82–90.
30. Dietl MM, Palacios JM (1991) Phylogeny of tachykinin receptor localization in the vertebrate central nervous system: apparent absence of neurokinin-2 and neurokinin-3 binding sites in the human brain. Brain Res 539: 211–222.
31. Caberlotto L, Hurd YL, Murdock P, Wahlin JP, Melotto S, et al. (2003) Neurokinin 1 receptor and relative abundance of the short and long isoforms in the human brain. Eur J Neurosci 17: 1736–1746.
32. Harrison S, Geppetti P (2001) Substance p. Int J Biochem Cell Biol 33: 555–576.
33. O'Shaughnessy CT, Connor HE (1993) Neurokinin NK1 receptors mediate plasma protein extravasation in guinea-pig dura. Eur J Pharmacol 236: 319–321.
34. Malcangio M, Bowery NG (1994) Effect of the tachykinin NK1 receptor antagonists, RP 67580 and SR 140333, on electrically-evoked substance P release from rat spinal cord. Br J Pharmacol 113: 635–641.
35. Lever IJ, Grant AD, Pezet S, Gerard NP, Brain SD, et al. (2003) Basal and activity-induced release of substance P from primary afferent fibres in NK1 receptor knockout mice: evidence for negative feedback. Neuropharmacology 45: 1101–1110.
36. Barry CM, Helps SC, den Heuvel C, Vink R (2011) Characterizing the role of the neuropeptide substance P in experimental subarachnoid hemorrhage. Brain Res 1389: 143–151.
37. Jiang MH, Chung E, Chi GF, Ahn W, Lim JE, et al. (2012) Substance P induces M2-type macrophages after spinal cord injury. Neuroreport 23: 786–792.
38. Freedman J, Post C, Kahrstrom J, Ohlen A, Mollenholt P, et al. (1988) Vasoconstrictor effects in spinal cord of the substance P antagonist [D-Arg, D-Trp7,9 Leu11]-substance P (Spantide) and somatostatin and interaction with thyrotropin releasing hormone. Neuroscience 27: 267–278.
39. Yashon D, Bingham WG, Jr., Faddoul EM, Hunt WE (1973) Edema of the spinal cord following experimental impact trauma. J Neurosurg 38: 693–697.
40. Kwon BK, Curt A, Belanger LM, Bernardo A, Chan D, et al. (2009) Intrathecal pressure monitoring and cerebrospinal fluid drainage in acute spinal cord injury: a prospective randomized trial. J Neurosurg Spine 10: 181–193.
41. Flanders AE, Spettell CM, Friedman DP, Marino RJ, Herbison GJ (1999) The relationship between the functional abilities of patients with cervical spinal cord injury and the severity of damage revealed by MR imaging. AJNR Am J Neuroradiol 20: 926–934.
42. Leypold BG, Flanders AE, Burns AS (2008) The early evolution of spinal cord lesions on MR imaging following traumatic spinal cord injury. AJNR Am J Neuroradiol 29: 1012–1016.
43. Bozzo A, Marcoux J, Radhakrishna M, Pelletier J, Goulet B (2011) The role of magnetic resonance imaging in the management of acute spinal cord injury. J Neurotrauma 28: 1401–1411.
44. Koyanagi I, Iwasaki Y, Isu T, Akino M, Abe H (1989) Significance of spinal cord swelling in the prognosis of acute cervical spinal cord injury. Paraplegia 27: 190–197.
45. Shepard MJ, Bracken MB (1999) Magnetic resonance imaging and neurological recovery in acute spinal cord injury: observations from the National Acute Spinal Cord Injury Study 3. Spinal Cord 37: 833–837.
46. Maikos JT, Shreiber DI (2007) Immediate damage to the blood-spinal cord barrier due to mechanical trauma. J Neurotrauma 24: 492–507.
47. Noble LJ, Wrathall JR (1987) The blood-spinal cord barrier after injury: pattern of vascular events proximal and distal to a transection in the rat. Brain Res 424: 177–188.
48. Jaeger CB, Blight AR (1997) Spinal cord compression injury in guinea pigs: structural changes of endothelium and its perivascular cell associations after blood-brain barrier breakdown and repair. Exp Neurol 144: 381–399.
49. Whetstone WD, Hsu JY, Eisenberg M, Werb Z, Noble-Haeusslein LJ (2003) Blood-spinal cord barrier after spinal cord injury: relation to revascularization and wound healing. J Neurosci Res 74: 227–239.

50. Nyberg F, Sharma HS (2002) Repeated topical application of growth hormone attenuates blood-spinal cord barrier permeability and edema formation following spinal cord injury: an experimental study in the rat using Evans blue, ([125])I-sodium and lanthanum tracers. Amino Acids 23: 231–239.
51. Mao L, Wang HD, Pan H, Qiao L (2011) Sulphoraphane enhances aquaporin-4 expression and decreases spinal cord oedema following spinal cord injury. Brain Inj 25: 300–306.
52. Kimura A, Hsu M, Seldin M, Verkman AS, Scharfman HE, et al. (2010) Protective role of aquaporin-4 water channels after contusion spinal cord injury. Ann Neurol 67: 794–801.

12

Thoracic Rat Spinal Cord Contusion Injury Induces Remote Spinal Gliogenesis but Not Neurogenesis or Gliogenesis in the Brain

Steffen Franz[1¶], Mareva Ciatipis[1¶], Kathrin Pfeifer[2], Birthe Kierdorf[2], Beatrice Sandner[1], Ulrich Bogdahn[2], Armin Blesch[1], Beate Winner[3], Norbert Weidner[1*]

1 Spinal Cord Injury Center, Heidelberg University Hospital, Heidelberg, Germany, **2** Department of Neurology, University of Regensburg, Regensburg, Germany, **3** IZKF Junior Group III and BMBF Research Group Neuroscience, Interdisciplinary Center for Clinical Research, Nikolaus-Fiebiger Center for Molecular Medicine, Friedrich-Alexander University-Erlangen-Nürnberg, Erlangen, Germany

Abstract

After spinal cord injury, transected axons fail to regenerate, yet significant, spontaneous functional improvement can be observed over time. Distinct central nervous system regions retain the capacity to generate new neurons and glia from an endogenous pool of progenitor cells and to compensate neural cell loss following certain lesions. The aim of the present study was to investigate whether endogenous cell replacement (neurogenesis or gliogenesis) in the brain (subventricular zone, SVZ; corpus callosum, CC; hippocampus, HC; and motor cortex, MC) or cervical spinal cord might represent a structural correlate for spontaneous locomotor recovery after a thoracic spinal cord injury. Adult Fischer 344 rats received severe contusion injuries (200 kDyn) of the mid-thoracic spinal cord using an Infinite Horizon Impactor. Uninjured rats served as controls. From 4 to 14 days post-injury, both groups received injections of bromodeoxyuridine (BrdU) to label dividing cells. Over the course of six weeks post-injury, spontaneous recovery of locomotor function occurred. Survival of newly generated cells was unaltered in the SVZ, HC, CC, and the MC. Neurogenesis, as determined by identification and quantification of doublecortin immunoreactive neuroblasts or BrdU/neuronal nuclear antigen double positive newly generated neurons, was not present in non-neurogenic regions (MC, CC, and cervical spinal cord) and unaltered in neurogenic regions (dentate gyrus and SVZ) of the brain. The lack of neuronal replacement in the brain and spinal cord after spinal cord injury precludes any relevance for spontaneous recovery of locomotor function. Gliogenesis was increased in the cervical spinal cord remote from the injury site, however, is unlikely to contribute to functional improvement.

Editor: Simone Di Giovanni, Hertie Institute for Clinical Brain Research, University of Tuebingen, Germany

Funding: Additional financial support came from the German Federal Ministry of Education and Research (BMBF, 01GQ113), the Bavarian Ministry of Education and Culture, Sciences and the Arts in the framework of the Bavarian Molecular Biosystems Research Network, and the Interdisciplinary Center for Clinical Research (University Hospital of Erlangen). The authors acknowledge financial support by "Deutsche Forschungsgemeinschaft and Ruprecht-Karls-Universität Heidelberg" within the funding program Open Access Publishing. The funders had no role in study design, data collection and analysis, decision to publish, or preparation of the manuscript.

* Email: norbert.weidner@med.uni-heidelberg.de

¶ These authors contributed equally to this work.

Introduction

Spinal cord injury (SCI) with complete axonal transection precludes any degree of sensorimotor or autonomous functional recovery [1,2]. In contrast, neurological and consecutively functional recovery is consistently observed in individuals with incomplete SCI, reflected by conversion in the American Spinal Injury Association Impairment Scale and by gains in respective functional assessments, such as the Spinal Cord Independence Measure and the Walking Index for Spinal Cord Injury [3–5]. The observed recovery should not be called "spontaneous", since patients with SCI undergo intense rehabilitation programs intended to promote functional recovery.

The exact structural correlates contributing to functional improvement in incomplete SCI have yet to be determined. It has been shown that axonal sprouting and synaptic rearrangements above and below the injury site in rodent and primate models contribute to recovery of function [6–10]. Whether intrinsic neural cell replacement remote from the injury site underlies the recovery process, at least in part, is yet unknown.

Adult neurogenesis - the generation of new neurons in the adult brain - represents a continuously occurring process in the dentate gyrus of the hippocampus (HC) and in the subventricular zone (SVZ), the latter of which demonstrates subsequent migration and neuronal differentiation in the olfactory bulb in animals and humans [11–13]. Several studies have documented the generation [14,15] and integration of newborn neurons into complex neuronal networks in neurogenic regions of the rodent and primate central nervous system (CNS) [16–18]. Neurons undergoing apoptotic cell death in the motor cortex (MC) following a highly selective cortical lesion appear to be replaced by newborn neurons, some with the capacity to extend axons as far as the cervical spinal cord in adult mice [17]. If remote neuronal cell death is a significant consequence of SCI, as previously indicated [19], neuronal replacement, as described in a proof of concept study [17], could contribute to spontaneous recovery observed in incomplete SCI.

In the injured adult spinal cord, neuronal and glial cell death occurs in the vicinity of and remote from the lesion site [20]. However, in the intact or injured adult spinal cord, cell replacement has only been described for glial cells, whereas neurogenesis has not been convincingly demonstrated and seems unlikely [21–29]. For spontaneous recovery after SCI, glial replacement might play a role in the context of oligodendroglial turnover and remyelination of axons, which survive to some degree even in clinically complete SCI subjects [30]. In spinal cord regions remote from the injury site, the relevance of glial cell replacement for spontaneous functional recovery has yet to be demonstrated.

In the present study, we hypothesized that spontaneous functional recovery observed in spinal cord contused adult rats is linked to relevant neuronal or glial cell replacement in cortical, subcortical, or spinal regions. To address this question, adult female rats underwent thoracic spinal cord contusions followed by intraperitoneal bromodeoxyuridine (BrdU) injections in order to visualize newborn cells. Animals were assessed in terms of locomotor function over 6 weeks after SCI. Thereafter, newly generated cells and their differentiation patterns were assessed in the MC, SVZ, corpus callosum (CC), HC, and cervical spinal cord.

Materials and Methods

Ethics Statement

Experiments were carried out in accordance with the European Communities Council Directive (86/609/EEC) and institutional guidelines. The animal protocol was approved by the District Government of Upper Palatinate (Permit Number: 54-2531.1-33/05). All surgical procedures were performed using a cocktail of ketamine, xylazine, and acepromazine, as defined below. All efforts were made to minimize discomfort.

Animal Subjects and Experimental Groups

Twenty female adult Fischer 344 rats (Charles River Germany GmbH, Sulzfeld, Germany) weighing between 160 and 180 g were used. All animals were housed in groups of 5 on a 12-h light/dark cycle with access to food and water *ad libitum*. For experimental purposes, the animals were separated into two groups (injured and control group), 10 animals each. All animals of the injured group received a spinal contusion, as described below. Animals of the control group did not undergo any surgical intervention.

Surgical Procedures and BrdU injections

Rats were deeply anesthetized by intramuscular injection of ketamine (62.5 mg/kg; 100 mg/l; WDT, Garbsen, Germany), xylazine (3.125 mg/kg; 20 mg/ml; Serumwerk Bernburg AG, Germany), and acepromazine (0.625 mg/kg; 13.56 mg/ml; Sanofi-Ceva, Düsseldorf, Germany). Animals received a laminectomy at Th10. Following fixation of the adjacent Th9 and Th11 vertebral body to suspend the target region, a standardized thoracic spinal contusion (200 kDyn) was applied using an Infinite Horizon Impactor (Precision Systems & Instrumentation, Lexington, KY, USA), as described [31,32]. Following the injury, muscle layers were sutured and the skin was closed. Post-interventional care included manual voiding of the bladder twice a day for the first 10 days, subcutaneous injections of cotrimoxazole (10 mg/kg; Ratiopharm, Ulm, Germany) to avoid bladder infections, and administration of analgesics (buprenorphine; 0.03 mg/kg max. twice a day) as needed. From day 4 to day 14, animals of both experimental groups received daily intraperitoneal injections of BrdU (50 mg/kg KG; 10 mg/ml in 0.9% saline). The prolonged period of BrdU injections was chosen to follow the fate of dividing cells in non-neurogenic regions, where a very limited number of cells undergoing neuronal differentiation was expected.

Functional Testing

Locomotor function was assessed by two observers independently using the modified 12-point Basso, Beattie & Bresnahan (BBB) open field locomotor scale on post-op days 1, 8, 15, 22, 29, 36, and 40 [33,34].

Tissue Processing

Six weeks post-operatively, rats were deeply anesthetized as described above and transcardially perfused with 0.9% saline solution, followed by 4% paraformaldehyde in 100 mM phosphate buffered saline (PBS). Brains and spinal cords were dissected, post-fixed with 4% paraformaldehyde overnight, and subsequently submersed in 30% sucrose at 4°C for at least 24 h. Brains were cut into 40 µm coronal sections on a sliding microtome (Leica, Germany), with every 12th section (480 µm intervals) processed for immunolabeling. A 5 mm block of spinal cord was excised at cervical level C4 and cut into 35 µm coronal sections with a cryostat (Leica, Germany). Every 10th section (350 µm intervals) was processed for immunolabeling. Brain and spinal cord sections were stored at −20°C in cryoprotectant solution (25% glycerol, 25% ethylene glycol, and 0.1 M phosphate buffer, pH 7.4).

Immunolabeling

For immunolabeling, free-floating brain and spinal cord sections were treated with 0.6% H_2O_2 in Tris-buffered saline (TBS: 0.15 M NaCl, 0.1 M Tris–HCl, pH 7.5) for 30 min. After rinsing in TBS, free-floating sections were incubated in 0.6% H_2O_2 for 30 min, washed again, and incubated for 1 h in 50% formamide/2xSSC (0.3 M NaCl, 0.03 M sodium citrate) at 65°C. Sections were rinsed in 2x SSC, incubated for 30 min in 2 M HCl at 37°C, and rinsed for 10 min in 0.1 M boric acid (pH 8.5). Following extensive washes in TBS, sections were blocked with a solution composed of TBS, 0.2% fish skin gelatin (Sigma-Aldrich, Germany), 1% bovine serum albumin (Biomol, Hamburg, Germany), and 0.1% Triton X-100 (Sigma-Aldrich, Germany) for 1 h followed by overnight incubation with the primary antibody at 4°C. On the following day, sections were washed extensively and incubated with biotin-conjugated species-specific secondary antibodies (Dianova, Hamburg, Germany and Vector Laboratories, Burlingame, USA) for 1 h, followed by incubation with a peroxidase–avidin complex solution (Vectastain Elite ABC kit; Vector Laboratories, Burlingame, USA). The peroxidase activity of immune complexes was visualized with a solution of TBS containing 0.25 mg/ml 3, 3′-diaminobenzidine (Vector Laboratories, Burlingame, USA), 0.01% H_2O_2, and 0.04% $NiCl_2$. Sections were mounted on gelatin coated slides and coverslipped in Neo-Mount (Merck, Darmstadt, Germany).

For the analysis of neuronal and glial differentiation, immunofluorescence labeling techniques were performed. For immunofluorescence labeling including BrdU antibodies, the DNA denaturation steps required for BrdU immunohistochemical detection were performed as described above. A combination of rat anti-BrdU and appropriate neuron- or glia-specific antibodies were applied in TBS-donkey serum for 24 h at 4°C. Fluorophorlabeled secondary antibodies, as defined below. After several washes in TBS, sections were mounted on slides and coverslipped with ProLong®Antifade (Molecular Probes).

The following primary antibodies were used: rat anti-BrdU antibody (1/500; Harlan SeraLab, Loughborough, UK), goat anti-doublecortin (DCX; 1/1000, Santa Cruz Biotechnology, Dallas, TX, USA), mouse anti-NeuN (1/500, Chemicon, Temecula, CA), rabbit anti-glial fibrillary acidic protein (GFAP) (1/1000, Dako, Hamburg, Germany), and mouse anti-adenomatous-polyposis-coli (APC)-protein (1/500; Calbiochem, Darmstadt, Germany), rabbit anti-NG2 (1:200; Chemicon, Temecula, CA, USA), and rabbit anti-ionized calcium binding adapter molecule 1 (IBA1) (1:500; Wako, Richmond, VA, USA). Immunoreactivity was visualized using Rhodamin-conjugated anti-rat (1/500; Dianova, Hamburg, Germany), Alexa 488–conjugated anti-goat (1/1000; Molecular Probes, Karlsruhe, Germany), Cy5-conjugated anti-rabbit (1/500; Dianova, Hamburg, Germany), and Alexa 488–conjugated anti-mouse (1/1000; Molecular Probes, Karlsruhe, Germany). All Alexa secondary antibodies were of donkey origin.

Early postmitotic neurons were identified by DCX immunoreactivity. Newly generated mature neurons were visualized by co-localization of BrdU and NeuN, astroglial cells by co-localization of BrdU with GFAP, oligodendrocytes by co-labeling of BrdU with APC in the absence of GFAP labeling, glial progenitor cells by co-labeling of BrdU with NG2 and activated microglia by co-localization of BrdU with IBA1 [35–40].

Counting Procedures

For quantification of the brightfield BrdU and DCX immunohistochemistry, a systematic unified random counting procedure, similar to the optical dissector [41], was used as described previously [42]. Every 12th brain section and every 10th spinal cord section were selected from each animal and analyzed for BrdU or DCX positive cells in the MC (7 sections per animal), SVZ (3 sections per animal), CC (5 sections per animal), HC (6 sections per animal) and cervical spinal cord (14 sections per animal).

The reference volume was determined by tracing the areas using a semi-automatic stereology system (Stereoinvestigator, MicroBrightField, Colchester, VT, USA) using a light microscope (Leica, Wetzlar, Germany). Newly generated cells (BrdU positive) and neurons (DCX positive) were counted exhaustively on each section in the SVZ, CC, HC, and MC. Within the HC only the dentate gyrus was included in the analysis. For analysis of the CC and SVZ the total extent according to the respective anatomical borders was chosen. The MC was defined as follows [43]: anterior-posterior from +3,7 to +1,6 mm, dorso-ventral was defined by a horizontal line drawn between the most dorsal edge of the cortex in each hemisphere (dorsal border) and another horizontal line drawn through the genu corpus callosum (ventral border). Within the spinal cord, BrdU positive cells were separately quantified in the region of the central canal, as well as in the surrounding parenchyma. The sums of BrdU and DCX positive cells of each section within the different brain and spinal cord regions were multiplied by a factor of 12 and 10, respectively, and are presented as absolute numbers.

Analysis of immunofluorescently labeled sections was performed using laser confocal microscopy (Leica TCS-NT). Co-localization of BrdU positive cells with respective differentiation markers in the spinal cord was determined by analyzing specimens of 5 animals with the highest number of BrdU positive cells in each group. 40 BrdU positive cells per animal – 20 cells in the ventral and 20 cells in the dorsal part of a horizontal spinal cord section (divided by a line through the central canal) – were randomly analyzed. Adjacent to the central canal, 40 BrdU positive cells were selected and also immunolabeled with differentiation markers. Co-localization for GFAP, APC, NG2 and IBA1 was confirmed, once the differentiation marker was spatially associated with BrdU nuclear labeling through subsequent optical sections in the z-axis. Co-localized cells are presented as percentage of BrdU positive cells. Total numbers were then calculated by multiplying the amount of BrdU positive cells with the respective ratios.

Statistical Analysis

All data are presented as mean values ± standard error of the mean (SEM). For intra-individual comparison of BBB scores in injured animals at two particular times of observation, one-way repeated measures ANOVA including Bonferroni post-hoc-test were applied. For all further inter-individual comparisons between injured and control animals, an unpaired t-test was used. A value of $p<0.05$ was considered significant ($p<0.05$ = *; $p<0.01$ = **; $p<0.001$ = ***). For statistical analysis, Prism software (Prism GraphPad Software, USA) was used.

Results

Spontaneous recovery of locomotor function after contusion spinal cord injury in adult rats

A standardized thoracic spinal contusion (200 kDyn) at T10 level induced complete paresis of both hindlimbs in all animals one day post-injury (Fig. 1). Two animals died within 24 h after surgery. Prior to surgery, none of the animals showed noticeable gait impairment. At post-op day 8, locomotor function substantially improved to an average BBB score of 5.9±1.6, ($p<0.0001$) compared to day 1 (Fig. 1). Animals displayed coordinated hindlimb movement with partial body weight support. Compared to BBB scores at day 8, locomotor function further improved at day 40, showing spontaneous functional recovery with nearly unimpaired walking patterns (BBB score 11.1±0.5; $p<0.0001$; Fig. 1).

Cell proliferation and neurogenesis

Effects of thoracic SCI on cell renewal in the brain (MC, SVZ, CC, HC) and cervical spinal cord of adult rats were assessed by counting BrdU positive cells 42 days post-injury (animals received BrdU injections between post-op day 4 and 14). No difference was observed in the number of newly generated cells between intact and injured animals in any of the brain regions investigated (MC, SVZ, CC, HC; Fig. 2).

DCX immunoreactive cells representing early post-mitotic neurons were only detectable in the SVZ and HC, as expected (Fig. 3). In both regions, quantification did not reveal any difference between intact and injured rats (SVZ: 2842±201 versus 3060±140; HC: 1062±67 versus 1007±58). In the MC, we analyzed on average 290 BrdU positive cells per animal and did not identify any BrdU/NeuN positive cell, indicating that no persisting new neurons were generated in this area following SCI (data not shown).

In contrast, BrdU positive cells were significantly increased in injured animals compared to intact animals in the cervical spinal cord, both in the spinal parenchyma and in the region of the central canal (101.5±24.1 versus 37.8±3.6, $p<0.05$; central canal: 14,4±2.9 versus 4.7±1.3, $p<0.05$; Fig. 4 A-E). The differentiation pattern within the spinal cord was further analyzed by examining the co-localization of BrdU with the astroglial marker GFAP, the oligodendroglial marker APC (Fig. 4F-J), the glial progenitor cell marker NG2 and the microglial marker IBA1 (Fig. 5). Glial cell renewal was observed only in the spinal

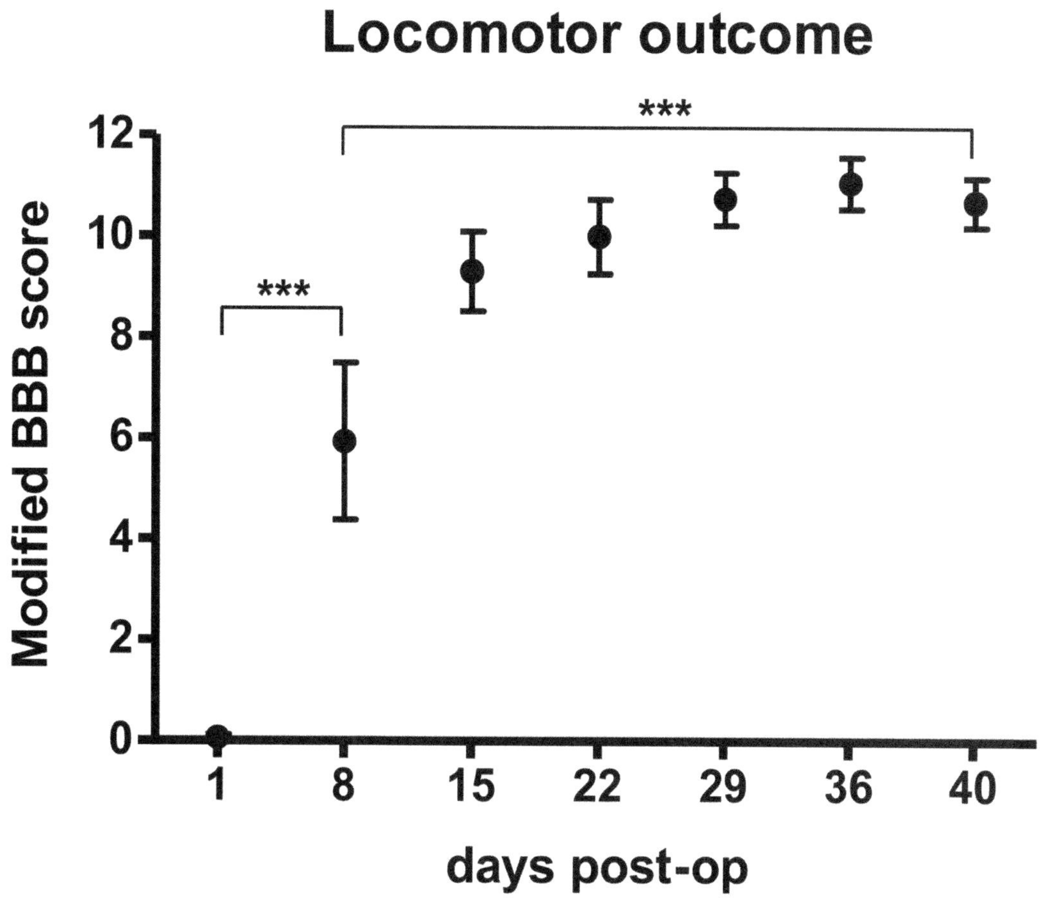

Figure 1. Spontaneous recovery of locomotion. Postoperative assessment of the modified 12-point BBB open field locomotor rating scale in 8 adult rats after a 200 kDyn mid-thoracic spinal cord contusion. Animals were monitored weekly starting day 1 post-injury until post-op day 40.

parenchyma of the cervical spinal cord. In the ependymal layer around the central canal, BrdU positive nuclei could not be co-localized with any of the tested glial markers (data not shown). The proportion of newborn cells displaying astro-/oligodendroglial, glial progenitor, or microglial differentiation was similar in the cervical spinal cord of injured versus intact animals (BrdU/GFAP co-localized cells: 35.5±3% versus 36±2.2%; BrdU/APC co-localized, GFAP negative cells: 7.5±0.8% vs. 8.0±1.5%; BrdU/NG2 co-localized cells: 14.5±5.1% vs. 15.0±2.4%; BrdU/IBA1 co-localized cells: 30.0±3.8% vs. 23.5±2.3%). Considering the significant difference in the number of BrdU positive cells, the absolute numbers of astroglial, oligodendroglia, glial progenitor cells, and microglia were significantly increased in the cervical spinal cord of injured animals (BrdU/GPAP co-localized cells: 36.0±3.8 vs. 13.6±0.9; $p<0.05$; BrdU/APC co-localized cells: 7.6±1.0 vs. 3.0±0.6, $p<0.05$; BrdU/NG2 co-localized cells: 14.7±3.5 vs. 5.7±0.5, $p<0.05$; BrdU/IBA1 co-localized cells: 30.4±7.2 vs. 8.9±0.8, $p<0.005$; Fig. 4F, Fig. 5A,E). There was no detectable DCX immunoreactivity in the cervical spinal cord, both in intact and injured animals (data not shown).

Discussion

The present study investigated cell proliferation/neurogenesis in remote CNS areas following a contusion injury that closely reflects human spinal cord pathology. Rats show robust spontaneous recovery of locomotor function, which is not paralleled by neurogenesis in the MC or CC. Moreover, neurogenesis is not altered in SCI rats compared to uninjured animals in the SVZ and HC. Interestingly, increased glial cell renewal can be observed in the cervical spinal cord remote from the thoracic lesion site. The functional relevance of the latter finding has yet to be determined.

The only other published study that analyzed supraspinal neurogenesis in spinal cord injured rats identified persistent depression of neurogenesis in the HC over 90 days after a cervical hemisection injury in adult rats [44]. In contrast, the mid-thoracic contusion SCI in the present study did not alter neurogenesis in the HC. The divergent findings may be explained by the different lesion level (cervical versus thoracic) and/or the different lesion paradigms, which likely effect axon pathways communicating with higher brain regions differentially.

Neuronal renewal should only be relevant for spontaneous functional recovery if the respective disease causes neuronal degeneration and cell death that contributes to functional impairment. For example, cell death represents an indisputable pathophysiological hallmark underlying functional impairment in ischemic stroke [45,46]. In contrast, neuronal cell death has a limited impact on functional decline in SCI, where the transection of long distance motor, sensory, and autonomous axon pathways defines the clinical phenotype [47,48]. Whether spinal cord axon transection results in neuronal cell death in the brain remains controversial. After a rat dorsal column transection, substantial degeneration of corticospinal neurons, as determined by the expression of apoptotic markers in layer V of the MC, has been

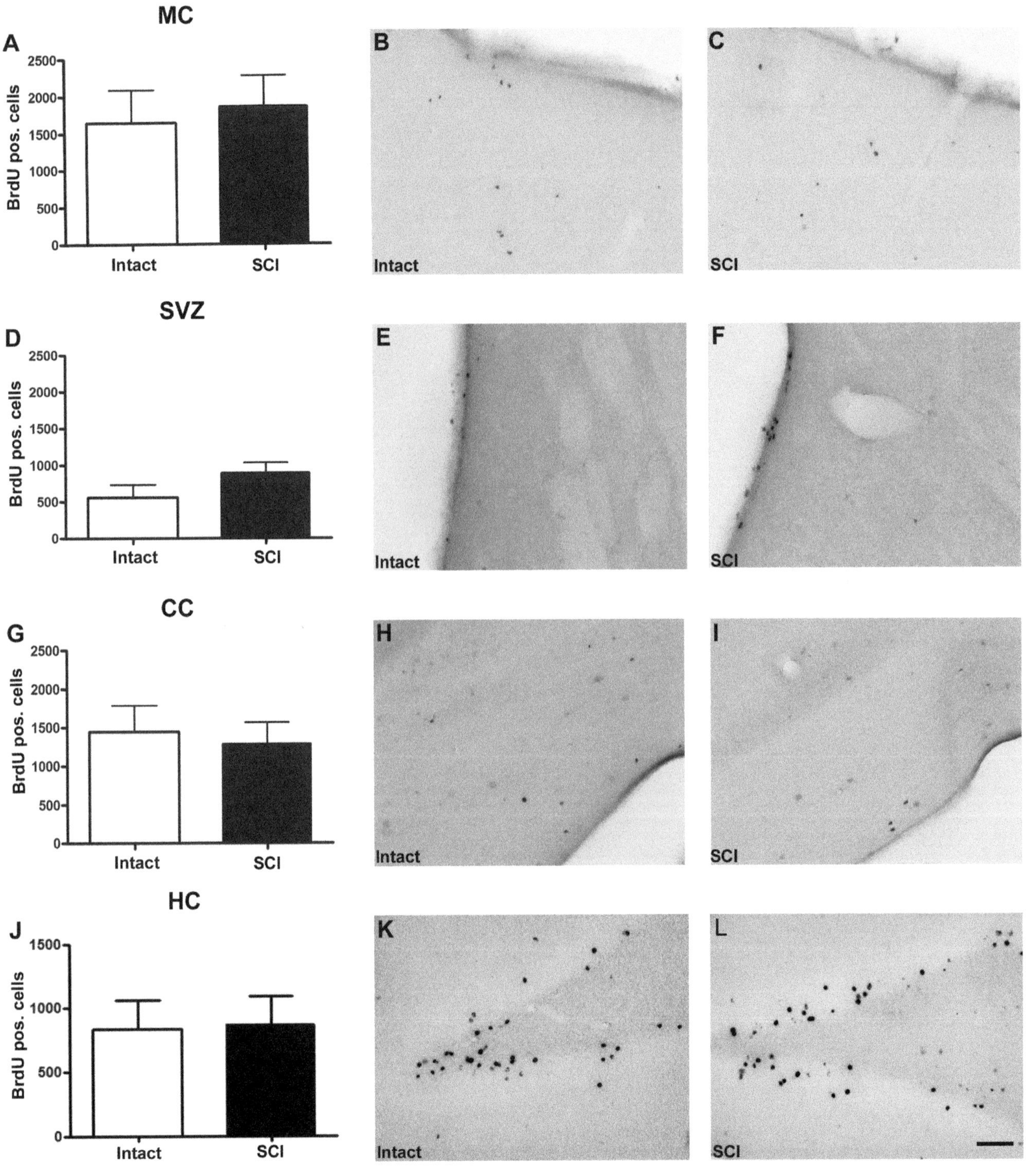

Figure 2. Post SCI cell renewal in motor cortex, subventricular zone, corpus callosum and hippocampus. (A, D, G, J) Quantification of BrdU positive cells in control (Intact) versus spinal cord injured (SCI) animals in the motor cortex (MC; A), subventricular zone (SVZ; D), corpus callosum (CC; G) and hippocampus (HC; H). Brightfield micrographs display cell renewal represented by BrdU immunoreactive nuclei in the MC (B, C), SVZ (E, F), CC (H, I) and HC (K, L) of control (Intact; B, E, H, K) and injured animals (C, F, I, L). Scale bar: 50 μm in (L).

reported within 2 weeks after injury [19]. In contrast, corticospinal axon quantification at the brainstem level following thoracic and cervical rat contusion SCI could not identify a significant decline of axon profiles, suggesting that cell death of corresponding neurons does not occur [49]. A more recent study from the same group employing an identical lesion model and identical assessments to determine pyramidal neuron cell death, as reported by Hains et al, could not replicate the finding of cortical neuronal death following rat SCI [50]. In human SCI subjects, atrophy of the corticospinal tract has been reported by magnetic resonance

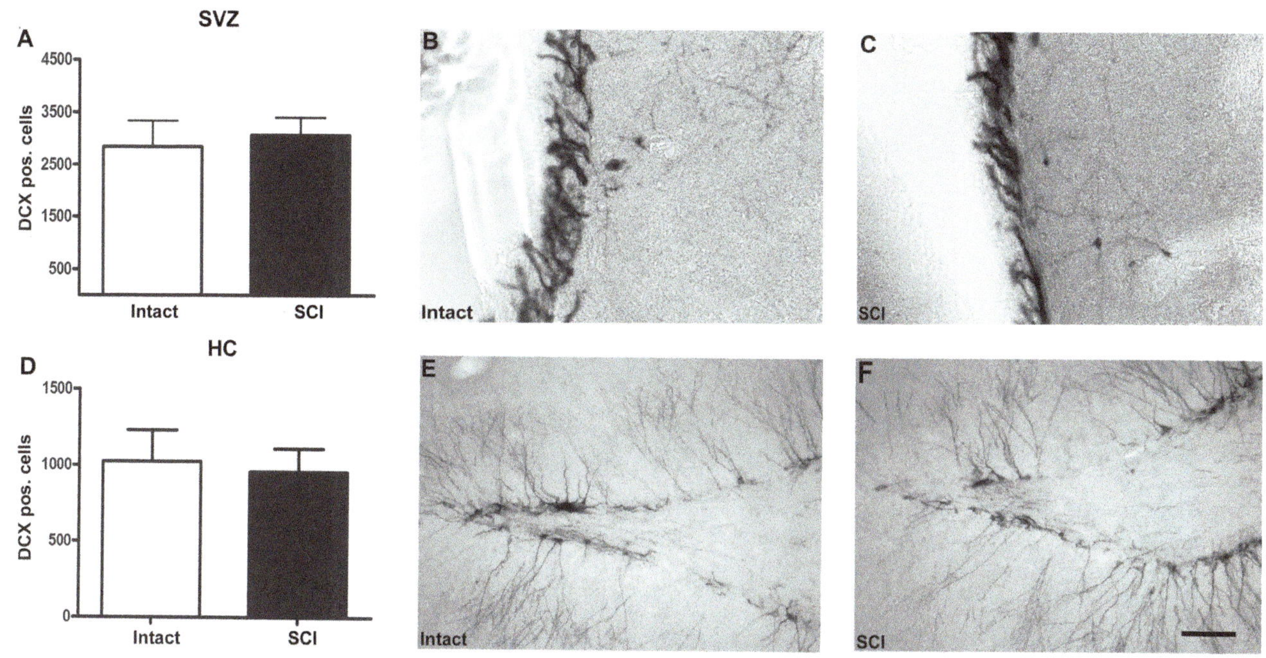

Figure 3. Neurogenesis in the subventricular zone and hippocampus. (A, D) Quantification of DCX immunoreactive cells in the subventricular zone (SVZ; A) and hippocampus (HC; D) in control (Intact) versus spinal cord injured (SCI) animals. Brightfield micrographs display representative section of DCX-expressing neuroblasts in the SVZ (B, C) and HC (E, F) of control (B, E) and spinal cord injured animals (C, F). Scale bar: 100 μm.

imaging. However, the limited resolution of MRI does not allow counting of individual axons. The observed atrophy could have been caused by degeneration of glial cells or shrinkage of corticospinal neurons/axons [51], rather than axon depletion due to pyramidal neuron cell death as the morphological substrate [52].

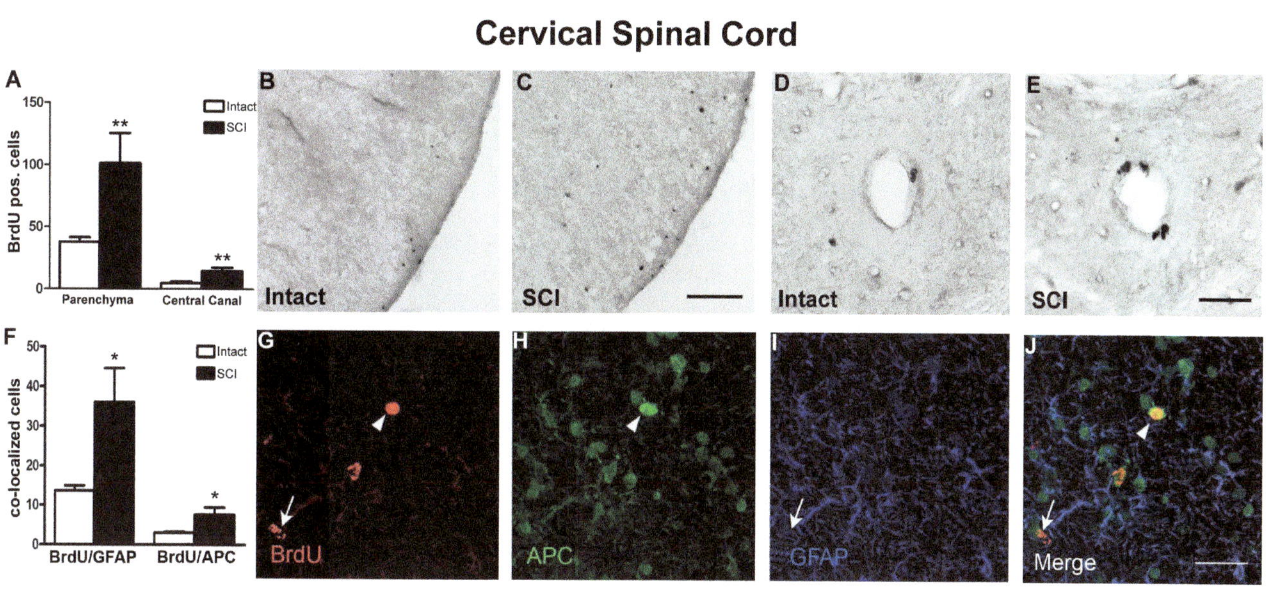

Figure 4. Post SCI cell renewal in the cervical spinal cord. Coronal spinal cord sections were analyzed in the parenchyma and around the central canal. (A) Quantification of BrdU positive surviving newborn cells in the spinal parenchyma and around the central canal of intact and SCI animals. BrdU positive nuclei in the lateral white matter (B, C) and in the ependymal layer of the central canal (D, E) of intact and injured animals (SCI). (F) Quantification of BrdU positive cells expressing GFAP representing astroglia; BrdU positive cells co-localizing with APC, but negative for GFAP, were counted as oligodendrocytes. (G-J) Immunofluorescent labeling for (G) BrdU (red), (H) APC (green) and (I) GFAP (blue) in a coronal cervical spinal cord section of an injured animal taken from the ventral gray matter. (J) Merged image of (G-I). Co-localization of BrdU with GFAP indicates astroglial differentiation (arrow), whereas BrdU/APC positive cells that are GFAP-negative represent oligodendrocytes (arrowhead). Scale bars: 100 μm in (C), 50 μm in (E), 34.1 μm in (J).

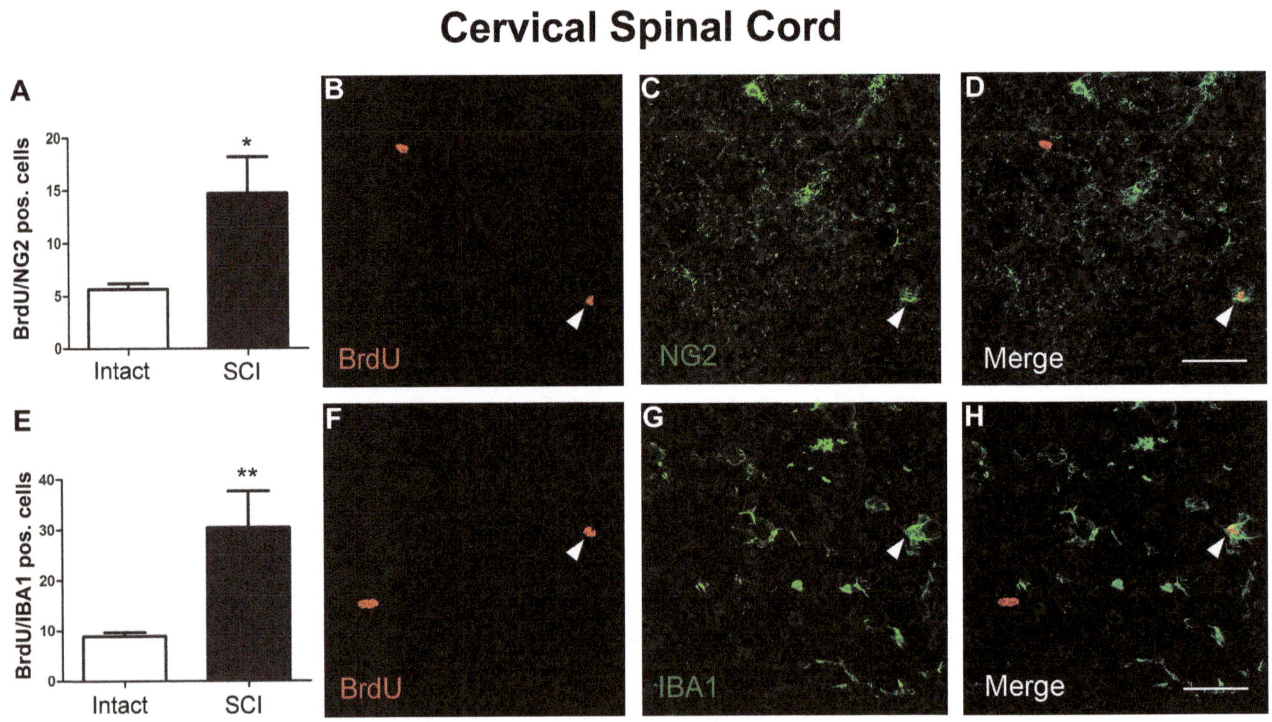

Figure 5. Post SCI glial progenitor cell and microglial renewal in the cervical spinal cord. (A) Quantification of BrdU positive cells expressing NG2 and thus representing glial progenitor cells. (B-D) Immunofluorescent labeling for (B) BrdU (red) and (C) NG2 (green). (D) Merged image of (B, C) indicating a co-localization of BrdU and NG2 (arrowhead). (E) Quantification of BrdU positive cells expressing IBA1 and thus representing newborn microglia. (F-H) Immunofluorescent labeling for (F) BrdU (red) and (G) IBA1 (green). (H) Merged image of (F, G) indicating a co-localization of BrdU and IBA1 (arrowhead). Scale bars: 60 μm in (D) and 45 μm in (H).

Irrespective of the debate regarding cell death of pyramidal neurons other factors may have contributed to the failure to detect cortical neurogenesis after SCI. The only study that has so far reported replacement of lost cortical neurons in adult mammals following a CNS lesion used a highly specific, limited injury model - apoptotic cell death via chromophore photoactivation. The first newborn mouse neurons projecting axons to the cervical spinal cord were detected at 12 weeks, peaking at the latest investigated time point – 56 weeks post cortical lesion. Overall, the number of detected newborn neurons was very small, between 1–6 neurons per mm^3 [17]. In the present study, the maximum time between neural progenitor generation and analysis of neuronal fate (BrdU/NeuN co-localization) was much shorter - 38 days (42 days post-injury survival minus 4 days post-injury start of BrdU administration). The time window of 38 days after BrdU injection in the present study should have been sufficient to detect at least DCX positive immature neuroblasts in the MC or in the primary neurogenic sites – the SVZ. Alternatively, the quantity of SVZ neurogenesis destined to replace cortical neurons might be too low to be identifiable in the current experimental setting.

The failure to demonstrate neurogenesis in the adult spinal cord confirms numerous previous reports [22–29]. Cell proliferation and reactive gliogenesis have been shown in regions close to the lesion site [24,35,53]. As sources of glial renewal cells around the central canal, NG2 positive glial progenitor cells in the white and grey matter and mature GFAP expressing astrocytes have been identified [54]. The observed glial cell replacement is paralleled by ongoing glial cell death in spinal cord regions, not only adjacent but also remote from the injury site [20,55,56]. In monkeys, sites of oligodendrogliogenesis correlate with demyelinated areas suggesting that replaced oligodendroglia contribute to remyelination and possibly functional recovery in incomplete SCI [57]. In the present study, glial replacement (astroglia, oligodendroglia, microglia) in the cervical spinal cord exceeded gliogenesis compared to uninjured control animals. It is conceivable that remote areas of demyelination become spontaneously remyelinated via endogenous oligodendroglial replacement. Whether remote demyelination or potential remyelination by replaced oligodendroglia influence the functional outcome, cannot be determined at this point. Astroglial renewal immediately at the spinal cord lesion site is attributed to reactive astrogliosis, which seals off the injury site from the surrounding spinal cord. The relevance of astroglial turnover observed at remote spinal cord levels has yet to be defined. Wallerian degeneration of ascending sensory projections at cervical spinal cord level represents a potential trigger, which might explain enhanced microglial cell recruitment following thoracic SCI.

Conclusion

The true functional relevance of the observed glial replacement in spinal regions distant from the injury site is unknown. However, considering the robust spontaneous recovery in contrast to the moderate cell replacement activities in the cervical spinal cord, it is unlikely that endogenous cell replacement contributes to spontaneous functional improvement in incomplete SCI.

Acknowledgments

We thank Julianne McCall for proofreading the manuscript.

Author Contributions

Conceived and designed the experiments: NW BW. Performed the experiments: SF MC KP BK BS. Analyzed the data: NW BW SF MC BS. Contributed reagents/materials/analysis tools: NW BW AB UB. Wrote the paper: NW SF MC. Revised the manuscript critically for important intellectual content: AB BW UB. Provided the final approval of the version to be published: NW BW AB.

References

1. Lu P, Blesch A, Graham L, Wang Y, Samara R, et al. (2012) Motor axonal regeneration after partial and complete spinal cord transection. J Neurosci 32: 8208–8218.
2. Ramón y Cajal S (1928) Degeneration and regeneration of the nervous system. London: Oxford University Press.
3. Fawcett JW, Curt A, Steeves JD, Coleman WP, Tuszynski MH, et al. (2007) Guidelines for the conduct of clinical trials for spinal cord injury as developed by the ICCP panel: spontaneous recovery after spinal cord injury and statistical power needed for therapeutic clinical trials. Spinal Cord 45: 190–205.
4. Swash M (1998) Outcomes in neurological and neurosurgical disorders. Cambridge: Cambridge University Press. xvi,612p p.
5. Spiess MR, Muller RM, Rupp R, Schuld C, van Hedel HJ (2009) Conversion in ASIA impairment scale during the first year after traumatic spinal cord injury. J Neurotrauma 26: 2027–2036.
6. Rosenzweig ES, Courtine G, Jindrich DL, Brock JH, Ferguson AR, et al. (2010) Extensive spontaneous plasticity of corticospinal projections after primate spinal cord injury. Nat Neurosci 13: 1505–1510.
7. Basso DM, Beattie MS, Bresnahan JC (1996) Graded histological and locomotor outcomes after spinal cord contusion using the NYU weight-drop device versus transection. Exp Neurol 139: 244–256.
8. Muir GD, Whishaw IQ (1999) Complete locomotor recovery following corticospinal tract lesions: measurement of ground reaction forces during overground locomotion in rats. Behav Brain Res 103: 45–53.
9. Weidner N, Ner A, Salimi N, Tuszynski MH (2001) Spontaneous corticospinal axonal plasticity and functional recovery after adult central nervous system injury. Proc Natl Acad Sci U S A 98: 3513–3518.
10. Ballermann M, Fouad K (2006) Spontaneous locomotor recovery in spinal cord injured rats is accompanied by anatomical plasticity of reticulospinal fibers. Eur J Neurosci 23: 1988–1996.
11. Sanai N, Nguyen T, Ihrie RA, Mirzadeh Z, Tsai HH, et al. (2011) Corridors of migrating neurons in the human brain and their decline during infancy. Nature 478: 382–386.
12. Eriksson PS, Perfilieva E, Bjork-Eriksson T, Alborn AM, Nordborg C, et al. (1998) Neurogenesis in the adult human hippocampus. Nat Med 4: 1313–1317.
13. Spalding KL, Bergmann O, Alkass K, Bernard S, Salehpour M, et al. (2013) Dynamics of hippocampal neurogenesis in adult humans. Cell 153: 1219–1227.
14. Magavi SS, Leavitt BR, Macklis JD (2000) Induction of neurogenesis in the neocortex of adult mice. Nature 405: 951–955.
15. Gould E, Reeves AJ, Graziano MS, Gross CG (1999) Neurogenesis in the neocortex of adult primates. Science 286: 548–552.
16. Nakatomi H, Kuriu T, Okabe S, Yamamoto S, Hatano O, et al. (2002) Regeneration of hippocampal pyramidal neurons after ischemic brain injury by recruitment of endogenous neural progenitors. Cell 110: 429–441.
17. Chen J, Magavi SS, Macklis JD (2004) Neurogenesis of corticospinal motor neurons extending spinal projections in adult mice. Proc Natl Acad Sci U S A 101: 16357–16362.
18. Arvidsson A, Collin T, Kirik D, Kokaia Z, Lindvall O (2002) Neuronal replacement from endogenous precursors in the adult brain after stroke. Nat Med 8: 963–970.
19. Hains BC, Black JA, Waxman SG (2003) Primary cortical motor neurons undergo apoptosis after axotomizing spinal cord injury. J Comp Neurol 462: 328–341.
20. Crowe MJ, Bresnahan JC, Shuman SL, Masters JN, Beattie MS (1997) Apoptosis and delayed degeneration after spinal cord injury in rats and monkeys. Nat Med 3: 73–76.
21. Couillard-Despres S, Winner B, Schaubeck S, Aigner R, Vroemen M, et al. (2005) Doublecortin expression levels in adult brain reflect neurogenesis. Eur J Neurosci 21: 1–14.
22. Frisen J, Johansson CB, Torok C, Risling M, Lendahl U (1995) Rapid, widespread, and longlasting induction of nestin contributes to the generation of glial scar tissue after CNS injury. J Cell Biol 131: 453–464.
23. Horner PJ, Power AE, Kempermann G, Kuhn HG, Palmer TD, et al. (2000) Proliferation and differentiation of progenitor cells throughout the intact adult rat spinal cord. J Neurosci 20: 2218–2228.
24. Horky LL, Galimi F, Gage FH, Horner PJ (2006) Fate of endogenous stem/progenitor cells following spinal cord injury. J Comp Neurol 498: 525–538.
25. Meletis K, Barnabe-Heider F, Carlen M, Evergren E, Tomilin N, et al. (2008) Spinal cord injury reveals multilineage differentiation of ependymal cells. PLoS Biol 6: e182.
26. Sellers DL, Maris DO, Horner PJ (2009) Postinjury niches induce temporal shifts in progenitor fates to direct lesion repair after spinal cord injury. J Neurosci 29: 6722–6733.
27. Barnabe-Heider F, Goritz C, Sabelstrom H, Takebayashi H, Pfrieger FW, et al. (2010) Origin of new glial cells in intact and injured adult spinal cord. Cell Stem Cell 7: 470–482.
28. Sabelstrom H, Stenudd M, Reu P, Dias DO, Elfineh M, et al. (2013) Resident neural stem cells restrict tissue damage and neuronal loss after spinal cord injury in mice. Science 342: 637–640.
29. Lacroix S, Hamilton LK, Vaugeois A, Beaudoin S, Breault-Dugas C, et al. (2014) Central canal ependymal cells proliferate extensively in response to traumatic spinal cord injury but not demyelinating lesions. PLoS One 9: e85916.
30. Kakulas BA (1999) The applied neuropathology of human spinal cord injury. Spinal Cord 37: 79–88.
31. Scheff SW, Rabchevsky AG, Fugaccia I, Main JA, Lumpp JE Jr (2003) Experimental modeling of spinal cord injury: characterization of a force-defined injury device. J Neurotrauma 20: 179–193.
32. Weber T, Vroemen M, Behr V, Neuberger T, Jakob P, et al. (2006) In vivo high-resolution MR imaging of neuropathologic changes in the injured rat spinal cord. AJNR Am J Neuroradiol 27: 598–604.
33. Basso DM, Beattie MS, Bresnahan JC (1995) A sensitive and reliable locomotor rating scale for open field testing in rats. J Neurotrauma 12: 1–21.
34. Ferguson AR, Hook MA, Garcia G, Bresnahan JC, Beattie MS, et al. (2004) A simple post hoc transformation that improves the metric properties of the BBB scale for rats with moderate to severe spinal cord injury. J Neurotrauma 21: 1601–1613.
35. McTigue DM, Wei P, Stokes BT (2001) Proliferation of NG2-positive cells and altered oligodendrocyte numbers in the contused rat spinal cord. J Neurosci 21: 3392–3400.
36. Francis F, Koulakoff A, Boucher D, Chafey P, Schaar B, et al. (1999) Doublecortin is a developmentally regulated, microtubule-associated protein expressed in migrating and differentiating neurons. Neuron 23: 247–256.
37. Miller MW, Nowakowski RS (1988) Use of bromodeoxyuridine-immunohistochemistry to examine the proliferation, migration and time of origin of cells in the central nervous system. Brain Res 457: 44–52.
38. Imai Y, Ibata I, Ito D, Ohsawa K, Kohsaka S (1996) A novel gene iba1 in the major histocompatibility complex class III region encoding an EF hand protein expressed in a monocytic lineage. Biochem Biophys Res Commun 224: 855–862.
39. Ito D, Imai Y, Ohsawa K, Nakajima K, Fukuuchi Y, et al. (1998) Microglia-specific localisation of a novel calcium binding protein, Iba1. Brain Res Mol Brain Res 57: 1–9.
40. Yoo S, Wrathall JR (2007) Mixed primary culture and clonal analysis provide evidence that NG2 proteoglycan-expressing cells after spinal cord injury are glial progenitors. Dev Neurobiol 67: 860–874.
41. Gundersen HJ, Bendtsen TF, Korbo L, Marcussen N, Moller A, et al. (1988) Some new, simple and efficient stereological methods and their use in pathological research and diagnosis. Apmis 96: 379–394.
42. Winner B, Rockenstein E, Lie DC, Aigner R, Mante M, et al. (2007) Mutant alpha-synuclein exacerbates age-related decrease of neurogenesis. Neurobiol Aging.
43. Paxinos G, Watson C (2007) The rat brain in stereotaxic coordinates. Amsterdam; Oxford: Elsevier Academic. xxxi, ca. 420 p. p.
44. Felix MS, Popa N, Djelloul M, Boucraut J, Gauthier P, et al. (2012) Alteration of forebrain neurogenesis after cervical spinal cord injury in the adult rat. Front Neurosci 6: 45.
45. Small SL, Buccino G, Solodkin A (2013) Brain repair after stroke—a novel neurological model. Nat Rev Neurol 9: 698–707.
46. Boncoraglio GB, Bersano A, Candelise L, Reynolds BA, Parati EA (2010) Stem cell transplantation for ischemic stroke. Cochrane Database Syst Rev: CD007231.
47. Hillen BK, Abbas JJ, Jung R (2013) Accelerating locomotor recovery after incomplete spinal injury. Ann N Y Acad Sci 1279: 164–174.
48. Raineteau O, Schwab ME (2001) Plasticity of motor systems after incomplete spinal cord injury. Nat Rev Neurosci 2: 263–273.
49. Nielson JL, Sears-Kraxberger I, Strong MK, Wong JK, Willenberg R, et al. (2010) Unexpected survival of neurons of origin of the pyramidal tract after spinal cord injury. J Neurosci 30: 11516–11528.
50. Nielson JL, Strong MK, Steward O (2011) A reassessment of whether cortical motor neurons die following spinal cord injury. J Comp Neurol 519: 2852–2869.
51. Wannier T, Schmidlin E, Bloch J, Rouiller EM (2005) A unilateral section of the corticospinal tract at cervical level in primate does not lead to measurable cell loss in motor cortex. J Neurotrauma 22: 703–717.
52. Freund P, Weiskopf N, Ashburner J, Wolf K, Sutter R, et al. (2013) MRI investigation of the sensorimotor cortex and the corticospinal tract after acute spinal cord injury: a prospective longitudinal study. Lancet Neurol.
53. Zai LJ, Wrathall JR (2005) Cell proliferation and replacement following contusive spinal cord injury. Glia 50: 247–257.
54. McTigue DM, Sahinkaya FR (2011) The fate of proliferating cells in the injured adult spinal cord. Stem Cell Res Ther 2: 7.

55. Shuman SL, Bresnahan JC, Beattie MS (1997) Apoptosis of microglia and oligodendrocytes after spinal cord contusion in rats. J Neurosci Res 50: 798–808.
56. Siegenthaler MM, Tu MK, Keirstead HS (2007) The extent of myelin pathology differs following contusion and transection spinal cord injury. J Neurotrauma 24: 1631–1646.
57. Yang H, Lu P, McKay HM, Bernot T, Keirstead H, et al. (2006) Endogenous neurogenesis replaces oligodendrocytes and astrocytes after primate spinal cord injury. J Neurosci 26: 2157–2166.

13

Arylsulfatase B Improves Locomotor Function after Mouse Spinal Cord Injury

Myungsik Yoo[1], Muntasir Khaled[1], Kurt M. Gibbs[1], Jonghun Kim[1], Björn Kowalewski[2], Thomas Dierks[2], Melitta Schachner[1,3]*

1 W. M. Keck Center for Collaborative Neuroscience and Department of Cell Biology and Neuroscience, Rutgers University, Piscataway, New Jersey, United States of America, **2** Department of Chemistry, Biochemistry I, Bielefeld University, Universitätsstr Bielefeld, Germany, **3** Center for Neuroscience, Shantou University Medical College, Shantou, Guandong Province, People's Republic of China

Abstract

Bacterial chondroitinase ABC (ChaseABC) has been used to remove the inhibitory chondroitin sulfate chains from chondroitin sulfate proteoglycans to improve regeneration after rodent spinal cord injury. We hypothesized that the mammalian enzyme arylsulfatase B (ARSB) would also enhance recovery after mouse spinal cord injury. Application of the mammalian enzyme would be an attractive alternative to ChaseABC because of its more robust chemical stability and reduced immunogenicity. A one-time injection of human ARSB into injured mouse spinal cord eliminated immunoreactivity for chondroitin sulfates within five days, and up to 9 weeks after injury. After a moderate spinal cord injury, we observed improvements of locomotor recovery assessed by the Basso Mouse Scale (BMS) in ARSB treated mice, compared to the buffer-treated control group, at 6 weeks after injection. After a severe spinal cord injury, mice injected with equivalent units of ARSB or ChaseABC improved similarly and both groups achieved significantly more locomotor recovery than the buffer-treated control mice. Serotonin and tyrosine hydroxylase immunoreactive axons were more extensively present in mouse spinal cords treated with ARSB and ChaseABC, and the immunoreactive axons penetrated further beyond the injury site in ARSB or ChaseABC treated mice than in control mice. These results indicate that mammalian ARSB improves functional recovery after CNS injury. The structural/molecular mechanisms underlying the observed functional improvement remain to be elucidated.

Editor: Thomas H. Gillingwater, University of Edinburgh, United Kingdom

Funding: This study was supported by the New Jersey Commission for Spinal Cord Research and in part from Deutsche Forschungsgemeinschaft. Funders had no role in study design, data collection and analysis, decision to publish, or preparation of the manuscript.

Competing Interests: The authors have declared that no competing interests exist.

* E-mail: schachner@stu.edu.cn

Introduction

Unlike fish and many non-mammalian vertebrates, mammals show a very limited capacity for regeneration after acute and chronic injury of the adult central nervous system [1–4]. Several cellular and molecular mechanisms may underlie this limitation including a paucity of conducive, and an abundance of inhibitory contributions to the damaged tissue to heal and to renew functions operant before injury. Among molecules identified in many studies to inhibit growth are members of the chondroitin sulfate proteoglycan (CSPG) family, which are up-regulated in expression in the injured parts of the central nervous system [5–7]. CSPGs are mostly localized in the extracellular matrix and are major formative determinants during nervous system development [8–11]. Their importance in synaptic functions and plasticity in the adult is increasingly becoming recognized, particularly regarding the striking structures of perineuronal nets whose contributions to interneuronal activity have been mainly unresolved, but are thought to limit plasticity [12–14]. Production of CSPGs increases in injured spinal cords in astrogliotic tissues around the lesion site [15–17]. The glial scar resulting from astrogliosis is considered a mechanical and molecular barrier to growing axons from supraspinal nuclei in brainstem and somatosensory cortex [18,19].

Glycosaminoglycan (GAG) chains mediate the inhibitory activities of CSPGs. Sulfate additions appear to be crucial determinants of inhibitory activities of GAG chains. Four different types of chondroitin sulfate (CS) sulfation (4-*O*-sulfation, C4S; 6-*O*-sulfation, C6S; 2,6-*O*-sulfation, C2, 6S; 4,6-*O*-sulfation, C4, 6S) inhibit neurite outgrowth and affect intracellular signaling. C4S demonstrated to be the major contributor of inhibiting axon outgrowth at the spinal cord lesion site [20], while C6S, also presented to be an inhibitory determinant in CNS injury [21], by inhibiting cortical neuronal outgrowth, which was blocked by treatment with C6S binding peptides [22,23]. Interestingly, C6S may paradoxically play a permissive role for neuronal regeneration. C6S-sulfotransferase knockout mice have diminished nigrostriatal axonal regeneration, while peripheral axons are unaffected [24]. In agreement with this observation, up-regulation of C6S-sulfotransferase-1 facilitates Schwann cell migration in the injured sciatic nerve [25]. Recent studies show that C4, 6S has an inhibitory role in injured cortex where it (along with C2S, C6S, but not C4S) was up-regulated in peri-infarct gliotic tissue compared to uninjured cortex. In addition, C4, 6S strongly inhibits dorsal root ganglion neurite growth [26], while targeted knockdown of C4, 6S-sulfotransferase, using shRNA, mitigated CSPG-mediated inhibition [27]. CSPGs have seemingly multi-

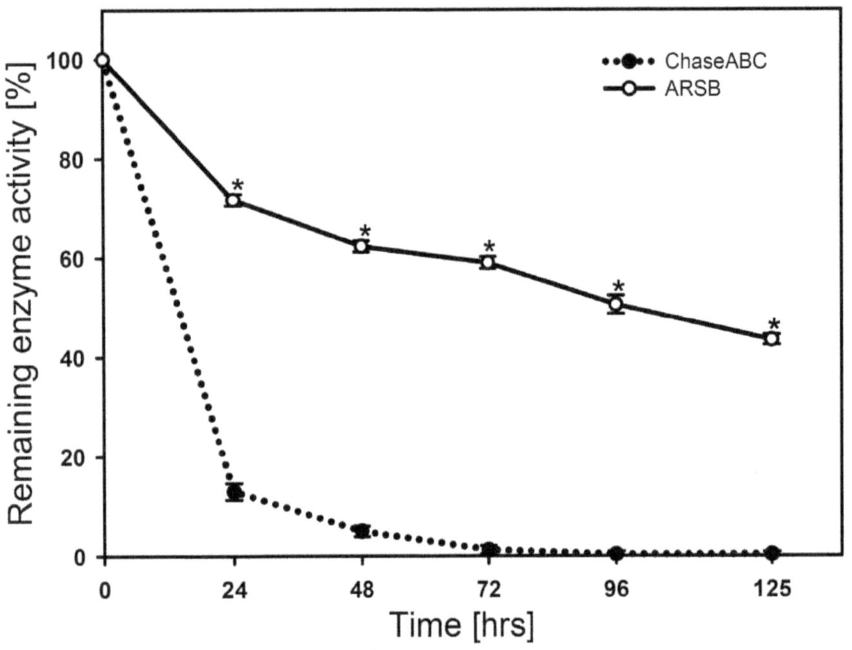

Figure 1. Thermostability of ARSB and ChaseABC. Stock solutions of each enzyme were incubated at 37°C/pH 6.8 for up to 125 hours. At the indicated time points aliquots were diluted into pre-warmed assay buffer (pH 8.0 for ChaseABC, pH 5.6 for ARSB) and subjected to activity determination (see Methods). Asterisks indicate significant differences between the groups $*p<0.001$ as assessed by t-Test. Data represent means ± SEM (n = 4).

functional roles but despite a few instances of growth permissiveness, the above-mentioned CSPGs have primarily been an obstacle to axon outgrowth.

The bacterial enzyme ChaseABC removes GAG chains of CSPGs [17,28,29]. The therapeutic potential of this enzyme has been repeatedly documented to promote locomotor recovery and axonal regrowth in different types of spinal cord injury paradigms in rodents [17,30,31], not only when applied by itself, but also in combination with other conducive agents, such as neurotrophins, stem cells, and the neural adhesion molecule L1 [32–34]. Furthermore, this enzyme is not only beneficial in acute stage of CNS injury, but in chronic spinal cord injury paradigms as well [3,35].

Treatment of spinal cord injured patients with ChaseABC has not yet reached clinical trials, possibly due in part to the potential immunogenicity of this bacterial protein and its chemical instability in injured tissues. Injured CNS develops a local acidic environment, of approximately pH 6.8 [36–38], while ChaseABC has an activity optimum pH of 8 [39–41]. In addition, ChaseABC loses activity at the mammalian body temperature of 37°C [40,42], and necessitates modification to increase its thermostability to remain active at that temperature [43]. Given the above characteristics of ChaseABC, we decided to probe the therapeutic potential of a less immunogenic and more chemically stable mammalian enzyme that removes sulfates and in particular, the C4S moieties from CSPGs in spinal cord injury. ARSB (N-acetylgalactosamine 4-sulfatase) lends itself to such analysis, since it has an acidic pH optimum [44] and is approved to treat patients with mucopolysaccharidosis type VI [45–47]. It functions in lysosomal removal of C4S groups from chondroitin and dermatan sulfate; these C4 sulfate groups, in extracellular CS, were shown to be the major structural determinant for axonal growth inhibition [20]. Recent findings report that ARSB is also localized in the extracellular matrix [48]. Here, we report that a one-time injection of human ARSB into the acute lesion site and in the close vicinity of this site in a mouse compression model of spinal cord injury leads to improved locomotor activity and re-growth/sprouting of descending axons. These observations encourage the expectation that human ARSB will be an added benefit to other modes of treatment for spinal cord injury and other injuries of the central nervous system in humans.

Results

4-O-sulfated GAG Abundance after Compression Injury and Injection of ARSB

We assessed the thermostability of ARSB in comparison to ChaseABC at 37°C and at the relevant pH range of 6.0 to 6.8. Under these conditions ARSB retained half of its activity even after 5 days, while ChaseABC at pH 6.8 lost approximately 90% of its activity within 24 hours, and was fully inactive after 3 days (**Fig. 1**); at pH 6.0 ChaseABC was completely inactived already after 24 hours (data not shown). We then investigated whether human ARSB would remove C4S immunoreactivity in sagittal sections of injured mouse spinal cord after directly injecting the enzyme after moderate compression injury into the spinal cord tissue at the lesion site and 0.5 mm rostral and caudal to the site. Five days after injection, immunofluorescent staining was performed on formaldehyde fixed tissue in sagittal sections, serially spaced 400 μm apart, comprising the lesion site and several micrometers (~100 μm) in its vicinity (**Fig. 2, Fig. S1**). An antibody specific for detection of C4S was used to show that spinal cord tissue treated with ARSB showed considerably less immunoreactivity than spinal cords treated with vehicle only (compare **Figs. 2a,c** with **Figs. 2b,d**). These observations indicate that after injection of ARSB, C4S immunoreactivity is reduced in the extracellular space under the physiological conditions of the host

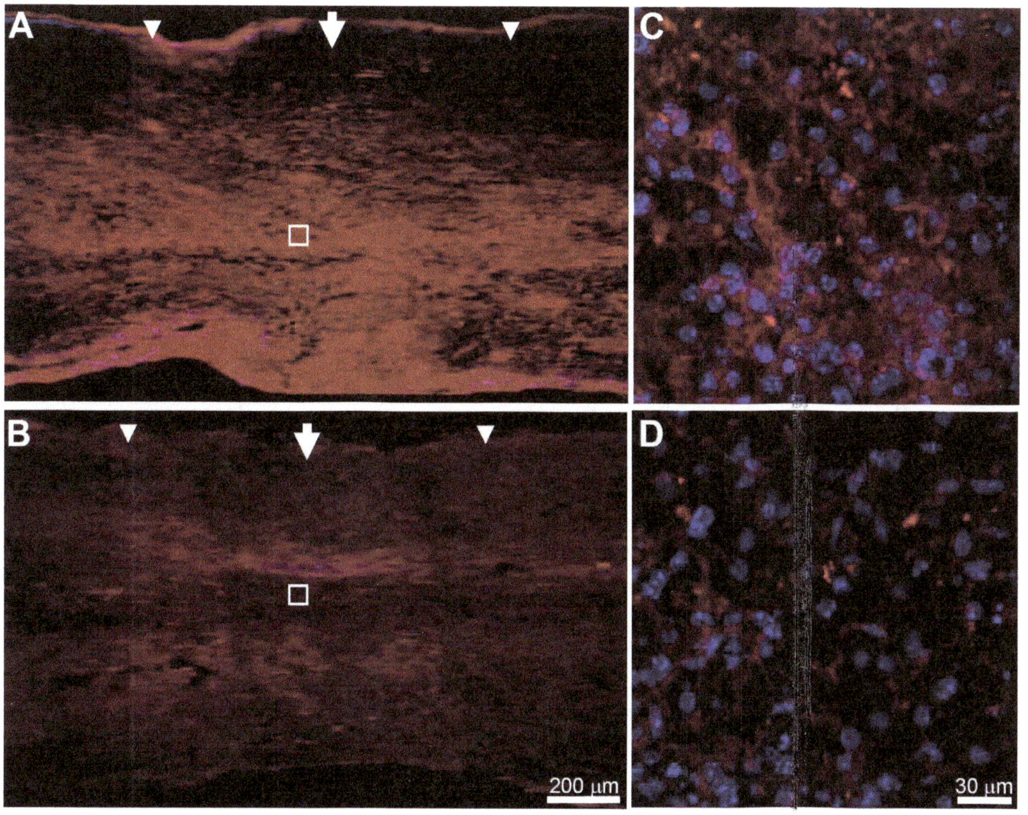

Figure 2. Chondroitin 4-*O*-sulfate (C4S) immunoreactivity is reduced at five days after ARSB injection after moderate compression-injury. Immediately after spinal cord injury, one µl of ARSB (10 U/ml) was injected at the injury site (arrow) and 0.5 mm rostral and caudal to this site (arrowheads). After 5 days, the mice were perfused, and sagittal spinal cord sections were analyzed by immunofluorescence using an antibody specific for C4S. C4S immunoreactivity is higher at the injury site in the buffer treated control mice (**A**) versus ARSB treated mice (**B**). (**C**) and (**D**) are higher magnifications of the insets in (**A**) and (**B**), respectively. Diamidino-phenylindole (DAPI, blue) was used for nuclear staining and merged with C4S immunoreactivity (**C,D**). Arrows and arrowheads indicate the injury site and injection sites, respectively.

tissue, either as a direct or indirect consequence of this enzyme activity.

Sulfated GAG Levels after Injection of ARSB and ChaseABC

We then compared the efficacy of C4S removal 9 weeks after injury between human ARSB and the bacterial enzyme ChaseABC treated mice, with equal enzymatic units injected per mouse, using the same injection protocol as for the immunofluorescent assessment five days after the injection of ARSB. In addition to the C4S-specific antibody, antibody CS56 (specific for both C4S and C6S) was used in parallel for immunofluorescent staining on consecutive spinal cord sagittal sections, and quantified with Image J software (**Figs. 3, 4**). In comparison to the tissue harvested from the vehicle only treated spinal cords, both enzymes removed C4S immunoreactivity significantly when the same quantities of enzyme units were injected, but ChaseABC reduced C4S immunoreactivity more effectively than ARSB. (For immunofluorescent images of sagittal sections, see **Figs. 3a–c**; and see **Fig. 3d** for the quantitative assessment of immunofluorescence intensity of each entire image in **Figs. 3a–c**). A similar result was obtained when immunofluorescent staining was performed with the GAG sulfate antibody CS56, which recognizes both C4S and C6S; both enzymes removed immunoreactivity significantly, but ChaseABC reduced immunoreactivity more efficiently than ARSB when assessed at 6 and 9 weeks after application (**Fig. 4a–f**).

Assessment of Locomotor Function

Two sets of experiments were performed to assess locomotor recovery after spinal cord injury and treatment with ARSB. The first experiment was designed to test whether injection of ARSB would enhance locomotor recovery by 6 weeks, compared to the control, in a moderate compression injury paradigm. Since this trial yielded promising results, we performed a second set of experiments using a severe compression injury paradigm including, for comparison, the bacterial enzyme ChaseABC. To test whether reduction of CS immunoreactivity at and around the lesion site would lead to better functional recovery, we next tested locomotor parameters weekly for 6 and 9 weeks after injury by comparing the vehicle only treated control mice to the enzyme treated mice (**Fig. 5**). The vehicle only treated mice showed spontaneous locomotor recovery within the expected range when scored by the BMS. Both ARSB and ChaseABC improved locomotor recovery, which became significantly different at 6 weeks after enzyme injection for ChaseABC, and at 7 weeks after enzyme injection for ARSB when compared to the control. It is noteworthy that no significant differences could be detected in the extent of locomotor recovery between ARSB and ChaseABC treated mice at the later time points after enzyme injection. In daily inspections of the injured mice, we detected no signs of autophagia or other indications of negative reactions to enzyme treatments.

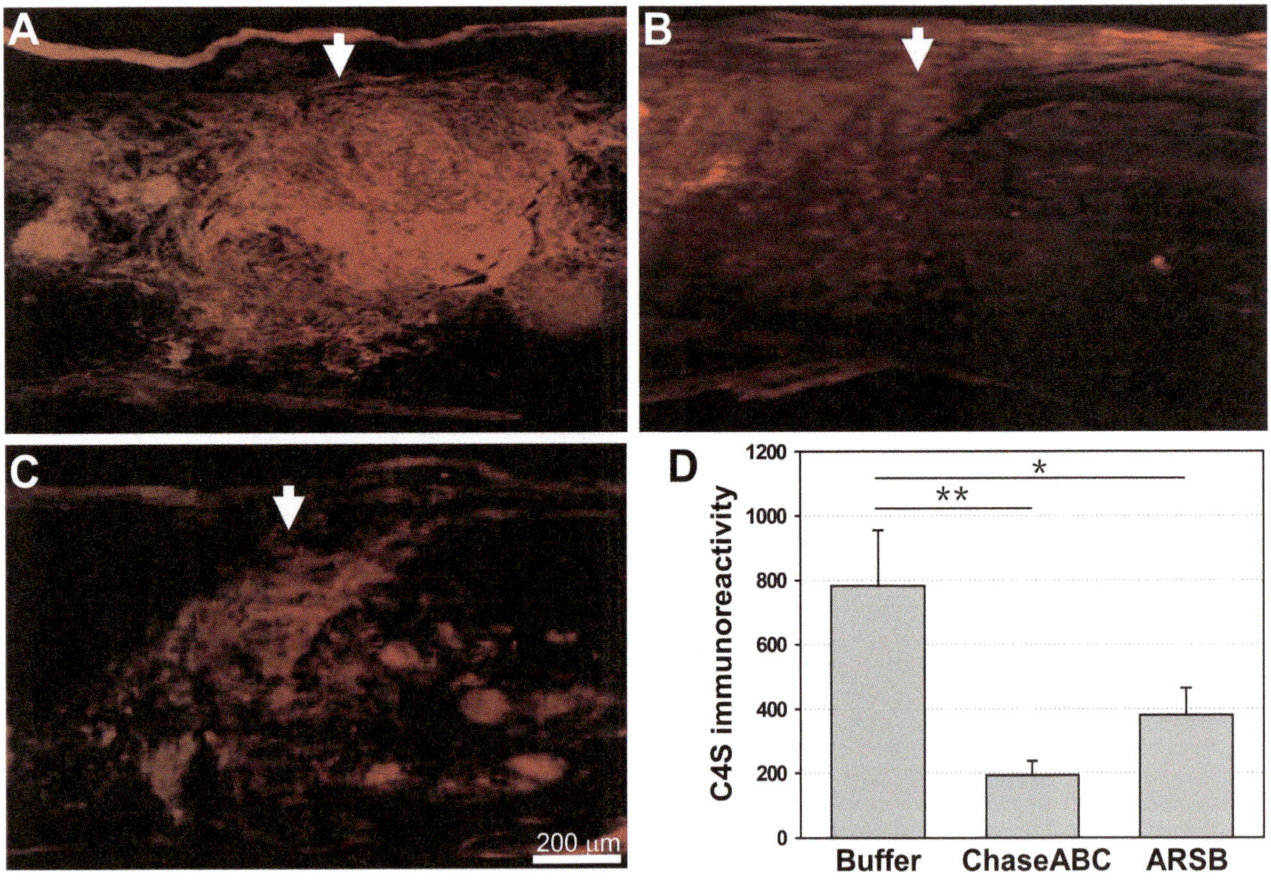

Figure 3. C4S immunoreactivity is reduced at 9 weeks after enzyme injection in severe compression injury. Immediately after spinal cord injury, one µl ChaseABC (10 U/ml), ARSB (10 U/ml) or buffer was injected at the injury site and 0.5 mm rostral and caudal to this site. After 9 weeks, the mice were perfused, and sagittal spinal cord sections were analyzed by immunofluorescence using an antibody specific for C4S. C4S immunoreactivity is more intense at the injury site in the buffer treated control mice (**A**) versus the ChaseABC (**B**) and ARSB (**C**) treated mice. Immunoreactivities of the entire images were quantified above threshold using Image J software (**D**). Mean fluorescence intensities of the area at 0.4 mm equidistant rostral and caudal to the center of the injury site show significantly less C4S immunoreactivity in ChaseABC and ARSB treated mice versus buffer treated control mice. Reduction of immunoreactivity is not significantly different between applications of ChaseABC versus ARSB. Arrows indicate the injury site. Asterisks indicate significant differences between the groups *$p<0.05$ and **$p<0.01$ as assessed by one-way ANOVA followed by Tukey's *post-hoc* analysis. Data represent means ± SEM (n = 4 mice).

Assessment of Glial Scar Size

As the glial scar is considered to be a mechanical and molecular barrier to axonal re-growth/sprouting, the size of the glial scar at the lesion site was investigated using an antibody against GFAP, which detects normal and activated astrocytes. In sagittal sections from spinal cords 6 and 9 weeks after enzyme injections, no differences were detectable between the three groups (**Fig. 6**).

Assessment of Serotonin Expressing Axons

Axons projecting from the brainstem are decisive contributors to locomotor functions when lesions are performed at the thoracic trunk level of the spinal cord. The immunoreactivities and lengths of serotonergic (5-HT) axons extending beyond the caudal margin of the injury site were measured by double immunostaining with 5-HT and neuronal intermediate filament-M (NF-M), 9 weeks after enzyme injection. Mice treated with ChaseABC tended to have more axons extending beyond the lesion site (**Fig. 7**). The difference between the groups of mice that had received either enzyme was not significant, but when compared to the vehicle control, the differences were significant. Mean fluorescent intensity of 5-HT immunoreactive axons penetrating into the caudal margin of the injury site was also higher for the ChaseABC treated mice than for the ARSB (**Fig. 7j**).

Assessment of Tyrosine Hydroxylase Expressing Axons

A different picture emerged when the tyrosine hydroxylase (TH) immunoreactive axons, which also originate from the brainstem, were analyzed (**Fig. 8**) by double immunofluorescent staining with NF-M. Application of either enzyme enhanced the lengths and numbers of TH immunoreactive axons beyond the lesion site 9 weeks after enzyme injection when compared to the control. The difference between the groups of mice that had received either enzyme was significant from one another as well as the vehicle control. Both enzymes showed more TH immunoreactive axons in the injury of caudal area when compared to the control when double immunostained (**Fig. 8c** versus **Fig. 8f** and **Fig. 8i**). Treatment with ARSB led to significantly more TH immunoreactive axons in and beyond the caudal margin of the injury site than treatment with ChaseABC (**Fig. 8j**).

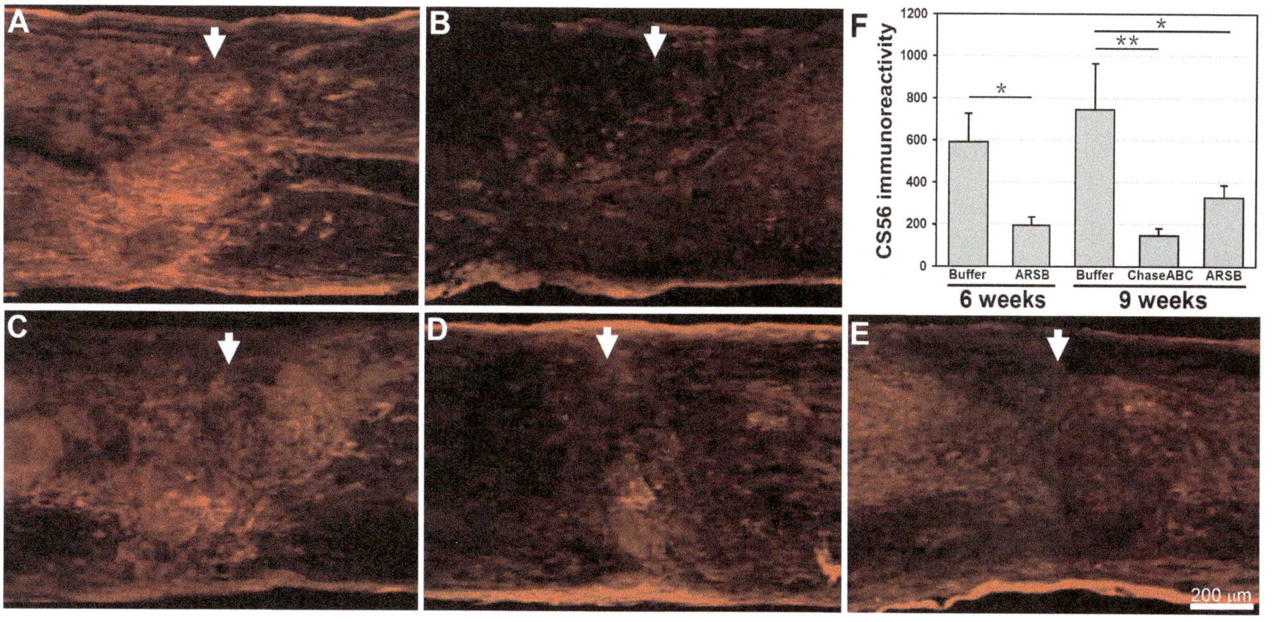

Figure 4. C4S and C6S immunoreactivities are reduced at 6 and 9 weeks after ARSB and ChaseABC treatment. Immediately after moderate (**A,B**) and severe (**C–E**) spinal cord injury, one µl ChaseABC (10 U/ml), ARSB (10 U/ml) or buffer was injected at the injury site and 0.5 mm rostral and caudal to this site. After 6 (**A,B**) and 9 weeks (**C–E**), the mice were perfused, and sagittal spinal cord sections were analyzed by immunofluorescence using the CS56 antibody reacting with C4S and C6S. Immunoreactivity is more intense at the injury site in the buffer treated control mice (**A,C**) versus the ChaseABC (**D**) and ARSB (**B,E**) treated mice. Immunoreactivities of the entire images were quantified above threshold using Image J software (**F**). Mean fluorescence intensities of the area at 0.4 mm equidistant rostral and caudal to the center of the injury site show significantly less expression of CSs in ChaseABC and ARSB treated mice versus buffer treated control mice. Reduction of immunoreactivity is not significantly different between applications of ChaseABC versus ARSB. Arrows indicate the injury site. Asterisks indicate significant differences between the groups $*p<0.05$ (ARSB) and $**p<0.01$ (ChaseABC) as assessed by one-way ANOVA followed by Tukey's *post-hoc* analysis. Data represent means ± SEM, (n = 3 mice).

Assessment of Microglia/Macrophages

Since the immune response is considered to be a major obstacle to the use of the bacterial form of the enzyme, the presence of activated microglia/macrophages was investigated using an antibody to the ionized calcium binding adaptor molecule 1 (Iba1). Iba1 positive microglia/macrophages persisted at the injury

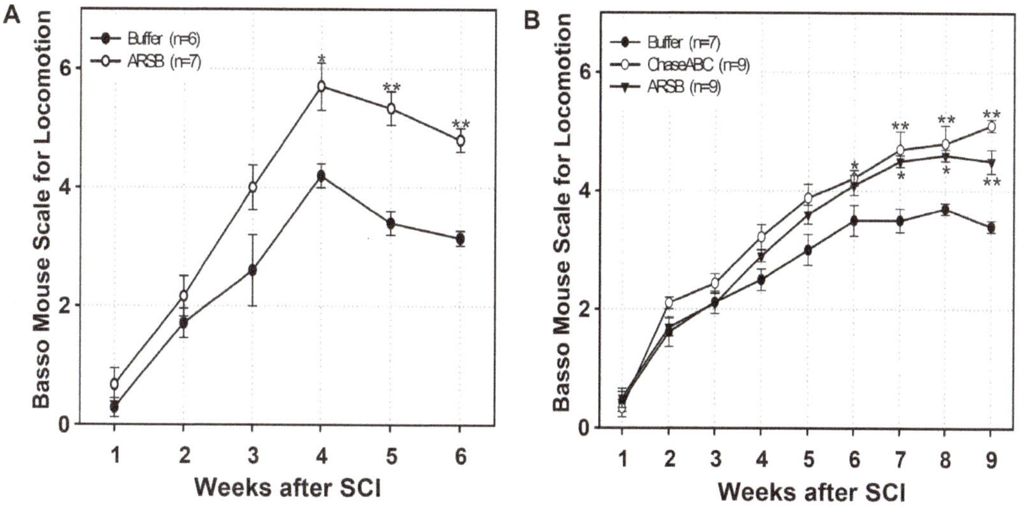

Figure 5. Functional recovery of ChaseABC or ARSB treated mice after moderate (A) and severe (B) compression. One µl ChaseABC (10 U/ml), ARSB (10 U/ml) or buffer was injected at the injury site and 0.5 mm rostral and caudal to this site. The Basso Mouse Scale for analysis of locomotor activity was used to score functional recovery up to 6 (**A**) and 9 (**B**) weeks after moderate and severe spinal cord injury (SCI), respectively. Asterisks indicate significant differences between the enzyme treated groups versus the buffer treated control group at the same time points ($*p<0.05$, $**p<0.01$). No significant difference is detectable between the ChaseABC and ARSB treated groups by one-way ANOVA followed by Tukey's *post-hoc* analysis. Data represent means ± SEM. Number of mice are indicated in brackets.

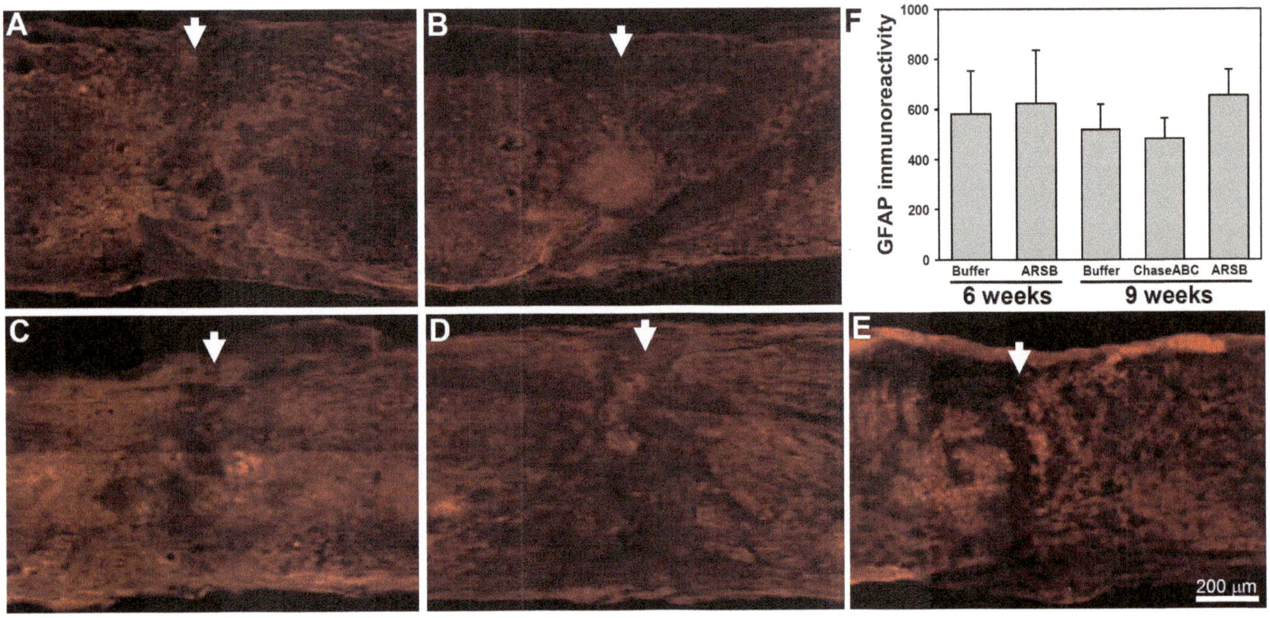

Figure 6. GFAP immunoreactivity is not different at 6 or 9 weeks after enzyme treatment. One µl of the ChaseABC (10 U/ml), ARSB (10 U/ml) or buffer was injected at the injury site and 0.5 mm rostral and caudal to this site after moderate and severe compression injury. After 6 (**A,B**) and 9 weeks (**C–E**), the mice were perfused, and sagittal spinal cord sections were analyzed by immunofluorescence for glial fibrillary acidic protein (GFAP). Photomicrographs show GFAP immunoreactivity at the injury site in the buffer treated control mice (**A,C**) versus ChaseABC (**D**) and ARSB (**B,E**) treated mice. Immunoreactive areas were quantified above threshold using Image J software (**F**). Mean fluorescence intensities of the area at 0.4 mm equidistant rostral and caudal to the center of the injury site are similar in all groups. Arrows indicate the injury site. One-way ANOVA followed by Tukey's *post-hoc* analysis indicates no difference between the groups ($p>0.9$). Data represent means ± SEM ($n=3$ mice).

site in the ChaseABC, but not the ARSB treated group, the latter being more similar to the buffer only control group (**Figs. 9a–c**). At the epicenter of the injury site, Iba1 positive cells can be observed in all treatment groups with significantly more microglia/macrophages detected after application of ChaseABC compared to the control or ARSB groups (**Fig. 9g**). Iba1 positive cells in all treatment groups displayed an "activated" morphology indicated by short, thick processes. However, the ChaseABC treated group had more Iba1 positive cells with amoeboid morphology than the buffer control and ARSB treated animals (**Figs. 9d–f**).

Discussion

Since ARSB would have considerable advantages over ChaseABC for therapeutic use in humans, we tested its performance in a rodent model of spinal cord injury. Indeed, we have demonstrated here that the human enzyme ARSB is more thermostable than the bacterial enzyme ChaseABC, and a one-time injection of ARSB immediately after injury enhanced locomotor recovery after both six weeks moderate and 9 weeks severe compression injury compared with buffer injected control mice. Immunofluorescent analysis suggests that functional effects are mediated by a reduction of C4S expression. Locomotor recovery was similar between mice injected with equal units of ARSB or ChaseABC, and both groups showed enhanced recovery relative to control mice. It is noteworthy that in both sets of experiments, serotonergic (5-HT) and tyrosine hydroxylase (TH) immunoreactive axons were more abundant beyond the injury of caudal area in the groups treated with ARSB and ChaseABC than in the control group. In addition, Iba1 immunoreactivity was significantly higher in the ChaseABC group than in the buffer control and ARSB treated groups at 9 weeks.

Improved Functional Recovery

Many investigators have documented that intraparenchymal ChaseABC injection enhances neurite outgrowth and improves locomotor recovery from the spinal cord injury in rodent paradigms [30–35,49–51]. In our study, we showed that ARSB enhanced locomotor function. Depending on the severity of the lesion, the beneficial effects of enzyme treated group were observed 4 or 7 weeks after moderate and severe cord compression injury, respectively. The first set of experiments treating moderate compression followed by injection of ARSB, revealed significantly better locomotor recovery than control mice at 4 weeks after injury. After severe injury and treatment with equal units of either bacterial ChaseABC or human enzyme ARSB, animals showed functional improvement after approximately 6 weeks, with no significant difference between the enzyme-treated groups. However, both enzyme-treated groups showed significant improvement over buffer-treated control mice. This delay over the first 3 weeks after severe compression injury can be attributed to injury severity, as control mice did not surpass a BMS score of 4. ChaseABC treated mice tended to show slightly, although not significantly better improvement relative to ARSB. This result may be because ChaseABC degrades GAG chain at the C4S and C6S, whereas ARSB degrades C4S without change of GAG chain. If confirmed in further experiments, this observation would raise the question of whether both C4S and C6S contribute to inhibition of neuritogenesis and functional remodeling of perineuronal nets. Like C4S, C6S increases in the spinal cord after injury [20] and inhibits axonal regeneration in cortical brain lesions [21]. However, other studies reported that C4S is neither up-regulated after cortical injury nor inhibitory to dorsal root ganglion axon outgrowth *in vitro*, and suggested C4, 6S (CS-E) is a potentially inhibitory molecule [26]. C6S binding peptides, obtained from

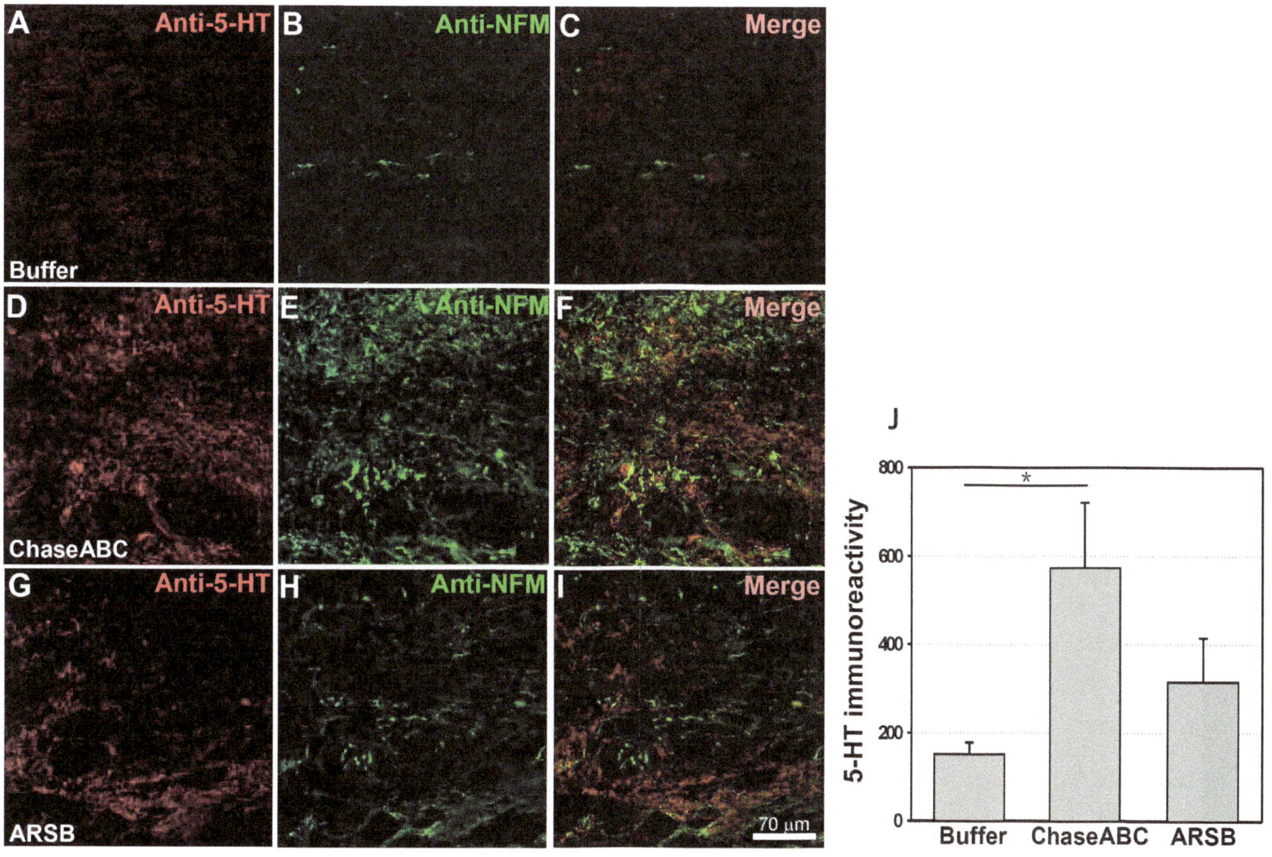

Figure 7. 5-HT immunoreactive axons are more abundant 9 weeks after enzyme treatment than in control mice. One μl ChaseABC (10 U/ml), ARSB (10 U/ml) or buffer was injected at the injury site and 0.5 mm rostral and caudal to this site in mice with severe compression injury. After 9 weeks, the mice were perfused, and sagittal spinal cord sections were analyzed by immunofluorescence. Double immunostaining for serotonin (5-HT) and neurofilament-M (NF-M) shows higher immunoreactivities caudal injury site in the ChaseABC (**D,E,F**) and ARSB (**G,H,I**) treated mice versus buffer treated control mice (**A,B,C**). (**A,D,G**) Immunostainings for 5-HT and (**B,E,H**) NF-M, and (**C,F,I**) merged for 5-HT with NF-M. 5-HT immunoreactive axons are seen beyond the injury site in the ChaseABC and ARSB injected mice. Immunoreactive areas were quantified above threshold using Image J software (**J**). Mean fluorescence intensity of the area between the injury site and 1 mm caudal to it is significantly higher in ChaseABC treated versus buffer treated control mice. Asterisk indicates significant differences between the groups *$p<0.05$ by one-way ANOVA followed by Tukey's *post-hoc* analysis. Data represent means ± SEM, (n = 5 mice).

a peptide phage display library, can block C6S and enhance cortical neurite outgrowth [22,23], suggesting an inhibitory role of C6S for cortical neurons. It is, however, also conceivable that application of ARSB is not as efficient as ChaseABC in changing GAG chain composition and/or that removal of GAG chain of C6S by ChaseABC may allow better access to the C4S specific antibody, thus yielding higher fluorescence intensity levels by immunohistochemistry using specific C4S antibody LY111 [52].

The chemical determination of CS chain structural changes due to ARSB application, in GAGs retrieved from live tissue, is not feasible with presently available methods of CS compositional analysis, since even with the most refined methods practiced in highly specialized laboratories [20,53] the tissue amounts needed would be overwhelming. Recently developed methods for heparan sulfate compositional analysis [54] await adaptation to CS analysis. Even if this method of analysis was available, interpreting the results would be problematic since ARSB, unlike ChaseABC, is not a lyase (chondroitinase), but acts as an exosulfatase [55,56] generating non-reducing end structures that may initiate unknown molecular interactions and signaling events. In fact the sulfation status of CS has been described to trigger several signaling pathways including pleiotrophin and HGF signaling during neuritogenesis [57]. It is noteworthy in this context to mention that addition of chondro-4-sulfatase, which like ARSB preferentially acts as an exo-4-sulfatase, to cultures of neurons in spot assays abolished the axon-repellent action of CS [20]. Analysis of CS structural changes due to ARSB is desirable, but the difficulty in interpreting any results obtained from such analysis is that application of ARSB into the injured tissue most probably leads to additional cellular and molecular consequences that are likely to be indirectly caused by ARSB activity at any time point after injury. In addition, such consequences may involve regulation (expression, release or activation) of endogenous biosynthetic or degradative enzymes as part of feedback mechanisms, in analogy to biosynthetic heparan sulfate remodeling, which has been described as a consequence of extracellular desulfation [58]. It should further be taken into consideration that presently, from the combined reports available, it is not yet clearly resolved which CS sulfation patterns are regeneration prohibitive or promoting. Thus, the aim of the present study was not to characterize the structure of the GAG chains resulting from the action of ARSB, but to determine the possibility to use a clinically approved enzyme in a central nervous system injury animal model.

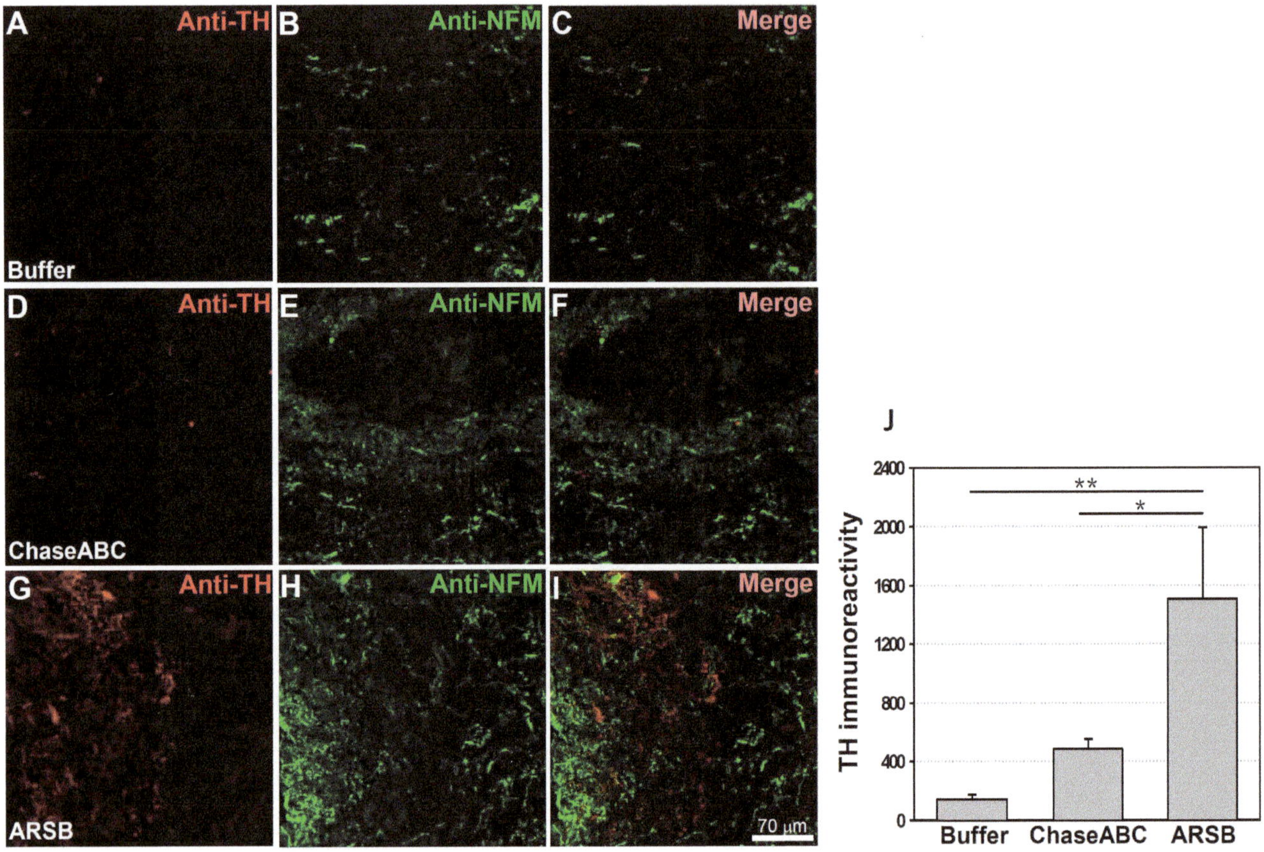

Figure 8. Tyrosine hydroxylase (TH) immunoreactive axons are more abundant 9 weeks after enzyme treatment than in control mice. One μl ChaseABC (10 U/ml), ARSB (10 U/ml) or buffer was injected at the injury site and 0.5 mm rostral and caudal of this site in mice with severe compression injury. After 9 weeks, the mice were perfused, and sagittal spinal cord sections were analyzed by immunofluorescence. Double immunostaining for TH and neurofilament-M (NF-M) shows higher immunoreactivities caudal to the injury site in the ChaseABC (**D,E,F**) and ARSB (**G,H,I**) treated mice versus the buffer treated control mice (**A,B,C**). (**A,D,G**) Immunostainings for TH and (**B,E,H**) NF-M, and (**C,F,I**) merged for TH with NF-M. Immunoreactive areas were quantified above threshold using Image J software (**J**). Mean fluorescence intensity of the area between the injury site and 1 mm caudal to it shows significantly higher immunofluorescence intensity in ARSB versus buffer treated control and ChaseABC treated mice. Asterisks indicate significant differences between the groups $*p<0.05$ and $**p<0.01$ as assessed by one-way ANOVA followed by Tukey's *post-hoc* analysis. Data represent means ± SEM, (n = 4 mice).

Some relationships between CSPGs, ChaseABC, axonal regeneration, and functional recovery are well documented, but the mechanisms of different CSPGs are not well understood. A recent study showed that CSPG production starts after breakdown of the blood brain barrier, mediated by the TGF-β/Smad pathway triggered by blood fibrinogen [59] and various Smad isoforms differentially regulate different CSPGs [60]. The build up of CSPG around the injury site serves as a growth-inhibiting signal for axons, and is also required for infiltrating immune cells to promote healing processes. This was demonstrated by CSPGs interacting with monocytes to stimulate their differentiation to M2 macrophages (anti-inflammatory) that secrete interleukin 10 (IL-10) and matrix metalloproteinase 13 (MMP13) to dissolve CSPGs, and attempt to resolve inflammation [61,62]. Thus, it is clear that CSPGs have differential effects on multiple cell types, and future experiments examining these effects in greater detail should be enlightening.

Glial Scar Formation after Injury

Many investigators have focused on formation of the "glial scar" after spinal cord injury. The "scar" is thought to be both a molecular barrier, via the expression of inhibitory molecules, and physical barrier that prevents axonal re-growth. It is also thought to regulate interactions between central nervous parenchyma and the blood brain barrier, preventing spread of cellular damage and minimizing infection [63]. Previous studies [34,49] have shown that glial scar size did not differ between experimental groups at 6 and 9 weeks after both moderate and severe spinal cord injury. However, quantification of GFAP immunoreactivity in the present study indicated increased astrogliosis after injury, as also reported previously [19,64].

Serotonin- and Tyrosine Hydroxylase-immunoreactive Axons

Serotonergic (5-HT) and tyrosine hydroxylase (TH) immunoreactive neurons are able to regenerate after spinal cord injury (for more recent publications, see papers by Alilain, et al. and Hawthorne, et al.) [65,66]. When 5-HT positive neurons were transplanted into an injured rodent spinal cord, they elongated and integrated into the CNS parenchyma leading to functional recovery [63]. We show here that both types of axons do indeed penetrate into and extend beyond the injury site. However, whereas TH immunoreactive axons extend beyond the lesion site slightly better after application of ARSB than after application of

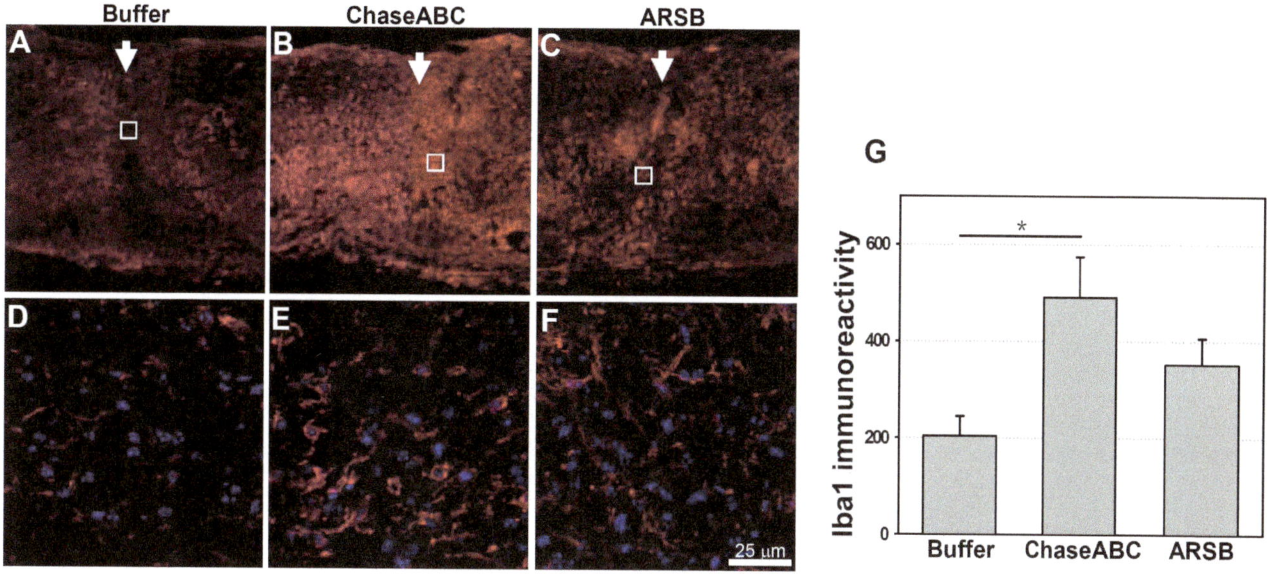

Figure 9. Iba1 immunoreactive microglia/macrophages are more abundant 9 weeks after ChaseABC treatment than in control mice. One µl ChaseABC (10 U/ml), ARSB (10 U/ml) or buffer was injected at the injury site and 0.5 mm rostral and caudal to this site in mice after severe compression. After 9 weeks, the mice were perfused, and sagittal spinal cord sections were analyzed by immunofluorescence. Immunoreactivity for Iba1 is less intense at the injury site in the buffer treated control mice (**A**) versus ChaseABC (**B**) or ARSB (**C**) treated mice. (**D**) (**E**) and (**F**) are higher magnifications of the insets in (**A**) (**B**) and (**C**), respectively, showing more microglia/macrophages with activated, amoeboid morphology in the area between the injury site and 1 mm caudal to it of mice treated with ChaseABC (**E**) or ARSB (**F**) versus the buffer treated control mice (**D**). Immunoreactive areas were quantified above threshold using Image J software (**G**). Mean fluorescence intensities at 0.4 mm equidistant rostral and caudal to the center of the injury site shows significantly higher immunoreactivity for Iba1 in ChaseABC treated mice versus buffer treated control mice. Arrows indicate the injury site. Diamidino-phenylindole (DAPI, blue) was used for nuclear staining and merged with Iba1 immunostaining (**D,E,F**). Asterisk indicates a significant difference between the groups $^*p<0.05$ as assessed by one-way ANOVA followed by Tukey's *post-hoc* analysis. Data represent means ± SEM, (n = 3 mice).

ChaseABC, application of ChaseABC resulted in considerably longer 5-HT axonal lengths 9 weeks after severe compression injury than after application of ARSB. We interpret these results as indicating that 5-HT and TH immunoreactive axons respond differently to the different types of enzyme action on CSs. Yet, in the overall assessment of locomotor function this difference does not appear to play a significant role.

Microglia/Macrophage Response after Enzyme Treatment

A robust and persistent inflammatory response occurs in the spinal cord after injury, with microglia/macrophages playing an important role in pathology and repair. These cells generally exacerbate injury and lead to poor recovery from CNS injury [67,68], but some investigators [64] have found otherwise. In the present study, the ChaseABC treated group differed significantly from vehicle controls and the ARSB treated groups when assayed for Iba1 positive microglia/macrophages (see **Fig. 9**). Interestingly, the ChaseABC group showed a greater number of macrophages with amoeboid morphology, suggesting that there is more active phagocytosis at 9 weeks after injury and treatment with ChaseABC, than with ARSB or control buffer. This difference is possibly due to eliciting a strong microglia/macrophage mediated immune response to the bacterial enzyme or resulting from GAG chain degradation from the extracellular environment of perineuronal net.

Major advantages of ARSB include its long-term stability at physiological temperature and increased enzymatic activity at acidic pH, which are clearly superior to the values for ChaseABC (**Fig. 1**). As local tissue acidification due to CNS injury stimulates ARSB activity, but reduces ChaseABC activity, ARSB is well suited for use in mammals. An additional and equally important advantage of ARSB over ChaseABC is its reduced immunogenicity in the mammalian host. Lastly, we demonstrate that a one-time injection of ARSB is sufficient to promote functional recovery. Taken together, these advantages make ARSB a particularly attractive candidate for treating not only spinal cord injury. In order to unravel the cascade of events finally leading to improved recovery, CSPG degradation as the proposed underlying mechanism will need to be confirmed in future experiments.

Materials and Methods

Production, Purification and Determination of Enzymatic Activity of Human ARSB and Bacterial ChaseABC

ARSB was expressed and purified to homogeneity as described [69]. The enzyme preparation used had a specific activity of 34 U/mg at a protein concentration of 0.35 mg/ml. We determined enzyme activity by using the artificial substrate pNCS (p-nitrocatechol sulfate dipotassium salt; Sigma, St. Louis, MO) following reported protocols [70,71]. Protease-free ChaseABC (Seikagaku, Tokyo, Japan) from Proteus vulgaris was assayed after a modified method [29]. The reaction buffer consisted of 40 mM Tris, 40 mM sodium acetate and 0.01% (w/v) BSA at a pH of 8.0. Briefly, 20 µl of the enzyme solution were added to 100 µl of pre-warmed chondroitin sulfate substrate (Sigma, from shark cartilage, dissolved at a concentration of 4 mg/ml in reaction buffer) in a Greiner UV-Star microplate. The increasing absorbance at 232 nm was assayed continuously for 25 min at 37°C, thus allowing activity calculation from the slope of the time course (absorbance/time). The temperature stability of ChaseABC and human ARSB was assessed at pH 6.0 (in 20 mM MES, 150 mM NaCl) and at pH 6.8 (20 mM MOPS, 150 mM NaCl) by incubating these solutions at 37°C for different times (up to five days, as given in the figure), before measuring enzyme activity at pH 5.5 (ARSB) or pH 8.0 (ChaseABC), as described above.

Animals

Eight-week-old C57BL/6 female mice were purchased from the Charles River Laboratories (Wilmington, MA). All experimental procedures were approved by the Animal Care and Facilities Committee of Rutgers, The State University of New Jersey. The mice were anesthetized with Ketamine-Xylazine (see details below) and subjected to spinal cord compression after a laminectomy. After spinal cord injury, the animals were maintained in the core animal facility at the Division of Life Science and the W.M. Keck Center for Collaborative Neuroscience. After surgery, the mice were kept on a warm mat (35°C) for several hours to prevent hypothermia and were thereafter singly housed in a temperature- and humidity-controlled room with water and standard food provided *ad libitum*. The bladders of the animals were manually voided once or twice daily if the bladder is manually palpable. The animals were euthanized under anesthesia and transcardially perfused with 4% paraformaldehyde to fix the tissues for histological and other analyses.

We performed two sets of experiments. In the first set, 7 mice received moderate compression injury and one intraspinal injection of human ARSB in Tris-buffered saline, pH 7.3 (TBS), the optimal buffer for enzyme stability. An additional 6 mice received TBS as vehicle control. In the second set, 9 mice received ARSB, the bacterial enzyme ChaseABC (Seikagaku, Tokyo, Japan), and 7 mice received TBS vehicle only as control. The mice were assessed for locomotor activity for 6 weeks in the first set and 9 weeks in the second set.

Surgery and Intraspinal Injection

After anaesthetizing the mice with an intraperitoneal injection of Ketamine (160 mg/kg (Butler Schein Animal Health, Chicago, IL) and Xylazine (24 mg/kg, Butler Schein Animal Health, Chicago, IL), 0.1 ml of 0.125% Bupivacaine (Hospira, Inc., Lake Forest, IL) was injected around the incision site to provide local anesthesia. A three cm skin incision along the median line on the back of the animals was made. Laminectomy was performed with Mouse Laminectomy Forceps (Fine Science Tools, Heidelberg, Germany) at the T7–T9 level, followed by a mechanically controlled compression injury using a mouse spinal cord compression device [72–74]. This device contains a pair of watchmaker forceps sterilized by a bead sterilizer, mounted onto a metal block attached to a stereotaxic frame and automated with regard to the force and time of compression by an electromagnetic device. The spinal cord was compressed for 0.5 seconds for the moderate compression injury and 1 second for the severe compression injury by a timed current through the electromagnetic drive. Injections were performed immediately after compression injury by inserting a 33-gauge needle connected to a 5 μl Hamilton syringe (Hamilton, Reno, NV) in a stereotactic micromanipulator (Narishige, New York, NY). ChaseABC, or ARSB (10 units/ml), or the control TBS solution was injected 1 mm deep into the cord midline (1 μl at the lesion center and 1 μl each at sites 0.5 mm rostral and caudal to the lesion center), with each injection lasting for 7 min. After injection, the skin was closed with wound clips.

Locomotor Assessment

We assessed locomotor function by the BMS score [74,75] one week before and every week after injury. For assessment of the BMS, the mice were allowed to move in an open field, 1 meter in diameter, for 5 min. The hindlimb movements were observed and scored according to the BMS scale by two expert and independent observers, blinded to the treatment. Statistical analyses were performed using repeated measures analysis of variance (one-way ANOVA), followed by Tukey's *post-hoc* test. The p values <0.05 were considered statistically significant.

Immunohistology

Animals were anaesthetized with an intraperitoneal injection of Ketamine and Xylazine followed by transcardial perfusion with 4% paraformaldehyde in phosphate-buffered saline, pH 7.3 (PBS), following vascular washout with PBS. After removing the spinal cords and cryoprotecting them by incubation in 20% sucrose solution overnight at 4°C, they were frozen and cut into 20-μm-thick serial, sagittal sections, including tissue rostral and caudal to the lesion site. The sections were mounted on microscope slides and saved at −80°C for immunofluorescent detection. The slides with sections of equivalent distance from the lesion center of each group were thawed to room temperature and then washed three times and blocked with 10% goat serum for 2 h at room temperature. Slides were incubated overnight at 4°C with mouse monoclonal anti-chondroitin sulfate antibody (CS56) (1:200, cat# C8035, Sigma-Aldrich, St. Louis, MO), mouse monoclonal anti-chondroitin-4-sulfate antibody (C4S) (1:100, cat# 270421, Seikagaku, Tokyo, Japan), and rabbit polyclonal antibodies to glial fibrillary acidic protein (GFAP) (1:200, cat# G4546, Sigma-Aldrich, St. Louis, MO), tyrosine hydroxylase (TH) (1:500, cat# AB152, Millipore, Temecula, CA), serotonin (5-HT) (1:400, cat# 10385, Abcam, Cambridge, MA) to Iba1 (1:800, Wako, Osaka, Japan) and to neurofilament-M (NF-M) (1:1000, cat# 13–0700, Invitrogen, Carlsbad, CA). For controls, non-immune mouse IgM and rabbit IgG were used as primary antibodies, which yielded no detectable signals (**Fig. S2**). Slides were washed three times with PBS and incubated with Alexa 555-conjugated goat anti-mouse IgG or Alexa 555-conjugated goat anti-rabbit IgG (1:800, Jackson Immunoresearch, West Grove, PA) for 2 h at room temperature. Sections were then washed with PBS, and some sections were incubated with diamidino-phenylindole (DAPI) for 10 min, rewashed with PBS, mounted with Aqua Poly/Mount medium (Polysciences Inc, Warrington, PA), and tile imaged with an Axiovert200 Fluorescence Live Cell Imaging Workstation (Zeiss).

Quantification of Immunofluorescence

Fluorescence intensities of spinal cord areas immunolabeled for CS56 ($n = 3$), C4S ($n = 4$), GFAP ($n = 3$), TH ($n = 4$), 5-HT ($n = 5$), and Iba1 ($n = 3$) were quantified using four sagittal sections spaced 400 μm apart, per condition. Photographic documentation was performed with the Axiovert200 Fluorescence Live Cell Imaging Workstation (Zeiss), AxioVision software (Zeiss) and Image J software. Both, immunostaining and imaging were performed under identical conditions by an experimenter blinded to the type of treatment. Staining intensity thresholds for each antibody were determined after all images were acquired to optimize the signal-to-noise ratio for each antibody. The threshold selected was 55 (within the full range of intensities extending from 0 to 255) for CS56-immunoreactivity (IR), 55 for C4S-IR, 55 for GFAP-IR, 40 for TH-IR, 40 for 5-HT-IR and 55 for Iba1-IR. The mean fluorescence intensity of the area of IR at 0.4 mm equidistant or 1 mm caudal from the center of the injury site with intensities higher than the thresholds stated above, were measured and normalized to total tissue areas.

Statistical Analysis

All numerical data are presented as group mean values with standard error of the mean (SEM). The statistical significance of BMS score and mean immunoreactivity intensity for each group was estimated by analysis of variance (one-way ANOVA), followed by Tukey's *post-hoc* test. The p values <0.05 were considered statistically significant.

Supporting Information

Figure S1 Chondroitin 4-O-sulfate (C4S) immunoreactivity is reduced by acute injection of ARSB after moderate compression injury. Immediately after spinal cord injury, one µl of ARSB (10 U/ml) was injected at the injury site (arrows) and 0.5 mm rostral and caudal to this site (arrowheads). After 5 days, the mice were perfused, and sagittal spinal cord sections were analyzed by immunofluorescence using an antibody specific for C4S. Except for the meninges, no immunoreactivity is detectable in sham-operated control animals (A). C4S immunoreactivity is higher at the injury site in the buffer-injected control mice (B) versus ARSB-injected mice (C).

Figure S2 Immunoreactivity of IgM and IgG isotype controls from non-immune mice (A) and rabbits (B), respectively. Fluorescence staining in sagittal sections at the injury site (arrow) and at the caudal and rostral injection sites (arrowheads) 9 weeks after control injected group, being less pronounced than the immunoreactivity seen with the specific immune antibodies as shown in **Fig. S1** and **Figs. 2**, **3**, **4**, and **6.**

Acknowledgments

We thank Joanne Tobacman for initial help with the enzyme assay, Eva Westendorf for quality control of ARSB preparations, Hock Ng and Sean O'Leary for animal care and technical assistance, and the Rutgers Animal Care and Facilities Committee for constant advice. We would also like to thank Dr. Wise Young for editorial advice. Melitta Schachner is New Jersey Professor of Spinal Cord Research.

Author Contributions

Conceived and designed the experiments: MY MS. Performed the experiments: MY MK JK BK. Analyzed the data: MY MK BK. Contributed reagents/materials/analysis tools: TD. Wrote the paper: MY MK MS KG.

References

1. Fawcett JW, Asher RA (1999) The glial scar and central nervous system repair. Brain Res Bull 49: 377–391.
2. Raineteau O, Schwab ME (2001) Plasticity of motor systems after incomplete spinal cord injury. Nat Rev Neurosci 2: 263–273.
3. Fehlings MG (2008) Repair of the chronically injured human spinal cord. J Neurosurg Spine 8: 205–206; discussion 206–207.
4. Fitch MT, Silver J (2008) CNS injury, glial scars, and inflammation: Inhibitory extracellular matrices and regeneration failure. Exp Neurol 209: 294–301.
5. McKeon RJ, Jurynec MJ, Buck CR (1999) The chondroitin sulfate proteoglycans neurocan and phosphacan are expressed by reactive astrocytes in the chronic CNS glial scar. J Neurosci 19: 10778–10788.
6. Asher RA, Morgenstern DA, Fidler PS, Adcock KH, Oohira A, et al. (2000) Neurocan is upregulated in injured brain and in cytokine-treated astrocytes. J Neurosci 20: 2427–2438.
7. Jones LL, Margolis RU, Tuszynski MH (2003) The chondroitin sulfate proteoglycans neurocan, brevican, phosphacan, and versican are differentially regulated following spinal cord injury. Exp Neurol 182: 399–411.
8. Brittis PA, Canning DR, Silver J (1992) Chondroitin sulfate as a regulator of neuronal patterning in the retina. Science 255: 733–736.
9. Silver J (1994) Inhibitory molecules in development and regeneration. J Neurol 242: S22–24.
10. Wilson MT, Snow DM (2000) Chondroitin sulfate proteoglycan expression pattern in hippocampal development: potential regulation of axon tract formation. J Comp Neurol 424: 532–546.
11. Cavalcante LA, Garcia-Abreu J, Mendes FA, Moura Neto V, Silva LC, et al. (2003) Sulfated proteoglycans as modulators of neuronal migration and axonal decussation in the developing midbrain. Braz J Med Biol Res 36: 993–1002.
12. Pizzorusso T, Medini P, Berardi N, Chierzi S, Fawcett JW, et al. (2002) Reactivation of ocular dominance plasticity in the adult visual cortex. Science 298: 1248–1251.
13. Deepa SS, Carulli D, Galtrey C, Rhodes K, Fukuda J, et al. (2006) Composition of perineuronal net extracellular matrix in rat brain: a different disaccharide composition for the net-associated proteoglycans. J Biol Chem 281: 17789–17800.
14. Carulli D, Rhodes KE, Fawcett JW (2007) Upregulation of aggrecan, link protein 1, and hyaluronan synthases during formation of perineuronal nets in the rat cerebellum. J Comp Neurol 501: 83–94.
15. Bovolenta P, Wandosell F, Nieto-Sampedro M (1991) Neurite outgrowth over resting and reactive astrocytes. Restor Neurol Neurosci 2: 221–228.
16. Fitch MT, Doller C, Combs CK, Landreth GE, Silver J (1999) Cellular and molecular mechanisms of glial scarring and progressive cavitation: in vivo and in vitro analysis of inflammation-induced secondary injury after CNS trauma. J Neurosci 19: 8182–8198.
17. Morgenstern DA, Asher RA, Fawcett JW (2002) Chondroitin sulphate proteoglycans in the CNS injury response. Prog Brain Res 137: 313–332.
18. Mukhopadhyay G, Doherty P, Walsh FS, Crocker PR, Filbin MT (1994) A novel role for myelin-associated glycoprotein as an inhibitor of axonal regeneration. Neuron 13: 757–767.
19. McKeon RJ, Hoke A, Silver J (1995) Injury-induced proteoglycans inhibit the potential for laminin-mediated axon growth on astrocytic scars. Exp Neurol 136: 32–43.
20. Wang H, Katagiri Y, McCann TE, Unsworth E, Goldsmith P, et al. (2008) Chondroitin-4-sulfation negatively regulates axonal guidance and growth. J Cell Sci 121: 3083–3091.
21. Properzi F, Carulli D, Asher RA, Muir E, Camargo LM, et al. (2005) Chondroitin 6-sulphate synthesis is up-regulated in injured CNS, induced by injury-related cytokines and enhanced in axon-growth inhibitory glia. Eur J Neurosci 21: 378–390.
22. Butterfield KC, Caplan M, Panitch A (2010) Identification and sequence composition characterization of chondroitin sulfate-binding peptides through peptide array screening. Biochemistry 49: 1549–1555.
23. Butterfield KC, Conovaloff A, Caplan M, Panitch A (2010) Chondroitin sulfate-binding peptides block chondroitin 6-sulfate inhibition of cortical neurite growth. Neurosci Lett 478: 82–87.
24. Lin R, Rosahl TW, Whiting PJ, Fawcett JW, Kwok JC (2011) 6-Sulphated chondroitins have a positive influence on axonal regeneration. PLoS One 6: e21499.
25. Liu J, Chau CH, Liu H, Jang BR, Li X, et al. (2006) Upregulation of chondroitin 6-sulphotransferase-1 facilitates Schwann cell migration during axonal growth. J Cell Sci 119: 933–942.
26. Gilbert RJ, McKeon RJ, Darr A, Calabro A, Hascall VC, et al. (2005) CS-4,6 is differentially upregulated in glial scar and is a potent inhibitor of neurite extension. Mol Cell Neurosci 29: 545–558.
27. Karumbaiah L, Anand S, Thazhath R, Zhong Y, McKeon RJ, et al. (2011) Targeted downregulation of N-acetylgalactosamine 4-sulfate 6-O-sulfotransferase significantly mitigates chondroitin sulfate proteoglycan-mediated inhibition. Glia 59: 981–996.
28. Lin R, Kwok JC, Crespo D, Fawcett JW (2008) Chondroitinase ABC has a long-lasting effect on chondroitin sulphate glycosaminoglycan content in the injured rat brain. J Neurochem 104: 400–408.
29. Prabhakar V, Capila I, Bosques CJ, Pojasek K, Sasisekharan R (2005) Chondroitinase ABC I from Proteus vulgaris: cloning, recombinant expression and active site identification. Biochem J 386: 103–112.
30. Yick LW, Cheung PT, So KF, Wu W (2003) Axonal regeneration of Clarke's neurons beyond the spinal cord injury scar after treatment with chondroitinase ABC. Exp Neurol 182: 160–168.
31. Bradbury EJ, Moon LD, Popat RJ, King VR, Bennett GS, et al. (2002) Chondroitinase ABC promotes functional recovery after spinal cord injury. Nature 416: 636–640.
32. Fouad K, Schnell L, Bunge MB, Schwab ME, Liebscher T, et al. (2005) Combining Schwann cell bridges and olfactory-ensheathing glia grafts with chondroitinase promotes locomotor recovery after complete transection of the spinal cord. J Neurosci 25: 1169–1178.
33. Kim BG, Dai HN, Lynskey JV, McAtee M, Bregman BS (2006) Degradation of chondroitin sulfate proteoglycans potentiates transplant-mediated axonal remodeling and functional recovery after spinal cord injury in adult rats. J Comp Neurol 497: 182–198.

34. Karimi-Abdolrezaee S, Eftekharpour E, Wang J, Schut D, Fehlings MG (2010) Synergistic effects of transplanted adult neural stem/progenitor cells, chondroitinase, and growth factors promote functional repair and plasticity of the chronically injured spinal cord. J Neurosci 30: 1657–1676.
35. Garcia-Alias G, Lin R, Akrimi SF, Story D, Bradbury EJ, et al. (2008) Therapeutic time window for the application of chondroitinase ABC after spinal cord injury. Exp Neurol 210: 331–338.
36. Vink R, McIntosh TK, Weiner MW, Faden AI (1987) Effects of traumatic brain injury on cerebral high-energy phosphates and pH: a 31P magnetic resonance spectroscopy study. J Cereb Blood Flow Metab 7: 563–571.
37. Huang PP, Young W (1994) The effects of arterial blood gas values on lesion volumes in a graded rat spinal cord contusion model. J Neurotrauma 11: 547–562.
38. Xiong ZG, Zhu XM, Chu XP, Minami M, Hey J, et al. (2004) Neuroprotection in ischemia: blocking calcium-permeable acid-sensing ion channels. Cell 118: 687–698.
39. Hamai A, Hashimoto N, Mochizuki H, Kato F, Makiguchi Y, et al. (1997) Two distinct chondroitin sulfate ABC lyases. An endoeliminase yielding tetrasaccharides and an exoeliminase preferentially acting on oligosaccharides. J Biol Chem 272: 9123–9130.
40. Prabhakar V, Capila I, Soundararajan V, Raman R, Sasisekharan R (2009) Recombinant expression, purification, and biochemical characterization of chondroitinase ABC II from Proteus vulgaris. J Biol Chem 284: 974–982.
41. Koshiishi I, Takenouchi M, Hasegawa T, Imanari T (1998) Enzymatic method for the simultaneous determination of hyaluronan and chondroitin sulfates using high-performance liquid chromatography. Anal Biochem 265: 49–54.
42. Tester NJ, Plaas AH, Howland DR (2007) Effect of body temperature on chondroitinase ABC's ability to cleave chondroitin sulfate glycosaminoglycans. J Neurosci Res 85: 1110–1118.
43. Lee H, McKeon RJ, Bellamkonda RV (2010) Sustained delivery of thermostabilized chABC enhances axonal sprouting and functional recovery after spinal cord injury. Proc Natl Acad Sci U S A 107: 3340–3345.
44. Wasserman SI, Austen KF (1976) Arylsulfatase B of human lung. Isolation, characterization, and interaction with slow-reacting substance of anaphylaxis. J Clin Invest 57: 738–744.
45. Munoz-Rojas MV, Horovitz DD, Jardim LB, Raymundo M, Llerena JC, Jr., et al. (2010) Intrathecal administration of recombinant human N-acetylgalactosamine 4-sulfatase to a MPS VI patient with pachymeningitis cervicalis. Mol Genet Metab 99: 346–350.
46. Harmatz P, Ketteridge D, Giugliani R, Guffon N, Teles EL, et al. (2005) Direct comparison of measures of endurance, mobility, and joint function during enzyme-replacement therapy of mucopolysaccharidosis VI (Maroteaux-Lamy syndrome): results after 48 weeks in a phase 2 open-label clinical study of recombinant human N-acetylgalactosamine 4-sulfatase. Pediatrics 115: e681–689.
47. Harmatz P, Whitley CB, Waber L, Pais R, Steiner R, et al. (2004) Enzyme replacement therapy in mucopolysaccharidosis VI (Maroteaux-Lamy syndrome). J Pediatr 144: 574–580.
48. Mitsunaga-Nakatsubo K, Kusunoki S, Kawakami H, Akasaka K, Akimoto Y (2009) Cell-surface arylsulfatase A and B on sinusoidal endothelial cells, hepatocytes, and Kupffer cells in mammalian livers. Med Mol Morphol 42: 63–69.
49. Iseda T, Okuda T, Kane-Goldsmith N, Mathew M, Ahmed S, et al. (2008) Single, high-dose intraspinal injection of chondroitinase reduces glycosaminoglycans in injured spinal cord and promotes corticospinal axonal regrowth after hemisection but not contusion. J Neurotrauma 25: 334–349.
50. Caggiano AO, Zimber MP, Ganguly A, Blight AR, Gruskin EA (2005) Chondroitinase ABCI improves locomotion and bladder function following contusion injury of the rat spinal cord. J Neurotrauma 22: 226–239.
51. Huang WC, Kuo WC, Cherng JH, Hsu SH, Chen PR, et al. (2006) Chondroitinase ABC promotes axonal re-growth and behavior recovery in spinal cord injury. Biochem Biophys Res Commun 349: 963–968.
52. Deepa SS, Yamada S, Fukui S, Sugahara K (2007) Structural determination of novel sulfated octasaccharides isolated from chondroitin sulfate of shark cartilage and their application for characterizing monoclonal antibody epitopes. Glycobiology 17: 631–645.
53. Yi JH, Katagiri Y, Susarla B, Figge D, Symes AJ, et al. (2012) Alterations in sulfated chondroitin glycosaminoglycans following controlled cortical impact injury in mice. J Comp Neurol 520: 3295–3313.
54. Skidmore MA, Guimond SE, Dumax-Vorzet AF, Yates EA, Turnbull JE (2010) Disaccharide compositional analysis of heparan sulfate and heparin polysaccharides using UV or high-sensitivity fluorescence (BODIPY) detection. Nat Protoc 5: 1983–1992.
55. Gorham SD, Cantz M (1978) Arylsulphatase B, an exo-sulphatase for chondroitin 4-sulphate tetrasaccharide. Hoppe Seylers Z Physiol Chem 359: 1811–1814.
56. Anson DS, Taylor JA, Bielicki J, Harper GS, Peters C, et al. (1992) Correction of human mucopolysaccharidosis type-VI fibroblasts with recombinant N-acetylgalactosamine-4-sulphatase. Biochem J 284 (Pt 3): 789–794.
57. Li F, Shetty AK, Sugahara K (2007) Neuritogenic activity of chondroitin/dermatan sulfate hybrid chains of embryonic pig brain and their mimicry from shark liver. Involvement of the pleiotrophin and hepatocyte growth factor signaling pathways. J Biol Chem 282: 2956–2966.
58. Lamanna WC, Frese MA, Balleininger M, Dierks T (2008) Sulf loss influences N-, 2-O-, and 6-O-sulfation of multiple heparan sulfate proteoglycans and modulates fibroblast growth factor signaling. J Biol Chem 283: 27724–27735.
59. Schachtrup C, Ryu JK, Helmrick MJ, Vagena E, Galanakis DK, et al. (2010) Fibrinogen triggers astrocyte scar formation by promoting the availability of active TGF-beta after vascular damage. J Neurosci 30: 5843–5854.
60. Susarla BT, Laing ED, Yu P, Katagiri Y, Geller HM, et al. (2011) Smad proteins differentially regulate transforming growth factor-beta-mediated induction of chondroitin sulfate proteoglycans. J Neurochem 119: 868–878.
61. Kigerl KA, Gensel JC, Ankeny DP, Alexander JK, Donnelly DJ, et al. (2009) Identification of two distinct macrophage subsets with divergent effects causing either neurotoxicity or regeneration in the injured mouse spinal cord. J Neurosci 29: 13435–13444.
62. Shechter R, Raposo C, London A, Sagi I, Schwartz M (2011) The glial scar-monocyte interplay: a pivotal resolution phase in spinal cord repair. PLoS One 6: e27969.
63. Bradbury EJ, Carter LM (2011) Manipulating the glial scar: chondroitinase ABC as a therapy for spinal cord injury. Brain Res Bull 84: 306–316.
64. Rolls A, Shechter R, Schwartz M (2009) The bright side of the glial scar in CNS repair. Nat Rev Neurosci 10: 235–241.
65. Alilain WJ, Horn KP, Hu H, Dick TE, Silver J (2011) Functional regeneration of respiratory pathways after spinal cord injury. Nature 475: 196–200.
66. Hawthorne AL, Hu H, Kundu B, Steinmetz MP, Wylie CJ, et al. (2011) The unusual response of serotonergic neurons after CNS Injury: lack of axonal dieback and enhanced sprouting within the inhibitory environment of the glial scar. J Neurosci 31: 5605–5616.
67. Giulian D, Robertson C (1990) Inhibition of mononuclear phagocytes reduces ischemic injury in the spinal cord. Ann Neurol 27: 33–42.
68. Popovich PG, Guan Z, Wei P, Huitinga I, van Rooijen N, et al. (1999) Depletion of hematogenous macrophages promotes partial hindlimb recovery and neuroanatomical repair after experimental spinal cord injury. Exp Neurol 158: 351–365.
69. Dierks T, Lecca MR, Schmidt B, von Figura K (1998) Conversion of cysteine to formylglycine in eukaryotic sulfatases occurs by a common mechanism in the endoplasmic reticulum. FEBS Lett 423: 61–65.
70. Porter MT, Fluharty AL, Kihara H (1969) Metachromatic leukodystrophy: arylsulfatase-A deficiency in skin fibroblast cultures. Proc Natl Acad Sci U S A 62: 887–891.
71. Knaust A, Schmidt B, Dierks T, von Bulow R, von Figura K (1998) Residues critical for formylglycine formation and/or catalytic activity of arylsulfatase A. Biochemistry 37: 13941–13946.
72. Curtis R, Green D, Lindsay RM, Wilkin GP (1993) Up-regulation of GAP-43 and growth of axons in rat spinal cord after compression injury. J Neurocytol 22: 51–64.
73. Steward O, Zheng B, Tessier-Lavigne M (2003) False resurrections: distinguishing regenerated from spared axons in the injured central nervous system. J Comp Neurol 459: 1–8.
74. Apostolova I, Irintchev A, Schachner M (2006) Tenascin-R restricts posttraumatic remodeling of motoneuron innervation and functional recovery after spinal cord injury in adult mice. J Neurosci 26: 7849–7859.
75. Basso DM, Fisher LC, Anderson AJ, Jakeman LB, McTigue DM, et al. (2006) Basso Mouse Scale for locomotion detects differences in recovery after spinal cord injury in five common mouse strains. J Neurotrauma 23: 635–659.

14

Reduced Inflammatory Phenotype in Microglia Derived from Neonatal Rat Spinal Cord versus Brain

Sam Joshva Baskar Jesudasan[1,2], Kathryn G. Todd[1,2], Ian R. Winship[1,2]*

1 Centre for Neuroscience, University of Alberta, Edmonton, Alberta, Canada, **2** Neurochemical Research Unit, Department of Psychiatry, University of Alberta, Edmonton, Alberta, Canada

Abstract

Microglia are the primary immune cells of the central nervous system (CNS). Membrane bound sensors on their processes monitor the extracellular environment and respond to perturbations of the CNS such as injury or infection. Once activated, microglia play a crucial role in determining neuronal survival. Recent studies suggest that microglial functional response properties vary across different regions of the CNS. However, the activation profiles of microglia derived from the spinal cord have not been evaluated against brain microglia in vitro. Here, we studied the morphological properties and secretion of inflammatory and trophic effectors by microglia derived from the brain or spinal cord of neonatal rats under basal culture conditions and after activation with lipopolysaccharide (LPS). Our results demonstrate that spinal microglia assume a less inflammatory phenotype after LPS activation, with reduced release of the inflammatory effectors tumor necrosis factor alpha, interleukin-1 beta, and nitric oxide, a less amoeboid morphology, and reduced phagocytosis relative to brain-derived microglia. Phenotypic differences between brain and spinal microglia are an important consideration when evaluating anti-inflammatory or immunomodulatory therapies for brain versus spinal injury.

Editor: Martin Stangel, Hannover Medical School, Germany

Funding: This research is funded by Alberta Innovates Health Solutions [IRW], the Heart and Stroke Foundation of Canada [IRW], the Natural Science and Engineering Research Council [IRW], Canadian Institutes of Health Research [KGT, IRW] and George and Dorthy Davey Endowment Fund for Brain Injury Research [KGT]. The funders had no role in study design, data collection and analysis, decision to publish, or preparation of the manuscript.

Competing Interests: The authors have declared that no competing interests exist.

* E-mail: iwinship@ualberta.ca

Introduction

Microglia are a unique population of cells in the central nervous system (CNS), constituting 5 to 15% of its total cell population, and were first identified by Rio-Hortega in 1932 [1–3]. As the resident immune cells of the brain and spinal cord, microglia are the front line of defense against invading pathogens and CNS injury [3]. In basal physiological conditions (i.e. prior to injury or activation), microglia have ramified morphology with long processes that monitor the extracellular environment surrounding the cells of the CNS [4]. After brain trauma or infection, microglia become activated and withdraw their processes to assume amoeboid and spherical morphologies [5]. Amoeboid microglia are capable of secreting anti-inflammatory factors, pro-inflammatory factors, prostaglandins, cytokines and reactive oxygen species [5–7]. These microglial effectors interact with surrounding neurons and other glial cells and can initiate trophic as well as toxic signaling pathways [5–7]. Upon further activation, microglia assume a spherical morphology and become predominantly phagocytic, acting to clear the CNS of dying cells and other debris [5–7].

Investigations of the role of microglia in CNS injury such as stroke demonstrate that the microglial response to injury is complex [8–13]. After injury to the brain, pro-inflammatory effectors such as nitric oxide (NO), tumor necrosis factor- alpha (TNF-α), interleukin-6 (IL-6) and IL-1 beta (IL-1β) are up-regulated within 24 hours and contribute to both neurotrophic and neurotoxic pathways [8–13]. Similarly, there is an acute increase in TNF-α, IL-1β and IL-6 in the spinal cord after spinal cord injury that contributes to cell death and lesion expansion [14,15]. As a major source for TNF-α, IL-1β, IL-6, and trophic factors including brain derived neurotrophic factor (BDNF), microglia are major contributors to increased levels of these cytokines after CNS injuries [6,12–14,16–22]. The consequences of altering the microglial response to injury are difficult to predict, as microglial effectors can have both trophic and toxic consequences after injury [6,12–14,16–22]. Nonetheless, several studies have examined the functional response profiles of microglia upon activation to define their secretory profile and morphological response to brain injury or infection [6,12–14,16–22].

Most studies investigating the functional activation profiles of microglia are done in brain microglia cultures (BM). Data from these studies have confirmed that microglia can secrete a wide variety of cytokines, with the amount and type of effector released varying with the nature of the activating stimulus. Activation with lipopolysaccharide (LPS) increases the release of TNF-α, IL-1β, IL-6 and nitric oxide (NO) in neonatal BM [18,23]. Recently, it was demonstrated *in vitro* that BM exposed to conditioned media collected from neurons subjected to moderate hypoxic injury were neuroprotective, but BM exposed to media collected from neurons subjected to severe hypoxic injury were neurotoxic [6]. These results and data showing severity dependent expression of cytokines by spinal microglia after spinal cord injury suggest that functional microglial response properties are dependent on the severity of neuronal injury [6,14].

In addition to a differential response to injury severity, microglia isolated from distinct regions of the brain have different effects on cell survival [18]. For example, activated microglia from cortex and hippocampus exhibit a neurotoxic profile relative to microglia from brainstem, striatum and thalamus [18]. TNF-α release by the microglia from cortex and hippocampus is significantly higher than that of other brain regions after activation with adenosine triphosphate [18]. Despite the observation that microglial effector profiles vary between regions in the brain, and the interest in understanding the role of microglia after spinal injury, very few studies have investigated activation profiles of microglia derived from the spinal cord (SCM) in culture [17,19]. In this study, we sought to characterize the morphological and secretory response profiles to an activating stimulus in SCM as compared to BM. To facilitate comparison, SCM and BM cultures were established from the same neonatal rat pups using a mild trypsinization protocol [24]. The primary microglia cultures were activated with the bacterial endotoxin lipopolysaccharide (LPS), an established and well-characterized activator of microglia [12,25–27]. The differences in the activation pattern of SCM and BM were then gauged by characterizing microglial morphology, cytokine release, nitric oxide release, and phagocytosis.

Materials and Methods

All animal protocols were conducted in accordance with Canadian Council on Animal Care Guidelines and approved by the Animal Care and Use Committee: Health Sciences for the University of Alberta.

Primary brain and spinal cord microglia cultures

Mixed glia cultures were prepared from brain and spinal cord of post-natal Day 1 Sprague-Dawley rats [6,28]. The meninges and blood vessels were removed from the brains and spinal cords, then tissue was finely minced and dissociated enzymatically by 0.25% Trypsin-EDTA for 20 minutes at 37°C. Trypsin was inactivated with Dulbecco Modified Eagle Medium/Ham's F12 (DMEM/F12; Gibco) containing 10% Fetal Bovine Serum (FBS; Gibco) and 2% Penicillin/Streptomycin (P/S; Gibco). The brain and spinal cord tissues were triturated mechanically in DMEM/F12 in 10% FBS+2% P/S and plated on poly-L-lysine coated 12 well plates at 1.7×10^7 cell/ml.

After 14–21 days *in vitro* (DIV), microglia were isolated by mild trypsinization [24]. Briefly, 0.25% Trypsin-EDTA was diluted in 1:3 ratio in DMEM/F12+2% P/S media was added to brain/spinal mixed primary culture and was incubated at 37°C in humidified 5% CO2 incubator for 20–50 mins. After aspirating out the diluted Trypsin-EDTA, DMEM/F12 with 10% FBS+2% P/S was added to the isolated microglia in the culture dish to inactivate trypsin and the culture dish was maintained at 37°C for 5 min. DMEM/F12 with 10% FBS was removed after 5 minutes and DMEM/F12 containing 2% P/S was added to the isolated brain microglia (BM) and spinal cord microglia (SCM). Isolated BM and SCM were allowed to recover in DMEM/F12 containing 2% P/S overnight prior to any treatment. For LPS activation, BM and SCM were treated with 1 µg/ml (final concentration in media) LPS for 24 hours. 24 hours after the LPS treatment the media from BM and SCM were assayed either for pro- and anti-inflammatory effectors released in the media, phagocytic activity or fixed with 10% formalin for morphometric analysis.

Immunocytochemistry

Immunocytochemistry was used to confirm culture purity and quantify microglia. Isolated brain and spinal microglia cultures were washed three times with phosphate buffered saline (PBS) and fixed with 10% formalin for 20 minutes. After three washes with PBS the cultured cells were permeabilized and blocked for 40 minutes with 0.1% Triton X-100 and 10% normal horse serum. Iba1 (ionized calcium binding adaptor molecule 1), a marker for microglia, was used to identify SCM and BM. Isolated brain and spinal microglia were incubated with a rabbit anti-Iba1 primary antibody (1:1000, Wako) at 4°C overnight. For immunofluorescent visualization of culture purity, the cultures dishes were then washed three times with PBS and incubated with an anti-rabbit Alexa 647 secondary antibody (1:200) for 1 hour at room temperature. After three washes, DAPI (4′, 6-diamidino-2-phenylindole in vectasheild mounting medium) was applied and a cover slip was mounted on top of cells. Negative controls without primary antibody were performed to rule out non-specific labeling by the secondary antibody. Epifluorescent images were acquired using Leica DMI 6000B microscope mounted with Leica DFC365 FX monochrome camera at 20X.

Microglia number was quantified by counting DAB (3,3′-Diaminobenzidine) positive cells. The procedure is similar to fluorescent immunocytochemistry up to the primary antibody incubation. After overnight incubation with primary antibody (rabbit anti-Iba1, 1:1000), the cultures were washed three times with PBS and labeled with a secondary antibody, biotinylated donkey anti-rabbit IgG (Santa Cruz, 1:200) for 1 hour at room temperature. After three washes the cultures were incubated with avidin-biotin complex (ABC staining kit, Thermo Scientific) for 30 minutes at room temperature. DAB was prepared in PBS containing 3% H_2O_2 and cultures were treated according to manufacturer protocols. Iba1 immunopositive cells after DAB visualization were counted in a field area of 0.785 mm^2 under 20x magnification and bright field illumination. Average SCM and BM counts (in four independent experiments) were determined from the average count in six such field areas in each of four wells of a 12 well culture plate. The total number of Iba1 immunopositive cells per well was counted using the following formula,

$$\begin{aligned}&Total\ number\ of\ SCM\ per\ well\\&=Average\ SCM\ counts\ per\ 0.785mm^2 X\ 483\end{aligned}$$

where 483 times the area of a field view is the total surface area of a single well in a 12 well culture dish. An unbiased observer verified SCM counts.

For morphology analysis, control and LPS activated Iba1 labeled microglia were counted from 6 fields acquired from three independent experiments. The images were acquired with DMI6000B Leica inverted microscope mounted with Leica DFC365 FX monochrome camera.

Nitric Oxide (NO) assay

NO in the media was assessed indirectly via its stable metabolite nitrite. 1 ml of media was collected after 24 hours after treatment or no treatment control. 100 µL of LPS treated or no treatment control media was added per well of 96-wellplate with 2 replicates per condition. 50 µL of 1% sulfanilamide (in 3 M HCl) was then added to the wells, followed by the equal volumes of 0.02% N-naphthylethylenediamine. The final mixture was read on a microplate reader at 540 nm (Molecular Devices SpectraMax M5).

Enzyme Linked Immunosorbent assays (ELISA)

A commercial ELISA kit was used to measure IL-1β and IL-6 in media (DuoSet, R&D Systems Minneapolis, USA)). ELISA procedures were carried out according to manufacturer protocols. For brain-derived neurotrophic factor (BDNF) ELISA, a competitive ELISA protocol was used. In brief, media and recombinant BDNF standards diluted in phosphate-buffered saline (PBS) were mixed 1:1 with goat anti BDNF (1:500, Santa Cruz, Texas, USA) and incubated with 96-well plates in the cold room overnight. This mixture was aspirated following incubation and the plates were washed three times with PBS. The plates were then blocked with the ELISA diluent (1% bovine serum albumin in PBS) for 1 h. After blocking, the plates were washed 3 times with PBS and incubated with anti goat IgG antibody conjugated to horseradish peroxidase (1:2000 in ELISA diluent, Santa Cruz, Texas, USA) for 30 min. The chromagen tetramethylbenzidine (Sigma, 0.027% in 0.82% sodium acetate, 0.36% citric acid and 40% methanol) was added to develop color. Upon development of the chromagen, 1.8 N sulfuric acid was added to stop the reaction, and the plates were read on microplate reader at 450 nm (Molecular Devices SpectraMax M5). All procedures were carried out at room temperature unless otherwise specified.

Multiplex bead based immunoassays for cytokines

Rat TNFα and IL-10 were quantified using BD Cytometric Bead Array kit (BD Biosciences, New Jersey, USA). Samples were prepared according to manufactures protocol. Briefly, 50 μL of control or LPS treated microglia culture media was added to 50 μL of multiplex capture beads (TNF-α, IL-10) in a v-bottom 96 well plate. The v-bottom 96 well plate was placed in an orbital shaker for 5 min at 500 rpm and then incubated at room temperature for 1 hr. 50 μL of phycoerythrin detection reagent was added to each sample in v-bottom 96 well plate and placed in an orbital shaker for 5 min at 500 rpm. The plate was then incubated at room temperature for 2 hr. The v-bottom 96 well plate was then centrifuged at 2000 g and supernatant was aspirated out. The multiplex capture beads in v-bottom 96 well plates were re-suspended in 150 μL of wash buffer and placed in a orbital shaker for 5 min at 500 rpm. The multiplex capture bead in wash buffer where then analyzed by BD FACSCantoII flow cytometer. Data analysis was done using FCAP Array software from BD Biosciences.

Phagocytosis Assay

Phagocytosis was measured using a fluorescent bead uptake assay [29]. Briefly, microglia were activated for 24 hours with LPS (1 μg/ml) and 2.5×10^6 carboxylate-modified 1 μm beads (per well, Sigma, Missouri, USA) were added to the LPS activated or control microglia for an hour. After incubation with these beads, the cells were washed with Hank's Balanced Salt Solution to wash away beads that were not phagocytized. BM and SCM were lysed in 1% Triton-X detergent and lysate was transferred to 96-well plate. Fluorescence emitted by cell lysate was measured using a microplate reader (Molecular Devices SpectraMax M5). The excitation and emission spectra of plate reader were set to 470 nm and 505 nm respectively. Negative controls were treated as above with the exception that cells with beads were maintained at 4 degrees Celsius.

Statistical Analysis

Results are represented as percentage of total population (morphology analyses), raw values normalized to total protein (NO, cytokines and trophic factors), and percentage over relative control (phagocytosis assay) ± standard error of mean. One-way ANOVA was used to determine main effect of treatment on BM and SCM followed by Newman-Keuls post hoc to test for significance between treatment groups. One-sample t-tests were performed to analyse significant changes in phagocytic activity between treatments and controls (as phagocytosis was normalized to control levels). n represents a single independent experiment (i.e an independent culture preparation) with a minimum of three technical replicates. Each technical replicate is a well in a 12 well culture plate, except for morphology studies where n represents a single well of an independent experiment. * represents $p<0.05$. All statistical analyses were done using Graphpad Prism version 5.

Results

Spinal cord microglia can be isolated by mild trypsinization

Mild trypsinization has been used successfully to isolate BM from neonatal mice [24], but its efficacy in isolating SCM had not been determined. To determine if mild trypsinization can isolate SCM from neonatal rat primary mixed glial populations, we applied 0.08% Trypsin-EDTA to 2–3 wk old primary mixed glial cultures derived from brain and spinal cord. The optimal incubation time required to isolate SCM was determined from mild trypsiniation durations of 20 min, 30 min, 40 min and 50 min. Twenty min of mild trypsiniztion produced the highest yield of SCM (Fig. 1A, B). SCM count decreased with increased duration in trypsin and at 40 min there was nearly a 60% loss of SCM compared to 20 min time point. The purity of BM and SCM cultures were assessed by immune labeling against Iba1 (a microglia/macrophage marker) and was found to be ≥95% for BM and SCM ($n=3$ independent experiments, see Fig.1A representative micrograph of SCM and BM).

Morphology of BM and SCM on activation with LPS (lipopolysacharide)

Lipopolysaccharide (LPS) is an endotoxin from gram-negative bacteria commonly used to activate immune cells. To evaluate if SCM and BM assume different morphology after activation, microglia were incubated overnight in 1 ug/ml LPS in media (DMEM with 2% P/S) for 24 hours. Ramified, amoeboid, and spherical morphological states were apparent in control (media alone) and activated microglia cultures from brain and spinal cord. Consistent with previous studies [6], morphological status was assigned based on the number of microglia processes: Microglia that have more than two primary processes (processes that are stemming from cell body of microglia are considered primary) were considered ramified, those with one process were considered amoeboid and those with no process extension were considered spherical. A significant effect of treatment group (BM control, BM LPS, SCM control, SCM LPS) was observed for the percentage of amoeboid and spherical morphologies ($F_{(3,8)}=14.32$ $p=0.0014$, $F_{(3,8)}=8.125$ $p=0.0082$, respectively), while a main effect on percentage of ramified microglia of BM and SCM narrowly missed statistical criterion for significance ($F_{(3,8)}=3.893$ $p=0.0551$) (Figure 2). Newman-Keuls post-hoc tests showed that LPS induced a significant increase in spherical morphology in BM (Fig. 2C, LPS 55.27%±4.12 vs. Control 27.99%±9.15, respectively $p<0.05$) and SCM (Fig. 2. LPS 60.72%±6.88 vs Control 28.27%±0.80 $p<0.05$), but the percentage of spherical microglia in basal or LPS-activated states was not significantly different between BM and SCM. Interestingly, LPS induced significantly less amoeboid morphology in SCM compared to SCM control microglia as well as LPS-activated BM (Fig.2B, SCM LPS

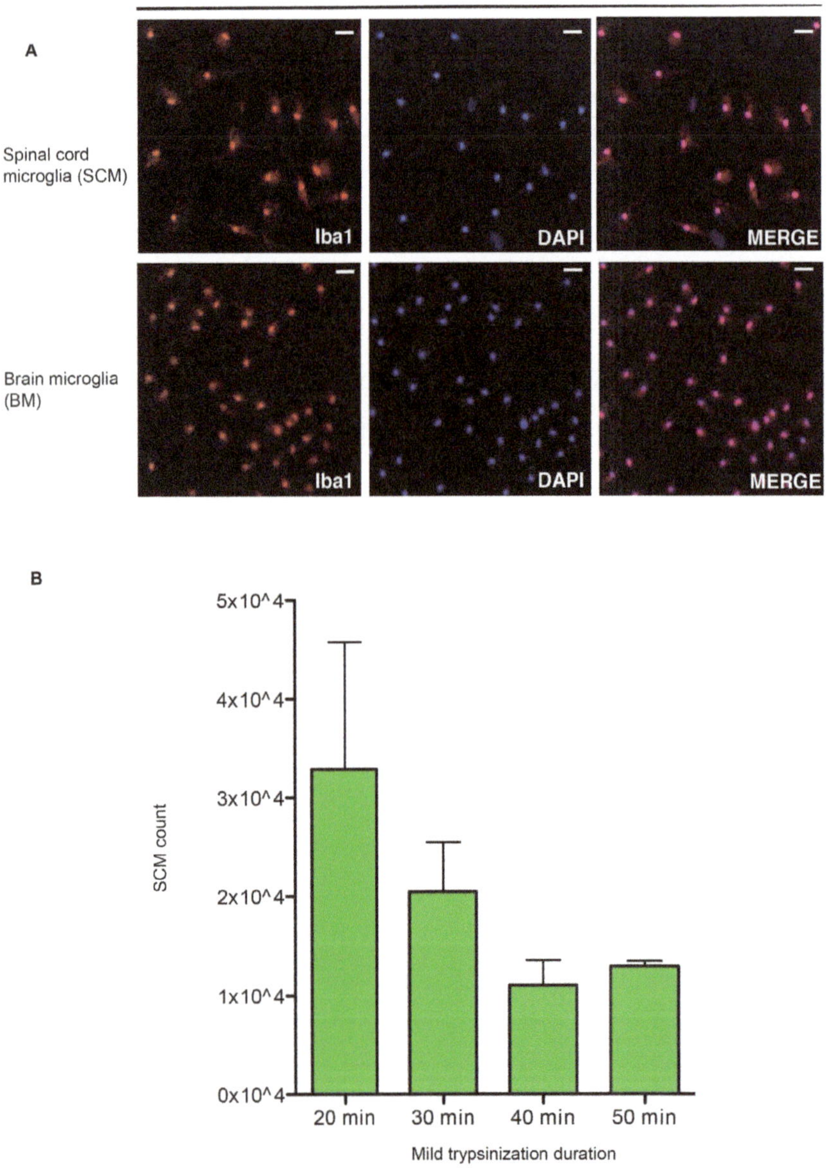

Figure 1. SCM isolation by mild trypsinization. (A) Representative micrograph of Iba1 labeled microglia derived from BM or SCM. Scale = 50 μm. (B) 20 minutes of mild trypsinization had the highest yield of SCM. SCM counts were quantified from average of 6 fields each from four wells of 12 well cell culture plate (n = 4 where n represent the number of independent experiments, where an independent experiment is a separate microglia preparation).

16.18%±0.86, SCM Control 37.50%±4.47, BM LPS 34.32%±3.04, $p<0.05$).

Secretion of pro-inflammatory and anti-inflammatory effectors by BM and SCM

TNF-α, IL-1β and NO are well-characterized pro-inflammatory effectors with established roles in inflammation and neurotoxicity after an injury to the CNS, and release of these inflammatory effectors by microglia varies with brain region of origin [5–7]. To determine if the release of inflammatory effectors differed between SCM and BM, microglia were activated with LPS (1 μg/ml) for 24 h. Relative changes in secreted levels of TNF-α, IL-1β and NO in media were measured using multiplex bead based flow cytometry for TNF-α, ELISA for IL-1β and the Greiss reaction assay for NO. One-way ANOVA identified a significant main effect of LPS treatment on the release of TNF-α ($F_{(3,16)} = 5.201$, $p = 0.0107$), IL-1β ($F_{(3,16)} = 4.21$, $p = 0.0225$) and NO ($F_{(3,24)} = 15.76$, $p = 0.0001$). Newman-Keuls post-hoc tests revealed that TNF-α, IL-1β and NO release by LPS-activated BM were significantly higher than basal release (Fig. 3A, 3B, 3C, TNF-α $p<0.05$; IL-1β $p<0.05$; NO $p<0.001$). LPS activated SCM showed a non-significant trend towards an increase in release of TNF-α, and TNF-α release from SCM was significantly less than BM ($p<0.01$). LPS did not induce significant release of IL-1β from SCM, and LPS-induced release was significantly reduced relative to BM ($p<0.05$). NO release was significantly increased in LPS activated SCM compared to SCM control ($p<0.05$); though it was still significantly less than LPS activated BM ($p<0.01$). No differences were found in the basal release of TNF-α, IL-1β or NO by BM vs. SCM. Notably, reduced release by SCM could not be explained

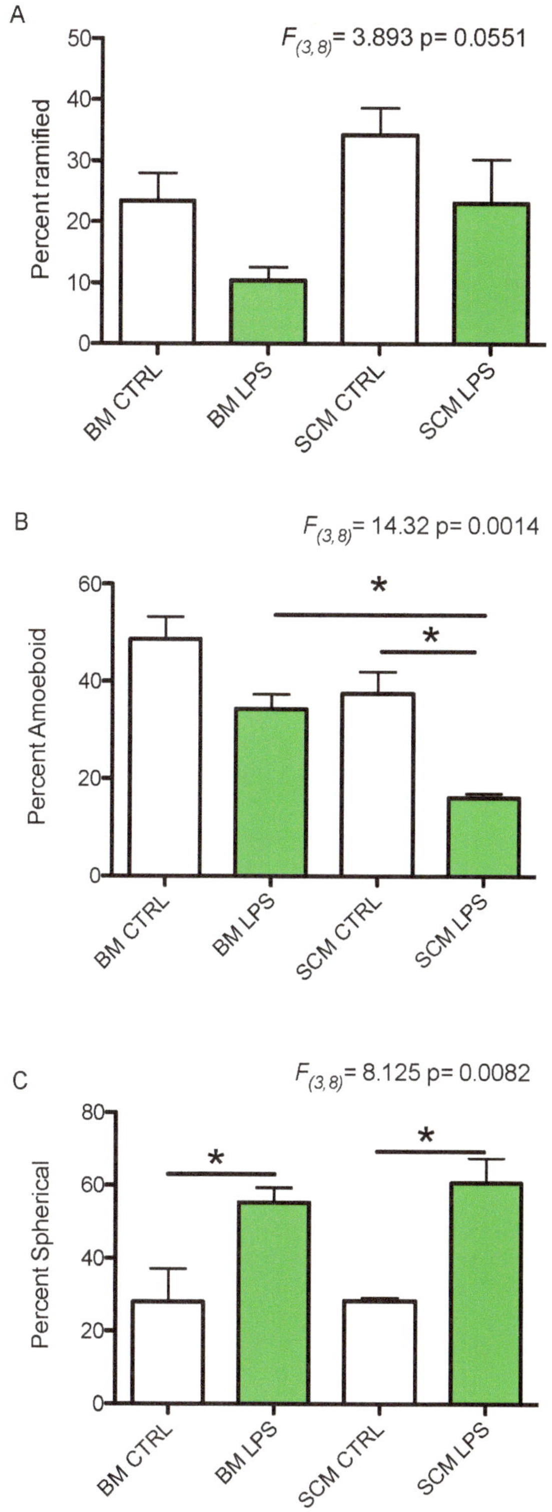

Figure 2. LPS mediated changes in morphology of SCM and BM. BM and SCM were activated with LPS to compare the differences in ramified, amoeboid and spherical morphologies. (A) A main effect of treatment group (BM control, BM LPS, SCM control, or SCM LPS) on the proportion of microglia with ramified morphology was not significant (ANOVA, $F_{(3,8)} = 3.893$, $p = 0.0551$). (B) A significant main effect of treatment on the percentage of amoeboid cells was found (ANOVA, $F_{(3,8)} = 14.32$, $p = 0.0014$). Notably, LPS activated SCM had significant lower percentage of amoeboid cells relative to SCM controls and LPS activated BM (Newman-Keuls post hoc test, n = 3, $p < 0.05$). (C) Treatment significantly altered the percentage of spherical cells (ANOVA, $F_{(3,8)} = 8.125$, $p = 0.00821$). LPS activated BM and SCM had a significant increase in spherical morphology relative to control conditions (Newman-Keul post hoc test, n = 3, $p < 0.05$). n represents the number of independent experiment with a minimum of three replicates. Bars represent percent morphology of cell ± s.e.m.

by differences in cell viability after LPS treatment. Tetrazolium dye (MTT (3-(4, 5-dimethylthiazol-2-yl)-2, 5-diphenyltetrazolium bromide), which is reduced to insoluble formazan only in cells with functional mitochondria, was used to assay the viability of microglia in culture. There was no significant difference in microglial viability between treatment groups (Method S1 and Figure S1).

BM are also capable of releasing IL-6, IL-10, and BDNF, well known mediators of inflammation and cell survival in CNS injury or disease [5–7]. Here, SCM and BM were treated with LPS (1 μg/ml in media) for 24 hours to determine if there are any differences in their release of IL-6, IL-10 and BDNF. Cytokine levels were evaluated by bead based flow cytometry for IL-10, ELISA for IL-6 and competitive ELISA for BDNF. One-way ANOVA showed a trend towards a main effect of treatment group on IL-6 release ($F_{(3,8)} = 3.632$, $p = 0.0642$) but not IL-10 ($F_{(3,16)} = 0.6086$, $p = 0.619$) or BDNF ($F_{(3,\ 8)} = 0.142$, $p = 0.932$) (Fig. 4).

LPS mediated phagocytosis in BM and SCM

Microglia can assume a phagocytic phenotype in response to activating stimuli. CNS diseases or injuries result in dying neurons and debris, which are cleared in part by phagocytic microglia [3,7]. Pro-inflammatory cytokines such as TNF-α have been shown to increase phagocytosis by microglia [3], and amoeboid and spherical microglial morphologies have been associated with phagocytic status [3,29]. LPS activation has been shown to increase phagocytic activity in previous studies of cultured BM. In this study, we compared the phagocytic activity of BM and SCM on activation with LPS (1 μg/ml in media) for 24 hours (Fig. 5). We show that LPS significantly increased the phagocytic activity of BM ($t_{(7)} = 2.815$, $p < 0.05$) but not SCM ($t_{(2)} = 1.336$, $p = 0.3132$).

Discussion

Summary

In this study, we show that SCM can be isolated from primary mixed glial cultures by mild trypsinization. Additionally, we show that the LPS-activated phenotype of SCM is different from that of BM. SCM microglia exhibited a significantly less amoeboid morphology relative to BM after LPS activation. In BM, LPS significantly increased the release of NO, TNF-α and IL-1β. Interestingly, LPS did not induce a statistically significant increase in the release TNF-α and IL-1β in SCM, and levels of all three of these pro-inflammatory cytokines in media from activated SCM were significantly reduced relative to BM. Conversely IL-6 and IL-10 release by LPS-activated SCM exhibited a non-significant trend towards higher release than BM. LPS activation was also associated with an increase in phagocytic activity of BM but not SCM. Overall, our findings suggest that SCM exhibit a less inflammatory and phagocytic phenotype than BM in response to activation with LPS. Interestingly, a recent *in vivo* study using fluorescence assisted cell sorting demonstrated that expression levels of the surface receptors CD45 and CD11b are higher in spinal microglia than brain microglia in naïve mice. In cells sorted three days after viral infection with Theiler's murine encephalomyelitis virus, surface receptors (including CD45, CD11b, CD40,

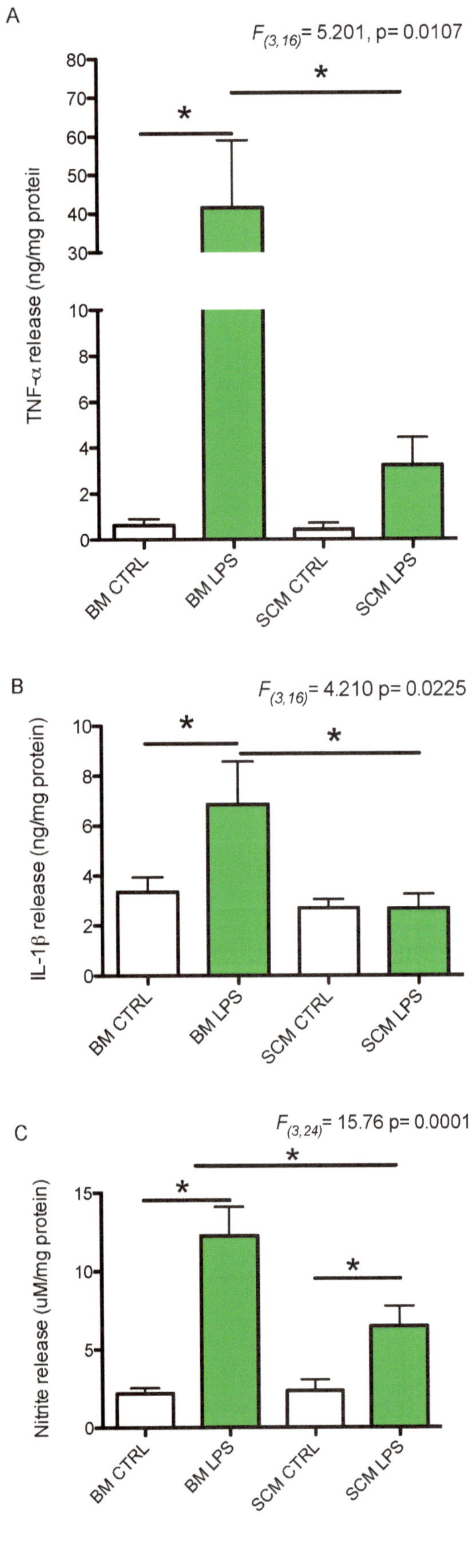

Figure 3. LPS mediated pro-inflammatory molecules release by SCM and BM. BM and SCM were activated with LPS to measure the difference in their pro-inflammatory molecules release. (A) A significant effect of treatment on TNF-α secretion between groups was observed (ANOVA, $F_{(3,16)} = 5.201$, $p = 0.0107$). LPS activated BM had significantly higher release of TNF-α compared to BM control and LPS activated SCM (Neuwman-Keuls post hoc test n = 5, $p < 0.05$). SCM had a trend towards increase in TNF-α on activation with LPS. (B) A significant effect of treatment was also observed for IL-1β secretion (ANOVA, $F_{(3,16)} = 4.210$, $p = 0.0225$). LPS BM had a significantly higher release of IL-1β compared to BM control and LPS activated SCM (Newman-Keul post hoc test n = 5, $p < 0.05$). We did not see any change in IL-1β release between LPS activated SCM and SCM control (Newman-Keul post hoc, n = 5, $p > 0.05$). (C) A significant main effect of treatment group on NO release was observed (ANOVA, $F_{(3,24)} = 15.76$, $p = 0.0001$). LPS induced a significant increase in release of NO by BM compared to BM control and LPS activated SCM (Newman-Keul post hoc, n = 7, $p < 0.05$). NO release by LPS activated SCM was significantly higher than that of SCM and BM controls (Newman-Keul post hoc, n = 7, $p < 0.05$). However, NO release by LPS activated SCM was significantly less than that of LPS activated BM (Newman-Keul post hoc, n = 7, $p < 0.05$). n represents the number of independent experiment with a minimum of three replicates. Bars represent cytokine or nitrite per milligram of total protein ± s.e.m.

CD80, CD86) were upregulated in spinal microglia compared to brain microglia [18,30]. Combined with our findings, these data suggest that the activating stimulus and local environment interact to determine the phenotypic response of microglia [18,30].

Isolation of spinal microglial culture via mild trypsinization

Regional heterogeneity (in morphology and cytokine release) of microglia within the CNS has been observed both *in vitro* and *in vivo* based on region of origin [14,18,21]. For example, microglia from neonatal cortex and hippocampus are more neurotoxic than those from striatum, thalami or brainstem [18]. Notably, microglia from neonatal striatum have a more ramified morphology (presence of extensive processes) and reduced release of pro-inflammatory effectors relative to cortical microglia. However, the morphological and functional heterogeneity of BM vs. SCM has not previously been assessed. Given that SCM can affect the fate of neurons during development and after spinal cord injury, an understanding of the functional response properties of spinal microglia is important. Primary SCM cultures are not common in the literature and have not been characterized to the extent of BM primary cultures [6,27,31–33]. Mild trypsinization (0.05%–0.12% Trypsin EDTA) is an established protocol for isolation of primary BM, with higher yields than isolation via shaking, but has not been well validated for use in SCM [24]. Here, we demonstrate that mild trypsinization can also be used to isolate microglia from mixed glial cultures derived from neonatal rat spinal cord tissue.

Morphology and phagocytic activity of BM and SCM

In the undisturbed CNS, microglia typically assume a ramified morphology, with extensive processes extending from their soma [5–7]. These processes contain membrane sensors to detect activating agents in the surrounding microenvironment. Activation of microglia typically results in a transition to an amoeboid morphology and expression of genes regulating cytokine (inflammatory, anti-inflammatory, and trophic) expression. Continued or extreme activation may induce a spherical and phagocytic morphology [34]. Previously studies have demonstrated that there is region specific heterogeneity in BM morphology and the secretory profile of microglia isolated from different brain regions [18]. We did not find any significant difference between

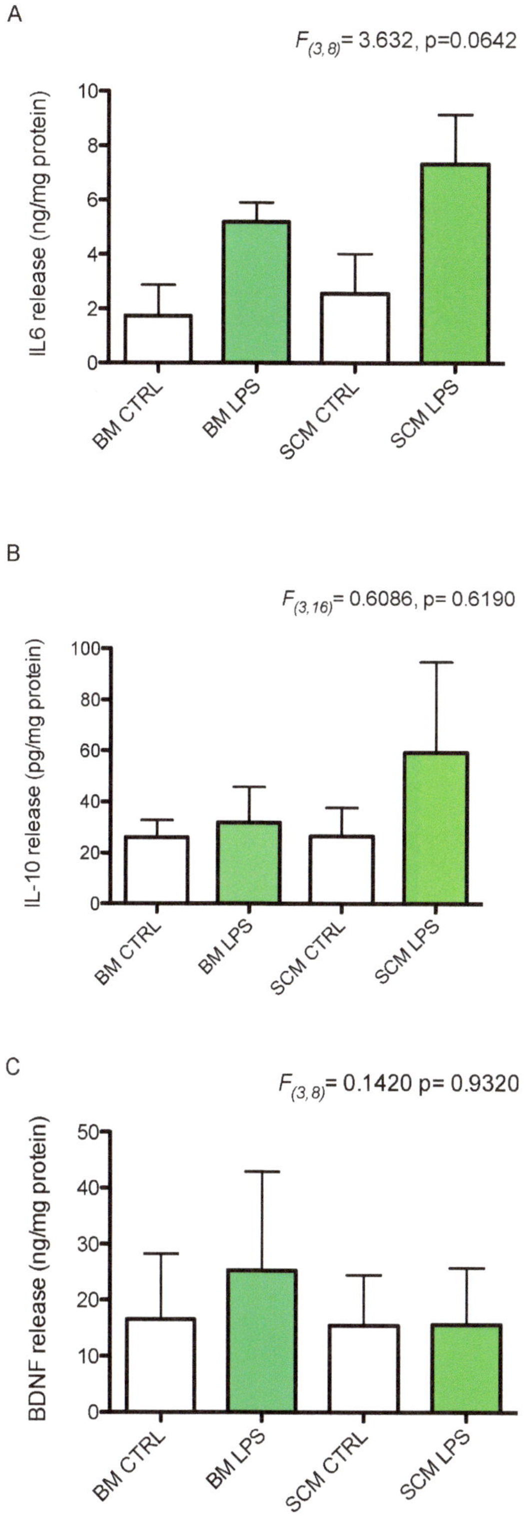

Figure 4. Release of IL-6, IL-10, and BDNF by SCM and BM under basal conditions and after LPS activation. BM and SCM were activated with LPS to measure the difference in their release of these cytokines and trophic factors. (A) There was no significant main effect of treatment group on IL-6 release (ANOVA, $F_{(3,8)} = 3.632$, $p = 0.0642$, $n = 3$) on IL-6 release. LPS activated BM and SCM exhibited a trend towards increased in release of IL-6 compared to their respective controls. Similarly, a significant main effect of treatment was not observed for either IL-10 release (B, ANOVA, $F_{(3,16)} = 0.6086$, $p = 0.6190$, $n = 5$) or BDNF release (C, ANOVA, $F_{(3,8)} = 0.1420$, $p = 0.9320$, $n = 3$). n represents the number of independent experiment with a minimum of three replicates. Bars represent cytokine or trophic factor per milligram of total protein ± s.e.m.

morphology of SCM and BM under basal conditions (Fig. 2). However, SCM exhibit less amoeboid morphology after LPS activation and a trend towards a persistent ramified morphology relative to BM. These morphological differences correlate with phagocytic activity of SCM and BM, where we see an increase in phagocytic activity in BM with increase in amoeboid and spherical form (Fig. 2, Fig. 5). Previous studies show that TNF-α can increase the phagocytic activity of microglia, while IL-10 can decrease phagocytic activity [26,34]. We show that TNF-α release is increased to a greater extent in LPS activated BM relative to SCM (IL-10 release is comparable between SCM and BM, Fig. 3, 4). These effector profiles are consistent with the reduced phagocytic activity of SCM (Fig. 5).

Cytokine Profile of BM and SCM

Cytokines play a major role in determining the outcome of CNS injuries and diseases and microglia are one of the primary sources of cytokines in the CNS. Moreover, microglia are a dynamic population of cell capable of being neurotoxic and or neurotropic depending on the severity of the injury [3,6,7,12–14,18,22,29,35,36]. It has been shown that TNF-α, IL-1β, NO, IL-6 are up-regulated after CNS injury [8–12,15,18,20,22,23,35,37]. However, the consequences of increased cytokine release are multifactorial. TNF-α exhibits both neurotoxic as well as neuroprotective actions after brain or spinal injury [38–43]. While up-regulation of TNF-α can exacerbate neuronal injury, genetic knockout of TNF-α or interference with TNF-α or TNF-α binding sites can increase neuronal tissue loss and reduce compensatory neuroplasticity after CNS injury

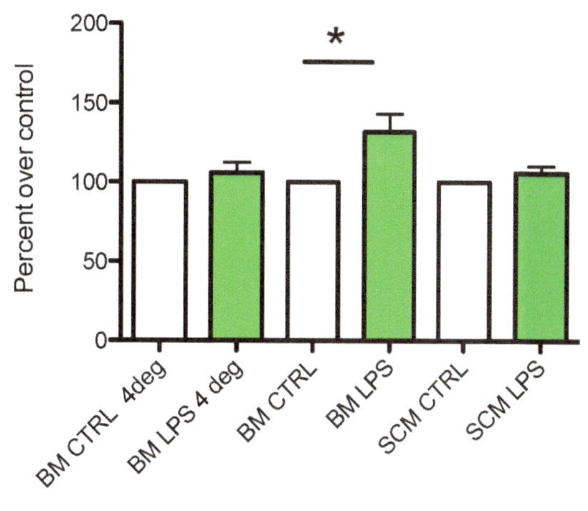

Figure 5. LPS mediated phagocytosis in SCM and BM. Phagocytosis was measured according to fluorescent intensity of cell lysate from control or LPS activation BM or SCM. Within each independent experiment, fluorescence was normalized to mean control values. LPS induced a significant increase in phagocytic activity of BM relative to control ($n = 8$, one sample t-test, $p < 0.05$) but did not induce any change in the phagocytic activity of SCM ($n = 3$, one sample t-test, $p > 0.05$). Phagocytic assays were performed at 4 degree Celsius as negative controls (i.e. a reduced phagocytosis condition) to confirm assay validity ($n = 5$). n represents the number of independent experiment with a minimum of three replicates.

[12,38–45]. IL-1β has a more typical inflammatory and neurotoxic profile, and inhibition of IL-1β reduces neuronal tissue damage after brain injury [6,9,14,23,37]. Similarly, NO is an inflammatory and neurotoxic mediator known to contribute the lesion growth in spinal cord injury, stroke, and brain injury by the reactive metabolite perioxynitrite [6,8,10,13,46]. As such, the relative reduction in the release of pro-inflammatory effectors (TNF-α, IL-1β and NO) by SCM relative to BM suggests that SCM might have a less neurotoxic profile after activation by LPS *in vitro*.

It is well known that IL-6 and IL-10 are upregulated after an injury or disease in CNS [15,22,36,47] and that microglia are capable of releasing IL-6 and IL-10 [19,20,25,48,49]. IL-6 has both pro- and anti-inflammatory actions, and is a major mediator of the brain's immune response to trauma or infection [48–50]. Conversely, IL-10 is associated with a primarily protective role after CNS injury [26,35,51,52]. IL-6 and IL-10 both down-regulate the expression of TNF-α and IL-1β and thereby reduce the neurotoxicity mediated by these pro-inflammatory cytokines [25,26,53–55]. Our data suggests that release of these mediators by BM and SCM is comparable, with a trend towards increased LPS mediated release of IL-10 and IL-6 by SCM relative to BM (Fig. 4). These data provide further support for the postulate that SCM exhibit a less inflammatory phenotype than BM after activation with LPS *in vitro*.

LPS has primarily been associated with a pro-inflammatory function due to its interactions with Toll like receptor 4 (TLR4). TLR4 is an essential component of the immune response and is known to up-regulate inflammatory cytokines via both myeloid differentiation primary-response protein 88 (MyD88) dependent and MyD88-independent pathways [56]. Activation of TLR4 MyD88-dependent pathway induces the production of TNF-α and IL-6 [56]. However, TLR4 MyD88-independent pathway, induces the production type 1 Interferon (IFN) gene products, but not TNF-α or IL-6, and mice deficient of MyD88 did not produce TNF-α and IL-6 [56]. Differences in the release of TNF-α by LPS activated SCM relative to BM (Fig. 3A) may therefore suggest differential weighting of the MyD88 dependent and independent pathways in BM and SCM.

Limitations. *In vitro* culture systems are a powerful reductionist model to study microglia in isolation. Commonly used activators such as LPS can act on receptors on other CNS cells including neurons and astrocytes. Hence, isolated microglia cultures improve resolution of microglial activation profiles without the interference from other CNS constituents. Nonetheless, *in vitro* models only mimic injury or inflammation found *in vivo*, and these simplified models *in vitro* may not reflect the whole spectrum of effectors involved *in vivo*. Notably, myelination is incomplete in day one neonatal rats and cultures, and this environmental difference prior to isolation may influence microglia phenotypes [57]. Similarly, recent studies show increased expression of purinergic receptors involved chemotaxis and phagocytosis in adult microglia relative to neonates [58–61]. Genes regulating factors cell adhesion, proliferation, migration, complement system activity, and transcription regulation also exhibited differential expression in adult vs. neonatal microglia [61]. Hence, microglia isolated from neonatal mixed glia preparation may not account for variances in response properties due to developmental state in microglia from different brain regions [60,61].

Conclusions. CNS microglia are a heterogeneous population of cells whose immune function is determined by local environment, severity of injury and age of the animal [6,14,18,60]. Our result suggests that SCM may be less pro-inflammatory on activation through the TLR4 pathway. These differences between microglial activation pathways in SCM as compared to BM are an important consideration in rationale design of immune-modulatory or anti-inflammatory therapies specific for spinal cord and brain injuries.

Supporting Information

Figure S1 BM, SCM viability after LPS treatment. Microglial viability was assessed via the MTT assay in four treatment groups (BM control, BM LPS, SCM control, or SCM LPS). There was no main effect of treatment group on microglial viability ($F_{(3,16)} = 0.8011$, $p = 0.5113$). $n = 5$ independent microglia culture preparations. Bars represent optical density (MTT absorbance) values per milligram of total protein ± s.e.m.

Method S1 Measurement of microglia viability.

Acknowledgments

We sincerely thank members of the Winship and Todd labs for critical discussion during the study and Ms. Dorothy Kratochwil-Otto for assistance with flow cytometry.

Author Contributions

Conceived and designed the experiments: SB KGT IRW. Performed the experiments: SB. Analyzed the data: SB KGT IRW. Contributed reagents/materials/analysis tools: KGT IRW. Wrote the paper: SB KGT IRW.

References

1. Giulian D, Baker TJ (1986) Characterization of ameboid microglia isolated from developing mammalian brain. The Journal of neuroscience: the official journal of the Society for Neuroscience 6: 2163–2178.
2. Rezaie P, Male D (1999) Colonisation of the developing human brain and spinal cord by microglia: a review. Microscopy research and technique 45: 359–382.
3. Aloisi F (2001) Immune function of microglia. Glia 36: 165–179.
4. Wake H, Moorhouse AJ, Jinno S, Kohsaka S, Nabekura J (2009) Resting microglia directly monitor the functional state of synapses in vivo and determine the fate of ischemic terminals. The Journal of neuroscience: the official journal of the Society for Neuroscience 29: 3974–3980.
5. Lai AY, Todd KG (2006) Hypoxia-activated microglial mediators of neuronal survival are differentially regulated by tetracyclines. Glia 53: 809–816.
6. Lai AY, Todd KG (2008) Differential regulation of trophic and proinflammatory microglial effectors is dependent on severity of neuronal injury. Glia 56: 259–270.
7. Kettenmann H, Hanisch UK, Noda M, Verkhratsky A (2011) Physiology of microglia. Physiological reviews 91: 461–553.
8. Kader A, Frazzini VI, Solomon RA, Trifiletti RR (1993) Nitric oxide production during focal cerebral ischemia in rats. Stroke 24: 1709–1716.
9. Hill JK, Gunion-Rinker L, Kulhanek D, Lessov N, Kim S, et al. (1999) Temporal modulation of cytokine expression following focal cerebral ischemia in mice. Brain Research 820: 45–54.
10. Castillo J, Rama R, Davalos A (2000) Nitric Oxide-Related Brain Damage in Acute Ischemic Stroke. Stroke 31: 852–857.
11. Clausen BH, Lambertsen KL, Meldgaard M, Finsen B (2005) A quantitative in situ hybridization and polymerase chain reaction study of microglial-macrophage expression of interleukin-1beta mRNA following permanent middle cerebral artery occlusion in mice. Neuroscience 132: 879–892.
12. Lambertsen KL, Clausen BH, Babcock AA, Gregersen R, Fenger C, et al. (2009) Microglia protect neurons against ischemia by synthesis of tumor necrosis factor. The Journal of neuroscience: the official journal of the Society for Neuroscience 29: 1319–1330.
13. Yenari MA, Kauppinen TM, Swanson RA (2010) Microglial activation in stroke: therapeutic targets. Neurotherapeutics: the journal of the American Society for Experimental NeuroTherapeutics 7: 378–391.
14. Yang L, Jones NR, Blumbergs PC, Van Den Heuvel C, Moore EJ, et al. (2005) Severity-dependent expression of pro-inflammatory cytokines in traumatic spinal

cord injury in the rat. Journal of clinical neuroscience: official journal of the Neurosurgical Society of Australasia 12: 276–284.
15. Smith PD, Puskas F, Meng X, Lee JH, Cleveland JC, et al. (2012) The Evolution of Chemokine Release Supports a Bimodal Mechanism of Spinal Cord Ischemia and Reperfusion Injury. Circulation 126: S110–S117.
16. Lai AY, Todd KG (2006) Microglia in cerebral ischemia: molecular actions and interactions. Canadian journal of physiology and pharmacology 84: 49–59.
17. Matsui T, Svensson CI, Hirata Y, Mizobata K, Hua XY, et al. (2010) Release of prostaglandin E(2) and nitric oxide from spinal microglia is dependent on activation of p38 mitogen-activated protein kinase. Anesthesia and analgesia 111: 554–560.
18. Lai AY, Dhami KS, Dibal CD, Todd KG (2011) Neonatal rat microglia derived from different brain regions have distinct activation responses. Neuron glia biology 7: 5–16.
19. Werry EL, Liu GJ, Lovelace MD, Nagarajah R, Hickie IB, et al. (2011) Lipopolysaccharide-stimulated interleukin-10 release from neonatal spinal cord microglia is potentiated by glutamate. Neuroscience 175: 93–103.
20. Green HF, Nolan YM (2012) GSK-3 mediates the release of IL-1beta, TNF-alpha and IL-10 from cortical glia. Neurochemistry international 61: 666–671.
21. Hua K, Schindler MK, McQuail JA, Forbes ME, Riddle DR (2012) Regionally distinct responses of microglia and glial progenitor cells to whole brain irradiation in adult and aging rats. PloS one 7: e52728.
22. Lambertsen KL, Biber K, Finsen B (2012) Inflammatory cytokines in experimental and human stroke. Journal of cerebral blood flow and metabolism: official journal of the International Society of Cerebral Blood Flow and Metabolism 32: 1677–1698.
23. Nakamura Y, Si QS, Kataoka K (1999) Lipopolysaccharide-induced microglial activation in culture: temporal profiles of morphological change and release of cytokines and nitric oxide. Neuroscience Research 35: 95–100.
24. Saura J, Tusell JM, Serratosa J (2003) High-yield isolation of murine microglia by mild trypsinization. Glia 44: 183–189.
25. Aderka D, Le JM, Vilcek J (1989) IL-6 inhibits lipopolysaccharide-induced tumor necrosis factor production in cultured human monocytes, U937 cells, and in mice. J Immunol 143: 3517–3523.
26. Broderick C, Duncan L, Taylor N, Dick AD (2000) IFN-gamma and LPS-mediated IL-10-dependent suppression of retinal microglial activation. Investigative ophthalmology & visual science 41: 2613–2622.
27. Durafourt BA, Moore CS, Zammit DA, Johnson TA, Zaguia F, et al. (2012) Comparison of polarization properties of human adult microglia and blood-derived macrophages. Glia 60: 717–727.
28. Siao CJ, Tsirka SE (2002) Tissue plasminogen activator mediates microglial activation via its finger domain through annexin II. The Journal of neuroscience: the official journal of the Society for Neuroscience 22: 3352–3358.
29. Hu X, Li P, Guo Y, Wang H, Leak RK, et al. (2012) Microglia/macrophage polarization dynamics reveal novel mechanism of injury expansion after focal cerebral ischemia. Stroke 43: 3063–3070.
30. Olson JK (2010) Immune response by microglia in the spinal cord. Annals of the New York Academy of Sciences 1198: 271–278.
31. Olson JK, Miller SD (2004) Microglia initiate central nervous system innate and adaptive immune responses through multiple TLRs. J Immunol 173: 3916–3924.
32. Gingras M, Gagnon V, Minotti S, Durham HD, Berthod F (2007) Optimized protocols for isolation of primary motor neurons, astrocytes and microglia from embryonic mouse spinal cord. Journal of neuroscience methods 163: 111–118.
33. Yip PK, Kaan TK, Fenesan D, Malcangio M (2009) Rapid isolation and culture of primary microglia from adult mouse spinal cord. Journal of neuroscience methods 183: 223–237.
34. von Zahn J, Moller T, Kettenmann H, Nolte C (1997) Microglial phagocytosis is modulated by pro- and anti-inflammatory cytokines. Neuroreport 8: 3851–3856.
35. Diab A, Zhu J, Xiao BG, Mustafa M, Link H (1997) High IL-6 and low IL-10 in the central nervous system are associated with protracted relapsing EAE in DA rats. Journal of neuropathology and experimental neurology 56: 641–650.
36. Jin R, Yang G, Li G (2010) Inflammatory mechanisms in ischemic stroke: role of inflammatory cells. Journal of leukocyte biology 87: 779–789.
37. Tarkowski E, Rosengren L, Blomstrand C, Wikkelso C, Jensen C, et al. (1995) Early intrathecal production of interleukin-6 predicts the size of brain lesion in stroke. Stroke 26: 1393–1398.
38. Sriram K, Matheson JM, Benkovic SA, Miller DB, Luster MI, et al. (2002) Mice deficient in TNF receptors are protected against dopaminergic neurotoxicity: implications for Parkinson's disease. FASEB journal: official publication of the Federation of American Societies for Experimental Biology 16: 1474–1476.
39. Wang X, Feuerstein GZ, Xu L, Wang H, Schumacher WA, et al. (2004) Inhibition of tumor necrosis factor-alpha-converting enzyme by a selective antagonist protects brain from focal ischemic injury in rats. Molecular pharmacology 65: 890–896.
40. Taylor DL, Jones F, Kubota ES, Pocock JM (2005) Stimulation of microglial metabotropic glutamate receptor mGlu2 triggers tumor necrosis factor alpha-induced neurotoxicity in concert with microglial-derived Fas ligand. The Journal of neuroscience: the official journal of the Society for Neuroscience 25: 2952–2964.
41. Takeuchi H, Jin S, Wang J, Zhang G, Kawanokuchi J, et al. (2006) Tumor necrosis factor-alpha induces neurotoxicity via glutamate release from hemichannels of activated microglia in an autocrine manner. The Journal of biological chemistry 281: 21362–21368.
42. Oshima T, Lee S, Sato A, Oda S, Hirasawa H, et al. (2009) TNF-alpha contributes to axonal sprouting and functional recovery following traumatic brain injury. Brain Res 1290: 102–110.
43. Taoufik E, Valable S, Muller GJ, Roberts ML, Divoux D, et al. (2007) FLIP(L) protects neurons against in vivo ischemia and in vitro glucose deprivation-induced cell death. The Journal of neuroscience: the official journal of the Society for Neuroscience 27: 6633–6646.
44. Araki E, Forster C, Dubinsky JM, Ross ME, Iadecola C (2001) Cyclooxygenase-2 inhibitor ns-398 protects neuronal cultures from lipopolysaccharide-induced neurotoxicity. Stroke 32: 2370–2375.
45. Centonze D, Muzio L, Rossi S, Cavasinni F, De Chiara V, et al. (2009) Inflammation triggers synaptic alteration and degeneration in experimental autoimmune encephalomyelitis. The Journal of neuroscience: the official journal of the Society for Neuroscience 29: 3442–3452.
46. Huang Z, Huang PL, Panahian N, Dalkara T, Fishman MC, et al. (1994) Effects of cerebral ischemia in mice deficient in neuronal nitric oxide synthase. Science 265: 1883–1885.
47. Woodroofe MN, Sarna GS, Wadhwa M, Hayes GM, Loughlin AJ, et al. (1991) Detection of interleukin-1 and interleukin-6 in adult rat brain, following mechanical injury, by in vivo microdialysis: evidence of a role for microglia in cytokine production. Journal of neuroimmunology 33: 227–236.
48. Ma TC, Zhu XZ (2000) Neurotoxic effects of interleukin-6 and sodium nitroprusside on cultured rat hippocampal neurons. Arzneimittel-Forschung 50: 512–514.
49. Cafferty WB, Gardiner NJ, Das P, Qiu J, McMahon SB, et al. (2004) Conditioning injury-induced spinal axon regeneration fails in interleukin-6 knock-out mice. The Journal of neuroscience: the official journal of the Society for Neuroscience 24: 4432–4443.
50. Leibinger M, Muller A, Gobrecht P, Diekmann H, Andreadaki A, et al. (2013) Interleukin-6 contributes to CNS axon regeneration upon inflammatory stimulation. Cell death & disease 4: e609.
51. Knoblach SM, Faden AI (1998) Interleukin-10 improves outcome and alters proinflammatory cytokine expression after experimental traumatic brain injury. Experimental neurology 153: 143–151.
52. Bethea JR, Nagashima H, Acosta MC, Briceno C, Gomez F, et al. (1999) Systemically administered interleukin-10 reduces tumor necrosis factor-alpha production and significantly improves functional recovery following traumatic spinal cord injury in rats. Journal of neurotrauma 16: 851–863.
53. Armstrong L, Jordan N, Millar A (1996) Interleukin 10 (IL-10) regulation of tumour necrosis factor alpha (TNF-alpha) from human alveolar macrophages and peripheral blood monocytes. Thorax 51: 143–149.
54. Ledeboer A, Breve JJ, Wierinckx A, van der Jagt S, Bristow AF, et al. (2002) Expression and regulation of interleukin-10 and interleukin-10 receptor in rat astroglial and microglial cells. The European journal of neuroscience 16: 1175–1185.
55. Erta M, Quintana A, Hidalgo J (2012) Interleukin-6, a major cytokine in the central nervous system. International journal of biological sciences 8: 1254–1266.
56. Akira S, Takeda K (2004) Toll-like receptor signalling. Nature reviews Immunology 4: 499–511.
57. Downes N, Mullins P (2013) The Development of Myelin in the Brain of the Juvenile Rat. Toxicologic pathology.
58. Haynes SE, Hollopeter G, Yang G, Kurpius D, Dailey ME, et al. (2006) The P2Y12 receptor regulates microglial activation by extracellular nucleotides. Nature neuroscience 9: 1512–1519.
59. Kurpius D, Nolley EP, Dailey ME (2007) Purines induce directed migration and rapid homing of microglia to injured pyramidal neurons in developing hippocampus. Glia 55: 873–884.
60. Lai AY, Dibal CD, Armitage GA, Winship IR, Todd KG (2013) Distinct activation profiles in microglia of different ages: a systematic study in isolated embryonic to aged microglial cultures. Neuroscience 254: 185–195.
61. Butovsky O, Jedrychowski MP, Moore CS, Cialic R, Lanser AJ, et al. (2014) Identification of a unique TGF-beta-dependent molecular and functional signature in microglia. Nature neuroscience 17: 131–143.

15

Molecular and Cellular Changes in the Lumbar Spinal Cord following Thoracic Injury: Regulation by Treadmill Locomotor Training

Hae Young Shin[1,2☯], Hyosil Kim[2,3☯], Min Jung Kwon[1,2], Dong Hoon Hwang[1,2], KiYoung Lee[2,3*], Byung Gon Kim[1,2,4*]

1 Department of Brain Science, Ajou University School of Medicine, Suwon, Republic of Korea, **2** Neuroscience Graduate Program, Department of Biomedical Sciences, Ajou University School of Medicine, Suwon, Republic of Korea, **3** Department of Biomedical Informatics, Ajou University School of Medicine, Suwon, Republic of Korea, **4** Department of Neurology, Ajou University School of Medicine, Suwon, Republic of Korea

Abstract

Traumatic spinal cord injury (SCI) often leads to debilitating loss of locomotor function. Neuroplasticity of spinal circuitry underlies some functional recovery and therefore represents a therapeutic target to improve locomotor function following SCI. However, the cellular and molecular mechanisms mediating neuroplasticity below the lesion level are not fully understood. The present study performed a gene expression profiling in the rat lumbar spinal cord at 1 and 3 weeks after contusive SCI at T9. Another group of rats received treadmill locomotor training (TMT) until 3 weeks, and gene expression profiles were compared between animals with and without TMT. Microarray analysis showed that many inflammation-related genes were robustly upregulated in the lumbar spinal cord at both 1 and 3 weeks after thoracic injury. Notably, several components involved in an early complement activation pathway were concurrently upregulated. In line with the microarray finding, the number of microglia substantially increased not only in the white matter but also in the gray matter. C3 and complement receptor 3 were intensely expressed in the ventral horn after injury. Furthermore, synaptic puncta near ventral motor neurons were frequently colocalized with microglia after injury, implicating complement activation and microglial cells in synaptic remodeling in the lumbar locomotor circuitry after SCI. Interestingly, TMT did not influence the injury-induced upregulation of inflammation-related genes. Instead, TMT restored pre-injury expression patterns of several genes that were downregulated by injury. Notably, TMT increased the expression of genes involved in neuroplasticity (Arc, Nrcam) and angiogenesis (Adam8, Tie1), suggesting that TMT may improve locomotor function in part by promoting neurovascular remodeling in the lumbar motor circuitry.

Editor: Subhabrata Sanyal , Biogen Idec, United States of America

Funding: This work was supported by the National Research Foundation of Korea (NRF) grant funded by the Korea government (MSIP) (NRF-2009-0069522, NRF-2009-0081466, and NRF-2012R1A5A2051429 to BGK; NRF-2013R1A2A2A04013317 to KYL). The funders had no role in study design, data collection and analysis, decision to publish, or preparation of the manuscript.

Competing Interests: The authors have declared that no competing interests exist.

* E-mail: kiylee@ajou.ac.kr (KYL); kimbg@ajou.ac.kr (BGK)

☯ These authors contributed equally to this work.

Introduction

Patients with moderate to severe traumatic spinal cord injury (SCI) almost invariably suffer from life-long deficits in locomotion. This locomotor dysfunction can be attributed to severance of connections between motor centers in the brain and the lumbar spinal cord. Currently, there is no pharmacological or biological therapeutic option clinically proven to improve locomotor function. The lack of effective treatments in part reflects overwhelming obstacles to promotion of axonal connection between the two motor centers.

An alternative approach is to train intrinsic spinal locomotor circuitry generating rhythmic spontaneous hindlimb movements [1–3]. Treadmill locomotor training (TMT) is employed to train and activate locomotor circuits located in the lumbar spinal cord by providing sensory afferent stimulation [4,5]. First established in spinalized cats [6,7], the effectiveness of TMT has been demonstrated in rodent models with variable injury severities and training regimens [8]. A recent study showed that epidural stimulation can effectively reactivate the lumbar motor circuitry to become more sensitive to sensory inputs provided by treadmill training (TMT) [9], raising a hope that TMT in combination with electrical stimulation and/or pharmacological neuromodulation [10] could be an effective therapeutic option to improve locomotor function after SCI [11].

Despite documented effects of TMT in animal models, the molecular and cellular mechanisms mediating "below-level" locomotor recovery are not fully understood. Several studies have suggested that elevated neurotrophin levels in the lumbar spinal cord mediate exercise-induced neuroplasticity [12]. However, there is no study that has systematically investigated molecular changes regulated by TMT. Gene expression profiling by microarray has been used in rodent SCI models to systematically reveal cellular and molecular processes leading to spinal cord degeneration and repair [13–15]. The current study employed the microarray strategy to examine gene expression changes in the lumbar motor regions following thoracic contusive SCI at the time points when spontaneous locomotor recovery is observed. Moreover, we compared gene expression patterns in the lumbar spinal cord regions between animals with and without TMT to search for molecular factors mediating TMT-induced locomotor recovery.

Materials and Methods

Animals and study design

A total of 81 Adult female Sprague Dawley rats (250~300 g, aged from 9 to 12 weeks old) were used in this study. All animal protocols were approved by the Institutional Animal Care and Use Committee of Ajou University School of Medicine. As a preliminary study to determine time points for microarray study, 8 injured animals each with or without TMT underwent behavioral examination (see below for detailed methods). For microarray analysis, animals were randomly assigned to four groups: 1) animals subjected to laminectomy alone (sham operation) (N = 3), 2) animals subjected to contusive injury and sacrificed 1 week after injury (N = 4), 3) animals subjected to contusive injury and sacrificed 3 weeks after injury (N = 4), 4) animals subjected to contusive injury and TMT beginning at 1 week and lasting until 3 weeks after injury (TMT of 2-week duration) (N = 4). To identify genes regulated by TMT independently of SCI, an additional group of animals (N = 3) was subjected to the sham operation and TMT of 2 week duration beginning at 1 week after the sham operation. Separate sets of animals were generated for verification experiments using RT-PCR and western blots (N = 4 for each group). Five animals for sham group, animals 3 weeks after injury with or without TMT were also generated for immunohistochemical studies. The number of animals in different experiments and the survival time points are provided in detail in Table 1.

Table 1. Number of animals in each group and at different time points for various experiments.

Experiment	Group	Survival		
		1 week	**3 week**	**8 week**
Behavior assessment	SCI			8
	SCI with TMT			8
Microarray	Sham	3		
	Sham + TMT		3	
	1 week injury	4		
	3 weeks injury		4	
	3 weeks injury + TMT		4	
Quantitative RT-PCR	Sham	4		
	1 week injury	4		
	3 weeks injury		4	
	3 weeks injury + TMT		4	
Western blot	Sham	4		
	1 week injury	4		
	3 weeks injury		4	
	3 weeks injury + TMT		4	
Histological assessment	Sham	5		
	3 weeks injury		5	
	3 weeks injury + TMT		5	

SCI: spinal cord injury, TMT: treadmill training.

Surgical procedures, TMT protocol, and behavioral assessment

To create contusive spinal cord injury model, animals were anesthetized with chloral hydrate (400 mg/kg, i.p.) during all surgical procedures. A dorsal laminectomy was performed at the ninth thoracic vertebral level (T9) to expose the spinal cord. Then animals were subjected to contusion injury by mechanical impact with a force of 200 kdyn using an Infinite Horizon Impactor (Precision System and Instrumentation, Lexington, KY, USA). Prophylactic antibiotics were administered by intraperitoneal injection on the day after each surgery, and bladder care was provided twice daily until spontaneous voiding resumed. TMT was performed in the Flat Treadmill System for rats with 4 channels (Model, IW-FT; IWOO Scientific Corporation, Seoul, Korea). Each channel consists of a 14 cm by 45 cm runway with an electrical stimulator installed at the end of the runway. Electric shocks of 1.2 mA were applied when an animal was not walking and displaced to the end of its runway. Typically, electric shocks were required several times on the first day of training, but were rarely applied after a few days. Although animals could not perform fully weight-supported plantar stepping when TMT was initiated at 1 week after injury, they were able to walk without auxiliary support at a slow speed (5 meters per minute). As locomotion was improved, the belt speed was gradually increased to 12 meters per minute during the first week and maintained at this level until the end of training. TMT was performed daily for 14 days with each session lasting 30 minutes. Locomotor recovery was assessed using the Basso, Beattie, and Bresnahan (BBB) locomotor rating scale. BBB test was carried out by observers blinded to the treatment conditions. BBB test was performed on each animal on the day following contusion and once a week thereafter until 8 weeks after.

RNA isolation for microarray

On the day of sacrifice, animals were anesthetized with an overdose of chloral hydrate and briefly perfused with ice-cold saline to remove blood components from the tissue. Spinal cord tissue containing the epicenter and the entire length below was quickly dissected. The dissected spinal cord was cut at the beginning of the lumbar enlargement, and the lumbar spinal cord block extending 1 cm distal to the initial cut was collected. This tissue block contained the rostral portion of the sacral segments but not the conus medullaris. Care was taken to remove the stubs of the lumbosacral roots attached to the cord. Dissected lumbar spinal cord blocks were frozen rapidly and stored at −70°C until use. Total RNA was isolated using an RNeasy Microarray Tissue Mini kit (Qiagen, Hilgen, Germany) in accordance with the manufacturer's instructions. The concentration of the RNA samples was quantified using a Nanodrop 1000 (Thermo Fisher Scientific, Wilmington, DE, USA). RNA quality was assessed using a Bioanalyzer 2100 (Agilent technologies Inc., Santa Clara, CA, USA), and RNA samples with RNA integrity number (RIN) higher than 7.5 were judged as acceptable. All of the samples prepared in our study had RIN value higher than 8.

Microarray analysis

For each sample, 6 µg of RNA were used as input into the Affymetrix procedure as recommended by the manufacturer's protocol (http://www.affymetrix.com). Briefly, 6 µg of total RNA was converted to double-strand cDNA using oligo (dT) primer incorporating a T7 promoter. Amplified RNA (cRNA) was generated from the double-stranded cDNA template though an IVT (in-vitro transcription) reaction and purified with the Affymetrix sample cleanup module. After fragmentation, RNA was hybridized to the arrays containing over 22,500 probe sets. After hybridization, the chips were stained and washed in a Genechip Fluidics Station 450 and the microarray signals were scanned by using a Genechip Array scanner 3000 7G. The robust multi-array average approach with a quantile normalization algorithm was applied to extract probe-level expression intensities of genes.

Data analysis

For gene-level expression, we calculated the mean value of the probe-level intensities for each gene. Differentially expressed genes were identified when individual genes met the following two conditions: 1) there was at least a 1.5-fold change in expression level of the genes between groups and 2) there was a statistically significant difference in the expression level using Student's t-test ($p<0.05$). Pathway and Gene Ontology-based functional enrichment analysis using DAVID (the Database for Annotation, Visualization and Integrated Discovery) [16] was employed by using differentially expressed genes from each pair-wise comparison among sham, injury, and TMT groups (cut-off threshold of significance: $p<0.1$). For clustering analysis, the k-means clustering algorithm implemented in the MEV (Multi Experiment View) software package [17] was applied to the genes that were differentially expressed between the 3 week post-injury and TMT groups. To identify and visualize the injury-related protein network modules, we used Cytoscape software version 2.8.3 [18]. For the rat protein-protein interactions we compiled diverse databases including BIND, BIND_t, BioGRID, CORUM, DIP, HPRD, IntAct, MINT, MPPI, OPHID, InnateDB, and MatrixDB. We also included human protein-protein interactions after converting human proteins to rat proteins using human-rat orthologs of the InParanoid database [19]. Our microarray data have been deposited in the NIH Gene Expression Omnibus database with accession code GSE52763.

Quantitative reverse transcription polymerase chain reaction (RT-PCR)

Expression changes of genes of interest were verified by quantitative real-time RT-PCR. Total RNA was extracted from lumbar spinal cords using Trizol (Qiagen, Hilgen, Germany) according to the manufacturer's protocol. Oneµg of RNA was reverse transcribed to cDNA using a standard reverse transcription protocol. Oneµl of cDNA was added to SYBR Green Master Mix (Dakara, Otsu, Shiga, Japan) containing primer pairs at 10 pM. Primer sequences are listed in Table 2. Quantitative real-time PCR was performed according to the manufacturer's protocol using a 7500 Real-Time PCR System (Applied Biosystems, Foster City, CA, USA). Cycling conditions were 94°C for 30s, 53°C ~ 64°C for 31s, and 72°C for 60s with a total of 34 cycles. Melting curves were generated after the last extension step, and Ct values were calculated by the Applied Biosystems 7500 software. Ct values of target genes were normalized to the housekeeping gene 18Sr and analyzed using the $2^{-\Delta\Delta Ct}$ method [20]. Using the $2^{-\Delta\Delta Ct}$ method, the data are presented as the fold change in gene expression normalized to an endogenous reference gene and relative to the control.

Table 2. Primer sequences used for real time RT-PCR.

Gene	5′ primer (Forward)	3′ primer (Reverse)
18S rRNA	CGGCTACCACATCCAAGGAA	TGCTGGCACCAGACTTGCCCTC
Galectin3	AGCCCAACGCAAACAGTATC	GGCTTCAACCAGGACCTGTA
C3	CAGCAGACCTCAGTGACCAA	GCCTCTTCTCTAGGCCGAAT
C1qa	GGCCTAGAAGCATCATAG-AACACGA	CACTCCACTGTGTCTTCATCAGCTC
C1qb	GGCCTAGAAGCATCATAGAA-CACGA	CACTCCACTGTGTCTTCATCAGCTC
Timp1	ACAGGTTTCCGGTTCGCCGCC	CTGCAGGCAGTGATGTGCAA
Itgb2	AAGGGAGTCATGGAGTGTGG	TCACTTTGTTGGGGATGTCA
March6	AGGGACCACAATGTTTCTGC	GGAAGCCAGAGCATCAGAAG
Kdm4c	GCCCATGACTGTGAAGGAGT	CGCACTCTTCTTCAACCACA
Frg1	TCCAGTCCTCCAGAGCAGTT	GCCATCTTCCCATCTTGAAA
Adam8	GCAGCCAGGTTGACCTAGAG	ATTCATGACAACAGGCACCA
Nrcam	GGCAGCAAAGAAGAATGGAG	CTTGGGTCGCAATATCCACT
Arc	CTGAGATGCTGGAGCACGTA	GCCTTGATGGACTTCTTCCA
Tie1	AAGGTCACACACACGGTGAA	CATTTTGGAGCTGCAGTTGA

Tissue processing and immunohistochemistry

Rats were anesthetized with an overdose of chloral hydrate and perfused with phosphate buffered saline (PBS) followed by 4% paraformaldehyde (PFA) in 0.2 M phosphate buffer. The spinal cord tissues was separated and post-fixed in 4% PFA for 2 hours, followed by cryoprotection in a graded series of sucrose solutions. For lumbar spinal cord tissue, 20 µm thick transverse cryosections were made in a 1:10 series. Tissue sections were mounted onto Superfrost plus slides (Fisher Scientific, Pittsburgh, PA, USA), and stored at −20°C until use. For immunohistochemistry, tissue sections were treated with 10% normal goat serum and 0.3% triton X-100 for one hour, and then primary antibodies dissolved in the same blocking solution were applied at 4°C overnight. The primary antibodies were rabbit anti-Iba1 (1:500; Wako, LA, CA, USA), mouse anti-synaptotagmin (1:500; Chemicon, Temecula, CA, USA), rabbit anti-C3 (1:100; MP Biomedicals, Aurora, OH, USA), mouse anti-CD11b (1:500; Serotec, Oxford, UK), and mouse anti-MAP2 (1:500; Sigma, St Louis, MO, USA). Tissue sections were washed thoroughly and then incubated with appropriate secondary antibodies tagged with Alexa Fluor 488 or 594 (1:500; Molecular Probes, Eugene, OR, USA) for one hour at room temperature. Coverslips were mounted onto the slides with glycerol-based mounting medium (Biomeda, Foster City, CA, USA). Images were taken using a FV 300 confocal microscope (Olympus, Tokyo, Japan). For brightfield imaging of Iba1 immunostaining, transverse spinal cord sections were treated with 10% hydrogen peroxide to quench endogenous peroxidase activity. After rinsing and blocking, slides were incubated with rabbit anti-Iba1 (1:500; Wako, LA, CA, USA) at 4°C overnight in a humid chamber. Tissue sections were rinsed and incubated with biotinylated goat anti-rabbit IgG secondary antibody (1:400), and the antigen-antibody reaction was visualized using a Vectastain Elite ABC kit (Vector, Burlingame, CA) with a Vector SG peroxidase substrate kit (Vector, Burlingame, CA). Eriochrome cyanine staining was used to define the boundary of gray and white matter.

Western blot

Lumbar spinal cord tissue blocks were dissected using the same methods as for the microarray experiment. The tissue blocks were homogenized in ice-cold lysis buffer containing 20 mM Tris-HCl (pH 7.5), 1 mM EDTA, 5 mM $MgCl_2$, 1 mM dithiothreitol, 0.1 mM phenylmethylsulfonyl fluoride, and a protease inhibitor cocktail (Pierce, Rockford, IL, USA). The tissue homogenate was centrifuged at 10,000 rpm for 15 min at 4̊C, and the protein concentration of the supernatant was measured using a Bradford assay. Equal amounts of proteins were resolved by SDS-PAGE and transferred to a PVDF membrane (Millipore, Bedford, MA). The membrane was blocked in Tris-buffered saline (TBS) containing 5% BSA and probed with rabbit anti-Arc (1:500; Santa Cruz, Dallas, USA) and rabbit anti-Adam8 (1:500; Millipore, Bedford, MA, USA). After washing, the membranes were incubated for 2 hrs at room temperature with secondary antibodies (goat anti-rabbit, 1:3000; Cell Signaling, Danvers, MA, USA). All blots were probed with antibodies against β-actin (1:20000; Sigma, St Louis, MO, USA) to normalize differences in loading amount.

Quantitative image analysis

For unbiased stereological evaluation of the number of microglia in the lumbar spinal cord sections, Iba1-positive cells were counted using an Olympus BX51 Microscope coupled with Stereo Investigator 8 software (MBF Bioscience, Williston, VT, USA). Cell counting was performed using one out of 10 serial slides (inter-section interval in one slide was 200 μm). In one slide, every 4th section was used for counting (section sampling fraction, ssf = 1/40). Iba1- positive cells within optical dissectors placed randomly in regions of interest were counted using stereological criteria. Lumbar spinal cord was delineated using a 4x objective, and optical dissectors consisting of an inclusion and an exclusion line were randomly placed. Based on the eriochrome myelin staining, white matter and gray matter were delineated separately. The sampling grid dimensions were $200 \times 200\ \mu m^2$ and the counting grid was $120 \times 120\ \mu m^2$, resulting in an area sampling fraction (asf) of 0.36. Using a dissector height of 12 μm, height sampling fraction (hsf) was 0.67 (12/18) with the average postprocessing section thickness 18 μm. Actual counting was performed using 40x magnification. A total of 5 animals from each group were used for quantification. To quantify the proportion of microglia and synaptotagmin co-localization, a total of three sections were chosen per each animal (5 animals per group). Five regions of interest were captured from the same transverse sections at 63x magnification using an LSM 510 confocal laser-scanning microscope. Counting of synaptotagmin puncta colocalizing with Iba1 immunoreactivity was performed in a single optical plane. The total number of colocalized synaptotagmin puncta was divided by the microglia number obtained in all 15 images (5 images per section, 3 sections).

Statistical methods

Statistical analysis was performed using GraphPad Prism software version 5.0 (San Diego, CA). Unpaired Student's t-tests or one-way ANOVA followed by Tukey's post-hoc test was used to compare group means at single time points. Repeated measures two-way ANOVA was used to compare differences in BBB locomotor scores over different time points. Numerical values in all the graphs are presented as mean ± SEM.

Results

TMT improved locomotor recovery after thoracic SCI

We first documented positive effects of our treadmill training (TMT) protocol on locomotor recovery after contusive thoracic SCI. Animals showed rapid locomotor recovery during the first week regardless of TMT (Figure. 1). Recovery in control animals (without TMT) measured using the BBB locomotor score was rapid until around 3 weeks, after which only minimal improvement was observed. Animals with TMT exhibited enhanced locomotor recovery beginning at 2 weeks and continued to show higher quality overground locomotion (Figure. 1). The locomotor improvement induced by TMT was statistically significant compared to control animals ($p<0.001$ by repeated measures two-way ANOVA). To gain an insight on the molecular mechanisms at the spinal level underlying the locomotor recovery, we performed gene expression profiling in the lumbar motor region where the spinal locomotor center is located. Seventh day after injury was chosen as an early time point because animals typically showed rapid locomotor improvement around this time. We also chose 21st day as a late time point when spontaneous locomotor recovery began to plateau and the effects of our TMT protocol became evident (Figure. 1). We first analyzed gene expression patterns in the lumbar motor region following thoracic SCI (T9 level) at these two time points.

Gene expression profiling in the lumbar spinal cord below the lesion

Contusive SCI led to an upregulation of almost 300 genes in the lumbar motor region at either 1 or 3 weeks after injury, 161 of which were upregulated at both time points (Figure. 2A). The number of downregulated genes at 1 week was smaller than that for upregulation at the same time point (Figure. 2B). However, the number of downregulated genes at 3 weeks was comparable to that for upregulated genes at the same time point. Intriguingly, the number of genes downregulated only at the 3- week time point was larger than that of genes downregulated only at 1 week, suggesting that more widespread transcriptional depression occurred by the later time point. Complete lists of genes that were differentially expressed in the lumbar motor regions after thoracic SCI are provided in Tables S1-3. Gene ontology analysis revealed that genes related to development, neuronal elements (such as axon, neuronal projection, and growth cone), neurotransmitter transport, metabolic process, and angiogenesis were preferentially downregulated at the 3-week time point (Figure. 2F). At the 1-week time point, genes involved in metabolic functions (cellular biosynthetic process, regulation of metabolic process), developmental process, and synapse were downregulated (Figure. 2D). Notably, genes related to synaptic function, such as Grin1 (encoding NMDA receptor subunit 1), Arc, Grm7 (encoding metabotropic glutamate receptor 7), and Syt6 (encoding synaptotagmin-6), were significantly downregulated at both 1 and 3 weeks (Figure. 2H).

The most striking finding in the expression profiling was the upregulation of genes with functions in immune processes and/or inflammatory reactions (Figure. 2C, 2E, and 2G). Biological processes related to this category include regulation of immune responses, immune cell (B cell, T cell, and leukocytes) proliferation and differentiation, cytokine production, the complement system, and inflammatory signaling pathways. Some of the genes related to inflammatory processes were upregulated at either 1 or 3 weeks after injury, but the majority of these genes were upregulated at both time points. We focused our analysis on the inflammation-related genes that showed robust (more than 2-fold) upregulation

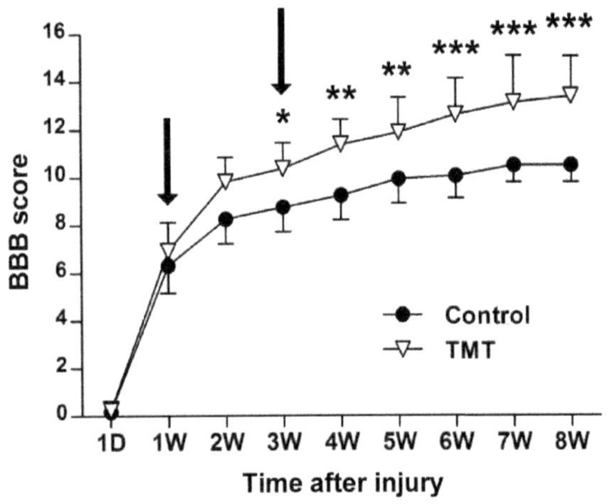

Figure 1. Treadmill training promotes locomotor recovery following contusive injury. Locomotor recovery was assessed by Basso, Beattie, and Bresnahan (BBB) locomotor scoring over the 8-week period after thoracic contusive injury. Animals subjected to treadmill training (TMT) showed enhanced locomotor recovery compared to those without TMT (control group). Arrows indicate the two time points chosen for microarray gene analysis. *, **, and *** indicate $p<0.05$, $p<0.01$, and $p<0.001$, respectively, by Bonferroni post-hoc tests following repeated measures two-way ANOVA. N = 8 animals per group.

at both time points (Table 3). Galectin3 (Lgals3), which is selectively expressed in microglial cells after SCI and thought to contribute to secondary injury [15,21], showed the most robust upregulation at both time points. Genes encoding markers for immune cells such as CD68, CD86, CD45 (Ptprc), and CD53 [22–24], were also upregulated. Matrix metalloproteinases (MMPs) regulate post-injury inflammation in the spinal cord contributing to diverse pathological outcomes [25]. We found that the Timp1 gene, an endogenous tissue inhibitor of metalloproteinases, was potently upregulated.

Particularly intriguing was the upregulation of several molecules that comprise components of the complement system. Of these, C3 showed the most robust upregulation (more than 4-fold and 3-fold at 1 and 3 weeks, respectively). All three subunits of C1q complexes and C2 were also robustly upregulated. When the changes in gene expression were mapped on a diagram of the protein interaction network of the complement pathway, most of the complement components that participate in a cascade (both classical and alternative) leading to activation of C3 showed increased expression (Figure. 3). In contrast, the complement components that participate in the assembly of membrane attack complex were not significantly changed. C3 activation plays a pivotal role in opsonization of pathogens which are then recognized by complement receptors on macrophages and ultimately phagocytosed [26]. Itgb2 (intergrin beta-2 subunit, CD18), which is a component of complement receptor 3 (CR3) and mediates C3-CR3 interaction in the phagocytic process [26], was also significantly upregulated (Table 3). Expression of the Serping1 (C1 inhibitor) and Complement factor H (Cfh) genes, encoding complement control proteins regulating the classical and alternative pathways [27], respectively, were increased as well (Table 3 and Figure. 3).

Robust upregulation of the Galectin3, C3, C1qa, C1qb, Itgb2 and Timp1 genes was verified by real-time RT-PCR (Figure. 4). For these inflammation-related genes upregulated by SCI, we compared expression levels between animals with or without TMT (at the 3-week time point). Microarray data showed that the elevated levels of expression of inflammation-related genes were maintained in the animals subjected to TMT (Table 3). Real-time RT-PCR also showed that the expression of the principal genes related to inflammation was not appreciably affected by TMT, except Galectin3 where a slight, but significant decrease in expression level was observed in animals with TMT (Figure. 4).

Potential roles of microglial cells in the lumbar spinal cord below the lesion

The increased expression of galectin3 and the myeloid cell marker CD68 suggested that microglia might increase in number in the lumbar motor region following thoracic SCI. Indeed, immunohistochemical staining showed a marked increase in the number of Iba1-positive microglia at 3 weeks after SCI (Figure. 5A-B). The increase in microglia number was not restricted to the white matter, where Wallerian degeneration of descending axons injured at the epicenter is expected to provoke active inflammation at around this time point [28], but was also observed in the gray matter. Stereological counting showed a comparable number of microglial cells in the gray and white matter (Figure. 5G and 5H). The increase in the number of microglia was not affected by TMT in either gray or white matter.

In the ventral gray matter at the lumbar level, Iba1-positive microglial cells were located near MAP2-positive neuronal cell bodies or dendritic neuropil (Figure. 5D-F), suggesting that intimate interactions between neurons and microglia could occur. Several studies have demonstrated roles of microglia in remodeling synaptic circuits during development or disease [29–31]. The complement cascade has also been implicated in synaptic remodeling [32], and a recent study showed that the interaction between neuronal C3 and microglial CR3 mediates the engulfment of synaptic puncta during development [29]. The microglial cells located in the ventral gray matter were positive for another CR3 component, CD11b (Figure. 6A and 6B). We also observed increased C3 protein around neuronal cell bodies and in the neuropil areas (Figure. 6D and 6E). Therefore, we tested the possibility that increased microglial activity in the ventral gray matter is involved in the removal of synaptic structures following SCI at the thoracic level. Synaptotagmin immunopositive puncta colocalizing with Iba1 immunoreactivity were considered as engulfed presynaptic material (Figure. 6G). The number of engulfed presynaptic puncta was almost three times higher at 3 week after injury in animals with SCI than in sham-operated controls (Figure. 6H and 6J). TMT for 2 weeks did not influence the expression of CR3 in microglia or C3 in neurons, or the number of engulfed synaptotagmin positive puncta (Figure. 6C, 6F, 6I, and 6J), suggesting that the potential synaptic remodeling mediated by microglia is unlikely to be regulated by TMT.

Regulation of the injury-induced gene expression profiles by TMT

To examine the effects of TMT on gene expression after injury, expression profiles were compared at 3 weeks after injury in animals with and without TMT. To exclude genes that are regulated by TMT independently of SCI, we compared gene expressions between sham operated animals with and without TMT. A total of 146 genes (60 upregulated and 86 downregulated) were regulated by TMT irrespective of SCI (Table S4). Five out of the 146 gene were found to be differentially expressed between animals at 3 weeks after injury with and without TMT (1 upregulated and 4 downregulated). Therefore, these 5genes were excluded from the analysis on TMT-regulated genes in the lumbar spinal cord after SCI.

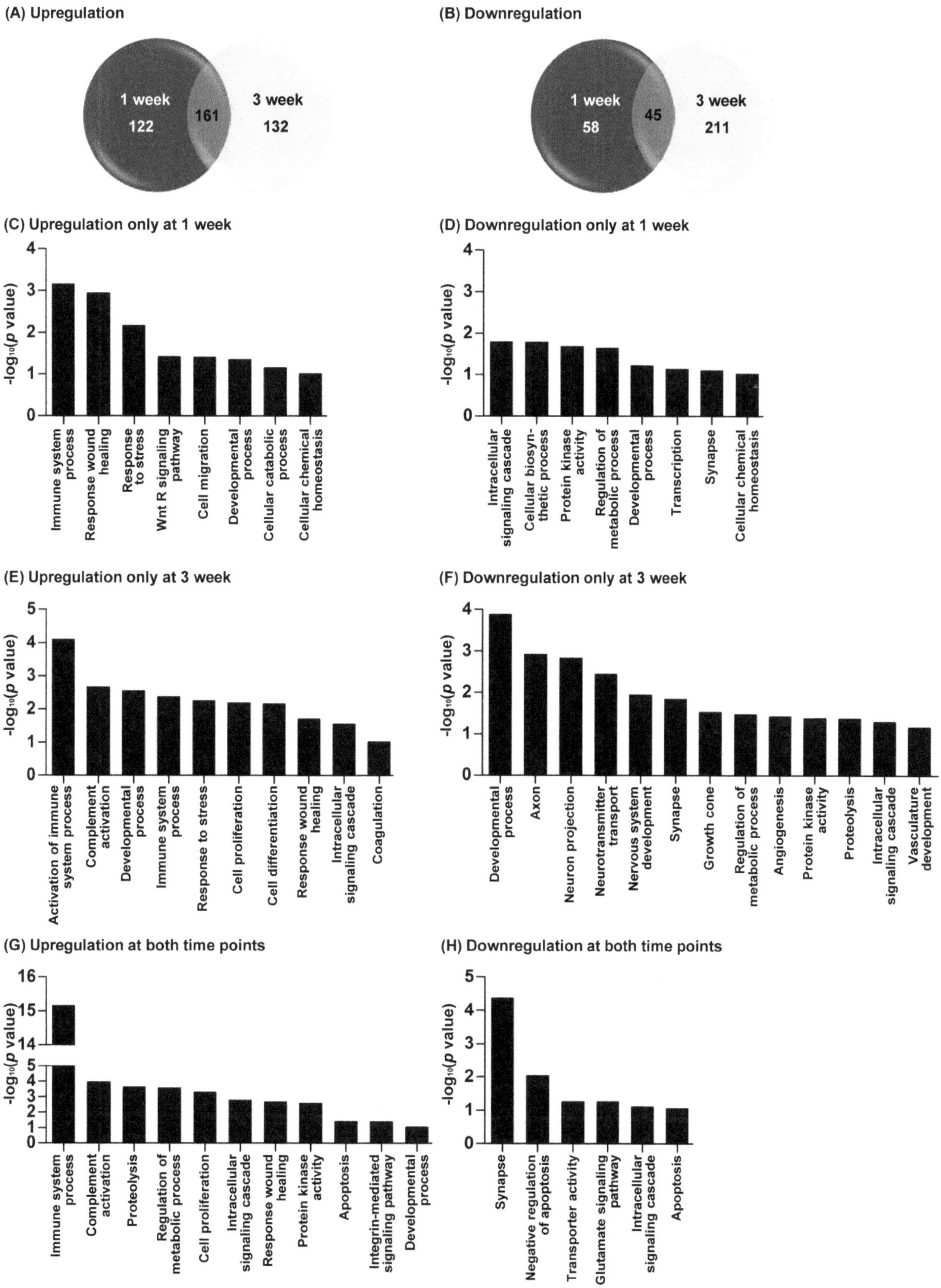
(A) Upregulation
1 week
122
161
3 week
132
(B) Downregulation
1 week
58
45
3 week
211
(C) Upregulation only at 1 week
-log10(p value)
Immune system process
Response wound healing
Response to stress
Wnt R signaling pathway
Cell migration
Developmental process
Cellular catabolic process
Cellular chemical homeostasis
(D) Downregulation only at 1 week
-log10(p value)
Intracellular signaling cascade
Cellular biosyn-thetic process
Protein kinase activity
Regulation of metabolic process
Developmental process
Transcription
Synapse
Cellular chemical homeostasis
(E) Upregulation only at 3 week
-log10(p value)
Activation of immune system process
Complement activation
Developmental process
Immune system process
Response to stress
Cell proliferation
Cell differentiation
Response wound healing
Intracellular signaling cascade
Coagulation
(F) Downregulation only at 3 week
-log10(p value)
Developmental process
Axon
Neuron projection
Neurotransmitter transport
Nervous system development
Synapse
Growth cone
Regulation of metabolic process
Angiogenesis
Protein kinase activity
Proteolysis
Intracellular signaling cascade
Vasculature development
(G) Upregulation at both time points
-log10(p value)
Immune system process
Complement activation
Proteolysis
Regulation of metabolic process
Cell proliferation
Intracellular signaling cascade
Response wound healing
Protein kinase activity
Apoptosis
Integrin-mediated signaling pathway
Developmental process
(H) Downregulation at both time points
-log10(p value)
Synapse
Negative regulation of apoptosis
Transporter activity
Glutamate signaling pathway
Intracellular signaling cascade
Apoptosis

Figure 2. Gene expression profile changes in the lumbar spinal cord at 1 and 3 weeks after thoracic spinal cord injury. (A-B) The number of genes differentially expressed (A, upregulated or B, downregulated) at 1 or 3 weeks after injury compared to sham operated animals. Venn diagrams show the total number of differentially expressed genes at 1 (dark gray circle) and 3 weeks (light gray circle) after injury. The number in the area of overlap of the two circles indicates the number of genes whose expression changed at both time points. (C-H) Gene ontology (GO)-based functional enrichment analysis using DAVID software. GO terms significantly ($p<0.1$) enriched in the following groups of genes are shown on the X-axis; upregulation only at 1 week (C), downregulation only at 1 week (D), upregulation only at 3 week (E), downregulation only at 3 week (F), upregulation at both time points (G), downregulation at both time points (H). Log_{10}- transformed p values are shown on the Y-axis.

Compared to the gene expression level at 3 weeks after injury, 9 genes were significantly downregulated in animals subjected to the 2-week TMT protocol (from 1 to 3 week). These genes are related to transcriptional activity, protein degradation, and cell-to-cell communication (Table 4). A much larger number of genes were upregulated by TMT; the expression of 49 genes was significantly upregulated in animals with TMT compared to those without TMT. The majority of these upregulated genes are involved in transcriptional activity, metabolism and biosynthesis, intracellular signaling, synapse, and angiogenesis (Table 4). Using the k-means clustering algorithm, genes regulated by TMT were classified into different clusters based on changes in gene expression pattern by injury and TMT. Of the downregulated genes, the majority belonged to cluster 1, 2 or 3, in which gene expression levels

Table 3. Inflammation-related genes that were upregulated by more than 2-fold at both 1 and 3 weeks after SCI.

Gene symbol	Gene full name	Log2 (fold change)		
		1 week	3 week	TMT
Lgals3	lectin, galactoside-binding, soluble, 3	2.53	3.41	3.34
C3	complement component 3	2.25	1.64	1.62
Cd68	Cd68 molecule	2.20	2.61	2.58
Cd86	Cd86 molecule	2.20	2.61	1.39
Aif1	allograft inflammatory factor 1	2.13	1.73	1.77
Timp1	TIMP metallopeptidase inhibitor 1	2.11	1.87	1.63
Ly86	lymphocyte antigen 86	2.03	1.34	1.44
Cfh	complement factor H	1.74	1.88	1.76
Ptprc	protein tyrosine phosphatase, receptor type, C (CD45)	1.74	1.14	1.30
Blnk	B-cell linker (Ly57)	1.72	1.60	1.72
Tifab	TRAF-interacting protein with forkhead-associated domain, family member B	1.66	1.16	1.35
Csf3r	colony stimulating factor 3 receptor (granulocyte)	1.63	1.30	1.42
Hmox1	heme oxygenase (decycling) 1	1.59	1.06	0.83
Klhl6	kelch-like family member 6	1.53	1.04	1.01
Pycard	PYD and CARD domain containing	1.44	1.11	1.19
C1qb	complement component 1, q subcomponent, B chain	1.44	1.49	1.46
Itgal	integrin, alpha L	1.42	1.14	1.54
Nckap1l	NCK associated protein 1 like (Hem1)	1.42	1.18	1.04
Ptpn6	protein tyrosine phosphatase, non-receptor type 6 (Shp1)	1.38	1.29	1.23
Fcgr2a/2b	Fc fragment of IgG, low affinity lia/b, receptor (CD32)	1.36	1.51	1.76
Cd53	Cd53 molecule	1.34	1.25	1.36
C1qa	complement component 1, q subcomponent, A chain	1.33	1.46	1.37
C2	complement component 2	1.33	1.40	1.16
Inpp5d	inositol polyphosphate-5-phosphatase D (Ship1)	1.26	1.21	1.16
Csf1r	colony stimulting factor 1 receptor	1.26	1.10	1.28
Mall	mal, T-cell differentiation protein-like	1.18	1.37	1.41
Anxa3	annexin A3	1.15	1.00	1.13
Mrc2	mannose receptor, C type 2	1.13	1.36	1.21
Cyba	cytochrome b-245, alpha polypeptide (p22-phox)	1.12	1.11	1.23
C1qc	complement component 1, q subcomponent, C chain	1.10	1.04	1.18
Itgb2	integrin, beta 2	1.03	1.29	1.36
Ifitm1	interferon induced transmembrane protein 1	1.01	1.28	0.80

TMT = treadmill locomotor training.

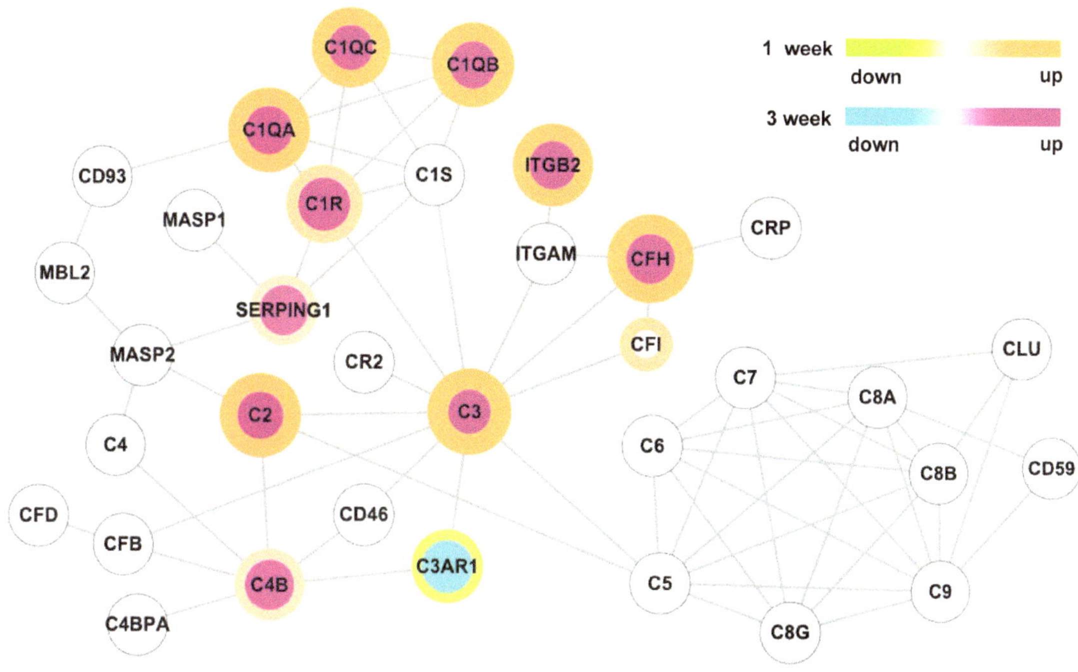

Figure 3. The complement pathway protein-protein interaction network. Nodes represent proteins and lines represent physical interactions between them. The color of the node indicates the fold-change in gene expression at 3 weeks relative to that in the control sham group. The color of the node border indicates the fold-change in expression at 1 week relative to that in the control sham group. Color scales are shown in the upper right. The fold-changes were log_2-transformed and only genes that showed significantly different expressions ($p<0.05$ by Student's t-test and absolute fold-change > 1.5) were color-mapped.

tended to increase after injury but to decrease with TMT (Figure. 7A and 7B). We chose three genes in these clusters and verified the microarray results by real-time RT-PCR. The expression of the March6 gene, encoding a ring finger family E3 ubiquitin ligase, was increased at 1 and 3 weeks after SCI, but TMT reversed the expression to the pre-injury level (Figure. 7C). An epigenetic modifier Kdm4c (also known as Jmjd2c), which possesses histone demethylase activity (H3K9) [33], showed a similar pattern of gene expression (Figure. 7D). The Frg1 gene is inappropriately overexpressed in facioscapulohumeral muscular dystrophy [34] and thought to function in mRNA splicing [35]. Frg1 showed robust upregulation at the 3-week time point and complete normalization by TMT (Figure. 7E).

Genes upregulated by TMT were classified into 5 clusters. The expression of genes in cluster 1 was not obviously changed by injury but markedly increased by TMT (Figure. 8A and 8B). A larger number of genes showed a variable degree of downregulation by injury with TMT inducing either reversal to the pre-injury level (clusters3 and 5) or an increase above the control value (clusters 2 and 4) (Figure. 8A and 8B). In general, TMT tended to upregulate the expression of genes in functional classes corresponding to the functional classes of genes that were downregulated by injury. For example, genes related to metabolism and biosynthesis were downregulated by injury (Figure. 2), and TMT upregulated 9 genes belonging to this functional category (Table 4). Genes with functions in synapse and angiogenesis were also downregulated by injury (Figure. 2). TMT upregulated synapse-related genes such as Arc, Nrcam, and Nlgn1. Similarly, the angiogenesis-related genes Tie1 and Adam8 were significantly upregulated by TMT.

To confirm the trend of TMT-induced restoration of gene expression observed in the microarray experiments, a combination of real-time PCR and western blotting was used. First, the expression pattern of two of the genes related to synapse function, Arc and Nrcam (neural cell adhesion molecule), was examined. Arc is a well-characterized immediate-early gene with a function in homeostatic plasticity at the synapse [36]. Real-time RT-PCR showed that the level of Arc gene expression tended to decrease at 1 and 3 weeks after SCI, and TMT significantly increased the mRNA expression above the pre-injury level (Figure. 8C). Arc expression was also examined at the protein level. We found that the Arc protein level substantially decreased at 3 weeks after SCI and tended to get normalized by TMT (Figure. 9A and 9B). Real-time RT-PCR also showed that the Nrcam mRNA level tended to decrease at 3 weeks after SCI and to increase to slightly above the pre-injury level with TMT (Figure. 8D), consistent with the microarray result.

The TMT-induced changes in expression of two genes with functions in angiogenesis were also validated. Adam8 is selectively expressed in endothelial cells and is associated with angiogenesis at the epicenter in a mouse SCI model [37]. Tie1 is an endothelial specific tyrosine kinase and known to play a regulatory role in angiopoietin1-dependent angiogenesis [38]. Real-time RT-PCR revealed robust reduction of Adam8 gene expression at the 3-week time point (Figure. 8E). The Adam8 gene expression was substantially restored close to the pre-injury level with TMT. Consistent with the gene expression data, we found that Adam8 protein exhibited a marked decrease at 3 weeks, and TMT resulted in an increase of the Adam8 protein level (Figure. 9C and 9D). TMT-induced significant upregulation of the Tie1 gene was also verified by real-time RT-PCR (Figure. 8F).

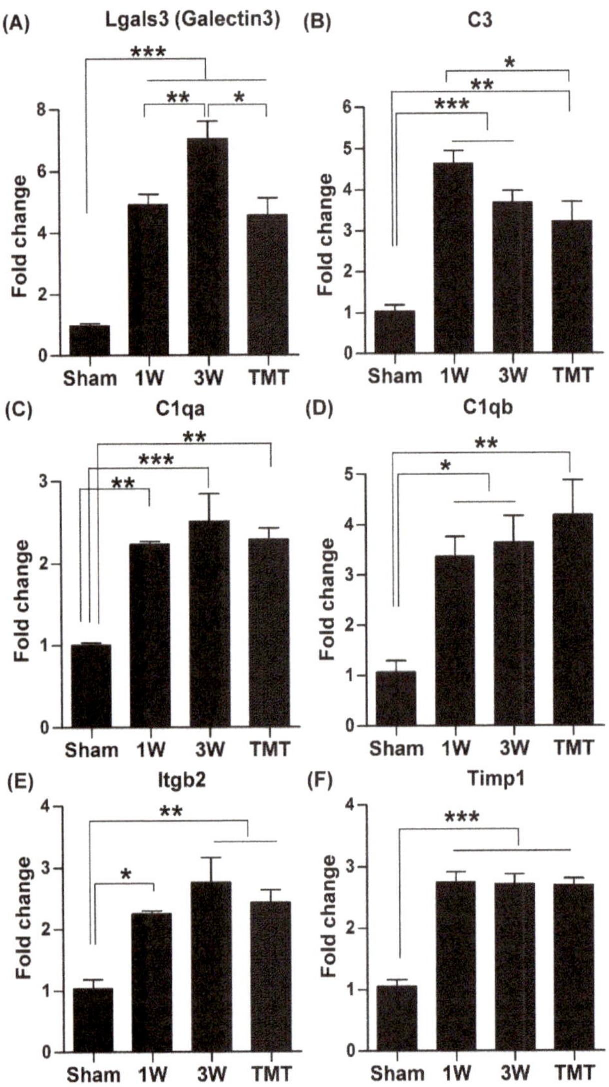

Figure 4. Validation of microarray data for inflammation-related genes using real time RT-PCR. (A-F) Quantification graphs of real-time RT-PCR for Lgals (Galectin3) (A), C3 (Complement component 3) (B), C1qa (complement component 1, q subcomponent, A chain) (C), C1qb (complement component 1, q subcomponent, B chain) (D), Itgb2 (integrin, beta 2, complement receptor 3 subunit) (E), and Timp 1 genes (F) in the sham operated group (sham), animals 1 week (1W), 3 weeks (3W) after injury without treadmill training (TMT), and with TMT. N = 4 animals for each group. *, **, and *** represent $p<0.05$, $p<0.01$, and $p<0.001$, respectively, by one way ANOVA followed by Tukey's post-hoc analysis. Error bars represent SEM.

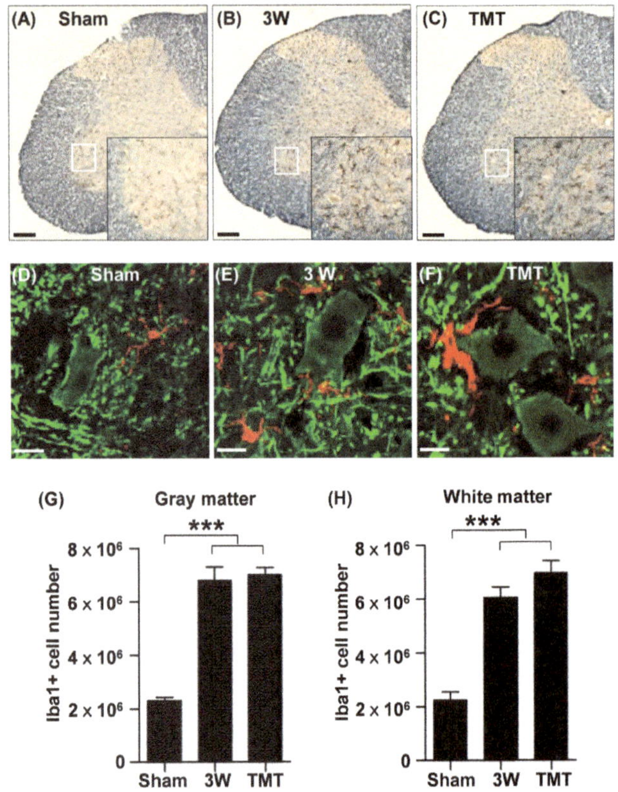

Figure 5. Microglia markedly increased in number in the lumbar motor region following thoracic SCI. (A-C) Representative images of lumbar spinal cord sections stained with an antibody recognizing the microglial marker Iba1 (dark brown) antibody in sham operation (A), at 3 weeks (3W) after injury (B), and at 3W after injury with treadmill training (TMT) (C). Immunostained sections were counterstained with eriochrome cyanine to differentiate the gray matter and white matters. Insets are magnified images of the regions in the white boxes in the ventral gray matter. Scale bars represent 100 μm. (D-F) Representative images of lumbar spinal cord sections colabeled with Iba1 (red) and MAP2 (green) antibodies in sham operation (D), at 3W after injury (E), and at 3W after injury with TMT (F). Note that Iba1 positive microglial cells are frequently associated with MAP2 positive neurons and dendritic neuropil areas. Scale bars represent 20 μm. (G-H) Quantification of stereological counting of Iba1-positive microglial cells in the gray matter (G) and white matter (H) of the lumbar spinal cord. *** represent $p<0.001$ by one-way ANOVA followed by Tukey's post-hoc analysis. N = 5 for each group. Error bars represent SEM.

Discussion

In this study, we characterized the patterns of gene expression changes in the lumbar spinal cord following thoracic contusive SCI with or without TMT, an intervention to promote locomotor recovery. Our data showed robust upregulation of inflammation-related genes at both 1 and 3 weeks after injury. Consistent with the gene expression changes, the number of microglial cells in the lumbar motor region substantially increased. Further experiments suggested potential roles of the complement components and microglial cells in synaptic remodeling of the lumbar motor circuit. Comparison of gene expression profiles between animals with or without TMT showed that the upregulation of inflammation-related genes was not appreciably affected by TMT. However, TMT frequently restored the expression levels of genes that were downregulated by injury. Notably, TMT increased the expression of genes involved in neuroplasticity and angiogenesis, suggesting that promoting neurovascular remodeling may in part be a mechanism by which TMT contributes to locomotor recovery.

The microarray method has been employed in many studies to profile gene expression changes in the spinal cord following SCI [13–15,39–44]. Most of these studies have focused on the gene expressions only at the epicenter or at the distal segment immediately adjacent to the epicenter where secondary tissue degeneration could be observed. To the authors' knowledge, only one study has examined transcriptional changes in a region sufficiently caudal to the epicenter (T8 in that study) to include the lumbar locomotor circuit, although it was not explicitly stated whether they intended to sample the lumbar motor region [45].

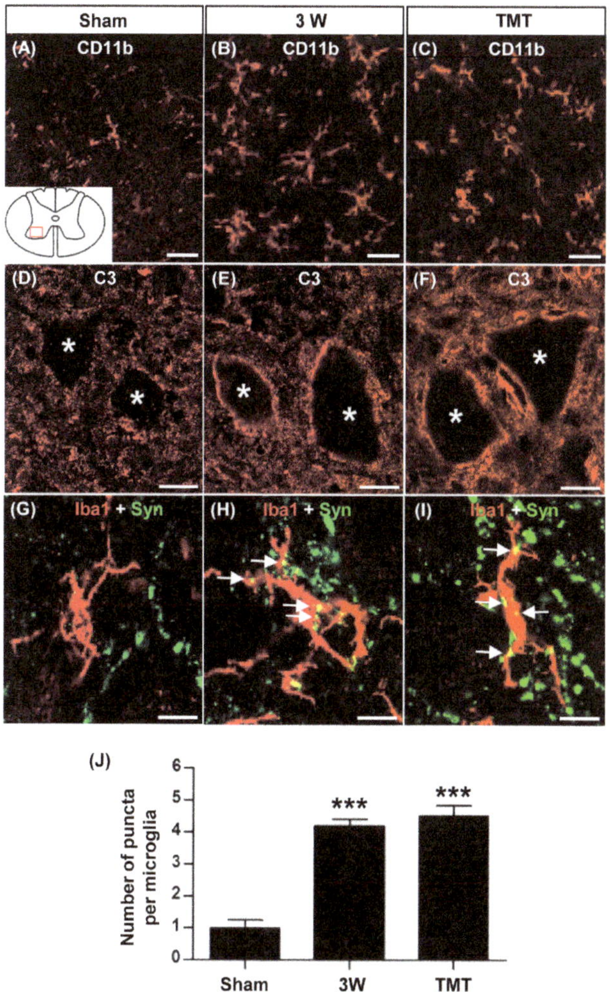

Figure 6. Involvement of microglial cells in synaptic remodeling in the lumbar motor region following thoracic spinal cord injury. (A-I) Representative images of transverse spinal cord sections from sham operated animals (A, D, G), animals at 3 weeks (3W) after injury (B, E, H), and animals at 3W after injury with treadmill training (TMT) (C, F, I). (A-C) Sections were stained with antibodies against CD11b (subunit of complement receptor 3). (D-F) Sections were stained with antibodies against C3 (complement component 3). Asterisks indicate cell bodies of ventral motor neurons. (G-I) Representative images of sections colabeled with Iba1 (red) and synaptotagmin (Syn; green). Each image consists of only a single optical plane. Double-labeled punctate signals (yellow) were considered as engulfed synaptic puncta (indicated by white arrows). The diagram inset in (A) shows the approximate location of regions of interest (red-boxed region within the ventral horn) for all the images. All scale bars represent 10 μm. (J) Quantification of the number of colocalized synaptic puncta per microglia. N = 5 animals for each group. *** represents $p<0.001$ by one-way ANOVA followed by Tukey's post-hoc analysis. Error bars represent SEM.

The pattern of gene expression changes in our study was similar to that in the caudal segment at comparable time points after SCI reported in the study by Aimone et al. (2004). The majority of the transcriptome changes in their study were not specific to the caudal segment but followed a similar pattern at the epicenter and rostral segment, suggesting that the global trend of gene expression changes spread rostrocaudally irrespective of functional distinction at different segmental regions. It is worth reporting that expressions of genes known to be highly specific for the peripheral nerves (such as P0 and PMP22) were observed in our samples despite our efforts to remove the root components during the dissection of spinal cord tissues. A caveat remains, therefore, that some of gene expression profiles found in microarray may result from transcriptional changes in the peripheral nerve.

In our study, the most robust changes were observed in genes related to immune processes or inflammation, including genes involved in immune cell differentiation and proliferation, inflammatory signaling pathways, cytokines, and the complement system. As mentioned above, the increases in expression of inflammation-related genes observed in previous studies occurred diffusely along the spinal cord: in the epicenter, adjacent regions, and rostrocaudal segments quite distant from the epicenter [15,45]. Therefore, the robust upregulation of inflammation-related genes observed in our study is unlikely to be specific to the caudal segment below the lesion site or the lumbar motor circuit.

A notable observation in our study was the robust and concurrent upregulation of the components of an early complement cascade leading to C3 activation (Figure. 3). Activation of the complement system around the injury site may facilitate phagocytic cell removal of dead cells or participation in the secondary degeneration of neural cells [46,47]. In addition, formation of the membrane attack complex (C5b-9) may induce neural cell death [48,49]. We observed persistent upregulation of the early complement pathway in the lumbar motor region where there is no overt tissue degeneration. In contrast, the complement components involved in the formation of membrane attack complex was not activated, whereas it was reported that they are strongly activated at the epicenter after SCI [49]. This suggests that the activation of the early complement pathway in the caudal region may serve functions different from those at the epicenter. Recent studies have suggested that activation of the complement system may promote elimination of synapses by microglial phagocytosis [29,32]. Our data revealed microglial activation in the gray matter in close proximity to ventral motor neurons and their dendritic processes. We further showed that neurons in the ventral horn upregulated C3 and microglial cells in the vicinity of motor neurons were strongly positive for CD11b, a subunit of the CR3 receptor, which, upon binding of C3, stimulates phagocytic activity in microglial cells [26]. Therefore, we speculated that activated microglia near motor neurons after SCI may participate in the remodeling of synaptic structures in a manner similar to that in which they are involved in synaptic pruning during neural circuit formation [29]. Indeed, the number of synaptic puncta colocalizing with the microglial marker was substantially increased in the lumbar motor region after SCI. However, the synaptic pruning by microglia in the previous study was activity-dependent [29], whereas the extent of synapse elimination in our study was not affected by TMT, which supposedly increases neural activity of the locomotor circuit in the lumbar motor region. It remains to be determined whether the synaptic remodeling elicited by injury in the mature CNS is independent of activity or whether changes in neural activity in response to TMT were not strong enough to affect the removal of synaptic elements by microglia.

When the effects of TMT on gene expression after SCI were examined, TMT did not significantly influence the expression of inflammation-associated genes that were robustly upregulated SCI. However, a trend towards reversal of other SCI-induced gene expression changes was observed. A large number of genes that were downregulated after SCI were upregulated by TMT and vice versa (Figure. 7 and 8). The majority of TMT-induced changes were upregulations, implying that a principal molecular mechanism mediating TMT-induced locomotor recovery is to

Table 4. A list of genes that were regulated by treadmill locomotor training.

Functional group	Gene symbol	Gene full name
Cell communication	Jag1	jagged1
	Odz2	teneurin transmembrane protein 2
Ubiquitination & proteosome	March6	membrane-associated ring finger (C3HC4) 6
	Klhdc5	kelch domain containing 5
Transcription & epigenetics	Frg1	FSHD regions gene 1
	Kdm4c	lysine (K)-specific demethylase 4C (Jmjd2c)
Metabolism	Glod5	glyoxalase domain containing 5
	Cox6c-ps1	cytochrome c oxidase subunit VIc, pseudogene
Proliferation	Dis3l2	DIS3 mitotic control homolog (S. cerevisiae)-like 2
Immune & inflammation	Stat5b	signal transducer and activator of transcription 5B
	Icoslg	inducible T-cell co-stimulator ligand
	Crlf2	cytokine receptor-like factor 2
Intracellular signaling	Grb10	growth factor receptor bound protein 10
	Arhgap32	Rho GTPase activating protein 32
	Arfgef2	ADP-ribosylation factor guanine nucleotide-exchange factor 2 (brefeldin A-inhibited)
	Pde2a	phosphodiesterase 2A, cGMP-stimulated
	Farp2	FERM, RhoGEF and pleckstrin domain protein 2
	Tbc1d10b	TBC1 domain family, member 10b
	Raph1	ras association (RalGDS/AF-6) and pleckstrin homology domains 1
	Fkbp14	FK506 binding protein 14
	Ppp1r1b	protein phosphatase 1, regulatory (inhibitor) subunit 1B
Transcription & DNA repair	Fubp3	far upstream element (FUSE) binding protein 3
	Usf2	upstream transcription factor 2, c-fos interacting
	Pias1	protein inhibitor of activated STAT, 1
	Aqr	aquarius homolog (mouse)
	Mkl1	megakaryoblastic leukemia (translocation) 1
	Ints3	integrator complex subunit 3
	Zfp709	zinc finger protein 709
	Polb	polymerase (DNA directed), beta
Synapse	Nrcam	neuronal cell adhesion molecule
	Arc	activity-regulated cytoskeleton-associated protein
	Nlgn1	neuroligin 1
	Gja4	gap junction protein, alpha 4 (connexin-37)
Metabolism & biosynthesis	Retsat	retinol saturase (all trans retinol 13,14 reductase)
	Mtmr1	myotubularin related protein 1
	Slc13a3	solute carrier family 13 (sodium-dependent dicarboxylate transporter), member 3
	Chst12	carbohydrate (chondroitin 4) sulfotransferase 12
	Immt	inner membrane protein, mitochondrial
	Cyb5a	cytochrome b5 type A (microsomal)
	Bckdha	branched chain ketoacid dehydrogenase E1, alpha polypeptide
	Bcat1	branched chain amino acid transaminase 1, cytosolic
Angiogenesis	Adam8	ADAM metallopeptidase domain 8
	Tie1	tyrosine kinase with immunoglobulin-like and EGF-like domains 1
Apoptosis	Stk17b	serine/threonine kinase 17b (Drak2)
Translation	Gatc	glutamyl-tRNA(Gln) amidotransferase, subunit C
	Zc3h14	zinc finger CCCH-type containing 14
Cytoskeleton	Epb4.1	erythrocyte protein band 4.1
	Capg	capping protein (actin filament), gelsolin-like
	Myo1e	myosin 1E

Table 4. Cont.

Functional group	Gene symbol	Gene full name
Lysosome	Laptm4a	lysosomal protein transmembrane 4 alpha
Ubiquitination & proteosome	Ngly1	N-glycanase 1 (PNGase)
	Dcaf8	DDB1 and CUL4 associated factor 8 (Wdr42a)
Proliferation	Spag5	sperm associated antigen 5
Neuropeptide	Sst	Somatostatin
Undetermined	Dd25	hypothetical protein Dd25
	Samd10	sterile alpha motif domain containing 10
	Trim26	tripartite motif-containing 26
	Rnase4	ribonuclease, RNase A family 4

restore transcriptional activities of the genes of which expression levels are decreased by SCI. Intriguingly, however, we observed a distinct group of genes showing obvious upregulation by injury and normalization by TMT (Figure. 7). Overexpression of Frg1, a gene whose expression is altered in facioscapulohumeral muscular dystrophy, results in aberrant alternative pre-mRNA splicing associated with a muscular dystrophy phenotype in transgenic mice [35]. This suggests that high Frg1 gene expression after SCI

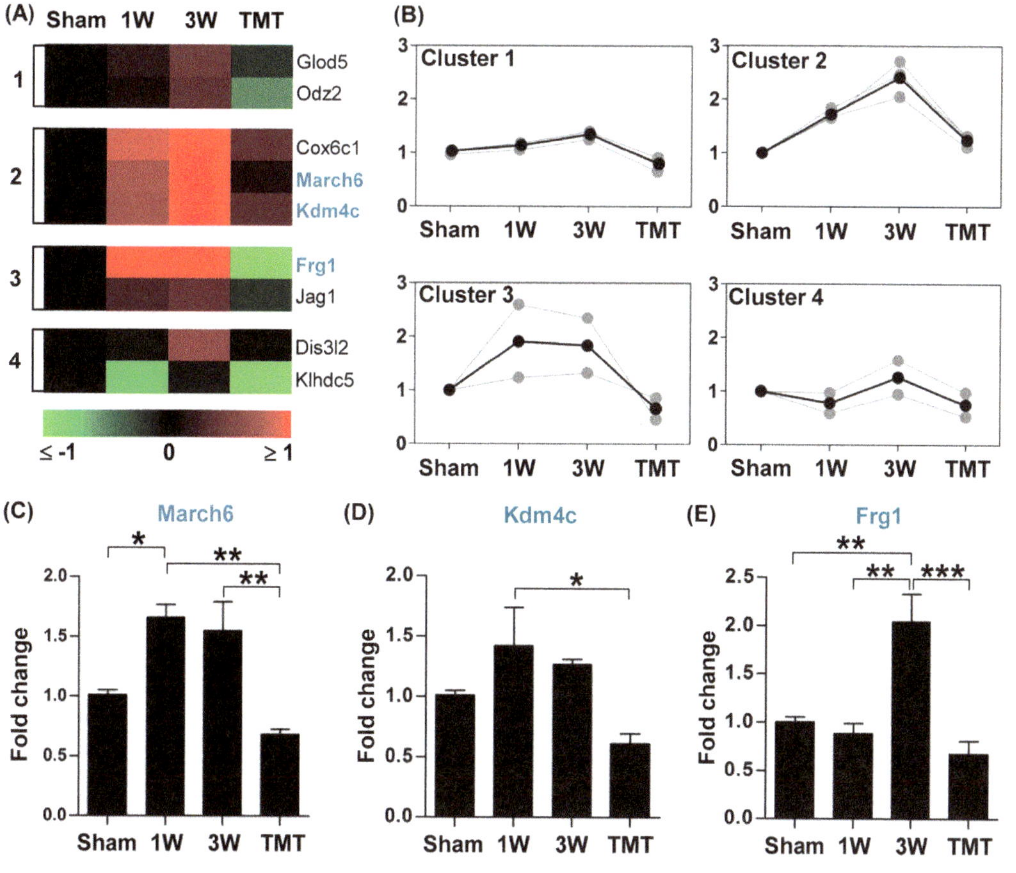

Figure 7. Genes downregulated by treadmill training. (A) Color-coded heatmaps of gene expression levels for genes whose expression was lower with treadmill training (TMT) than without TMT at 3 week after injury. Fold changes in gene expression level relative to the sham group expression level were $\log_2$-transformed and color-coded based on the color scale shown at the bottom. Genes were grouped into 4 clusters using a k-means clustering algorithm. The numbers shown at the left side of the heatmaps indicate the cluster indexes to which the genes belong. Genes for which validation data are represented are shown in blue. (B) Expression patterns of genes in each cluster. Gray lines indicate expression levels of individual genes and black lines indicate the average expression level of all genes in the cluster. Numbers on the Y-axis indicate $\log_2$-transformed fold changes relative to the expression level in the sham group. (C-E) Graphs of real-time RT-PCR results for genes selected from the list in (A) (shown in blue). N = 4 animals for each group. *, **, and *** represent $p<0.05$, $p<0.01$, and $p<0.001$, respectively, by one-way ANOVA followed by Tukey's post-hoc analysis. Error bars represent SEM.

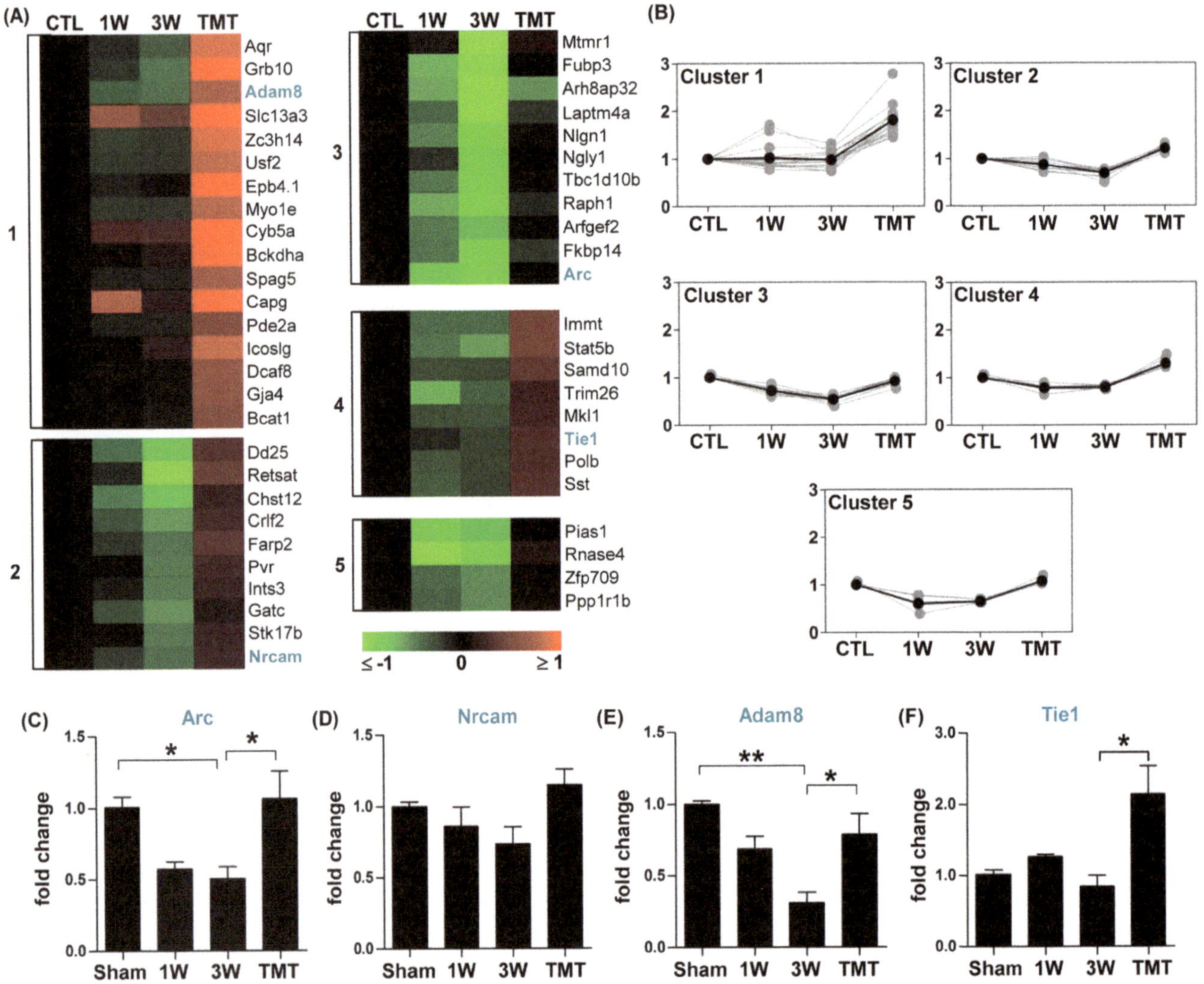

Figure 8. Genes upregulated by treadmill training. (A) Color-coded heatmaps of gene expression levels for the genes whose expression was higher with treadmill training (TMT) than without TMT at 3 weeks after injury. Fold changes in gene expression level relative to the sham group expression level were log_2-transformed and color-coded based on the color scale shown at the bottom. Genes were grouped into 5 clusters using a k-means clustering algorithm. The numbers shown at the left side of heatmaps indicate the cluster indexes to which the genes belong. Genes for which validation data are presented are shown in blue. (B) Expression patterns of genes in each cluster. Gray lines indicate expression levels of individual genes and black lines indicate the average expression level of all genes in the cluster. Numbers on the Y-axis indicate log_2-transformed fold changes relative to the expression level in the sham group. (C-F) Graphs of real-time RT-PCR results for genes selected from the list in (A) (shown in blue). N = 4 animals for each group. *, **, and *** represent $p<0.05$, $p<0.01$, and $p<0.001$, respectively, by one-way ANOVA followed by Tukey's post-hoc analysis. Error bars represent SEM.

may lead to a gain of dysfunction caused by altered transcription after abnormal splicing activity. In a similar vein, inappropriately augmented Kdm4c or March6 expression also may entail cellular dysfunction by dysregulating the methylation status of histones [33] or by altering ubiquitin-mediated proteolysis, respectively. TMT not only enhances locomotor recovery but also ameliorates dysfunctions including allodynia [50] and spasticity [51]. It is conceivable that normalizing inappropriate upregulation of these genes may contribute to the attenuation by TMT of such SCI-induced dysfunctions.

Gene expression profiling in the lumbar motor regions at 3 weeks revealed reduced transcriptional activities of genes related to neural functions (neural development, axon, synapse, neurotransmitter transport, etc), angiogenesis (including endothelial cell development), and metabolic processes (Figure. 2). These findings indicate that inadequate functions in these processes may in part be responsible for the limited extent of spontaneous locomotor recovery. In other words, restoring optimal functions in these processes may promote locomotor recovery following SCI. In agreement with this notion, TMT restored the expression of many genes involved in these processes to their pre-injury levels or boosted their expression to even higher than their control levels. These findings my provide clues as to potential mechanisms mediating TMT-induced locomotor recovery. Of the genes that were upregulated by TMT, we were particularly interested in genes involved in neuroplasticity and angiogenesis. Nrcam (neural cell adhesion molecule) has been shown to play a role in synaptic plasticity, neuritogenesis, and synaptogenesis [52–54]. Therefore, restoration of Nrcam expression by TMT may ensure an adequate level of plasticity after injury. Arc, also known as Arg3.1, is not

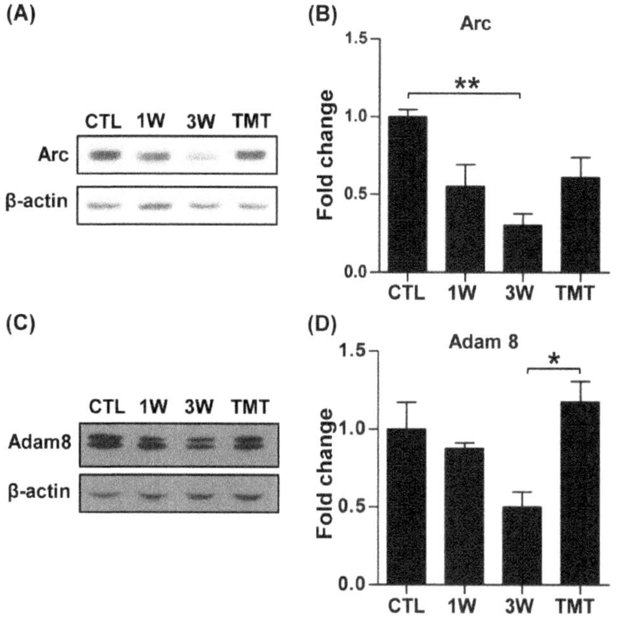

Figure 9. Validation of changes in protein expression from the Arc and Adam8 genes. (A, C) Representative western blots of Arc (A) and Adam8 (C). β-actin was used to normalize differences in loading amounts. (B, D) Quantification graphs of Arc (B) and Adam8 (D) western blots. Data are presented as fold-changes relative to the normal protein expression level after normalization with β-actin. N = 3 to 4 animals for each group. * and ** represent $p<0.05$ and $p<0.01$, respectively, by one-way ANOVA followed by Tukey's post-hoc analysis.

only involved in plasticity of synaptic strength (long-term potentiation or depression) but also in structural plasticity of dendritic spines [55–58]. Therefore, a decrease in the basal Arc level may lead to dysregulated spine remodeling occurring caudal to the injury level [59]. Furthermore, Arc has been implicated in regulating the homeostatic plasticity that maintains the neuronal threshold of excitability in response to chronic changes in synaptic activity [36]. For example, a loss of Arc leads to excess network hyperexcitability [58]. Decreased expression of Arc in the lumbar motor regions after SCI may contribute in part to the dysregulated spinal cord excitability that is responsible for functional disabilities observed in patients with SCI [60,61]. Together, this suggests that restoration of the level of Arc by TMT may contribute to improvement of locomotor function via multiple mechanisms.

TMT also upregulated the expression of the angiogenesis-related genes Adam8 and Tie1. It was recently reported that Adam8 is upregulated selectively in endothelial cells in the spinal cord and may regulate angiogenesis after SCI [37]. In particular, Adam8 may play a role in neovascularization by regulating ectodomain shedding of membrane proteins related to angiogenesis [62,63]. Tie1 is known to be an important regulator of angiopoietin-1 signaling in angiogenesis and vascular maintenance [64]. Based on these known functions, TMT-induced upregulation of Adam8 and Tie1 may promote vascular remodeling in the lumbar motor regions after SCI. A previous *in vivo* imaging study demonstrated a dynamic vascular remodeling in the lesioned spinal cord [65]. It is conceivable that a similar vascular remodeling process occurs in the lumbar motor region below the lesion, and that the vascular remodeling is one of the principal biological processes that are substantially influenced by TMT.

Together, our data showing that TMT concurrently upregulates neuroplasticity genes and angiogenesis genes suggests that TMT may contribute to locomotor recovery through promotion of neurovascular remodeling in the lumbar motor region. This notion is particularly intriguing because neural circuit formation and angiogenesis are thought to share common mechanisms [66]. It is possible that this shared signaling during development may be reactivated following injury. Indeed, dynamic neurovascular interactions have been observed in lesioned spinal cord [65]. Further studies will be needed to identify these developmentally linked signals that regulate neurovascular remodeling in the lumbar motor region thereby mediating locomotor recovery following SCI.

Supporting Information

Table S1 A list of genes that were differentially expressed only at 1-week time point.

Table S2 A list of genes that were differentially expressed only at 3-week time point.

Table S3 A list of genes that were differentially expressed only at 3-week time point.

Table S4 A list of genes that were differentially regulated by treadmill training in sham- operated animals.

Author Contributions

Conceived and designed the experiments: HYS KYL HK BGK. Performed the experiments: HYS HK MJK DHH. Analyzed the data: HYS KYL HK BGK. Wrote the paper: HYS KYL HK BGK.

References

1. MacKay-Lyons M (2002) Central pattern generation of locomotion: a review of the evidence. Phys Ther 82: 69–83.
2. Dobkin BH (2004) Neurobiology of rehabilitation. Ann N Y Acad Sci 1038: 148–170.
3. Rossignol S, Frigon A (2011) Recovery of locomotion after spinal cord injury: some facts and mechanisms. Annu Rev Neurosci 34: 413–440.
4. Edgerton VR, Tillakaratne NJ, Bigbee AJ, de Leon RD, Roy RR (2004) Plasticity of the spinal neural circuitry after injury. Annu Rev Neurosci 27: 145–167.
5. Roy RR, Harkema SJ, Edgerton VR (2012) Basic concepts of activity-based interventions for improved recovery of motor function after spinal cord injury. Arch Phys Med Rehabil 93: 1487–1497.
6. Barbeau H, Rossignol S (1987) Recovery of locomotion after chronic spinalization in the adult cat. Brain Res 412: 84–95.
7. de Leon RD, Hodgson JA, Roy RR, Edgerton VR (1998) Locomotor capacity attributable to step training versus spontaneous recovery after spinalization in adult cats. J Neurophysiol 79: 1329–1340.
8. Battistuzzo CR, Callister RJ, Callister R, Galea MP (2012) A systematic review of exercise training to promote locomotor recovery in animal models of spinal cord injury. J Neurotrauma 29: 1600–1613.
9. Harkema S, Gerasimenko Y, Hodes J, Burdick J, Angeli C, et al. (2011) Effect of epidural stimulation of the lumbosacral spinal cord on voluntary movement, standing, and assisted stepping after motor complete paraplegia: a case study. Lancet 377: 1938–1947.
10. Courtine G, Gerasimenko Y, van den Brand R, Yew A, Musienko P, et al. (2009) Transformation of nonfunctional spinal circuits into functional states after the loss of brain input. Nat Neurosci 12: 1333–1342.
11. Edgerton VR, Roy RR (2012) A new age for rehabilitation. Eur J Phys Rehabil Med 48: 99–109.
12. Gomez-Pinilla F, Ying Z, Roy RR, Molteni R, Edgerton VR (2002) Voluntary exercise induces a BDNF-mediated mechanism that promotes neuroplasticity. J Neurophysiol 88: 2187–2195.

13. Velardo MJ, Burger C, Williams PR, Baker HV, Lopez MC, et al. (2004) Patterns of gene expression reveal a temporally orchestrated wound healing response in the injured spinal cord. J Neurosci 24: 8562–8576.
14. Di Giovanni S, Knoblach SM, Brandoli C, Aden SA, Hoffman EP, et al. (2003) Gene profiling in spinal cord injury shows role of cell cycle in neuronal death. Ann Neurol 53: 454–468.
15. Byrnes KR, Garay J, Di Giovanni S, De Biase A, Knoblach SM, et al. (2006) Expression of two temporally distinct microglia-related gene clusters after spinal cord injury. Glia 53: 420–433.
16. Huang da W, Sherman BT, Lempicki RA (2009) Bioinformatics enrichment tools: paths toward the comprehensive functional analysis of large gene lists. Nucleic Acids Res 37: 1–13.
17. Saeed AI, Bhagabati NK, Braisted JC, Liang W, Sharov V, et al. (2006) TM4 microarray software suite. Methods Enzymol 411: 134–193.
18. Smoot ME, Ono K, Ruscheinski J, Wang PL, Ideker T (2011) Cytoscape 2.8: new features for data integration and network visualization. Bioinformatics 27: 431–432.
19. O'Brien KP, Remm M, Sonnhammer EL (2005) Inparanoid: a comprehensive database of eukaryotic orthologs. Nucleic Acids Res 33: D476–480.
20. Livak KJ, Schmittgen TD (2001) Analysis of relative gene expression data using real-time quantitative PCR and the 2(-Delta Delta C(T)) Method. Methods 25: 402–408.
21. Pajoohesh-Ganji A, Knoblach SM, Faden AI, Byrnes KR (2012) Characterization of inflammatory gene expression and galectin-3 function after spinal cord injury in mice. Brain Res 1475: 96–105.
22. Maecker HT, Todd SC, Levy S (1997) The tetraspanin superfamily: molecular facilitators. FASEB J 11: 428–442.
23. Slavik JM, Hutchcroft JE, Bierer BE (1999) CD28/CTLA-4 and CD80/CD86 families: signaling and function. Immunol Res 19: 1–24.
24. Holness CL, Simmons DL (1993) Molecular cloning of CD68, a human macrophage marker related to lysosomal glycoproteins. Blood 81: 1607–1613.
25. Zhang H, Chang M, Hansen CN, Basso DM, Noble-Haeusslein LJ (2011) Role of matrix metalloproteinases and therapeutic benefits of their inhibition in spinal cord injury. Neurotherapeutics 8: 206–220.
26. van Lookeren Campagne M, Wiesmann C, Brown EJ (2007) Macrophage complement receptors and pathogen clearance. Cell Microbiol 9: 2095–2102.
27. Rodriguez de Cordoba S, Esparza-Gordillo J, Goicoechea de Jorge E, Lopez-Trascasa M, Sanchez-Corral P (2004) The human complement factor H: functional roles, genetic variations and disease associations. Mol Immunol 41: 355–367.
28. George R, Griffin JW (1994) Delayed macrophage responses and myelin clearance during Wallerian degeneration in the central nervous system: the dorsal radiculotomy model. Exp Neurol 129: 225–236.
29. Schafer DP, Lehrman EK, Kautzman AG, Koyama R, Mardinly AR, et al. (2012) Microglia sculpt postnatal neural circuits in an activity and complement-dependent manner. Neuron 74: 691–705.
30. Paolicelli RC, Bolasco G, Pagani F, Maggi L, Scianni M, et al. (2011) Synaptic pruning by microglia is necessary for normal brain development. Science 333: 1456–1458.
31. Schafer DP, Stevens B (2010) Synapse elimination during development and disease: immune molecules take centre stage. Biochem Soc Trans 38: 476–481.
32. Stevens B, Allen NJ, Vazquez LE, Howell GR, Christopherson KS, et al. (2007) The classical complement cascade mediates CNS synapse elimination. Cell 131: 1164–1178.
33. Whetstine JR, Nottke A, Lan F, Huarte M, Smolikov S, et al. (2006) Reversal of Histone Lysine Trimethylation by the JMJD2 Family of Histone Demethylases. Cell 125: 467–481.
34. Gabellini D, Green MR, Tupler R (2002) Inappropriate gene activation in FSHD: a repressor complex binds a chromosomal repeat deleted in dystrophic muscle. Cell 110: 339–348.
35. Gabellini D, D'Antona G, Moggio M, Prelle A, Zecca C, et al. (2006) Facioscapulohumeral muscular dystrophy in mice overexpressing FRG1. Nature 439: 973–977.
36. Shepherd JD, Rumbaugh G, Wu J, Chowdhury S, Plath N, et al. (2006) Arc/Arg3.1 mediates homeostatic synaptic scaling of AMPA receptors. Neuron 52: 475–484.
37. Mahoney ET, Benton RL, Maddie MA, Whittemore SR, Hagg T (2009) ADAM8 is selectively up-regulated in endothelial cells and is associated with angiogenesis after spinal cord injury in adult mice. J Comp Neurol 512: 243–255.
38. Singh H, Tahir TA, Alawo DO, Issa E, Brindle NP (2011) Molecular control of angiopoietin signalling. Biochem Soc Trans 39: 1592–1596.
39. Byrnes KR, Washington PM, Knoblach SM, Hoffman E, Faden AI (2011) Delayed inflammatory mRNA and protein expression after spinal cord injury. J Neuroinflammation 8: 130.
40. Ghasemlou N, Lopez-Vales R, Lachance C, Thuraisingam T, Gaestel M, et al. (2010) Mitogen-activated protein kinase-activated protein kinase 2 (MK2) contributes to secondary damage after spinal cord injury. J Neurosci 30: 13750–13759.
41. De Biase A, Knoblach SM, Di Giovanni S, Fan C, Molon A, et al. (2005) Gene expression profiling of experimental traumatic spinal cord injury as a function of distance from impact site and injury severity. Physiol Genomics 22: 368–381.
42. Hashimoto M, Koda M, Ino H, Yoshinaga K, Murata A, et al. (2005) Gene expression profiling of cathepsin D, metallothioneins-1 and -2, osteopontin, and tenascin-C in a mouse spinal cord injury model by cDNA microarray analysis. Acta Neuropathol 109: 165–180.
43. Di Giovanni S, Faden AI, Yakovlev A, Duke-Cohan JS, Finn T, et al. (2005) Neuronal plasticity after spinal cord injury: identification of a gene cluster driving neurite outgrowth. FASEB J 19: 153–154.
44. Carmel JB, Galante A, Soteropoulos P, Tolias P, Recce M, et al. (2001) Gene expression profiling of acute spinal cord injury reveals spreading inflammatory signals and neuron loss. Physiol Genomics 7: 201–213.
45. Aimone JB, Leasure JL, Perreau VM, Thallmair M (2004) Spatial and temporal gene expression profiling of the contused rat spinal cord. Exp Neurol 189: 204–221.
46. Cowell RM, Plane JM, Silverstein FS (2003) Complement activation contributes to hypoxic-ischemic brain injury in neonatal rats. J Neurosci 23: 9459–9468.
47. Galvan MD, Luchetti S, Burgos AM, Nguyen HX, Hooshmand MJ, et al. (2008) Deficiency in complement C1q improves histological and functional locomotor outcome after spinal cord injury. J Neurosci 28: 13876–13888.
48. Bellander BM, Bendel O, Von Euler G, Ohlsson M, Svensson M (2004) Activation of microglial cells and complement following traumatic injury in rat entorhinal-hippocampal slice cultures. J Neurotrauma 21: 605–615.
49. Anderson AJ, Robert S, Huang W, Young W, Cotman CW (2004) Activation of complement pathways after contusion-induced spinal cord injury. J Neurotrauma 21: 1831–1846.
50. Hutchinson KJ, Gomez-Pinilla F, Crowe MJ, Ying Z, Basso DM (2004) Three exercise paradigms differentially improve sensory recovery after spinal cord contusion in rats. Brain 127: 1403–1414.
51. Adams MM, Hicks AL (2011) Comparison of the effects of body-weight-supported treadmill training and tilt-table standing on spasticity in individuals with chronic spinal cord injury. J Spinal Cord Med 34: 488–494.
52. Luthl A, Laurent JP, Figurov A, Muller D, Schachner M (1994) Hippocampal long-term potentiation and neural cell adhesion molecules L1 and NCAM. Nature 372: 777–779.
53. Kiryushko D, Kofoed T, Skladchikova G, Holm A, Berezin V, et al. (2003) A synthetic peptide ligand of neural cell adhesion molecule (NCAM), C3d, promotes neuritogenesis and synaptogenesis and modulates presynaptic function in primary cultures of rat hippocampal neurons. J Biol Chem 278: 12325–12334.
54. Cambon K, Hansen SM, Venero C, Herrero AI, Skibo G, et al. (2004) A synthetic neural cell adhesion molecule mimetic peptide promotes synaptogenesis, enhances presynaptic function, and facilitates memory consolidation. J Neurosci 24: 4197–4204.
55. Messaoudi E, Kanhema T, Soule J, Tiron A, Dagyte G, et al. (2007) Sustained Arc/Arg3.1 synthesis controls long-term potentiation consolidation through regulation of local actin polymerization in the dentate gyrus in vivo. J Neurosci 27: 10445–10455.
56. Plath N, Ohana O, Dammermann B, Errington ML, Schmitz D, et al. (2006) Arc/Arg3.1 is essential for the consolidation of synaptic plasticity and memories. Neuron 52: 437–444.
57. Korb E, Finkbeiner S (2011) Arc in synaptic plasticity: from gene to behavior. Trends Neurosci 34: 591–598.
58. Peebles CL, Yoo J, Thwin MT, Palop JJ, Noebels JL, et al. (2010) Arc regulates spine morphology and maintains network stability in vivo. Proc Natl Acad Sci U S A 107: 18173–18178.
59. Tan AM, Waxman SG (2012) Spinal cord injury, dendritic spine remodeling, and spinal memory mechanisms. Exp Neurol 235: 142–151.
60. Frigon A, Rossignol S (2006) Functional plasticity following spinal cord lesions. Prog Brain Res 157: 231–260.
61. Norton JA, Bennett DJ, Knash ME, Murray KC, Gorassini MA (2008) Changes in sensory-evoked synaptic activation of motoneurons after spinal cord injury in man. Brain 131: 1478–1491.
62. Guaiquil VH, Swendeman S, Zhou W, Guaiquil P, Weskamp G, et al. (2010) ADAM8 is a negative regulator of retinal neovascularization and of the growth of heterotopically injected tumor cells in mice. J Mol Med (Berl) 88: 497–505.
63. Dreymueller D, Pruessmeyer J, Groth E, Ludwig A (2012) The role of ADAM-mediated shedding in vascular biology. Eur J Cell Biol 91: 472–485.
64. Singh H, Hansen TM, Patel N, Brindle NP (2012) The molecular balance between receptor tyrosine kinases Tie1 and Tie2 is dynamically controlled by VEGF and TNFalpha and regulates angiopoietin signalling. PLoS One 7: e29319.
65. Dray C, Rougon G, Debarbieux F (2009) Quantitative analysis by in vivo imaging of the dynamics of vascular and axonal networks in injured mouse spinal cord. Proc Natl Acad Sci U S A 106: 9459–9464.
66. Carmeliet P, Tessier-Lavigne M (2005) Common mechanisms of nerve and blood vessel wiring. Nature 436: 193–200.

16

Pre-Evaluated Safe Human iPSC-Derived Neural Stem Cells Promote Functional Recovery after Spinal Cord Injury in Common Marmoset without Tumorigenicity

Yoshiomi Kobayashi[1,2]⁹, Yohei Okada[1]⁹, Go Itakura[1,2], Hiroki Iwai[1,2], Soraya Nishimura[1,2], Akimasa Yasuda[1], Satoshi Nori[1], Keigo Hikishima[2,3], Tsunehiko Konomi[1,2], Kanehiro Fujiyoshi[4], Osahiko Tsuji[5], Yoshiaki Toyama[1], Shinya Yamanaka[6], Masaya Nakamura[1]*, Hideyuki Okano[2]*

1 Department of Orthopedic Surgery, School of Medicine, Keio University, Tokyo, Japan, **2** Department of Physiology, School of Medicine, Keio University, Tokyo, Japan, **3** Central Institute for Experimental Animals, Kanagawa, Japan, **4** Department of Orthopedic Surgery, National Hospital Organization Murayama Medical Center, Tokyo, Japan, **5** Department of Orthopedic Surgery, Saitama Social Insurance Hospital, Saitama, Japan, **6** Center for iPS Cell Research and Application (CiRA), Kyoto, Japan

Abstract

Murine and human iPSC-NS/PCs (induced pluripotent stem cell-derived neural stem/progenitor cells) promote functional recovery following transplantation into the injured spinal cord in rodents. However, for clinical applicability, it is critical to obtain proof of the concept regarding the efficacy of grafted human iPSC-NS/PCs (hiPSC-NS/PCs) for the repair of spinal cord injury (SCI) in a non-human primate model. This study used a pre-evaluated "safe" hiPSC-NS/PC clone and an adult common marmoset (*Callithrix jacchus*) model of contusive SCI. SCI was induced at the fifth cervical level (C5), followed by transplantation of hiPSC-NS/PCs at 9 days after injury. Behavioral analyses were performed from the time of the initial injury until 12 weeks after SCI. Grafted hiPSC-NS/PCs survived and differentiated into all three neural lineages. Furthermore, transplantation of hiPSC-NS/PCs enhanced axonal sparing/regrowth and angiogenesis, and prevented the demyelination after SCI compared with that in vehicle control animals. Notably, no tumor formation occurred for at least 12 weeks after transplantation. Quantitative RT-PCR showed that mRNA expression levels of human neurotrophic factors were significantly higher in cultured hiPSC-NS/PCs than in human dermal fibroblasts (hDFs). Finally, behavioral tests showed that hiPSC-NS/PCs promoted functional recovery after SCI in the common marmoset. Taken together, these results indicate that pre-evaluated safe hiPSC-NS/PCs are a potential source of cells for the treatment of SCI in the clinic.

Editor: Kenji Hashimoto, Chiba University Center for Forensic Mental Health, Japan

Funding: This work was supported by grants from Grants-in-Aid for Scientific Research from Japan Society for the Promotion of Science (SPS) and the Ministry of Education, Culture, Sports, Science, and Technology of Japan (MEXT); the Project for Realization of Regenerative Medicine; and Support for Core Institutes for iPS Cell Research from the MEXT; Japan Science and Technology–California Institute for Regenerative Medicine collaborative program; "Funding Program for World-leading Innovative R&D on Science and Technology (FIRST Program); the Kanrinmaru project from Keio University; Research Fellowships for Young Scientists from JSPS; Keio Gijuku Academic Development Funds; by a Grant-in-Aid for the Global COE program from MEXT to Keio University; and by a Grant-in-Aid for Scientific Research on Innovative Areas (Comprehensive Brain Science Net- work) from the Ministry of Education, Science, Sports and Culture of Japan. The funders had no role in study design, data collection and analysis, decision to publish, or preparation of the manuscript.

Competing Interests: The authors have declared that no competing interests exist.

* E-mail: masa@a8.keio.jp (MN); hidokano@a2.keio.jp (HO)

⁹ These authors contributed equally to this work.

Introduction

Stem cell-based approaches, such as the transplantation of neural stem/progenitor cells (NS/PCs) into sites of damage, are promising therapies for the alleviation of various central nervous system disorders [1,2,3]. Previously, we demonstrated the effectiveness of NS/PC transplantation for the treating spinal cord injury (SCI) in rodents [4] and non-human primates [5]. Considering the differences in the anatomy and functions of the spinal cord between rodents and primates, it was crucial to obtain the proof of concept on the effectiveness of human fetal NS/PCs transplantation for SCI in non-human primates. Nevertheless, we are currently unable to progress toward testing the efficacy of NS/PCs in clinical trials involving humans because of ethical issues surrounding the use of fetus-derived cells. To overcome this hurdle, we have instead focused our efforts on induced pluripotent stem cells (iPSCs) [6,7] and have demonstrated the utility of "safe" NS/PC clones derived from murine and human iPSCs (iPSC-NS/PCs) in a rodent model of SCI [8,9].

The present pre-clinical study investigated the therapeutic potential of transplanting pre-evaluated NS/PCs (hiPS-NS/PCs) derived from the safe human iPSC clone, 201B7, into the injured spinal cord of a non-human primate, the adult common marmoset (*Callithrix jacchus*). Grafted hiPSC-NS/PCs survived and differentiated into all three neural lineages (i.e., neurons, astrocytes, and oligodendrocytes), with no evidence of tumor formation. Furthermore, hiPSC-NS/PCs prevented demyelination at the lesion epicenter and enhanced axonal sparing/regrowth and angiogenesis, thereby promoting functional recovery after SCI. These findings suggest that pre-evaluated safe hiPSC-NS/PCs are a promising source of cells for clinical intervention following SCI.

Materials and Methods

Animals

All interventions and animal care procedures were performed in accordance with the Laboratory Animal Welfare Act, the Guide for the Care and Use of Laboratory Animals (National Institutes of Health, USA), the Guidelines and Policies for Animal Surgery provided by the Animal Study Committee of the Central Institute for Experimental Animals and Keio University and the guidelines outlined by Weatherall Report,and were approved by the Animal Study Committee of Keio University (IRB approval number 09091-8). Adult female common marmosets (>2 y old) were purchased from a CLEA Japan (Tokyo, Japan). The animals were kept at 26°C with 65% humidity and illumination for 12 h/d. All the animals had free access to food and water in the cage.

Cell culture, neural induction, and lentivirus transduction

Cell culture and neural induction of hiPSCs (clone 201B7) were performed as described previously [10], with slight modifications. Briefly, hiPSCs (201B7) grown on gelatin-coated (0.1%) tissue culture dishes were maintained in standard ES cell medium and used for EB formation as described previously [10,11]. EBs were then enzymatically dissociated into single cells and cultured in suspension in serum-free media hormone mix (MHM) media for 10–14 days to allow the formation of neurospheres. Neurospheres were dissociated into single cells and then cultured in the same manner for passage. To assay the degree of differentiation, neurospheres were plated on poly-L-ornithine/fibronectin-coated cover glasses and allowed to differentiate for 10–12 days as previously reported [12]. The lentivirus was prepared and transduced into neurospheres according to previously described methods [9]. Briefly, the concentrated virus particles were added to the culture medium to infect the hiPSC-NS/PCs. 12 days later, human iPSC-derived primary neurospheres were dissociated and infected with lentivirus-expressing Venus fluorescent protein under the control of the elongation factor (EF) promoter (pCSII-EF-Venus). This vector enabled the detection of grafted cells as fluorescent Venus signals using anti-green fluorescent protein (GFP) antibody in fixed spinal-cord sections, since the Venus was originally modified from GFP [13]. This virus was obtained as previously reported [9]. "The titer of the concentrated virus was 1×10^8–2×10^8 transducing units per milliliter (TU/ml) when assayed using 293T cells, and infectivity was determined by fluorescence expression, which was analyzed using a FACSCalibur flow cytometer (Becton-Dickinson, Franklin, Lakes, NJ). The primary neurospheres were then passaged into secondary and tertiary neurospheres and used for transplantation.

Contusive SCI in common marmosets

Adult female common marmosets (*C. jacchus*; CLEA Japan Inc., Tokyo, Japan) were anesthetized with an intramuscular injection of ketamine (50 mg/kg; Sankyo Co., Ltd., Tokyo, Japan) and xylazine (5 mg/kg; Bayer AG, Leverkusen, Germany), followed by inhalation of isoflurane (Fluren; Abbott Japan Co., Ltd., Tokyo, Japan). A moderate contusive SCI was induced in 10 marmosets using a modified NYU (New York University) weight-drop device, as previously reported [5,14,15]. Briefly, a 17 g weight (3.5 mm in diameter) was dropped from a height of 50 mm onto the exposed dura mater at the C5 level. During the surgical procedures, the physiological condition of the experimental animals was continuously monitored by electrocardiogram, transcutaneous pulse oximetry (which estimates O_2 saturation), and both skin and rectal temperature. Nine days after injury, partially dissociated hiPSC-NS/PCs (approximately 1×10^6 cells/5 µl in cell culture medium without added growth factors) were injected into the lesion epicenter using a glass pipette fitted to a 25-ll Hamilton syringe and a microstereotaxic injection system (David Kopf Instruments, Tujunga, CA). An equal volume of phosphate buffered saline (PBS) was injected into the lesion site for vehicle control common marmosets.

The animals were placed in a temperature-controlled chamber until thermoregulation was reestablished. Manual bladder expression was carried out twice a day until voiding reflexes were reestablished. Paralyzed animals were given adequate amounts of food and water until they recovered their ability to ingest food and water without assistance. Thereafter, they had free access to food and water in the cage.

All animals received daily ampicillin (100 mg/kg; Meiji Seika Kaisha, Ltd., Tokyo, Japan) for 1 week after cell transplantation and subcutaneous cyclosporine injections (10 mg/kg; Novartis, Basel, Switzerland) until they were sacrificed for analysis. At 12 weeks after cell engraftment, animals were anesthetized by intramuscular administration of a mixture of ketamine (50 mg/kg; Sankyo Lifetech Co., Ltd., Tokyo, Japan), xylazine (5 mg/kg; Bayer, Leverkusen, Germany), and atropine (0.02–0.05 mg/kg; Mitsubishi Tanabe Pharma Corporation, Osaka, Japan) prior to magnetic resonance imaging (MRI) scanning. Once anesthetized, the animals were given a mixture of oxygen and 1.5–2.0% isoflurane (Abbott Japan, Tokyo, Japan) via a tracheal intubation tube at a constant rate using an artificial respirator (SN-480-7; Shinano, Tokyo, Japan). The animals were placed on their side in a specially designed body holder (Qualita Ltd., Saitama, Japan). During the scan, the physiological condition of the experimental animals was continuously monitored by electrocardiogram, transcutaneous pulse oximetry and both skin and rectal temperature. Animals were given replacement fluids both before and after the scan. After MRI scanning, animals were euthanized in a humane manner via deep anesthesia (intravenous sodium pentobarbital, 100 mg/kg) for histological analysis. All procedures were approved by the Ethics Committee of Keio University (Tokyo, Japan) and were in accordance with the Guide for the Care and Use of Laboratory Animals (National Institutes of Health, Bethesda, MD).

Open field test

All behavioral tests were performed from the time of the initial injury up until 12 weeks after SCI. The original open field rating scale was used to evaluate open field locomotion, as described previously [16]. Briefly, all marmosets were individually tested for 5 min on the floor and then in the cage to obtain the overall score (maximum 30 points). During the open field test, marmosets were encouraged by slight tapping if they remained stationary for longer than 15 seconds. In cases of borderline locomotor performance or disagreement between examiners, scores indicating the greater deficit were assigned. The test was performed three times a week up until 4 weeks after SCI, and once a week thereafter. All lower limb and trunk movements except those that were obviously part of a reflex (i.e., spastic extensive bilateral flexion or extension of the hip, knee, and ankle joint) were assessed to obtain the lower limb and trunk score (maximum 10 points). The movements of each bilateral upper limb were separately assessed to obtain the upper limb score, which was defined as the mean of the two independent upper limb scores (maximum 20 points).

Bar grip test

The motor function of the upper extremities was evaluated using a bar grip strength test, which examines the animal's gripping reflex (the motion undertaken when attempting to grasp an object placed before the animal). The test was performed three times per day, and the maximal daily grip strength was expressed as a percentage of the pre-injury grip strength before SCI [14].

Cage climbing test

The cage climbing test was developed to evaluate the coordination of the fore and hind limbs. A seven-point scale (from 0 to 6) was used to evaluate the motor coordination of each common marmoset over a period of 3 min. The evaluations were conducted twice a day from immediately before the injury up until 12 weeks after the injury.

Magnetic resonance imaging

From the viewpoint of the pre-clinical trial, it is critical to evaluate the effect of hiPSC-NS/PCs on the injured spinal cord non-invasively. Therefore, MRI, which enables pathogenic events such as hemorrhage, edema, and cavity formation to be assessed non-invasively [17,18], was performed at 12 weeks after cell transplantation. MRI was performed by using a 7.0-Tesla superconducting magnet (Bruker Biospin GmbH, Ettlingen, Germany) fitted with a 62 mm inner diameter volume coil under general anesthesia. T2-weighted imaging and Myelin mapping were performed as previously described [19,20]. Briefly, the non-Gaussian profile for molecular diffusion was directly estimated by performing a Fourier transformation of the data gained from a pulsed gradient spin-echo (PGSE) sequence [21,22]. An in-house IDL® program was used to perform this analysis. Myelin maps were reconstructed from normalized leptokurtic diffusion data. PGSE sequences were performed using the following parameters: repetition time (TR)/echo time (TE) = 3500 ms/37.8 ms; matrix = 256×192; field of view (FOV) = 40×40 mm^2; and slice thickness = 1.5 mm. Myelin map-positive myelinated area was quantified using ImageJ software (version 1.29, http://rsbweb.nih.gov/ij/) (n = 5 for each group).

Histological Analysis

Twelve weeks after cell engraftment, each animal was anesthetized and intracardially perfused with 4% paraformaldehyde (PFA, pH 7.4). Spinal cord tissues were removed, post-fixed in 4% PFA, and immersed overnight in 10% sucrose followed by 30% sucrose. The cord was then embedded in Optimal Cutting Temperature (OCT) compound and sectioned on a cryostat at 20 µm to obtain axial sections. The sections were stained with H-E for general histological examination and with luxol fast blue (LFB) or eriochrome cyanine (EC) to evaluate the extent of the myelination/demyelination after SCI. To quantify the cells of interest in H-E-, LFB-, and EC- stained sections, we obtained images of the stained sections by fluorescence microscopy (BZ-9000; Keyence), manually outlined them, and quantified them using Dynamic cell count BZ-HIC software. The threshold values were maintained at a constant level for all analyses using BZ-HIC. To quantify the area of the cystic cavity, we captured H-E images at the lesion epicenter in axial sections at 100× magnification (n = 5 per group). To quantify the LFB- and EC-positive areas, we automatically captured four regions in axial sections (at the lesion epicenter and 2, 4, and 6 mm rostral and caudal to the epicenter) at 400× magnification (n = 3 per group). To quantify the RT97 positive fibers, the axial sections were scanned at the lesion epicenter, and at 2, 4, and 6 mm rostral and caudal to the epicenter at 400× magnification (n = 5 for each group). To quantify the CaMK-IIα positive fibers, the dorsal corticospinal tract (CST) areas were captured in axial sections of the lesion epicenter at 400× magnification (n = 4 for each group). To quantify the CGRP positive fibers, the dorsal horn areas were captured in axial sections of the 6 mm roatral and caudal to the epicenter at 400× magnification (n = 3 for each group). To quantify the Iba-1-positive areas in axial sections of the lesion epicenter, we captured at the lesion epicenter in axial sections at 10× magnification (n = 3 for each group). For the quantification of PECAM-1 positive blood vessels area, the axial sections were captured at the lesion epicenter at 100× magnification (n = 5 for the transplantation group and 4 for the control group). To quantify the proportion of each cell phenotype *in vivo*, we selected representative mid-sagittal sections and automatically captured five regions within 1 mm rostral and caudal to the lesion epicenter at 200× magnification. Venus-positive engrafted and phenotypic marker-positive cells were counted in each section (n = 4 per group).

Tissue sections were stained with the following primary antibodies: anti-green fluorescent protein (GFP, rabbit IgG, 1:200; Frontier Institute Co., Ltd., Hokkaido, Japan), anti-GFP (goat IgG, 1:200; Rockland Immunochemicals, Gilbertsville, PA), anti-β-tubulin isotype III (βIII tubulin, Tuj1, mouse IgG, 1:1,000; Sigma Chemical Co., St. Louis, MO), anti-HNu (mouse IgG, 1:500; Chemicon, Temecula, CA), anti-NeuN (mouse IgG, 1:200; Chemicon), anti-glial fibrillary acidic protein (GFAP) (rabbit IgG, 1:200; Dako, Carpinteria, CA), anti-GFAP (guinea pig IgG, 1:200; Advanced ImmunoChemical, Long Beach, CA), anti-GFAP (rat IgG, 1:200; Invitrogen, Carlsbad, CA), anti-Olig1 (mouse IgG, 1:200; R&D Systems, Minneapolis, MN), anti-human-specific Nestin protein (rabbit IgG, 1:200; described previously, refs. [5,9,23,24]), anti-Ki-67 (rabbit IgG, 1:500; Novocastra), anti-NF-200 (RT97 monoclonal antibody, mouse IgG, 1:200; Chemicon), anti-PECAM-1 (rat IgG, 1:50; BD Bioscience Pharmingen, San Diego, CA), anti-CaMK-IIα (CaMK-IIα, mouse IgG, 1:100; Invitrogen) anti-calcitonin gene-related peptide (CGRP, rabbit IgG, 1:1,000; Affinity), and anti-Iba-1 (rabbit IgG, 1:200; Wako)

Images were obtained via fluorescence microscopy with a BZ-9000 fluorescence microscope (Keyence, Woodcliff Lake, NJ) or by confocal laser scanning microscopy with a LSM700 Laser Scanning Microscope (Carl Zeiss Microscopy, GmbH, Munich, Germany).

For immunohistochemistry with RT97, spinal cord tissues were first exposed to 0.3% H_2O_2 for 30 min at room temperature to inactivate endogenous peroxidases. The tissues were then reacted with a biotinylated secondary antibody (Jackson ImmunoResearch Laboratories, West Grove, PA). Immunohistochemical signals were enhanced using the Vectastain ABC kit (Vector Labs, Burlingame, CA). Nuclei were stained with Hoechst 33258 (10 µg/mL; Sigma), a DNA-specific fluorochrome.

RNA Isolation and RT-PCR

Gene expression profiling of hiPSC-NS/PCs and hDFs was performed *in vitro* to evaluate the mRNA expression levels of trophic factors related to axonal regrowth and angiogenesis (NT3, NT4, CNTF, and vascular endothelial growth factor [VEGF]). RNA was isolated from each cell type using TRIzol (Invitrogen) according to the manufacturer's instructions. Total RNA (1 µg) was treated with TURBO DNase (Ambion Life Technologies, Grand Island, NY) and then reverse transcribed using oligo (dT) primers and SuperScript III (Invitrogen). Quantitative mRNA expression levels for the trophic factor-related genes were simultaneously analyzed (n = 2 for each cell type) using quantitative RT-PCR arrays using TaqMan Array Fast (Applied Biosystems) according to the manufacturer's instructions. The following commercially available primers against human DNA sequences (Applied Biosystems, Carlsbad, CA) were useed: GAPDH-Hs99999905_m1, NTF3-Hs00267375_s1, NTF4-Hs01921834_s1, ZFP91-CNTF-Hs00173456_m1, and

VEGFA-Hs00900058_m1. The mRNA expression level for each factor was normalized to the level of glyceraldehyde 3-phosphate dehydrogenase (GAPDH) mRNA. The mRNA expression data for the hiPSC-NS/PCs were then calculated as the amount of mRNA for each factor relative to the amount in hDFs.

Statistical Analysis

All data are reported as the mean ± SEM. For all histological examinations, an unpaired two-tailed Student's t-test was used for single comparisons between the transplantation and vehicle control groups. The results of the open field test, bar grip test, and cage climbing test were analyzed using a Mann-Whitney U-test. In each case, *$p<0.05$ and **$p<0.01$ were considered to be statistically significant.

Results

Grafted hiPSC-NS/PCs survive and differentiate into all three neural lineages without becoming tumorigenic

A moderate contusive SCI was induced at cervical level 5 (C5) in adult common marmosets as reported previously [14]. Nine days after injury, human iPSC-NS/PCs (1×10^6 cells/5 μl) were transplanted into the injured spinal cord in the transplantation group. In the vehicle control group, PBS was injected instead of cells. At 12 weeks post-engraftment, hematoxylin-eosin (HE) staining showed that cystic cavity formation was prominent in the vehicle control group compared with the transplantation group (Fig. 1A). A significant difference in the size of the transverse area of the cystic cavity at the lesion epicenter was observed between the two groups (Fig. 1B). Notably, no evidence of tumor formation was observed in any of the animals in the transplantation group at 12 weeks after cell engraftment (Fig. 1A, B).

Immunostaining for Oct4, a marker for undifferentiated pluripotent stem cells [25], revealed that undifferentiated iPSCs were all positive for Oct4 (Fig. 1. C-1). On the other hand, no Oct4-positive cells were observed among the grafted human nuclear protein (HNu)-positive hiPSC-NS/PCs (Fig. 1. C-2). We also performed immunostaining for the proliferation marker Ki-67 to determine the level of proliferation of the grafted cells. The percentage of HNu-positive cells that were also Ki-67-positive was 0.55±0.08% (Fig. 1. C-3). Indeed, grafted hiPSC-NS/PCs survived around the lesion epicenter in the host spinal cord and differentiated into mature neuronal nuclei (NeuN)-positive neurons, GFAP-positive astrocytes, and oligodendrocyte transcription factor 1 (Olig1)-positive oligodendrocyte progenitor cells (Fig. 1D-1–D-3). Quantitative analyses revealed that the population of differentiated cells within the host spinal cord consisted of 52.0±3.7% NeuN-positive cells, 30.8±1.9% GFAP-positive cells, 26.5±7.8% Olig1-positive cells, and 23.9±2.8% Nestin-positive cells (Fig. 1D-4). In contrast, hiPSC-NS/PCs primarily differentiated into βIII-tubulin-positive neurons (98.7±0.9%) *in vitro* (Fig. 1E).

Transplantation of hiPSC-NS/PCs prevents demyelination after SCI

Next, LFB and EC staining were performed to evaluate the effect of hiPSC-NS/PC transplantation on the extent of demyelination/remyelination after SCI. Severe demyelination was evident in the central and posterior parts of the lesion site in both the transplantation group and the vehicle control group, whereas an area of spared myelination was prominent at the rim of the injured spinal cord in the transplantation group (Fig. 2A). Quantification of the myelinated areas in the lesion sites revealed significant differences between the transplantation and control groups at 12 weeks after cell engraftment (Fig. 2B).

Conventional MRI and Myelin map imaging of the spinal cord were conducted at 12 weeks after cell transplantation as described previously [19,20] (Fig. 3A). T2-weighted images (T2WIs) showed that an intramedullary high-signal intensity area at the lesion site was prominent in the vehicle control group, which was significantly larger than the comparable area in the transplantation group (Fig. 3B). These findings are consistent with the quantitative data discussed above regarding the increased transverse area of the cystic cavity at the lesion epicenter in the vehicle control relative to the transplantation group (Fig. 1B). Furthermore, the Myelin map showed that the overall myelin-positive area at the lesion epicenter was significantly larger in the transplantation group than in the control group (Fig. 3C). These results are also consistent with the quantitative data shown in Fig. 2B regarding the differences in the size of the LFB- and EC-positive transverse myelinated areas between the two groups.

Grafted hiPSC-NS/PCs enhance axonal sparing/regrowth and angiogenesis

To evaluate the impact of grafted hiPSC-NS/PCs on axonal sparing/regrowth, immunostaining for neurofilament-200 (NF-200, Fig. 4A-1) and α-CaM (Ca^{2+}/calmodulin-dependent) kinase II (CaMK-IIα, Fig. 4B-1) was performed. NF-200 (detected by monoclonal antibody RT97) is a marker for mature, large-diameter axons, and CaMK-IIα is a marker for descending motor axons. Immunostaining analysis revealed a greater number of RT97-positive areas at the lesion epicenter as well as at sites adjacent to the lesion in the transplantation group relative to the vehicle control group (Fig. 4A-1). Moreover, quantitative analysis demonstrated that the overall RT97-positive area was larger in the transplantation group than in the control group (Fig. 4A-2). The CaMK-IIα-positive area at the lesion epicenter was also significantly larger in the transplantation group than in the control group at 1 week after SCI. Contusive SCI resulted in a significant decrease in the size of the CaMK-IIα–positive area at the lesion site, which was followed by a slight, but not statistically significant, increase in the control group 12 weeks after SCI. The size of the CaMK-IIα-positive area 12 weeks after SCI was significantly increased in the transplantation group. There was a significant difference in the CaMK-IIα-positive area at the lesion epicenter between the transplantation and the control groups (Fig. 4B-2). Furthermore, We investigated the distribution of calcitonin gene-related peptide (CGRP) fibers, which are involved in peripheral and spinal pain mechanisms [9,26,27,28], to examine the effect of hiPSC-NS/PCs in pain afferents entering the dorsal horn of the spinal cord both above and below the injured spinal segments (Fig. 4C-1). There were no significant differences in the size of the CGRP-positive areas in lamina III between the hiPSC-NS/PCs and the control group (Fig. 4C-2).

Immunohistochemical analysis for platelet endothelial cell adhesion molecule-1 (PECAM-1) was next performed to evaluate the effects of hiPSC-NS/PC transplantation on angiogenesis after SCI (Fig. 5A-1). A significantly larger number of PECAM-1-positive blood vessels per unit area were observed at the lesion epicenter in the transplantation group compared with the vehicle control group (Fig. 5A-2). Taken together, the results of the immunohistochemical study suggest that the transplanted hiPSC-NS/PCs mediated regeneration and/or sparing of axons and generation of new blood vessels in our injury model.

Human dermal fibroblasts (hDFs) are the original cell source of the hiPSC-NS/PCs used in this study. Quantitative RT-PCR of the cultured hiPSC-NS/PCs and hDFs revealed that mRNA

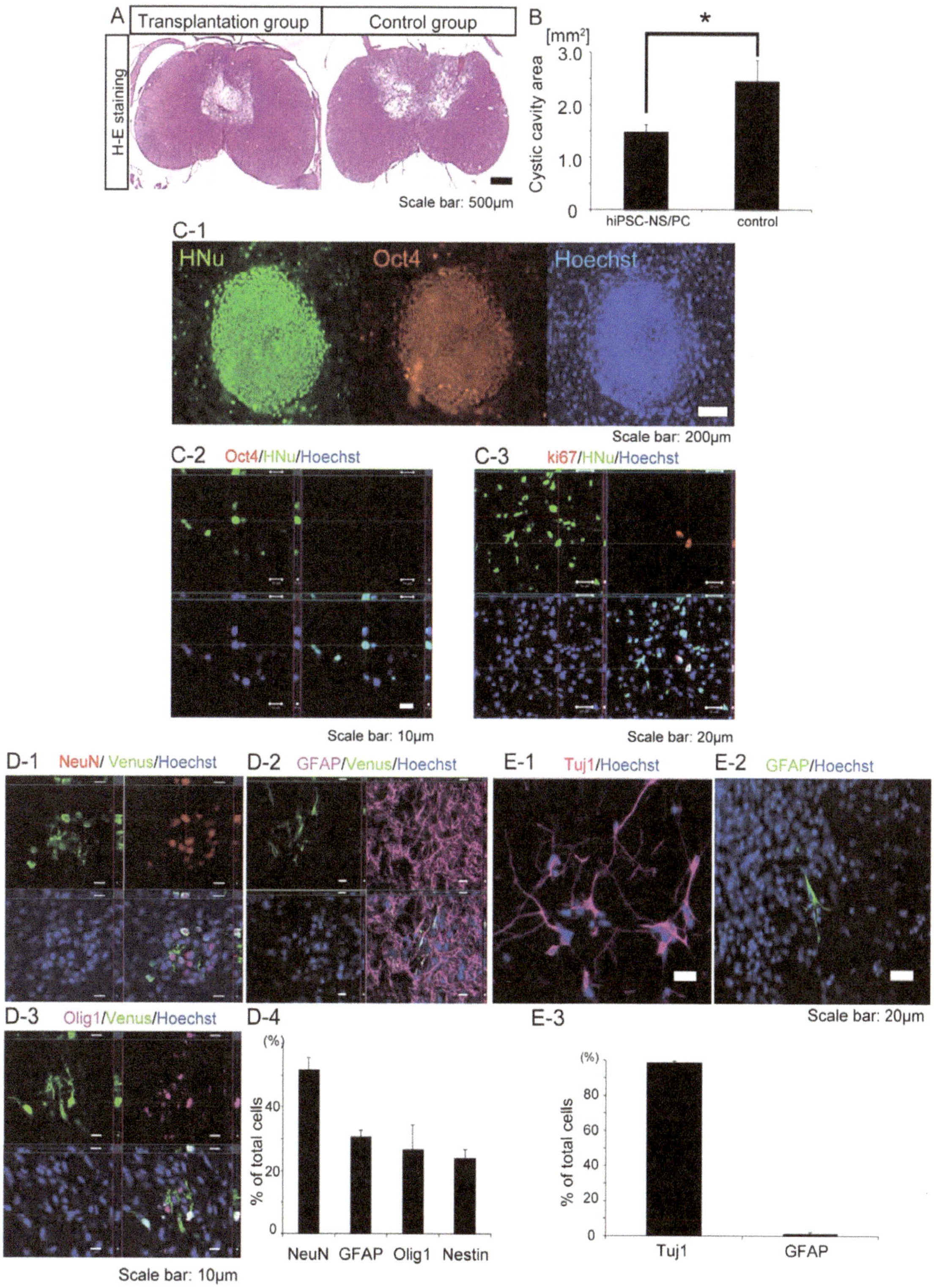

Figure 1. Grafted hiPSC-NS/PCs differentiate into three neural lineages without tumor formation in the injured spinal cord. (A) Representative H-E stained images of axial sections at the lesion epicenter at 12 weeks (84 days) after cell transplantation. No tumor formation was observed in the hiPSC-NS/PC-transplanted group during this time. H-E staining showed that cystic cavity formation at the lesion epicenter was prominent in the vehicle control group compared with the transplantation group, whereas there was no clear difference in the transverse area of the injured spinal cord. (**B**) Quantification of the cystic cavity area. Data represent the mean ± the SEM (n = 5 for each group, $*p<0.05$). (**C**) Immunostaining for Oct4 and Ki-67. (**C-1**) All colonies of undifferentiated iPSCs were positive for Oct4, a marker of undifferentiated ESCs and iPSCs. (**C-2**) Grafted hiPSC- NS/PCs yielded no Oct4-positive following transplantation into the injured spinal cord. (**C-3**) The percentage of HNu-positive cells that were also Ki-67-positive was 0.55±0.08%. (**D**) Differentiation of grafted hiPSC-NS/PCs. (**D-1-3**) Representative images of Venus-positive grafted hiPSC-NS/PCs immunostained with antibodies against NeuN to detect mature neurons, GFAP to detect astrocytes, and Olig1 to detect

oligodendrocyte progenitor cells. (**D-4**) Percentages of cell type-specific, marker-positive cells among the Venus-positive grafted hiPSC-NS/PCs at 12 weeks post-engraftment. (**E**) In vitro differentiation of hiPSC-NS/PCs. (**E-1, 2**) Representative images of hiPSC-NS/PCs immunostained with antibodies against βIII-tubulin to detect neurons, and GFAP to detect astrocytes. (**E-3**) Percentages of cell type-specific marker-positive cells among the hiPSC-NS/PCs 10 days after the initiation of cell differentiation in vitro.

expression levels of human neurotrophic factors associated with axonal growth and survival of host neurons (i.e., neurotrophin (NT) 3, NT4, and ciliary neurotrophic factor (CNTF)) [29,30,31] were significantly higher in cultured hiPSC-NS/PCs than in cultured hDFs (Fig. 5B). The mRNA expression level for the human pro-angiogenic factor, VEGF [32] was also elevated in cultured hiPSC-NS/PCs. Thus, secretion of NT3, NT4, CNTF, and VEGF may contribute to the regenerative properties of the transplanted stem cells after SCI.

Microglial activation and glial scar formation at 12 weeks after transplantation

We performed Iba1 staining to assess microglial activation and GFAP staining to assess glial scar formation. Iba1-positive microglia showed a more rounded shape in the control and transplantation groups than in the pre-injury sample (Fig. 6A-1). However, we could not detect the difference between control and transplantation groups, nor detect the apparent evidence of immunomodulation by the hiPSC-NS/PCs at this time point (12 weeks after transplantation) (Fig. 6A-2). There were no significant differences in the size of GFAP-positive areas between the hiPSC-NS/PCs and control groups (Fig. 6B).

Grafted hiPSC-NS/PCs promote functional recovery after SCI

Contusion SCI at the C5 level caused severe tetraplegia in the adult common marmosets. Tetraplegia was followed by gradual recovery of motor function, as reported previously [14]. Immediately after injury, all of the examined variables in the behavioral tests (the open field test, bar grip test, and cage climbing test) sharply decreased to a mean value of zero in the transplantation group and in the vehicle control group (Fig. 7).

Open field locomotion was evaluated by the original open field rating scale [16]. Briefly, all marmosets were individually tested for 5 min on the floor and then in the cage to obtain the overall score (maximum 30 points). Because this study used a severe central cord injury model rather than a complete injury model, the behavioral scores in the overall original open field rating scale gradually increased from zero and reached a plateau of ~21 in the transplantation group over the course of the experiment. The corresponding behavioral scores reached a plateau of ~13 in the vehicle control group (Fig. 7A-1). The results for the vehicle control group are consistent with the clinical course of central cord injury [33,34]. Significant differences were observed between the two groups in the overall open field behavioral scores at 8 weeks (56 days) following SCI and thereafter (Fig. 7A-1). Significant differences were also observed at 56 days following SCI and thereafter in the open field upper limb scores (Fig. 7A-2), and at 28 days following SCI and thereafter in the open field lower limb and trunk scores (Fig. 7A-3).

The bar grip strength of the forelimbs also increased from a mean value of zero over the course of the experiment and gradually reached a plateau of ~57% and ~40% of the pre-injury value in the transplantation group and the control group, respectively, at 12 weeks after injury (Fig. 7B). Similarly, the mean scores of the cage climbing test improved from zero to a value of 4 in the transplantation group and 2.8 in the vehicle

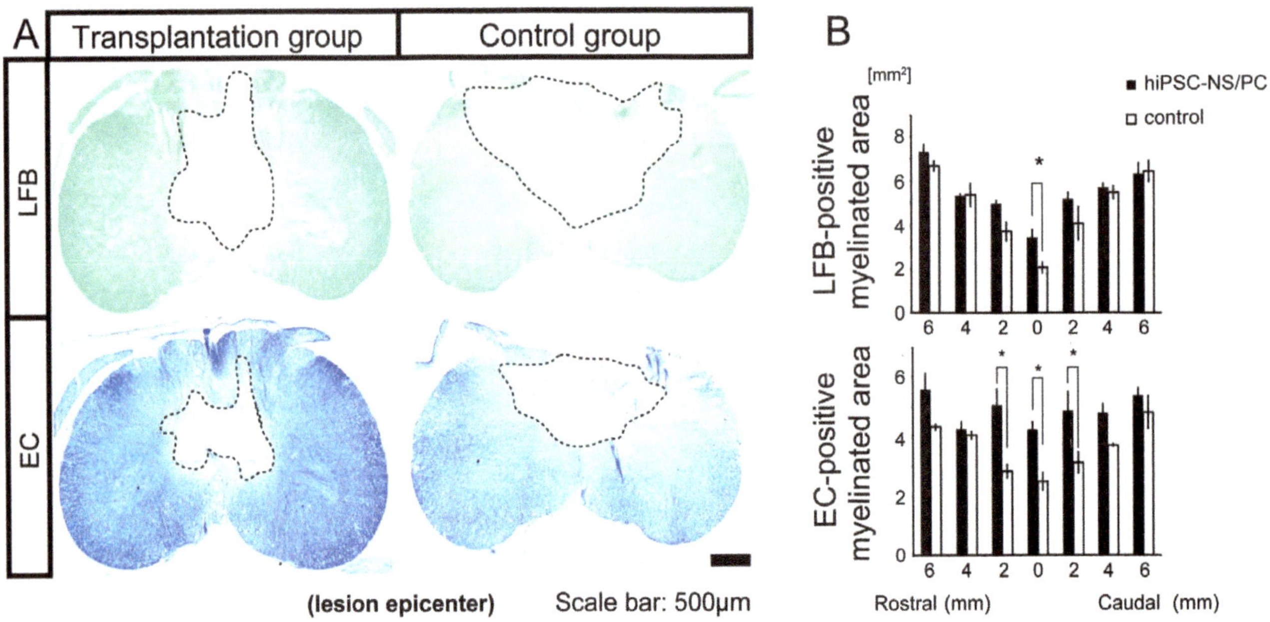

Figure 2. Grafted hiPSC-NS/PCs prevent demyelination after SCI. (**A**) Representative LFB- and EC-stained images of axial sections through the lesion epicenter at 12 weeks post-engraftment. The region enclosed by the dashed line indicates the demylinated area. (**B**) Quantification of the images revealed significant preservation in the size of the myelinated areas at the lesion epicenter in the transplantation group compared with the vehicle control group. Data represent the mean ± SEM (n = 3 per group, *p<0.05).

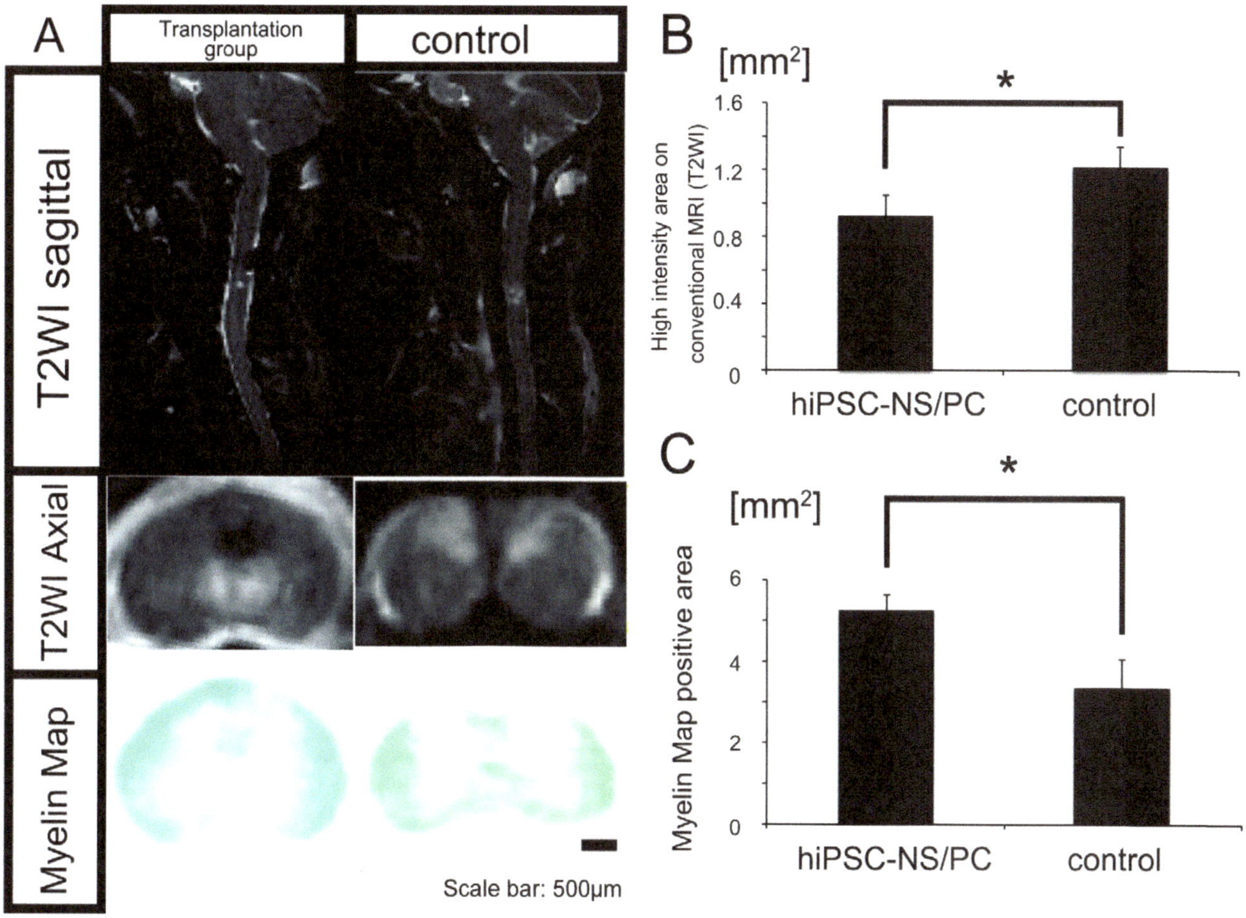

Figure 3. Conventional MRI and construction of a Myelin map. (**A**) MRI and Myelin map of the spinal cord was carried out at 12 weeks after cell engraftment. (**B**) T2WIs obtained by conventional MRI showed that the intramedullary high-signal intensity area at the lesion epicenter was prominent in the vehicle control group compared with the transplantation group. Data represent the mean ± SEM (n = 5 per group, *$p<0.05$). (**C**) The Myelin map-positive area was increased in the transplantation group relative to that in the control group. Data represent the mean ± SEM (n = 5 per group, *$p<0.05$).

control group (Fig. 7C). All of the examined values for the open field test, bar grip test, and cage climbing test were significantly different between the transplantation and vehicle control groups at 8 weeks following SCI and thereafter.

Discussion

Rationale for the level of injury, type of injury, and timing of the intervention

It is important that validated experimental approaches in animal models are improved to meet the needs of individuals with SCI and to advance the field of regenerative neuroscience [35]. Because the number of patients with cervical injuries is increasing [36], further work with cervical contusive/compressive SCI models is required in parallel with clinical trials. Therefore, we developed a cervical contusion SCI model in the common marmoset in the present study.

Previous reports show that transient severe inflammation occurs around the injured site during the acute phase of SCI when the levels of many inflammatory cytokines, which have neurotoxic or astrocyte-inducing effects (such as IL-1, IL-6, and TNF), increase and then decline sharply within 24 hr [37]. Therefore, the microenvironment of the injured spinal cord during the acute phase is not suitable for the survival or differentiation of grafted cells. In fact, the transplantation of NS/PCs 9 days after SCI results in mitogenic neurogenesis, whereas this does not occur when the transplantation is performed within a few days of SCI [4,38]. The chronic phase of SCI is unlikely to be a suitable period for therapeutic transplantation due to the formation of enlarged cysts and the development of glial scarring, which might inhibit axonal regeneration [39,40]. Based on these studies, we hypothesized that the subacute phase of SCI is the optimal time for NS/PC transplantation.

Differentiation potential of grafted hiPSC-NS/PCs

In our previous study [9], we evaluated the tumorigenicity of hiPSC-NS/PCs grafted into the injured spinal cords of NOD-Scid mice. Long-term observation after transplantation (3 months) revealed no tumorigenicity of NS/PCs derived from the 201B7 clone. Based on this finding, we consider 201B7-iPS to be a "safe clone". The present study evaluated the therapeutic potential of these pre-evaluated safe hiPSC-NS/PCs for SCI in adult common marmosets. The grafted hiPSC-NS/PCs differentiated into neurons, astrocytes, and oligodendrocyte progenitor cells *in vivo*, whereas hiPSCs predominantly differentiated into neurons *in vitro*. These findings were consistent with the results of the

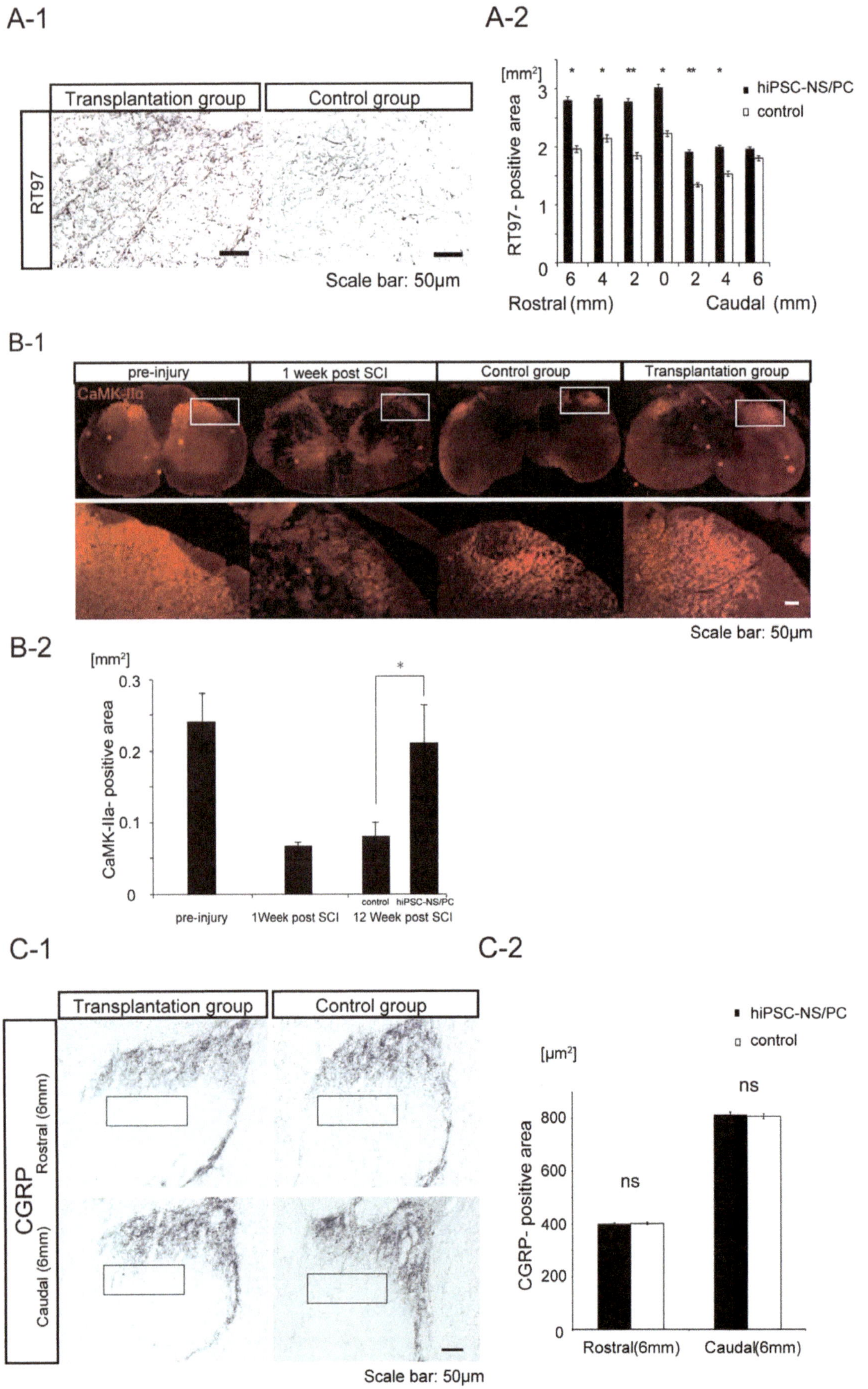
A-1
Transplantation group
Control group
RT97
Scale bar: 50μm
A-2
[mm²]
RT97- positive area
* * ** * ** *
hiPSC-NS/PC
control
Rostral (mm)
Caudal (mm)
B-1
pre-injury
1 week post SCI
Control group
Transplantation group
CaMK-IIα
Scale bar: 50μm
B-2
[mm²]
CaMK-IIa- positive area
control hiPSC-NS/PC
pre-injury
1Week post SCI
12 Week post SCI
C-1
Transplantation group
Control group
CGRP
Rostral (6mm)
Caudal (6mm)
Scale bar: 50μm
C-2
hiPSC-NS/PC
control
[μm²]
CGRP- positive area
ns
ns
Rostral(6mm)
Caudal(6mm)

Figure 4. Grafted hiPSC-NS/PCs spare descending motor axons but do not induce abnormal innervations of pain-related CGRP positive afferents after SCI. (**A-1**) Representative images of RT97-positive neurofilament staining in the ventral region of the spinal cord at the lesion epicenter at 12 weeks post-engraftment. (**A-2**) Quantification of RT97-positive areas at the lesion epicenter. The overall RT97-postive area was larger in the transplantation group than in the control group. Data represent the mean ± SEM (n = 5 per group, *$p<0.05$, **$p<0.01$). (**B-1**) Representative images of CaMK-IIα-positive descending motor axons in the dorsal corticospinal tract (CST) area of the lesion epicenter. (**B-2**) Quantification of CaMK-IIα-positive areas at the lesion epicenter. The overall CaMK-IIα-positive area was increased in the transplantation group compared with that in the control group at 1 week post SCI. Data represent the mean ± SEM (n = 4 for each group, *$p<0.05$). (**C-1**) Representative images of CGRP-positive fibers in the dorsal horn 6 mm rostral and caudal to the lesion epicenter. (**C-2**) Quantitative analysis of the CGRP-positive areas in the dorsal horn 6 mm rostral and caudal to the lesion epicenter. There were no significant differences in the size of the CGRP-positive areas in the dorsal horn between the transplantation and control groups. Data represent the mean ± the SEM (n = 3 per group.)

transplantation of hiPSC-NS/PCs into the injured spinal cord of immunodeficient mice, suggesting that inhibitory factors for neuronal maturation exist within the injured spinal cord. It is also possible that the oligodendrocytes differentiation factors are absent *in vitro*, but present in the injured spinal cord. By contrast, human fetus-derived NS/PCs primarily differentiated into astrocytes following transplantation into the injured spinal cord of common marmosets in an earlier study [5]. Although the microenvironment of the injured spinal cord is critical for the survival and differentiation of grafted NS/PCs [38], these findings suggest that the origin of the NS/PCs plays an important role in their differentiation phenotype following transplantation during the subacute phase of SCI.

Tumorigenicity of hiPSC-NS/PCs

Because one of the predominant concerns regarding hiPSC-based therapy is the potential tumorigenicity of the grafted cells, animals were observed for tumor formation for up to 12 weeks after cell transplantation. No histological evidence of tumor formation was found during this time in any of the animals; this result was also confirmed by conventional MRI. For example, Oct4 is required for maintaining the pluripotency of embryonic stem cells (ESCs) [25,41] and for generating iPSCs [6,7], but is potentially tumorigenic when expressed in grafted hiPSC-NS/PCs [42]. However, histological assessment revealed that the grafted hiPSC-NS/PCs were negative for Oct4. We also examined the amount of proliferation among the grafted cells by Ki-67 labeling. The percentage of HNu-positive cells that were Ki-67-positive cells was 0.55±0.08%. On the other hand, 23.9±2.8% of the grafted hiPSC-NS/PCs remained immature, as determined by their expression of Nestin within the host spinal cord at 12 weeks (84 days) after transplantation; the percentage of Nestin-positive hiPSC-NS/PCs was similar to that of human fetus-derived NSCs (25.2±2.9%) at 56 days after transplantation into the injured spinal cord of common marmosets [5]. Interestingly, when NS/PCs derived from the same hiPSC clone were grafted into the injured spinal cord of immunodeficient mice in our previous study [9], lower percentages of Nestin-positive hiPSC-NS/PCs were observed (10.7±2.2% at 56 days and 7.5±1.0% at 112 days after transplantation). Thus, differentiation of transplanted cells might

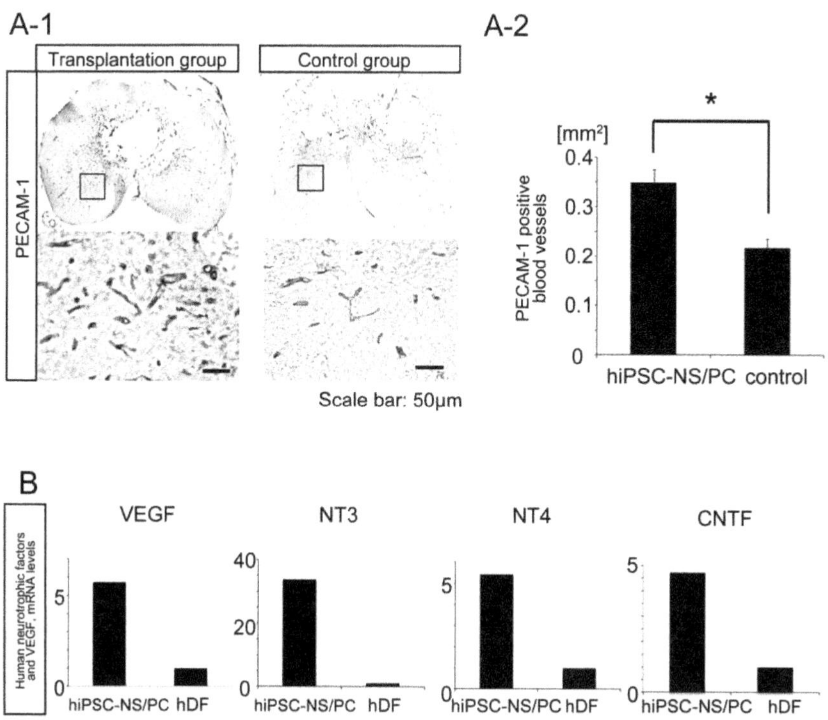

Figure 5. Grafted hiPSC-NS/PCs secrete neurotrophic factors and enhance angiogenesis after SCI. (**A-1**) Representative images of PECAM-1-positive blood vessels at the lesion epicenter. Scale bar: 50 μm. (**A-2**) Quantification of PECAM-1-positive blood vessels. The number of PECAM-1-positive blood vessels per unit area was higher in the transplantation group than in the control group. Data represent the mean ± SEM (n = 5 for the transplantation group and n = 4 for the control group, *$p<0.05$). (**B**) Quantitative RT-PCR and mRNA expression levels of VEGF and human neurotrophic factors. The expression levels of VEGF, NT3, NT4, and CNTF were all significantly higher in hiPSC-NS/PCs than in hDFs.

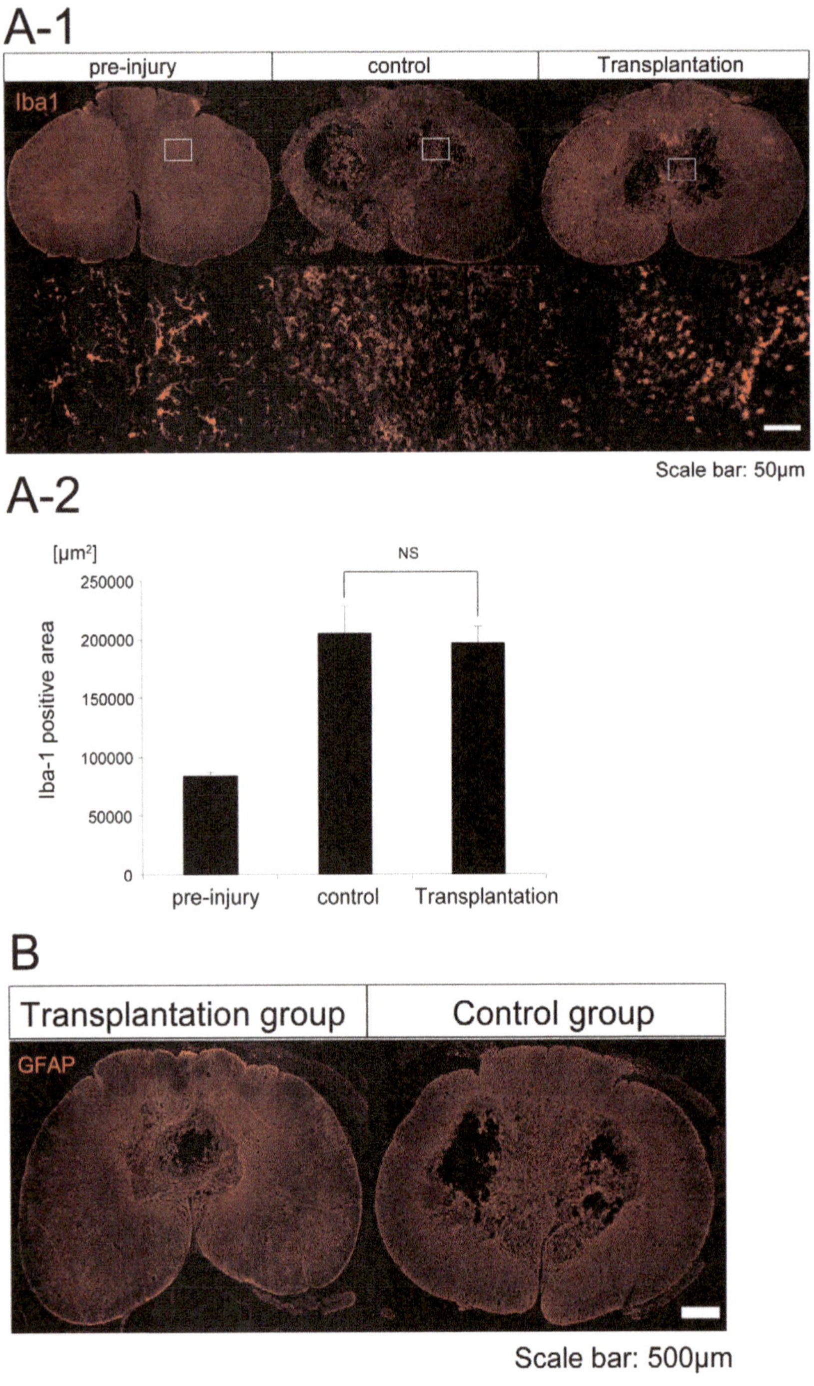

Figure 6. Microglial activation and glial scar formation at 12 weeks after transplantation. (A-1) Representative images of Iba1 staining in the spinal cord at the lesion epicenter at 12 weeks post-engraftment. Iba1-positive microglia showed a more rounded shape in the control and transplantation groups than in the pre-injury sample. (A-2) Quantification of the size of the Iba-1-positive area. The size of the Iba-1-positive area was not significantly different between control and transplantation groups at 12 weeks post-transplantation. (B) Representative GFAP-stained images of axial sections at the lesion epicenter at 12 weeks after cell transplantation. There were no significant differences in the size of GFAP-positive areas between the hiPSC-NS/PCs and the control groups.

be influenced not only by the origin of the NS/PCs, but also by species-specific differences in the microenvironment afforded by the host spinal cord. Strictly, we cannot exclude the risk of tumorigenesis derived from these Nestin-positive undifferentiated neural progenitor cells after 16 weeks post-transplantation. Thus, considering the fail safe system of future clinical trial, we should establish the selective ablation of the grafted-cell using such as the herpes simplex thymidine kinase (HSV-tk) and "suicide" gene system [43,44], if tumor formation occurred after human iPS-NS/PC transplantation.

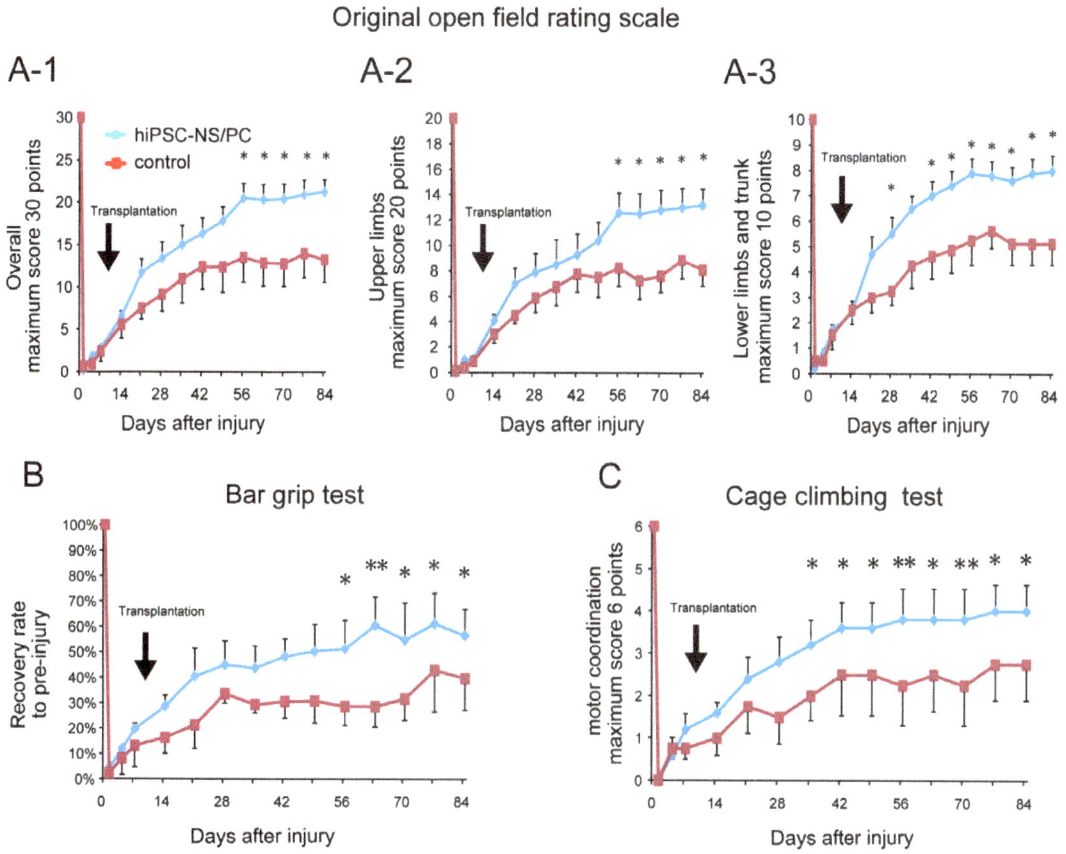

Figure 7. Grafted hiPSC-NS/PCs promote functional recovery after SCI. (**A-1**) Original open field rating scale (maximum 30 points). Immediately after injury, the score decreased to approximately zero for both groups. By 12 weeks after injury, the score had increased to a plateau of ~21 in the transplantation group and ~13 in the vehicle control group. Data represent the mean ± SEM (n = 5 animals for the transplantation group and n = 4 for the control group, *p<0.05). (**A-2**, **A-3**) Open field locomotor rating scale for the upper limbs (maximum 20 points) and the lower limbs and trunk (maximum 10 points). Data represent the mean ± SEM (n = 5 for the transplantation group and 4 for the control group, *p<0.05). (**B**) Bar grip test showing the time course of recovery of bar grip strength in the transplantation and the control groups. Each value indicates the percentage of pre-injury bar grip strength. Bar grip strength recovered gradually, reaching a plateau of ~57% versus ~40% of the pre-injury value in the transplantation group and the control group, respectively, by 12 weeks after injury. Data represent the mean ± SEM (n = 5 for the transplantation group and n = 4 for the control group, *p<0.05, **p<0.01). (**C**) Cage climbing test. The average test score was zero for both groups immediately after injury. By 12 weeks after injury, the mean score of the animals in the transplantation group had improved to 4, whereas the mean score of the animals in the control group had improved to 2.8. Data represent the mean ± the SEM (n = 5 for the transplantation group and n = 4 for the control group, *p<0.05, **p<0.01).

Mechanism of functional recovery after hiPSC-NS/PCs transplantation

Stem cell-based therapies for SCI could hypothetically affect histological and/or functional outcomes through a number of beneficial mechanisms, including axonal regeneration, local-circuitry reconstruction, neurotrophic effects, angiogenesis and immunomodulation, all of which have been reported to regenerate the damaged spinal cord in previous studies using rodent ESCs/iPSCs [8,9,45]. Compared with rodents, non-human primates such as common marmosets have distinct differences in terms of anatomy, functional neural pathways in the spinal cord, and immune responses. Although it is difficult to evaluate the functional recovery of the forelimbs in the rodents, this is possible in the SCI model of the non-human primates. Furthermore, to validate and predict the therapeutic effects of interventions used as human treatments, contusive injury is considered to be the most relevant to human SCI. Thus, the present study using common marmosets could be important for the pre-clinical evaluation of human iPSC therapy for human SCI.

The current study identified significantly larger areas at the lesion epicenter that were immunopositive for CaMK-IIα, NF-200, and PECAM-1 in the transplantation group relative to the vehicle control group, suggesting that the grafted hiPSC-NS/PCs increased axonal sparing/regrowth as well as angiogenesis after SCI. The details of mammalian central pattern generator (CPG), which is responsible for coordinated locomotor function, remain elusive although the spinal locomotor CPG is better characterized in rodents after functional recovery after SCI [46]. Furthermore, descending fibers from the motor cortex are more crucial for motor functions, including dexterous hand movements, in primates than in rodents [47]. The increased sparing/regrowth of the descending axons induced by hiPSC-NS/PCs may contribute to functional recovery after SCI. Furthermore, NT3, NT4, and CNTF encourage axonal sparing/regrowth after SCI [29,30,31,48,49] and VEGF enhances angiogenesis at the lesion site by promoting cell survival pathways and inhibiting cell death [50,51]. Importantly, cultured hiPSC-NS/PCs expressed significantly higher levels of NT3/4, CNTF and VEGF mRNA than hDFs, from which the hiPSCs were originally derived.

Transplanted NS/PCs not only promote replacement but also exert immunomodulatory and neuroprotective effects to prevent tissue damage [52,53]. Furthermore, undifferentiated NS/PCs persisting in the injured spinal cord can secrete trophic factors capable of protecting endogenous neural cells from cell death, preventing glial scar formation, and increasing endogenous re-myelination along with immunomodulatory molecules [52,53,54,55]. We performed Iba1 staining to assess microglial activation (Fig. 6A-1,A-2) and GFAP staining to assess glial scar formation (Fig. 6B). However, the size of the Iba1-positive area was not significantly different between control and transplantation groups, and there was no evidence of immunomodulation by hiPSC-NS/PCs at this time point (12 weeks after transplantation).

Previous studies demonstrated that the transplantation of oligodendrocyte progenitor cells derived from human ESCs can increase re-myelination after SCI in rodents [56]. Our recent study also revealed that remyelination was significant in terms of functional recovery after NS/PC transplantation into SCI mice [57]. In the present study, we confirmed that grafted hiPSC-NS/PCs survived in the host spinal cord and differentiated into Olig1-positive oligodendrocyte progenitor cells. However, the hiPSC-NS/PCs did not differentiate into mature myelin basic protein (MBP)-positive oligodendrocytes during the course of the experiment, perhaps because the period of observation was too short. By contrast, MRI and LFB and EC staining revealed that cell transplantation increased the size of the residual, or spared, myelination areas at the lesion site. These findings suggest that the grafted hiPSC-NS/PCs contributed to the preservation of myelin sheaths rather than to re-myelination after SCI. It is possible that mature oligodendrocytes appear at a later time-point, as oligodendrocyte progenitor cells were present in the grafted cells.

In conclusion, NS/PCs derived from the pre-evaluated safe human iPSC clone 201B7 survived and differentiated into three neural lineage cells within the injured spinal cord of adult common marmosets, with no evidence of tumor formation. The hiPSC-NS/PCs also contributed to significant functional recovery in this non-human primate model of SCI. Although hiPSCs hold great promise as a cell source for the study and treatment of human diseases and disorders [58,59], it is critical to carefully assess safety concerns prior to their use in the clinic [60]. In particular, hiPSCs generated using retroviruses show integration of the virus DNA into host chromosomes [61], which may lead to unpredictable genetic dysfunction. Therefore, further study using integration-free hiPSC [62,63,64,65,66,67,68,69,70,71]-derived NS/PCs is required to validate the safety of such cells for stem cell interventions following SCI.

Acknowledgments

We thank Drs. Y. Takahashi, M. Takano, M. Shinozaki, A. Iwanami, F. Renault-Mihara, S. Shibata, H. Shimada, F. Toyoda, T. Harada, S. Miyao, and H.J. Okano for technical assistance and scientific discussions; and all the members of the H.O. and S.Y. laboratories for encouragement and generous support. We also thank Dr. K. Takahashi for the undifferentiated iPS cells.

Author Contributions

Conceived and designed the experiments: YK YO YT MN HO. Performed the experiments: YK YO HI S. Nishimura KH TK KF. Analyzed the data: YK HI S. Nishimura AY TK KF MN. Contributed reagents/materials/analysis tools: YK YO GI HI S. Nishimura AY S. Nori KH TK KF OT SY. Wrote the paper: YK KH MN HO.

References

1. Gage FH (2000) Mammalian neural stem cells. Science 287: 1433–1438.
2. Bjorklund A, Lindvall O (2000) Cell replacement therapies for central nervous system disorders. Nature Neuroscience 3: 537–544.
3. Lindvall O, Kokaia Z (2006) Stem cells for the treatment of neurological disorders. Nature 441: 1094–1096.
4. Ogawa Y, Sawamoto K, Miyata T, Miyao S, Watanabe M, et al. (2002) Transplantation of in vitro-expanded fetal neural progenitor cells results in neurogenesis and functional recovery after spinal cord contusion injury in adult rats. Journal of Neuroscience Research 69: 925–933.
5. Iwanami A, Kaneko S, Nakamura M, Kanemura Y, Mori H, et al. (2005) Transplantation of human neural stem cells for spinal cord injury in primates. Journal of Neuroscience Research 80: 182–190.
6. Takahashi K, Yamanaka S (2006) Induction of pluripotent stem cells from mouse embryonic and adult fibroblast cultures by defined factors. Cell 126: 663–676.
7. Takahashi K, Tanabe K, Ohnuki M, Narita M, Ichisaka T, et al. (2007) Induction of pluripotent stem cells from adult human fibroblasts by defined factors. Cell 131: 861–872.
8. Tsuji O, Miura K, Okada Y, Fujiyoshi K, Mukaino M, et al. (2010) From the Cover: Therapeutic potential of appropriately evaluated safe-induced pluripotent stem cells for spinal cord injury. Proceedings of the National Academy of Sciences of the United States of America 107: 12704–12709.
9. Nori S, Okada Y, Yasuda A, Tsuji O, Takahashi Y, et al. (2011) Grafted human-induced pluripotent stem-cell-derived neurospheres promote motor functional recovery after spinal cord injury in mice. Proceedings of the National Academy of Sciences of the United States of America 108: 16825–16830.
10. Okada Y, Matsumoto A, Shimazaki T, Enoki R, Koizumi A, et al. (2008) Spatiotemporal recapitulation of central nervous system development by murine embryonic stem cell-derived neural stem/progenitor cells. STEM CELLS 26: 3086–3098.
11. Okada Y, Shimazaki T, Sobue G, Okano H (2004) Retinoic-acid-concentration-dependent acquisition of neural cell identity during in vitro differentiation of mouse embryonic stem cells. Developmental biology 275: 124–142.
12. Imaizumi Y, Okada Y, Akamatsu W, Koike M, Kuzumaki N, et al. (2012) Mitochondrial dysfunction associated with increased oxidative stress and alpha-synuclein accumulation in PARK2 iPSC-derived neurons and postmortem brain tissue. Molecular brain 5: 35.
13. Nagai T, Ibata K, Park ES, Kubota M, Mikoshiba K, et al. (2002) A variant of yellow fluorescent protein with fast and efficient maturation for cell-biological applications. Nature Biotechnology 20: 87–90.
14. Iwanami A, Yamane J, Katoh H, Nakamura M, Momoshima S, et al. (2005) Establishment of graded spinal cord injury model in a nonhuman primate: the common marmoset. Journal of Neuroscience Research 80: 172–181.
15. Yamane J, Nakamura M, Iwanami A, Sakaguchi M, Katoh H, et al. (2010) Transplantation of galectin-1-expressing human neural stem cells into the injured spinal cord of adult common marmosets. Journal of Neuroscience Research 88: 1394–1405.
16. Kitamura K, Fujiyoshi K, Yamane J-I, Toyota F, Hikishima K, et al. (2011) Human hepatocyte growth factor promotes functional recovery in primates after spinal cord injury. PloS one 6: e27706.
17. Ohta K, Fujimura Y, Nakamura M, Watanabe M, Yato Y (1999) Experimental study on MRI evaluation of the course of cervical spinal cord injury. Spinal cord 37: 580–584.
18. Metz GA, Curt A, van de Meent H, Klusman I, Schwab ME, et al. (2000) Validation of the weight-drop contusion model in rats: a comparative study of human spinal cord injury. Journal of neurotrauma 17: 1–17.
19. Fujiyoshi K, Tsuji O, Konomi T, Hikishima K, Yamada M, et al. (2011) q-space MR imaging depict demyelination after spinal cord injury in non-human primate. [abstract] 41st Annual Meeting Neuroscience 2011, Washington, DC 160.117/CC116.
20. Fujiyoshi K, Tsuji O, Hikishima K, Yamada M, Kitamura K, et al. (2009) q-space MR imaging depict demylination after spinal cord injury in non-human primate. [abstract] 39th Annual Meeting Neuroscience 2009, Chicago: 542.549/S546.
21. Cory DG, Garroway AN (1990) Measurement of translational displacement probabilities by NMR: an indicator of compartmentation. Magnetic resonance in medicine 14: 435–444.
22. Callaghan PT, Coy A, Macgowan D, Packer KJ, Zelaya FO (1991) Diffraction-Like Effects in Nmr Diffusion Studies of Fluids in Porous Solids. Nature 351: 467–469.
23. Nakamura Y, Yamamoto M, Oda E, Yamamoto A, Kanemura Y, et al. (2003) Expression of tubulin beta II in neural stem/progenitor cells and radial fibers during human fetal brain development. Laboratory investigation 83: 479–489.
24. Kanemura Y, Mori H, Kobayashi S, Islam O, Kodama E, et al. (2002) Evaluation of in vitro proliferative activity of human fetal neural stem/progenitor cells using indirect measurements of viable cells based on cellular metabolic activity. Journal of Neuroscience Research 69: 869–879.
25. Loh YH, Wu Q, Chew JL, Vega VB, Zhang W, et al. (2006) The Oct4 and Nanog transcription network regulates pluripotency in mouse embryonic stem cells. Nature genetics 38: 431–440.

26. Krenz NR, Weaver LC (1998) Sprouting of primary afferent fibers after spinal cord transection in the rat. Neuroscience 85: 443–458.
27. Krenz NR, Meakin SO, Krassioukov AV, Weaver LC (1999) Neutralizing intraspinal nerve growth factor blocks autonomic dysreflexia caused by spinal cord injury. The Journal of Neuroscience 19: 7405–7414.
28. Hofstetter CP, Holmstrom NA, Lilja JA, Schweinhardt P, Hao J, et al. (2005) Allodynia limits the usefulness of intraspinal neural stem cell grafts; directed differentiation improves outcome. Nature Neuroscience 8: 346–353.
29. Bradbury EJ, Khemani S, Von R, King, Priestley JV, et al. (1999) NT-3 promotes growth of lesioned adult rat sensory axons ascending in the dorsal columns of the spinal cord. The European journal of neuroscience 11: 3873–3883.
30. Shang A-J, Hong S-Q, Xu Q, Wang H-Y, Yang Y, et al. (2011) NT-3-secreting human umbilical cord mesenchymal stromal cell transplantation for the treatment of acute spinal cord injury in rats. Brain research 1391: 102–113.
31. McTigue DM, Horner PJ, Stokes BT, Gage FH (1998) Neurotrophin-3 and brain-derived neurotrophic factor induce oligodendrocyte proliferation and myelination of regenerating axons in the contused adult rat spinal cord. The Journal of Neuroscience 18: 5354–5365.
32. Leung DW, Cachianes G, Kuang WJ, Goeddel DV, Ferrara N (1989) Vascular endothelial growth factor is a secreted angiogenic mitogen. Science 246: 1306–1309.
33. Scivoletto G, Di Donna V (2009) Prediction of walking recovery after spinal cord injury. Brain research bulletin 78: 43–51.
34. van Middendorp JJ, Hosman AJ, Donders ART, Pouw MH, Ditunno JF, et al. (2011) A clinical prediction rule for ambulation outcomes after traumatic spinal cord injury: a longitudinal cohort study. Lancet.
35. Fehlings MG, Vawda R (2011) Cellular treatments for spinal cord injury: the time is right for clinical trials. Neurotherapeutics 8: 704–720.
36. Devivo MJ (2012) Epidemiology of traumatic spinal cord injury: trends and future implications. Spinal cord 50: 365–372.
37. Nakamura M, Houghtling RA, MacArthur L, Bayer BM, Bregman BS (2003) Differences in cytokine gene expression profile between acute and secondary injury in adult rat spinal cord. Exp Neurol 184: 313–325.
38. Okada S, Ishii K, Yamane J, Iwanami A, Ikegami T, et al. (2005) In vivo imaging of engrafted neural stem cells: its application in evaluating the optimal timing of transplantation for spinal cord injury. The FASEB journal 19: 1839–1841.
39. Okano H (2002) Stem cell biology of the central nervous system. Journal of Neuroscience Research 69: 698–707.
40. Okano H (2002) Neural stem cells: progression of basic research and perspective for clinical application. The Keio journal of medicine 51: 115–128.
41. Dhodapkar KM, Feldman D, Matthews P, Radfar S, Pickering R, et al. (2010) Natural immunity to pluripotency antigen OCT4 in humans. Proceedings of the National Academy of Sciences of the United States of America 107: 8718–8723.
42. Guo Y, Liu S, Wang P, Zhao S, Wang F, et al. (2011) Expression profile of embryonic stem cell-associated genes Oct4, Sox2 and Nanog in human gliomas. Histopathology 59: 763–775.
43. Schuldiner M, Itskovitz-Eldor J, Benvenisty N (2003) Selective ablation of human embryonic stem cells expressing a "suicide" gene. STEM CELLS 21: 257–265.
44. Eiges R, Schuldiner M, Drukker M, Yanuka O, Itskovitz-Eldor J, et al. (2001) Establishment of human embryonic stem cell-transfected clones carrying a marker for undifferentiated cells. Current biology 11: 514–518.
45. Fujimoto Y, Abematsu M, Falk A, Tsujimura K, Sanosaka T, et al. (2012) Treatment of a mouse model of spinal cord injury by transplantation of human induced pluripotent stem cell-derived long-term self-renewing neuroepithelial-like stem cells. STEM CELLS 30: 1163–1173.
46. Bradbury EJ, McMahon SB (2006) Spinal cord repair strategies: why do they work? Nature reviews Neuroscience 7: 644–653.
47. Lemon RN (2008) Descending pathways in motor control. Annual review of neuroscience 31: 195–218.
48. Ishii K, Nakamura M, Dai H, Finn TP, Okano H, et al. (2006) Neutralization of ciliary neurotrophic factor reduces astrocyte production from transplanted neural stem cells and promotes regeneration of corticospinal tract fibers in spinal cord injury. Journal of Neuroscience Research 84: 1669–1681.
49. Sundberg M, Skottman H, Suuronen R, Narkilahti S (2010) Production and isolation of NG2+ oligodendrocyte precursors from human embryonic stem cells in defined serum-free medium. Stem cell research 5: 91–103.
50. Kim HM, Hwang DH, Lee JE, Kim SU, Kim BG (2009) Ex vivo VEGF delivery by neural stem cells enhances proliferation of glial progenitors, angiogenesis, and tissue sparing after spinal cord injury. PloS one 4: e4987.
51. Lee HJ, Kim KS, Park IH, Kim SU (2007) Human neural stem cells over-expressing VEGF provide neuroprotection, angiogenesis and functional recovery in mouse stroke model. PloS one 2: e156.
52. Martino G, Pluchino S (2006) The therapeutic potential of neural stem cells. Nature reviews Neuroscience 7: 395–406.
53. Pluchino S, Quattrini A, Brambilla E, Gritti A, Salani G, et al. (2003) Injection of adult neurospheres induces recovery in a chronic model of multiple sclerosis. Nature 422: 688–694.
54. Butovsky O, Koronyo-Hamaoui M, Kunis G, Ophir E, Landa G, et al. (2006) Glatiramer acetate fights against Alzheimer's disease by inducing dendritic-like microglia expressing insulin-like growth factor 1. Proceedings of the National Academy of Sciences of the United States of America 103: 11784–11789.
55. Kokaia Z, Martino G, Schwartz M, Lindvall O (2012) Cross-talk between neural stem cells and immune cells: the key to better brain repair? Nature Neuroscience 15: 1078–1087.
56. Keirstead HS, Nistor G, Bernal G, Totoiu M, Cloutier F, et al. (2005) Human embryonic stem cell-derived oligodendrocyte progenitor cell transplants remyelinate and restore locomotion after spinal cord injury. The Journal of Neuroscience 25: 4694–4705.
57. Yasuda A, Tsuji O, Shibata S, Nori S, Takano M, et al. (2011) Significance of remyelination by neural stem/progenitor cells transplanted into the injured spinal cord. STEM CELLS 29: 1983–1994.
58. Wernig M, Zhao JP, Pruszak J, Hedlund E, Fu D, et al. (2008) Neurons derived from reprogrammed fibroblasts functionally integrate into the fetal brain and improve symptoms of rats with Parkinson's disease. Proceedings of the National Academy of Sciences of the United States of America 105: 5856–5861.
59. Hanna J, Wernig M, Markoulaki S, Sun CW, Meissner A, et al. (2007) Treatment of sickle cell anemia mouse model with iPS cells generated from autologous skin. Science 318: 1920–1923.
60. Okano H, Nakamura M, Yoshida K, Okada Y, Tsuji O, et al. (2012) Steps toward safe cell therapy using induced pluripotent stem cells. Circulation Research in press.
61. Wang W, Yang J, Liu H, Lu D, Chen X, et al. (2011) Rapid and efficient reprogramming of somatic cells to induced pluripotent stem cells by retinoic acid receptor gamma and liver receptor homolog 1. Proceedings of the National Academy of Sciences of the United States of America: 1–6.
62. Zhou H, Wu S, Joo JY, Zhu S, Han DW, et al. (2009) Generation of induced pluripotent stem cells using recombinant proteins. Cell Stem Cell 4: 381–384.
63. Kim D, Kim CH, Moon JI, Chung YG, Chang MY, et al. (2009) Generation of human induced pluripotent stem cells by direct delivery of reprogramming proteins. Cell Stem Cell 4: 472–476.
64. Shi Y, Do JT, Desponts C, Hahm HS, Scholer HR, et al. (2008) A combined chemical and genetic approach for the generation of induced pluripotent stem cells. Cell Stem Cell 2: 525–528.
65. Maherali N, Hochedlinger K (2009) Tgfbeta signal inhibition cooperates in the induction of iPSCs and replaces Sox2 and cMyc. Current Biology 19: 1718–1723.
66. Jia F, Wilson KD, Sun N, Gupta DM, Huang M, et al. (2010) A nonviral minicircle vector for deriving human iPS cells. Nature Methods 7: 197–199.
67. Hu K, Yu J, Suknuntha K, Tian S, Montgomery K, et al. (2011) Efficient generation of transgene-free induced pluripotent stem cells from normal and neoplastic bone marrow and cord blood mononuclear cells. Blood 117: e109–e119.
68. Rhee Y-H, Ko J-Y, Chang M-Y, Yi S-H, Kim D, et al. (2011) Protein-based human iPS cells efficiently generate functional dopamine neurons and can treat a rat model of Parkinson disease. The Journal of clinical investigation: 1–10.
69. Yu J, Hu K, Smuga-Otto K, Tian S, Stewart R, et al. (2009) Human induced pluripotent stem cells free of vector and transgene sequences. Science 324: 797–801.
70. Yusa K, Rad R, Takeda J, Bradley A (2009) Generation of transgene-free induced pluripotent mouse stem cells by the piggyBac transposon. Nature Methods 6: 363–369.
71. Kaji K, Norrby K, Paca A, Mileikovsky M, Mohseni P, et al. (2009) Virus-free induction of pluripotency and subsequent excision of reprogramming factors. Nature 458: 771–775.

17

Examination of the Combined Effects of Chondroitinase ABC, Growth Factors and Locomotor Training following Compressive Spinal Cord Injury on Neuroanatomical Plasticity and Kinematics

Olivier Alluin[1], Hugo Delivet-Mongrain[1]☯, Marie-Krystel Gauthier[2]☯, Michael G. Fehlings[3], Serge Rossignol[1], Soheila Karimi-Abdolrezaee[2,4]*

1 Multidisciplinary Team in Locomotor Rehabilitation of the Canadian Institutes of Health Research (CIHR) and Groupe de Recherche sur le Système Nerveux Central (GRSNC) of the Fonds de Recherche du Québec – Santé (FRQS), Department of Physiology, University of Montreal, Montreal, Quebec, Canada, **2** The Department of Physiology and Pathophysiology and the Spinal Cord Research Center, University of Manitoba, Winnipeg, Manitoba, Canada, **3** Department of Surgery and Spinal Program, University of Toronto; Toronto Western Research Institute, University Health Network, Toronto, Ontario, Canada, **4** Regenerative Medicine Program and Manitoba Institute of Child Health, Winnipeg, Manitoba, Canada

Abstract

While several cellular and pharmacological treatments have been evaluated following spinal cord injury (SCI) in animal models, it is increasingly recognized that approaches to address the glial scar, including the use of chondroitinase ABC (ChABC), can facilitate neuroanatomical plasticity. Moreover, increasing evidence suggests that combinatorial strategies are key to unlocking the plasticity that is enabled by ChABC. Given this, we evaluated the anatomical and functional consequences of ChABC in a combinatorial approach that also included growth factor (EGF, FGF2 and PDGF-AA) treatments and daily treadmill training on the recovery of hindlimb locomotion in rats with mid thoracic clip compression SCI. Using quantitative neuroanatomical and kinematic assessments, we demonstrate that the combined therapy significantly enhanced the neuroanatomical plasticity of major descending spinal tracts such as corticospinal and serotonergic-spinal pathways. Additionally, the pharmacological treatment attenuated chronic astrogliosis and inflammation at and adjacent to the lesion with the modest synergistic effects of treadmill training. We also observed a trend for earlier recovery of locomotion accompanied by an improvement of the overall angular excursions in rats treated with ChABC and growth factors in the first 4 weeks after SCI. At the end of the 7-week recovery period, rats from all groups exhibited an impressive spontaneous recovery of the kinematic parameters during locomotion on treadmill. However, although the combinatorial treatment led to clear chronic neuroanatomical plasticity, these structural changes did not translate to an additional long-term improvement of locomotor parameters studied including hindlimb-forelimb coupling. These findings demonstrate the beneficial effects of combined ChABC, growth factors and locomotor training on the plasticity of the injured spinal cord and the potential to induce earlier neurobehavioral recovery. However, additional approaches such as stem cell therapies or a more adapted treadmill training protocol may be required to optimize this repair strategy in order to induce sustained functional locomotor improvement.

Editor: Hatem E. Sabaawy, Rutgers-Robert wood Johnson Medical School, United States of America

Funding: This work was supported by the operating grants from the following: 1) the Craig H. Neilsen Foundation to SKA, MGF and SR; 2) the Christopher and Dana Reeve Foundation to SKA, MGF and SR; 3) the Manitoba Health Research Council (MHRC) to SKA; 4) the Canadian Institutes of Health Research (Sensorimotor Rehabilitation Research Team - SMRRT - grant and Canada Research Chair) to SR; 5) OA was supported by a postdoctoral fellowship from the Fonds de Recherche du Québec - Santé and Sensorimotor Rehabilitation Research Team - SMRRT; and 6) MGF is supported by the Halbert Chair in Neural Repair and Regeneration and by grants from the Krembil and Dezwirek Foundations. The funders had no role in study design, data collection and analysis, decision to publish, or preparation of the manuscript.

Competing Interests: The authors have declared that no competing interests exist.

* Email: soheila.karimi@med.umanitoba.ca

☯ These authors contributed equally to this work.

Introduction

Spinal cord injury (SCI) results in motor deficits below the level of injury that can be temporary or permanent, incomplete or complete depending on the severity of the lesion [1–4]. Recovery of locomotion is generally limited in SCI patients in spite of recent advances in clinical care and rehabilitation medicine [5]. Over the past years, various cellular and neurochemical repair strategies have been evaluated in experimental models of SCI for their efficacy in promoting neuroplasticity, axon regeneration, remyelination, and re-establishment of spinal circuitry to improve motor recovery following such injury [6–13]. Among these treatment strategies, targeting the inhibitory properties of chondroitin sulfate proteoglycans (CSPGs) located in the extracellular matrix of glial scar has shown promising potential in enhancing SCI repair [11,12,14–21].

Chondroitinase ABC (ChABC) facilitates the degradation of CSPGs in the injured spinal cord [12]. Therefore, over the past decade, ChABC has been utilized extensively in different models of SCI and in various combinatorial approaches to evaluate its impact in promoting functional repair and recovery [11,14,16,20,22,23]. Emerging evidence demonstrates that ChABC alone or in conjunction with growth factors, neurotrophins and/or cell-based treatments can promote structural repair and regeneration in the injured spinal cord [11–15,17,21,22,24,25]. ChABC treatment has also shown the potential to enhance locomotion in combination with other therapies in models of transection or compressive/contusive SCI [11,14,21].

ChABC in combination with cell therapies improves moderate recovery of function [11,14]. Studies by Fouad and colleagues showed that ChABC in synergy with a Schwann cell bridge and transplantation of olfactory ensheathing cells allowed recovery of function in rats after complete transection SCI [14]. We have also shown that degradation of CSPGs in the glial scar with ChABC was needed to improve the outcomes of transplanting neural precursor cells (NPCs) in chronic SCI [11] or efficient activation and oligodendrocyte replacement of endogenous spinal cord precursor cells in subacute SCI [15]. Sustained delivery of ChABC in combination with a growth factor (GF) cocktail containing EGF, FGF2 and PDGF-AA significantly increased the long-term survival and migration of transplanted NPCs in chronic compressive SCI [11]. Combined effects of ChABC, GFs and NPCs transplantation attenuated axonal die back in the corticospinal tract (CST) and enhanced sprouting of the CST and serotonergic fibers in the chronically injured spinal cord [11]. Moreover, we have shown that ChABC and GFs synergistically enhances the activation and oligodendrocyte differentiation of endogenous precursor cells after SCI and attenuated astrogliosis [15]. However, our functional testing showed that although ChABC, by itself, allowed substantial structural plasticity in the spinal cord, it was not sufficient to enhance locomotor recovery until it was combined with NPCs transplantation and *in vivo* infusion of GFs [11].

ChABC has been also used in combination with motor training in order to synergistically enhance activity dependent neuroplasticity and the recovery of locomotion in experimental models of SCI [16,20,26]. Current evidence indicates a limited efficiency of motor training in improving function in rodents or cats with incomplete SCI; contusive/compressive or hemisection [26–29]. In our recent work, kinematic analyses showed that regular motor training on treadmill did not improve the quality of spontaneous recovery of locomotion in rats with incomplete compressive SCI, although the rats regained impressive functional locomotion of the hindlimbs [27].

The aim of the present study was to evaluate whether combination of ChABC and growth factors (GFs) with daily treadmill training would synergistically enhance endogenous repair mechanisms and activity dependent functional plasticity, together allowing a significantly better recovery of hindlimb locomotion in rats with compressive SCI. We used neuroanatomical and kinematic analyses to assess neuroplasticity and functional recovery over a 7-week recovery period. Our findings show that this strategy promoted a significant degree of structural plasticity in corticospinal and serotonin-dependent pathways and that our pharmacological treatment mitigated the evolution of chronic peri-lesional astrogliosis and inflammation with a modest synergistic effects of treadmill training. Although an earlier return of locomotion was associated with an overall improvement of hindlimb angular excursions in the group treated with ChABC + GFs, this observation did not reach the statistically significant threshold needed to claim a difference between groups. Additionally, we observed an impressive locomotor recovery at the endpoint of study in all rats; however, the combinatorial approach had no additive long-term beneficial effects on the locomotor parameters studied with our stringent kinematic parameters.

Materials and Methods

All the neurobehavioural and neuroanatomical protocols in this study were performed based on approaches previously described by our group [6,11,15,27,30]. We used appropriate randomization and blinding in all neurobehavioural and histological techniques. Unbiased methodologies were used to undertake the neuroanatomical assessments. A list of abbreviations is provided in Table 1.

Animal care

A total number of 48 adult female Wistar rats (250–275 g) from Charles River Laboratory (Quebec, Canada) were used for different aspects of this study. Animals were housed in standard plastic cages at 22°C before spinal cord injury (SCI) and 25°C after SCI in a 12:12 h light/dark photoperiod. Food (Agribrands Purina, Ontario, Canada) and drinking water were available *ad libitum*. Hardwood sawdust bedding (PWI brand, Quebec, Canada) was used before SCI and then was replaced by soft paper bedding (Diamond Soft Bedding, Harlan Teklad) after SCI to prevent skin lesion. Animals were examined daily. After SCI, the bladder was expressed two times daily until the recovery of spontaneous bladder function occurred (between 7 and 14 days post-injury). All the animal procedures included in the present study were approved by the University of Manitoba and the University of Montreal Research Ethics Board and were conducted according to the Canadian Guide to the Care and Use of Experimental Animals (Canadian Council on Animal Care).

Experimental design and groups

After a one-week period of housing in the animal facility, rats were habituated to walk consistently on the treadmill at different speeds for three weeks. Afterwards, kinematic baselines were recorded for all rats during a second three-week period, and then SCI procedure was performed on each rat. One rat died during the surgery because of respiratory failure. Four days after SCI, rats were randomized into four experimental groups: 1) vehicle/untrained group ($n = 12$), 2) vehicle/trained group ($n = 12$), 3) ChABC+GFs/untrained group ($n = 11$), and 4) ChABC+GFs/trained group ($n = 12$). All SCI rats from groups 3–4 and 10 SCI rats from groups 1–2 (5 per group) underwent a second surgical procedure to infuse ChABC+GFs or vehicle via an intrathecal catheter connected to an Alzet osmotic minipump. After recovering from the implantation (2–3 days), kinematics was recorded weekly during 7 weeks for all rats of groups 3 and 4 and for 10 rats in groups 1 and 2 (5 per group). Finally, all the spinal cords were harvested for histology. Except for treadmill training sessions and data recording, all rats could move freely in their cage.

Table 1. List of abbreviations.

ChABC	Chondroitinase ABC
GFs	Growth factors (EGF + FGF-2+ PDGF-AA)
SCI	Spinal cord injury
CSPGs	Chondroitin Sulfate Proteoglycans
BBB	Basso, Beattie and Bresnahan rating scale
LFB/HE	Luxol Fast Blue and hematoxylin/Eosin
BDA	Biotin dextran amine
CST	Corticospinal tract
CV	Coefficient of Variation
PBS	Phosphate Buffer Saline
PFA	Paraformaldehyde
GFAP	Glial Fibrillary Acidic Protein
5-HT	Serotonin
ANOVA	Analyse Of Variance
SEM	Standard Error of the Mean
F subphase	First part of the swing phase (Flexion)
E1 subphase	Second part of the swing phase (Extension)

Treadmill apparatus and habituation

The treadmill belt was laid under a Plexiglas box (Length = 41 cm×Depth = 9.3 cm×Height = 14 cm) with a removable top. All rats were progressively familiarized to walk consistently on the treadmill at speeds ranging from 14 $m.min^{-1}$ (low) to 30 $m.min^{-1}$ (high) during the three weeks training program before SCI. Each session lasted 15 minutes and the number of sessions depended on the ability of each rat to perform the task. A soft plastic stick was used when necessary to stimulate the rats and induce appropriate locomotion by touching their hindquarters. Progressively, rats learned to walk freely and regularly in the locomotor device, using all four limbs at each speed of the range defined above.

Surgical procedures

All surgeries were performed in sterile conditions and under general gas anesthesia consisting in a mixture of O_2/isoflurane (2%) given through a mask integrated in a surgical stereotaxic frame. Immediately after surgery, rats were placed under a heating lamp until they fully recovered consciousness. Animals were given postoperative analgesia (50 µg/kg Temgesic, Schering-Plough, Hertfordshire, UK) and saline (3 ml) subcutaneously to prevent pain and dehydration, and then received antibiotics in drinking water (Clavamox drops, Pfizer Animal Health) for 1 week.

Thoracic Spinal Cord Injury. The aneurysm clip spinal compression model has been extensively described previously by our group [6,11,15,27,30–32]. Briefly, a midline incision was made at the thoracic vertebrae (T5-T9) and the skin and superficial muscles were retracted. The rats underwent a T6–T8 laminectomy and then, received a 23.8 g clip (Walsh Inc., Oakville, Ontario, Canada) compression injury for 1 min at the level of T7 of the spinal cord. Next, a piece of sterile absorbable gelatin sponge (1.5×1×0.7 cm, Gelfoam, Pfizer Inc.) was placed over the dura between T6–T8 and finally, muscles and skin were sutured. This injury produces moderately severe incomplete SCI with neurological outcomes of spastic paraparesis.

Administration of ChABC and Growth Factors. At four days post SCI, all rats were anesthetized using a mixture of O_2/isoflurane (2%) and then the injured spinal cord was carefully re-exposed using microsurgical techniques. ChABC (Seikagaku Corporation, Tokyo, Japan, 5 U/ml in saline plus 0.1% rat serum albumin) plus a cocktail of growth factors [GFs, including PDGF-AA (Sigma, 1 µg/100 µl), bFGF (Sigma, 3 µg/100 µl) and EGF (Sigma, 3 µg/100 µl) in a solution containing saline and 0.1% rat serum albumin] was infused for seven days using a subarachnoid catheter (Alzet, Rat IT, 0007741, 0.36 mm OD; 0.18 mm ID) connected to an osmotic minipump (Alzet pump model No.1007D, 0.5 µl/hr), as we have previously reported [6,33]. The catheter was inserted in the subarachnoid space around the injured area. Five rats in each vehicle group underwent identical surgical procedures but received saline plus 0.1% rat serum albumin). In our previous studies in the same model of SCI [11,15], we have extensively tested the efficacy of ChABC treatment in CSPG degradation. Using quantitative immunohistochemistry and slot blotting for CSPGs as well as 2B6 and C4S (detecting the degraded products of CSPGs), we have confirmed that one week ChABC treatment delivered at 3 days or 6 weeks post SCI can significantly degrade CSPGs after SCI. In our previous studies, our analysis at the end of one-week ChABC delivery with Alzet pump infusion has consistently confirmed a 60–75% reduction in CSPGs deposits and instead an 80% increase in C4S immunoreactivity (by-products of ChABC activity) in the matrix of subacute or chronic SCI [11,15].

BDA Anterograde tracing of the corticospinal tract (CST). Two weeks before the end of experiments, rats underwent anterograde tracing of the corticospinal tract (CST) with biotinylated dextran amine (BDA) (n = 3–6 rats/group). Under isoflurane anesthesia (as above), rats were positioned in a stereotaxic frame. BDA (10%, 10,000 MW; Invitrogen, Eugene, OR) was injected unilaterally into the left sensorimotor cortex at eight sites (0.5 µl per site) using the following coordinates (in reference to Bregma): (1) 1 mm anterior and 1 mm lateral; (2) 0.5 mm anterior and 1 mm lateral; (3) 1 mm posterior and 1 mm lateral; (4) 2.5 mm posterior and 1 mm lateral; (5) 0.5 mm posterior and 2 mm lateral; (6) 1.5 mm posterior and 2 mm lateral, (7) 1 mm anterior and 2.5 mm lateral, (8) 1.5 mm anterior and 2.5 mm lateral. Injections were made 1.2 mm from the surface of the cortex. Our previous studies have shown that the two weeks interval between BDA labeling and animal sacrifice is sufficient for anterograde labelling of the CST in thoracic regions [11,34].

Treadmill training program and kinematic recordings

Rats from groups 2 and 4 were all trained to walk on the motorized treadmill belt from 1 day to 7 weeks following SCI. The training program was performed 5 days/week and consisted in a walking session of 10 min daily on the treadmill at various speeds (from 14 to 26 $m.min^{-1}$) depending on the locomotor recovery level of each rat. Early after SCI, rats were incapable of autonomous hindlimb stepping, and were therefore stimulated by pinching the perineum. This evoked, in most cases, some hindlimb locomotion adapted to the belt speed but sometimes only flexion/extension alternation without plantar paw placement. During the training session, the belt speed was set at 14 $m.min^{-1}$ and the trunk of the animal was manually maintained to limit the lateral imbalance as long as the animal required perineal stimulation to walk. As soon as the rat was capable to walk without perineal stimulation, the belt speed was incremented in steps of 2 $m.min^{-1}$ every 2 minutes until the maximum speed tolerated by the rat was reached (*i.e.* in the range defined above). Throughout the recovery period, the trunk of the animals was manually supported when necessary.

Kinematic recordings. Kinematic baseline data were recorded at 14, 20 and 26 $m.min^{-1}$ for each rat to obtain control values. After SCI, the locomotor performance was evaluated weekly for 7 weeks until the maximum velocity that the animal could reach in the range defined above. Moreover, the untrained groups were assessed during short sessions to avoid the training effect of the evaluation itself. Kinematic recording method has been previously described in detail by our group [27]. Briefly, after shaving the left hindquarter of the rat, five markers were set on the skin of the lateral side at the level of ilium, greater trochanter, ankle joint, metatarsophalangeal joint and tip of the third toe. During the recording session, a left side view of the rat walking on the treadmill was captured using a high frequency numerical video camera (120 Hz). All the kinematics parameters were generated from the *x, y* coordinates of each marker and from the paw contact/lift events. Triangulation was used to extract the knee position from hip and ankle joint markers.

Definition of locomotion on treadmill. Since rats in each group exhibited different locomotor capability on treadmill at the end of the experiment, it was necessary to define simple criteria to include in kinematics analysis only animals capable of producing motor pattern considered as locomotor. Rats capable of performing at least 10 consecutive bilateral flexion-extension alternations of the hindlimbs with paw placement (plantar or dorsal) on the treadmill belt at 14 $m.min^{-1}$ were included in locomotion analysis. Rats that have not reached these criteria were considered not to have recovered locomotion.

Calculation of coordination. The method employed to evaluate the interlimb coordination has been described in detail previously [27] and gives an index of the neuronal coupling between each paw during locomotion. The coordination between fore- and hindlimbs (*i.e.* anteroposterior) as well as limbs from the same girdle (*i.e.* homologous) was calculated using the same method. Briefly, the coordination value of a given limb in a given step cycle represents the temporal position of the ground contact from this limb relative to the whole step cycle duration of the other limb. For instance, left hindlimbs homologous coordination value of 0.5 in a given step cycle means that ground contact of left hindlimb occurs at 50% of the right hindlimb step cycle duration.

Evaluation of individual variability. The method of individual variability assessment has been previously reported in detailed description [27]. Briefly, the coefficient of variation (CV) of every kinematic parameter was used to assess the intrinsic variability of each rat during locomotion. Since the analysis of locomotion of a given rat was based on consecutive sequences of several step cycles, each individual kinematic data at a given time point was an averaged value from the consecutive step cycles associated with a standard deviation. Thus, in the present study, the CV of a given parameter in a given rat at a given time point is the individual standard deviation expressed in percent of the mean of this parameter.

Tissue Processing and Neuroanatomical Analyses

Animal perfusion. At the end of experiments, animals were deeply anesthetized with sodium pentobarbital (80 mg/kg, intraperitoneal.) and then perfused transcardially with cold phosphate buffer saline (PBS, 0.1 M) followed by 4% paraformaldehyde (PFA) in 0.1 M PBS, pH 7.4. A two cm length of the spinal cord centered at the injury center was dissected and processed for different procedures as follows:

Frozen Sections. For cryotomy, the spinal cord were postfixed in the perfusion solution plus 10% sucrose overnight at 4°C, and then cryoprotected in 20% sucrose in PBS for 48 hr at 4°C. Then, the spinal cord centered at the injury site was dissected and embedded in mounting media (HistoPrep, Fisher Scientific) on dry ice. Cryostat sections (25 μm) were cut and stored at −80°C.

Vibratome sectioning. The spinal cords of the rats that underwent BDA anterograde labeling were postfixed in 4% PFA for overnight at 4°C, and then stored in PBS containing 0.1% sodium azide. The spinal cord were embedded in 10% low-temperature gelling agarose (Sigma), and 50 μm free floating serial transverse sections were cut on a vibratome (Leica) and collected in multi-well plates containing PBS plus 0.1% sodium azide.

Morphometric assessment of spinal cord lesion. Serial frozen spinal cord sections at 500 μm intervals were stained with myelin-selective pigment Luxol Fast Blue (LFB) and the tissue stain Hematoxylin-Eosin (HE) to identify the injury epicentre (N = 3–6 rats/group) as we reported previously [27,30]. Tissue sections displaying the largest proportion of cystic cavity compared with total cross-sectional area were taken to represent the epicentre of the injury. For analysis of tissue sparing and cavity formation after SCI, for each rat, we selected the spinal sections at epicentre and 1 mm and 2 mm rostral and caudal to the epicentre. The sections were stained with LFB-HE. We also immunostained the adjacent slide for astrocytes using an antibody against GFAP (rabbit, 1:1000, Dako) to precisely identify the borders of lesion cavity in each section. Reactive astrocytes surround the lesion area that includes the tissue debris and macrophages/microglia. Therefore, we used this criterion to differentiate the damaged tissue/debris within the lesion from the surrounding spared spinal cord tissue. The measurements were carried out in a blinded manner on coded slides using NIH ImageJ software (Media Cybernetics Inc., MD). Spared tissue was measured and normalized as a percentage of the total cross-sectional area of the spinal cord.

Immunohistochemical procedures and image analysis

For all immunohistochemical staining, the blocking solution contained 5% non-fat milk, 1% BSA and 0.3% Triton X-100 in 0.1 M PBS unless otherwise has been mentioned. The specificities of all antibodies were verified with both a negative control, omitting the primary antibody in our immunohistochemistry staining protocol, and a positive control, testing the antibody on tissues or cell preparations known to express the antigen.

GFAP and CD11b (OX42) immunostaining. Five transverse sections at epicentre and 1 mm and 2 mm rostral and caudal to the epicentre from each rat (N = 3–6 rats/group) were immunostained against GFAP and OX42 to assess astrocytic glial scar and macrophages/microglia, respectively. The frozen slides were air-dried at room temperature, and then were washed with PBS for 10 min. The sections were blocked and then incubated with primary antibodies. The following primary antibodies were used overnight at 4°C: rabbit anti-GFAP (1:1000, Dako) for astrocytes and mouse anti-CD11b (OX42, Serotec, 1:50). The slides were washed in PBS three times and then incubated with fluorescent Alexa 568 or 488 goat-anti mouse or anti-rabbit secondary antibodies (Invitrogen, 1:500) for 1 hr. The slides were coverslipped with Mowiol mounting medium containing DAPI to counterstain the nuclei. The images were taken using a Zeiss 710 laser confocal microscope or a Zeiss AxioVision microscope.

BDA visualization. We employed anterograde BDA labeling to study the sprouting of the CST fibers in the spinal gray matter as we described previously [11]. Three transverse vibratome sections (50 μm thickness) per animal at 5, 9 and 11 mm rostral to the injury site were selected for immunohistochemical processing to visualize BDA (N = 3–5/rats per group). One section per distance was processed for immunohistochemistry. Free-floating sections were incubated with the following reagents: 0.3% hydrogen peroxide (H_2O_2) in absolute methanol for 30 min at 4°C (using blocking solution as above), Vectastain AB (ABC Elite Kit, Vector Labs) in PBS containing 0.5% Triton X-10 according to manufacturer instructions for 2 hrs, 0.05% diaminobenzidine and 0.05% H_2O_2 in PBS for about 5 min. Sections were mounted onto slides and air-dried. Then, the slides were dehydrated through an alcohol series, cleared in xylene and coverslipped with Permount (Fisher Scientific).

5-HT immunostaining. Free-floating (50 μm thickness) at the injury epicenter and various distances relative to the injury epicenter: 1.5, 3 and 6 mm both rostrally and caudally were processed for immunohistochemistry for 5-HT (N = 3–6 rats/group). One section per distance was processed for immunohistochemistry. Sections were blocked and then incubated in anti-rabbit 5-HT antibody (1:10,000, ImmunoStar) for overnight at 4°C, and then Alexa 568 goat-anti rabbit secondary antibody (1:400, 2 hrs at room temperature) with three PBS washes after each step.

Image processing and analysis

In all neuroanatomical procedures, quantification was executed in an unbiased fashion by examiners blinded to the treatment groups based on the previously described methods by our group [6,11,15,27,30].

Immunohistochemical assessments of GFAP, CD11b (Ox42) and 5-HT. For immunodensity measurements of GFAP, CD11b (Ox42) and 5-HT, we imaged the entire cross section of the spinal cord at 10× primary objective using Mosaic tiling software (Zeiss). Then, using NIH Image analysis system (Image J), we traced entire cross section of the spinal cord and measured the relative density of GFAP, CD11b or 5-HT immunoreactivity as we performed previously [11] (N = 3–6 rats/group). Furthermore, we performed automatic thresholding for each image using NIH ImageJ software to determine the threshold for specific signal. After setting the threshold, the immunodensity above the threshold was automatically calculated. Background intensity from an area with no positive immunoreactivity was also subtracted from the intensity value to correct for non-specific reactions. Then, we divided the integrated density to the sample area to calculate the mean density per unit area. This calculation was performed to compensate for the different size of the region of interest in the spinal cord as we performed previously [11].

Assessment of axonal sprouting in the corticospinal tract. We performed anterograde BDA labeling to assess the sprouting of the CST fibers in the spinal gray matter as we described previously [11]. We normalized the intensity value of the BDA labeled collaterals in the gray matter to the intensity of BDA labeled fibers in the main CST to correct for inter-animal variation in the BDA labeling efficiency and/or the preservation of CST fibers. We imaged the dorsal columns of the spinal cord at 10×primary magnification using a Zeiss microscope at 5, 9 and 11 mm rostral to injury epicenter (N = 3–5/rats per group). In our SCI model, descending fibers of the CST are directly impacted by the injury and undergo Wallerian degeneration at and caudal to the injury epicenter. The axons in the rostral segment are also subjected to retrograde axonal degeneration or "die-back" as we described before [11].

Therefore, we selected rostral distances at 5 mm and further to the injury epicenter for our assessment of the CST fibers collateral sprouting. Using ImageJ Software, we measured the relative density of BDA immunoreactivity in the CST within the dorsal column. We employed automatic thresholding for each image using ImageJ software to determine the threshold for specific signal. The immunodensity above the threshold was quantified and the mean net density for BDA was calculated by dividing the immunointensity for BDA to the traced area. Background intensity from an area with no BDA positive immunoreactivity was also subtracted from the intensity value to correct for non-specific reactions. For collateral sprouting in spinal gray matter, we undertook the same approach as described above for BDA in the main CST to measure the relative intensity of BDA labeling within a the dorsal and intermediate gray matter. Then, we normalized the intensity value of the BDA labeled collaterals in the gray matter to the intensity of BDA labeled fibers of the main CST [11].

Statistical analysis

For neuroanatomical examinations and statistical intensity measurements, Two-Way ANOVA comparing groups and distances was used followed by post hoc pairwise multiple comparisons testing by the Holm-Sidak post hoc test. For kinematic analysis, individual data from each rat at every time point were averaged from a minimum of 10 consecutive locomotor cycles. Analysis of kinematic and regression data was performed using SigmaPlot program (Systat software Inc., San Jose, USA). Two-way ANOVA Repeated Measures was used to compare the effects of groups and delays on kinematics parameters followed by all pairwise multiple comparison (Holm-Sidak post hoc test) when ANOVA was significant. ANOVA was also used to test the linear regression between kinematic and neuroanatomical data. All the regressions analysis presented in this study have passed the normality test (Shapiro-Wilk) and the equal variance test. Non-parametric χ^2 with Yates correction and power test (α set at 0.05) or Fisher's exact test analysis were used to compare the distribution of rats capable or not to walk on treadmill at the different time points and velocity after SCI. Samples sizes were calculated to allow a 20% chance for a Type II error ($\beta \leq 0.2$). Grouped data are reported as mean ± SEM and the significance threshold for all statistical analysis was $p \leq 0.05$.

Results

Morphometric analysis of the spinal cord lesion

We first studied the effects of the treatments on tissue preservation and lesion following SCI. We quantified the extent of tissue sparing in spinal cord serial sections at five distances along the rostrocaudal length of the injured spinal cord centered at the injury epicenter as we described previously [27,30]. Representative photomicrographs of Luxol Fast Blue, hematoxylin and eosin-Y (LFB/HE) counterstained cross-sectional spinal cord sections are demonstrated for all treatment groups in Fig. 1A. Values representing the mean percentage of spared tissue for each examined distance in all experimental groups are summarized in Table 2. Our quantitative analysis showed no statistically significant difference in tissue sparing across the experimental groups suggesting that ChABC, GFs and training had no beneficial effects on attenuating tissue degeneration following injury.

Effects of ChABC, growth factors and daily exercise on the evolution of chronic astrogliosis and inflammation around the SCI lesion

We further investigated the influence of ChABC, GFs and daily treadmill training on the evolution of chronic reactive astrogliosis and inflammation within the spinal cord lesion. We quantified GFAP immunodensity (marking astrocytes) in spinal cord sections at the injury epicenter and at the peri-lesional areas around 1 mm and 2 mm rostral and caudal points to the epicenter (Fig. 2A–P, images depict representative sections at the epicenter and 1 mm rostral and caudal). Our data showed clear effects of ChABC and GFs attenuating astrogliosis, evident by reduced GFAP immunodensity, at the injury epicenter in the rats that received pharmacological treatments relative to untreated rats (Fig. 2Q, $*p<0.05$, two-way ANOVA, Holm-Sidak *post hoc*). Our analyses of the peri-lesional areas also showed a significantly reduced GFAP immunodensity in ChABC+GFs/trained group compared to the SCI vehicle/untrained group at 1 mm rostral and caudal points and compared to the SCI vehicle/trained group only at the 1 mm rostral distance (Fig. 2Q). These significant peri-lesional effects only present in ChABC+GFs/trained animals suggest a trend of synergy in our combinatorial strategy. Although there was a trend for reduced GFAP immunodensity in ChABC+GFs/trained group in comparison to the ChABC+GFs/untrained group, the difference between the two groups was not statistically significant. Interestingly, our examination also showed a significant attenuation in astrogliosis in ChABC+GFs/untrained group compared to the SCI vehicle/trained and SCI vehicle/untrained groups at the epicenter of the lesion (Fig. 2Q) which is in agreement with our previous results in a subacute SCI lesion after administration of ChABC+GFs [15]. Here, we did not observe any difference in lesional and peri-lesional astrogliosis between the two trained and untrained SCI vehicle groups as the result of treadmill motor exercise alone. Although, the differences between ChABC+GFs trained and untrained groups did not reach the significant level, the positive effects only obtained with the 3 combined treatments in the peri-lesional area suggest a potential moderate synergy. However, ChABC and GFs treatment seemed to be the key to induce the main effects.

Next, we studied how treatment with ChABC, GFs and training affect chronic inflammation assessed by the presence of macrophages/microglia within the lesional and peri-lesional regions (Fig. 3A–P, images depict representative sections at the epicenter and 1 mm rostral and caudal). Our neuroanatomical data at all the above-mentioned distances showed a significantly reduced macrophages/microglia in the chronic SCI lesion in the ChABC+GFs/trained group compared to the vehicle/untrained group and at the epicenter compared to the vehicle/trained group (Fig. 3R, $*p<0.05$, two-way ANOVA, Holm-Sidak *post hoc*). However, there was no significant difference between ChABC+GFs/trained and ChABC+GFs/untrained groups. Interestingly, rats in the ChABC+GFs/untrained group also showed less density of macrophages/microglia compared to the vehicle/untrained group that was significantly different at the epicenter and 1 mm rostral peri-lesional area, showing the effect of ChABC and GFs treatments on the reduction of inflammation process (Fig. 3Q, $*p<0.05$). This is also in agreement with our previous study that showed the positive effects of ChABC alone and in combination with GFs in attenuating lesional recruitment of macrophages/microglia in subacute SCI [15]. In the present chronic study, the significant reduction in macrophages/microglia at 2 mm rostral and 1 and 2 mm caudal to the epicenter only in ChABC+GFs/trained group suggests moderate synergistic effects of training with ChABC+GFs treatments.

ChABC, growth factors and daily training synergistically promote collateral sprouting of the corticospinal tract and serotonergic fibers after SCI

To assess whether our combined strategy would enhance neuroplasticity in the injured spinal cord, we studied the sprouting of two major descending pathways to the spinal cord: the corticospinal tract (CST) and serotonergic pathway. For studying the CST, we used anterograde BDA tracing to label the CST and its collateral fibers in the spinal cord (Fig. 4A–L). Of note, as we have shown previously, in our protocol to induce clip compressive SCI, the CST is disrupted by the injury and its axons caudal to the injury epicenter undergoes degeneration [11]. Moreover, CST axons proximal to the impact of injury are subject to axonal die-back and therefore are absent in rostral distances closer to the epicenter [11,35]. Accordingly, we examined the density of BDA labeling at starting at 5 mm distance rostral to the injury epicenter where the main CST is partially preserved following clip compression SCI [11]. To correct for inter-animal variation in the BDA labeling efficiency, we normalized the intensity of the BDA labeled collaterals in the gray matter to the intensity of BDA labeled main CST in the same section. Analysis of the dorsal and intermediate gray matter regions (boxed area depicted in Fig. 4A–L), at 5, 9 and 11 mm rostral points, revealed a significant increase in the density of BDA-labeled collaterals of the CST axons in the ChABC+GFs/trained group when compared to all other SCI experimental groups at 9 mm and to Vehicle/trained and untrained groups at 5 mm distances rostral to the lesion (Fig. 4M, $*p<0.05$, two-way ANOVA, Holm-Sidak *post hoc*). While the ChABC and GFs treatments together also demonstrated a non-significant trend toward a positive effect on promoting collateral sprouting of the CST in its target region at 5 mm rostral point, only the combination of these treatments with training was sufficient to significantly promote CST sprouting. Interestingly, in agreement with our previous reports with ChABC treatment, our combined strategy did not result in long distance axonal regeneration in the CST, as we did not detect any BDA traced CST fibers beyond the lesion [11].

We further examined the effects of ChABC+GFs/training on the plasticity of the descending serotonergic pathway that modulates neuronal activity and locomotion in the spinal cord [36–39]. In intact spinal cord, serotonergic fibers mainly terminate in the ventral and intermediate gray matter as well as lamina X and to lesser extent in the dorsal horn (Fig. 5A). As we reported previously, a sizable increase in serotonin immunoreactivity is seen in rostral white matter regions particularly in the lateral and dorsal

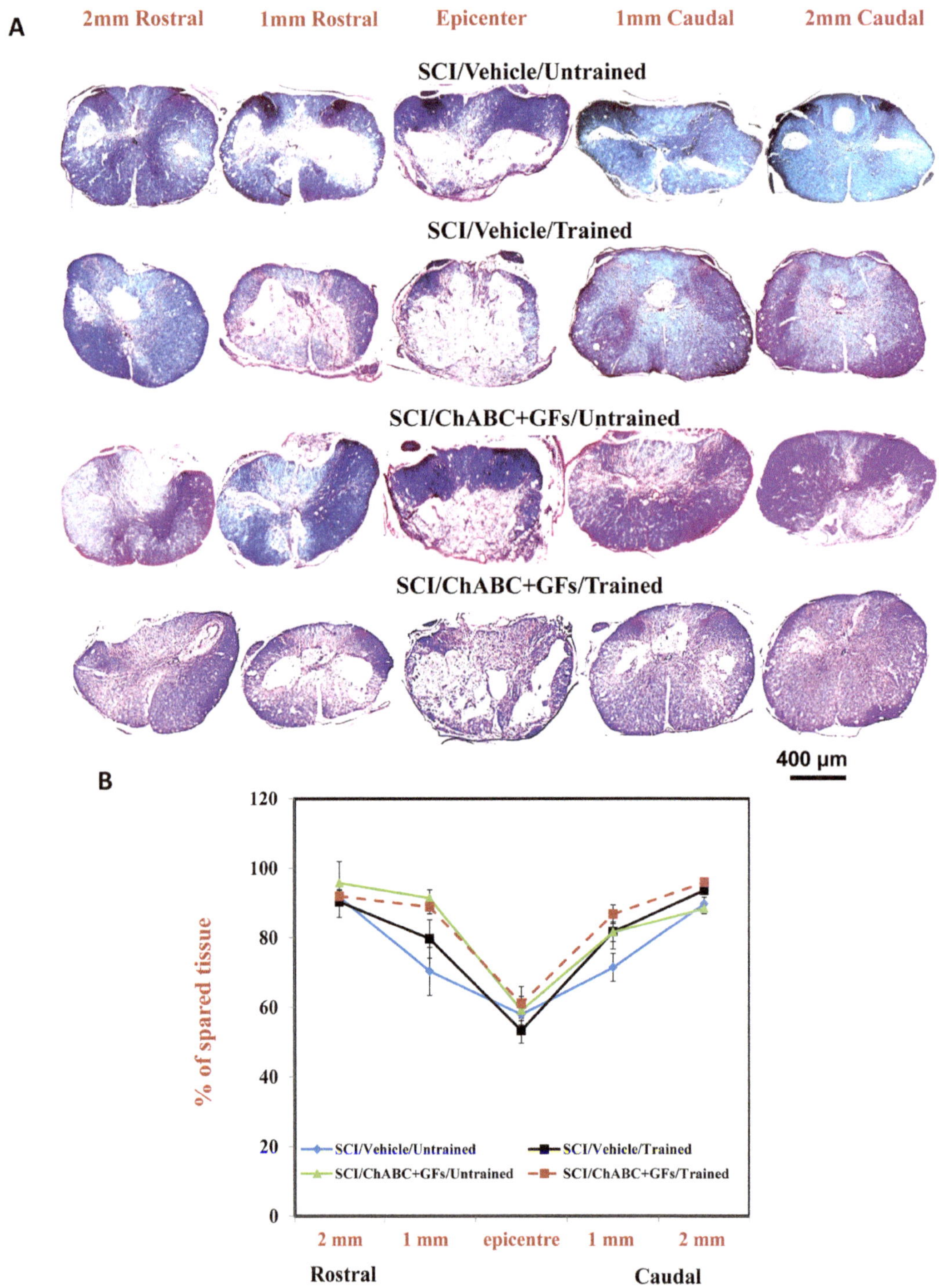

Figure 1. Morphometric analysis of the spinal cord lesion. (**A**) LFB/HE staining of cross sections of the injured spinal cord at various distances to the injury epicentre (both rostrally and caudally) is depicted for all experimental groups at seven weeks post-injury. The area of spared spinal cord tissue was traced and measured. (**B**) The percentage of spared tissue was calculated by normalizing the area of spared tissue to the total cross sectional area of the spinal cord. Although our quantitative analysis showed a positive trend in increasing tissue preservation in groups that received ChABC+GFs/Trained and ChABC+GFs/Untrained compared to Vehicle/Untrained counterpart in 1 mm rostral area, the difference was not statistically significant (Fig. 1B, Two-Way ANOVA, N = 3–6/group).

funiculi in our base-line SCI model (Fig. 5C) suggestive of spontaneous plasticity, increased expression of serotonin and/or accumulation of 5-HT in the serotonergic axons. Assessment of 5-HT immunodensity in multiple rostral and caudal distances to the injury epicenter (Fig. 5H) showed a significant increase in the density of serotonergic axons in ChABC+GFs/trained group (Fig. 5G) at all examined distances compared to both vehicle/untrained and vehicle/trained groups (Fig. 5C and E, $*p<0.05$). In addition, the 5-HT immunodensity was significantly increased in ChABC+GFs treated group with treadmill training relative to

Table 2. Percent of spared tissue.

Groups	2 mm rostral	1 mm rostral	Epicenter	1 mm caudal	2 mm caudal
SCI/Vehicle/Untrained	91.6±1.99	70.3±6.9	57.9±4.2	71.4±4	89.7±1.93
SCI/Vehicle/Trained	90.4±4.5	79.7±5.5	53.35±3.6	81.65±2.8	93.7±1
SCI/ChABC+GFs/Untrained	95.7±6.2	91.3±2.47	59.1±4.1	81.8±4.87	88.36±1.46
SCI/ChABC+GFs/Trained	91.9±1.95	88.8±1.91	61.03±4.8	86.8±2.65	95.91±0.6

Values are expressed as mean ± SEM.

the ChABC+GFs/untrained group (Fig. 5F, *$p<0.05$) at most distances excepted 1.5 mm rostral and caudal from the epicenter. On another hand, no difference was present between Vehicle/trained and Vehicle/untrained groups at all distances demonstrating a clear synergistic effect of the treadmill training with the pharmacological treatment toward an increase of 5-HT expression. Moreover, ChABC+GFs/untrained group showed a statistically significant elevation in 5-HT immunodensity at the epicenter as well as at 1.5 mm rostral and caudal points compared to both vehicle/untrained and vehicle/trained injured groups (Fig. 5H, *$p<0.05$). Serotonin density was also significantly higher at 3 mm rostral to the SCI epicenter in ChABC+GFs/untrained group compared to the vehicle/untrained counterpart. These findings collectively indicate that ChABC+GFs promote plasticity in serotonergic pathways and regular motor training enhances the magnitude of this response.

Recovery of kinematic parameters during treadmill locomotion

In accordance with our previous study on trained and untrained adult rats with a severe thoracic spinal cord clip compression [27], most of injured rats in the present study, regardless of treatment group, spontaneously recovered an impressive capability to generate efficient and coordinated hindlimb locomotor movements given the severity of the lesion. Consequently, the additional treadmill training provided during the 7-week recovery period failed to improve the locomotor parameters measured beyond this considerable spontaneous recovery at least at the end of experiment. In addition, none of the rats in the present study achieved full recovery in lateral balance during treadmill locomotion and only few animals recovered partial weight bearing (based on observations of the experimenters). Consequently, the trunk and/or tail of the rats were manually supported during treadmill training and/or kinematic recording sessions throughout the recovery period. The comparison of groups based on kinematic parameters indicated no significant effect of treadmill training throughout the recovery period. Consequently, to increase the statistical power and focus on the potential effects of ChABC + GFs treatment, the rats were then gathered in two groups: 1) ChABC + GFs treated and 2) vehicle treated animals. Figure 6 illustrates kinematic results of locomotor performance on treadmill from both groups before (*i.e.* baseline) and during the 7 weeks following SCI.

The data showed no significant difference between the two groups in the kinematics of locomotion on treadmill at later timepoints. Overall, although weight support and lateral balance remained deficient, when the trunks of the rats were supported they were capable of producing a well-defined and coordinated spontaneous locomotor pattern on the treadmill. In fact, throughout the recovery period, the step cycle length and duration were similar to the baseline (no significant difference; Fig. 6A and B). Interestingly, when the tail and/or trunk support provided by the experimenters was removed, the performance of the rats decreased drastically, they fell on the ground and they were then no longer capable of following the treadmill belt. This observation suggests that after severe compressive SCI, the absence of external postural adjustment, such as during free overground locomotion, could mask the capability of the spinal cord to produce full locomotor pattern.

Although the step cycle length was near-normal at week 7 (Fig. 6A), the parts of the locomotor cycle in front and in back of the vertical projection of the hip was respectively lower ($p\leq0.001$; Fig. 6C left part) and higher ($p\leq0.001$; Fig. 6C right part). As we reported previously [27], these data demonstrate that the locomotor movements of the hindlimbs shifted backwards. Nevertheless, despite the postural support, the knee joint movement remained affected 7 weeks after SCI (see knee angle excursion in Fig. 6F) and its amplitude was half of the baseline value all along the recovery period ($p\leq0.001$; Fig. 6D). To maintain the amplitude of the whole locomotor pattern, the animals compensated by increasing the ankle amplitude in similar proportion than the decrease of the knee ($p\leq0.001$; Fig. 6E). The angular excursions of the hindlimbs joints (*i.e.* hip, knee, ankle and MTP) during locomotion were very similar between treated and untreated groups 7 weeks after SCI (Fig. 6F right panel). In addition, though the amplitude of knee and ankle changed (Fig. 6D and E) the global shape of angles joints excursion during locomotion returned close to normal at the end of the post-lesion period (Fig. 6F, right panel compared to the left).

The shape of hindlimb instant velocity during the swing phase was changed 7 weeks after SCI. Even if the acceleration and the peak of velocity in the first 20% of the swing were close to normal (comparison of the first 20% of the normalized swing phase duration between top and bottom panel in Fig. 6G), the injured rats decelerated shortly after (from about 30%; Fig. 6G bottom panel) while normal rats maintained the maximum speed until about 45% of the swing (Fig. 6G top panel). These findings suggest that although the injured rats were capable of reaching the highest velocity of a normal swing phase (*i.e.* about 0.9 $m.s^{-1}$); they lost the ability to maintain this speed. In normal rats, the rebound of velocity in the last 20% of the swing corresponds to the final ankle extension just before the foot landing (Fig. 6G top panel). In injured rats, this rebound is lost 7 weeks after SCI (Fig. 6G bottom panel) due to the incapability of landing the foot far enough in front of the hip vertical projection as shown in the figure 6C.

Recovery of locomotor coordination

SCI rats in both ChABC + GFs and vehicle treated groups recovered the capability of generating locomotor pattern with the hindlimbs; however, they never recovered coupling between anterior and posterior paws while the coordination between both hindlimbs remained similar to the baseline (Figure 7). In normal

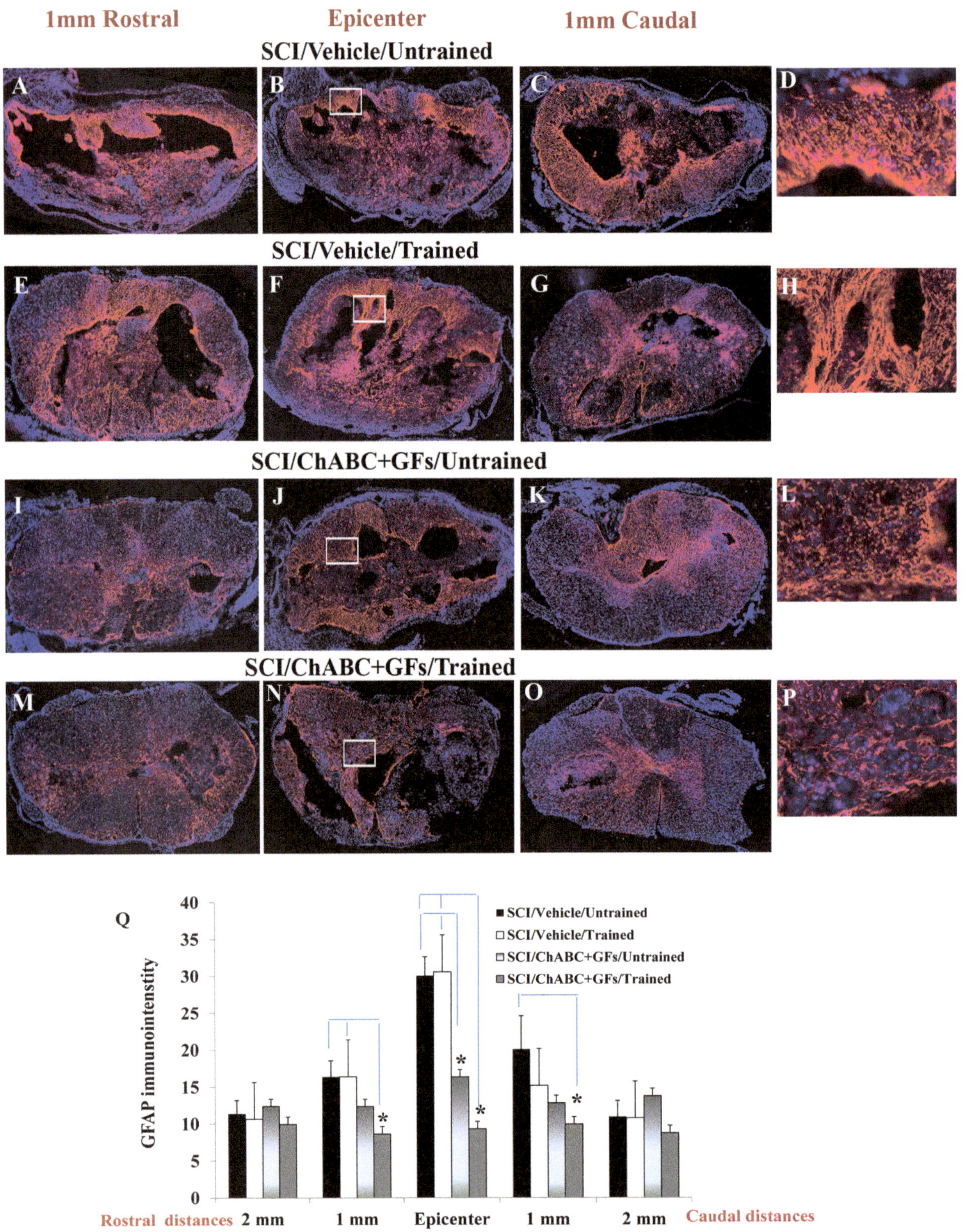

Figure 2. Effects of ChABC, GF and daily exercise on chronic astrogliosis after SCI. (**A–P**) Images show cross sections of the injured spinal cord immunostained for GFAP to mark astrocytes. Representative images from vehicle/untrained, vehicle/trained, ChABC+GFs/untrained and ChABC+ GFs/trained injured rats are depicted at various rostral and caudal distances to the lesion epicenter. Confocal images show an overall reduction in the expression of GFAP particularly in the surrounding parenchymal region in ChABC+GFs/untrained and ChABC+GFs/trained groups relative to both Vehicle/Untrained and Vehicle/Trained groups. Images in D, H, L, and P depict magnified areas inside the boxed regions identified in B, F, J and N, respectively. (**Q**) Our quantitative analysis of GFAP immunointensity confirmed a significant reduction in astrogliosis in the ChABC+GFs/trained group at the SCI epicenter as well as 1 mm rostral and caudal in comparison to the Vehicle treated groups. ChABC+GFs/untrained group also demonstrated

a significant decrease in GFAP immunoreactivity at the epicenter compared to both vehicle treated groups (Two-way ANOVA, *$p<0.05$, n = 3–6/group). Although ChABC+GFs/trained group consistently showed less astrogliosis compared to the ChABC+GFs/untrained counterpart, our statistical analysis showed no significant differences between the two groups.

rats, the frequency of each of the four limbs is the same during locomotion and the anteroposterior coordination value remains very stable around 0.3 all along the treadmill locomotor session (Fig. 7A). After SCI, the coupling between anterior and posterior girdles was lost and unrecovered for all rats all along the post-injury period. This is demonstrated by the progressive drift of the cumulated coordination value during treadmill locomotor sequence at the end of the recovery period (Fig. 7B). In fact, this continuous drift was due to the de-synchronization of the fore- and hindlimbs frequencies after SCI suggesting the loss of neuronal coupling between corresponding CPGs. However, although some fluctuations around the baseline value (*i.e.* 0.5) were present during the post-SCI period, rats have recovered the coordination between both hindlimbs 7 weeks after SCI (Fig. 7C).

Distribution of walking rats and quality of the locomotor pattern

Data related to the distribution of rats capable to walk on treadmill at different time points show a trend of an earlier recovery in ChABC + GFs group for the three studied velocities 14, 20 and 26 $m.min^{-1}$ (Fig. 8). Two weeks after SCI, only rats from ChABC + GFs group were capable of walking on the treadmill at all velocities (14 $m.min^{-1}$: 21.73%; 20 $m.min^{-1}$: 13.04%; 26 $m.min^{-1}$: 4.34%; Fig. 8A1, B1 and C1). Three weeks after SCI, the distribution of walking rats was still greater in the treated group at 14 $m.min^{-1}$ (ChABC: 47.82%; Vehicle: 20%: Fig. 8A1) and 20 $m.min^{-1}$ (ChABC: 43.47%; Vehicle: 10%: Fig. 8B1) while only rats from treated group were capable to walk on treadmill at 26 $m.min^{-1}$ (26.08%; Fig. 8C1). Four weeks after SCI the distribution of rats capable of walking on treadmill was similar between groups for the less challenging speed (14 $m.min^{-1}$; Fig. 8A1). However, the proportion of walking rats 4 weeks post-lesion remained greater in ChABC + GFs treated group for the highest speeds, 20 $m.min^{-1}$ (ChABC + GFs: 69.56%; Vehicle: 50%; Fig. 8B1) and 26 $m.min^{-1}$ (ChABC + GFs: 65.21%; Vehicle: 40%; Fig. 8C1). In addition, the comparison of angular excursions of the hip, knee, ankle and MTP from representative rats 3 weeks after the lesion shows clearly that the gait of ChABC + GFs treated rats was more regular and consequently the locomotor patterns was more efficient at 14 and 20 $m.min^{-1}$ (Fig. 8A3 and B3). In addition, at the same period, the ChABC + GFs treated rats still showed a very regular locomotor pattern at the highest and most challenging speed (Fig. 8C3). Four weeks following SCI, although the distribution of walking rats remained in favor of ChABC + GFs treated group at 20 and 26 $m.min^{-1}$ (Fig. 8B1 and C1), the organization of angular patterns became equivalent throughout the groups (Fig. 8B4 and C4).

Relationship between neuroanatomical parameters and kinematic performance

Since the kinematic data showed no significant effect of treatments on treadmill locomotor performances, the global regression analysis was performed by combining the data from all groups. This approach aimed to highlight the main relationships between behavioural outcomes and various neuroanatomical indices of spinal cord tract integrity at the end of experiment. Figure 9 depicts the significant relationships of kinematic parameters with the overall density of corticospinal tract (CST) fibers (BDA; Fig. 9A–D), serotonergic fibers (5-HT; Fig. 9E) and presence of macrophages/microglia cells (OX42; Fig. 9F) in the injured spinal cord. Our analyses showed that density of the CST fibers in the injured spinal cord was positively correlated with the variability of the foot position at the onset of the swing (*i.e.* foot lift; Fig. 9A). The feet lift occurring at the transition between stance and swing phases, and the length variability of both phases were also positively correlated with the presence of CST fibers (Fig. 9B–C). Consequently, the inconsistent foot lift position could explain the positive relationship between the presence of CST fibers and the variability of the whole step cycle length (Fig. 9D). Similarly, 5-HT expression in the SCI site was positively correlated with the variability of the foot velocity in the last part of the swing phase (*i.e.* hindlimb extension part named E1 subphase; Fig. 9E). Taken together, these results strongly suggest that the change in the gait variability measured over time in the present study represents a plasticity mechanism mediated at least in part by the corticospinal tract whereby there is an attempt to constantly adapt the step cycle compared to a more repetitive robot-like locomotor pattern mainly controlled by spinal circuits. Interestingly, the presence of OX42-positive macrophages/microglia, which is representative of the extent of inflammation, and the foot velocity in the first part of the swing phase (*i.e.* hindlimb flexion part named F subphase) were negatively interrelated at the end of experiment (Fig. 9F). These data suggest that the increase of inflammation in the spinal cord could be related to the decrease in movement velocity especially during swing phase.

Discussion

In the present study, we investigated the impact of combining daily motor training on treadmill with pharmacological treatment consisting of ChABC as well as growth factors (GFs), containing EGF, bFGF and PDGF-AA, on the structural plasticity of the spinal cord and the recovery of locomotion in rats with clip compression spinal lesion at T7. We report evidence of neuroanatomical spinal plasticity with the combined therapy and modest neurobehavioural effects as exhibited by a trend for an earlier (3–4 weeks after SCI) return of bilateral hindlimb locomotion after SCI in animals treated with ChABC + GFs. However, this combinatorial approach did not induce long-term functionally significant improvement of our specific kinematic parameters at the end of the 7-week recovery period.

Combinatorial treatment enhances neuroanatomical plasticity in the spinal cord

The use of ChABC and GFs therapy was based on our previous work that showed promising results when combined with neural precursor cell (NPCs) transplantation in promoting neuroplasticity and remyelination in chronic SCI [11]. ChABC and GFs therapy also enhanced endogenous oligodendrocyte replacement and attenuated astrocyte generation and pre-lesional glial scarring and inflammation when applied subacutely following SCI [15]. Our goal in the present study was to determine whether addition of a regular motor training regimen, as a clinically viable therapy, to the ChABC and GFs treatment would synergistically improve the recovery of locomotion after SCI by enhancing activity dependent plasticity in spinal circuitry. On day four after SCI, we delivered ChABC and GFs intrathecally for one week. This

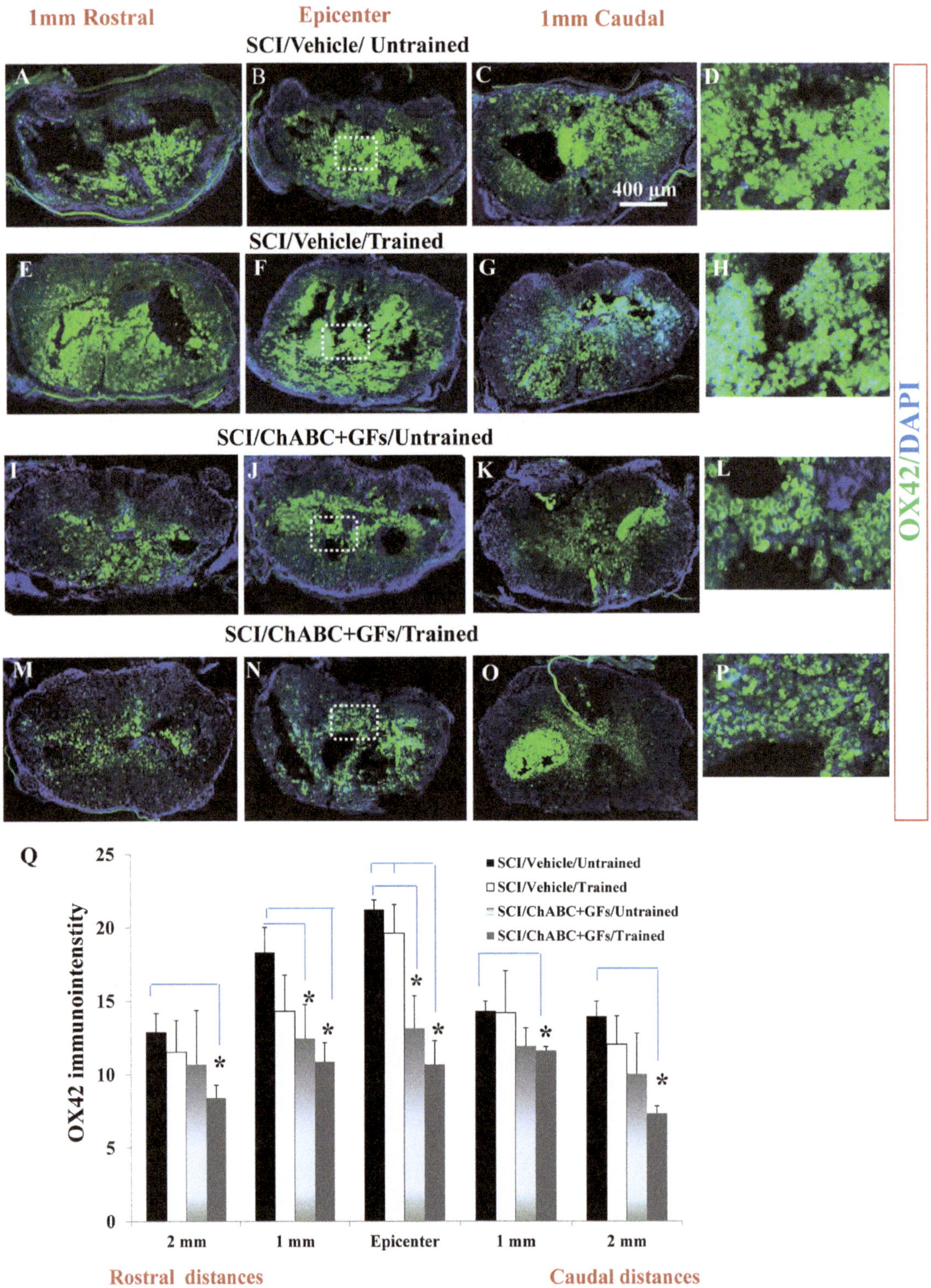

Figure 3. Effects of ChABC, GF and daily exercise on chronic presence of macrophages/microglia at the site of SCI lesion. (**A–P**) Confocal images showing the cross sections of the injured spinal cord immunostained for CD11b (OX42). Representative images from vehicle/untrained, vehicle/trained, ChABC+GFs/untrained and ChABC+GFs/trained injured rats are depicted at various rostral and caudal distances to the lesion epicenter. CD11b marks macrophages and microglia populations. Images in D, H, L, and P depict magnified areas inside the boxed regions identified in B, F, J and N, respectively. (**Q**) Our quantitative analysis of CD11b immunointensity showed reduced recruitment of macrophages/microglia in ChABC+GFs/trained group compared to the Vehicle/Untrained group at all distances and compared to the Vehicle/Trained group at the epicenter. Interestingly, ChABC+GFs/Untrained group also showed a significant reduction in CD11b immunoreactivity compared to the Vehicle/Untrained group at the injury epicenter (*$p<0.05$, Two way ANOVA, Holm-Sidak *post hoc,* N = 3–6/group).

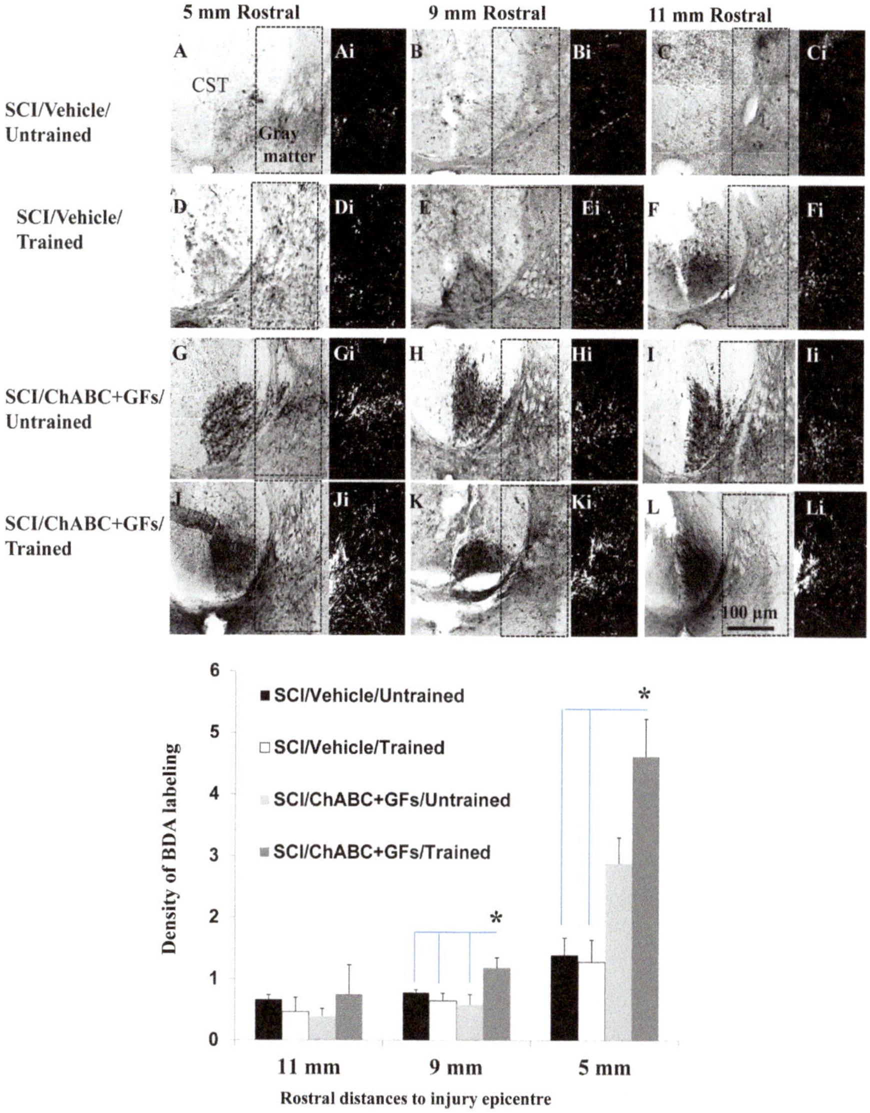

Figure 4. Synergistic effects of ChABC, GF and daily exercise enhance the collateral sprouting of the CST axons in the injured spinal cord. (**A–L**) Images of the BDA-labeled CST at 5, 9 and 11 mm rostral to the lesion are depicted in different experimental groups after unilateral injections of BDA into the sensorimotor cortex (Ai-Li). Inverted images were generated from the boxed region depicted in A–L for better visualization. BDA labeling was unilateral, so only contralateral CST is labeled. To correct for inter-animal variations in the BDA labeling efficiency, the intensity value of the BDA labeled collaterals in the gray matter were normalized to the intensity of BDA labeled fibers of the main CST. (**M**) Quantification of the areas depicted in Ai-Li at various distances revealed an increase in BDA density in the combined ChABC+GFs/trained treatment group compared to all other groups at 5 and 9 mm distances. Comparison of BDA-labeled collaterals among different injured groups also showed an increase in the density of BDA-labeled CST fibers in the ChABC+GFs/untrained group that was significantly higher than both vehicle treated groups at 5 mm rostral point to the SCI epicenter (*$p<0.05$, Two-way ANOVA, Holm-Sidak *post hoc*, N = 3–5).

delayed administration was specifically chosen for ChABC in SCI since: 1) CSPGs are highly upregulated and easily visualized within the spinal lesion at this time [15,40], 2) previous studies have shown the beneficial immunomodulatory effects of CSPGs in the acute phase of SCI [41], and 3) delayed therapies would facilitate a clinically relevant therapeutic time window of intervention for SCI. Our findings demonstrate that combining ChABC, GFs and daily exercise synergistically enhanced axonal plasticity in the descending CST and 5-HT spinal cord pathways. Additionally, the pharmacological treatment attenuated the evolution of astrocytic scar formation and chronic inflammation after SCI with a synergistic effect provided by treadmill training. These results are in general agreement with our previous studies in which we combined ChABC, GFs with NPC transplantation [11]. In fact, ChABC administration itself was sufficient to induce remarkable increase in collateral sprouting and/or preservation of the CST in rostral regions to the injury epicenter as well as sprouting of the serotonergic fibers within the lesional and peri-lesional areas [11]. Our neuroanatomical data here are also consistent with previous work by other groups indicating the overall positive impact of inhibiting CSPGs in improving injury microenvironment for repair and regeneration [16–18,22,42–45].

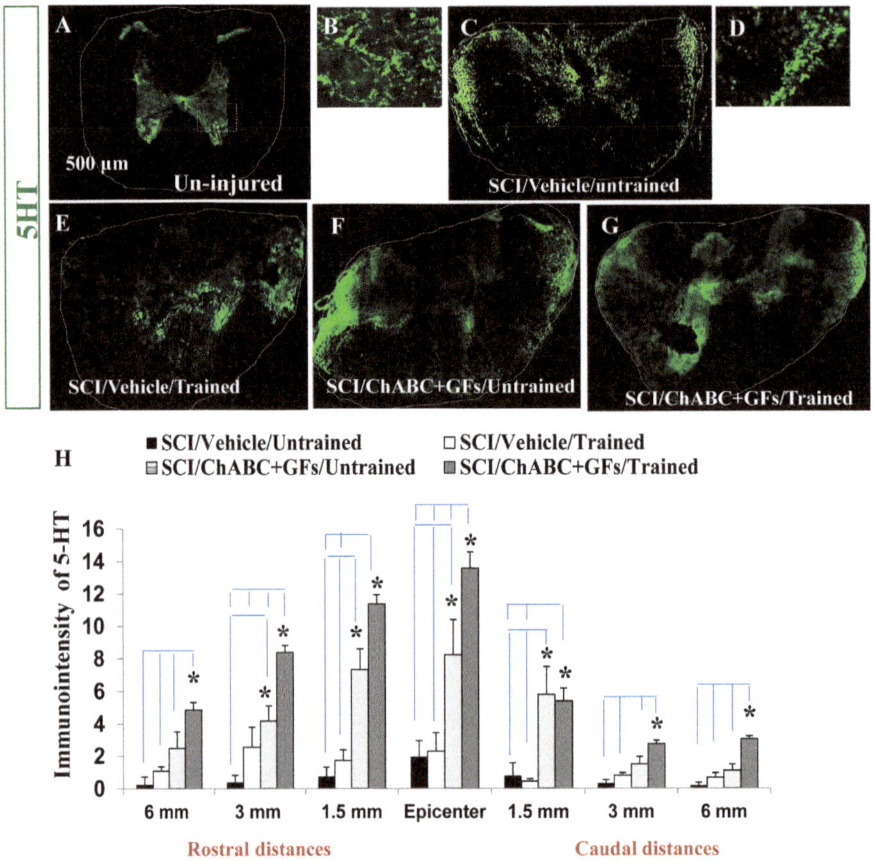

Figure 5. Combination of ChABC, GFs and training promotes plasticity of serotonergic fibers after SCI. (**A**) Transverse section of an uninjured spinal cord at mid-thoracic region demonstrates normal innervation pattern of serotonergic pathway (5-HT positive fibers) within the spinal cord. (**B**) Higher magnification of the boxed area in A shows the presence of serotonergic fibers in the gray matter areas representing of the signal that was quantified in our assessments. (C–G) At 7 weeks post-injury, 5-HT positive fibers in all experimental groups show significant changes in their localization (images shown for 1.5 mm rostral). In contrast to uninjured spinal cord, 5-HT immunoreactive fibers were sprouting in different regions of white matter in all injured groups. (**D**) Higher magnification of the boxed area in C shows the presence of serotonergic fibers in the white matter areas representing of the signal that was quantified in our assessments (H) Quantification of 5-HT immunointensity in the entire cross section of the spinal cord (traced areas in images) at various rostral and caudal distances revealed significantly increased level of 5-HT immunoreactivity in ChABC+ GFs/trained group compared to both vehicle treated group at all examined rostral and caudal distances (*$p<0.05$, Two-way ANOVA, Holm-Sidak *post hoc*, n = 3–6). Interestingly, at the epicenter and 1.5 mm rostral and caudal distances, the ChABC+GFs/untrained group also showed a significantly higher expression of 5-HT-immunoreactivity compared to the vehicle treated groups (*$p<0.05$, Two-way ANOVA, Holm-Sidak *post hoc*).

Absence of synergistic effects of treadmill training with ChABC and GF treatments on measurements of kinematic parameters at the end of the 7-week recovery period

Although the positive effects of ChABC administration on structural plasticity and regeneration in SCI has been established in the literature, its functional impact on specific motor patterns such as locomotion is still debated particularly in compressive/contusive models of SCI. To date, functional benefits of ChABC in SCI has been mainly achieved in partial transection models [12,13,16,18,19,22,44], and when ChABC was administered in more clinically-relevant models of SCI such as contusion and/or compression models as is the case in our study, its effects on functional recovery was minimal [11,43,46,47]. Recently, a study reported the transplantation of genetically modified Schwann cells to secrete endogenously D15A (neurotrophin mimicking the effects of NT-3 and BDNF) and ChABC in the injury site of rats with contusive SCI [21]. In agreement with our present and previous investigations [11], the data of this work showed a strong effect of the modified Schwann cells on the structural plasticity of the spinal cord (axonal regeneration, decrease of CSPGs, increase of myelination and 5-HT positive axons…) but a very moderate effect on the locomotor recovery (+0.5 improvement on the BBB scale compared to control group at the end of the experimental series lasting up to 14 weeks). Functional recovery with ChABC also seems to depend on the severity of SCI lesion. Caggiano and colleagues showed the positive effects of ChABC on hindlimb locomotor recovery only in rats with more severe compressive SCI [48]. Interestingly, in the same study, one experimental group with a moderate injury, comparable to the SCI severity in our present work, received no benefits on the recovery of locomotion from ChABC treatment [48].

Although, we show that rats in all experimental conditions had recovered the capability to generate fast, ample, coordinated and well-defined hindlimb locomotor movements on treadmill at the end of the 7 week recovery period and a trend of earlier return of locomotion in pharmacologically treated rats, our statistical analysis failed to detect any significant effects in treadmill trained animals (with or without pharmacological treatment). These results reinforce the conclusions of previous studies that showed

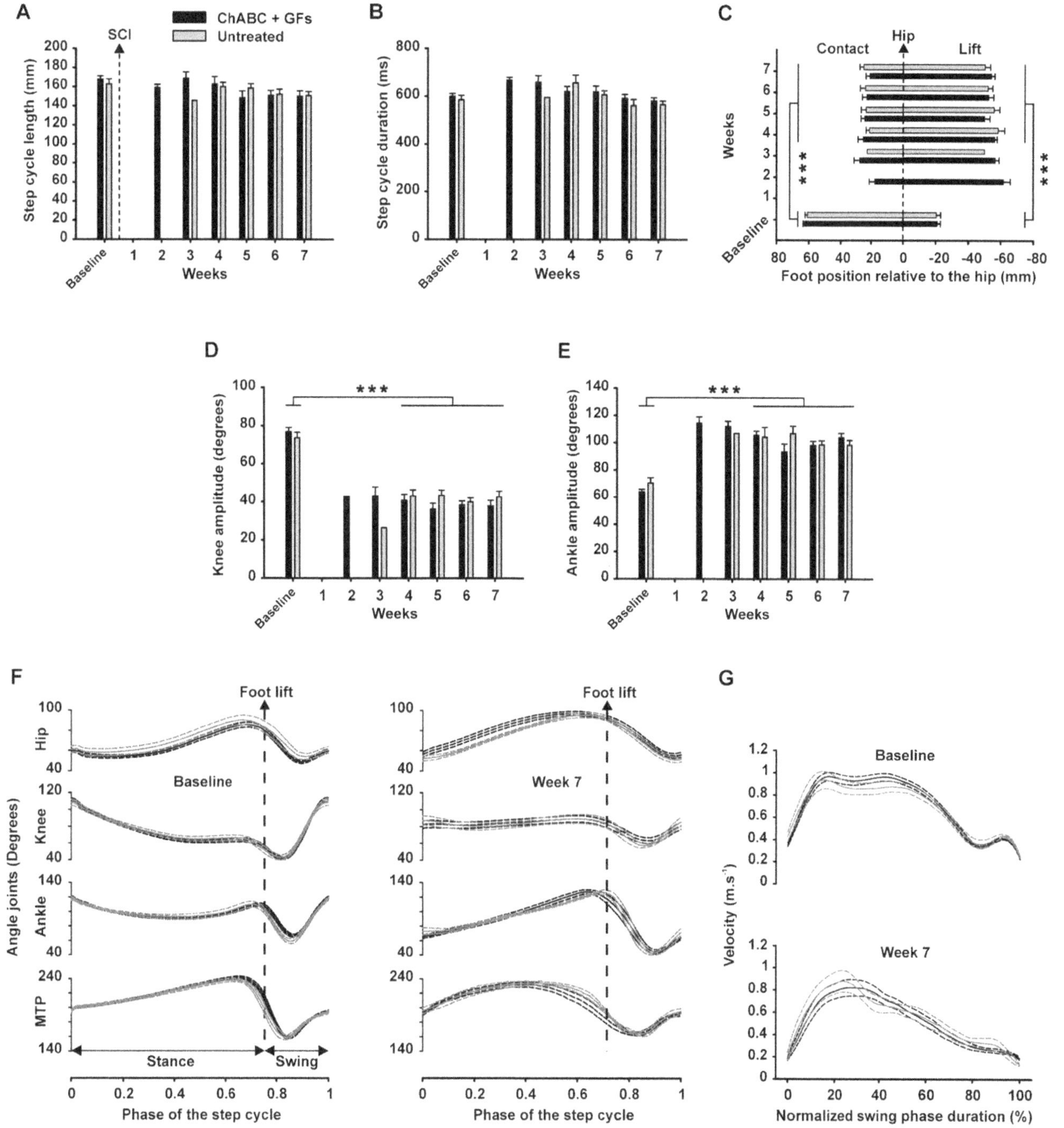

Figure 6. Kinematic analysis of locomotor patterns during the recovery period. Kinematic data were gathered in two groups (i.e. ChABC+ GFs and vehicle groups) and averaged before (baseline) and each week for 7 weeks after SCI. Because too few animals were capable to walk on treadmill during the three first weeks after SCI, statistical analysis were performed on baseline and week 4–7 only. (**A**) Mean length of the full step cycle (*i.e.* stance + swing phases) in millimeters is presented. (**B**) Mean duration of the full step cycle in milliseconds are shown. (**C**) Position of the foot contact (*i.e.* left part of the chart) and lift (*i.e.* right part) in millimeters relative to the vertical projection of the great trochanter are depicted (*i.e.* named hip in the chart and represented by the zero value). (**D**) Averaged amplitude of the knee joint in degrees and (**E**) averaged amplitude of ankle joint are presented. (**F**) Averaged angle excursions of the hip, knee, ankle and MTP, before (left panel) and 7 weeks after SCI (right panel) are shown. (**G**) Comparison of the averaged instant foot velocity (*i.e.* full lines) during swing phase before (top panel) and 7 weeks after SCI (bottom panel) for both groups, their respective SEM envelopes (*i.e.* dash line) are given. Symbol *** represent a significance threshold ≤0.001.

the absence of locomotor improvement in trained rats with incomplete SCI [27–29,49–51]. Interestingly, Caudle and colleagues report that when the hindlimbs of rats with mid thoracic contusion are immobilized on adapted wheelchair immediately after SCI, the overground locomotor performance of their hindlimbs decreases dramatically and then increases when the wheelchair is removed suggesting a substantial training effect of spontaneous locomotor movements [52]. Consequently, the

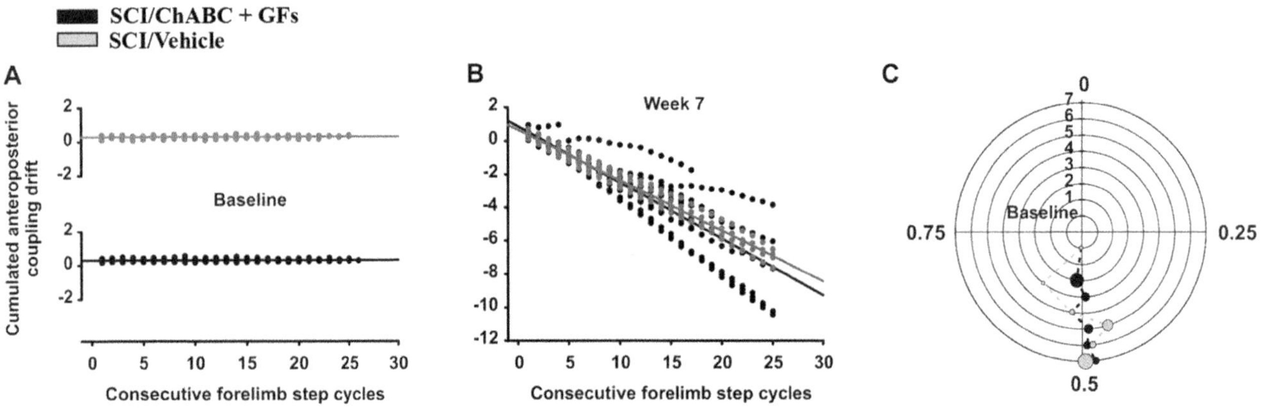

Figure 7. Limb coordination during locomotion. In **A** and **B**, coordination values plotted for each consecutive forelimb step cycle before and 7 weeks after SCI respectively. Usually the coordination measurement is expressed using polar coordinates. To simplify the representation of the coordination drift we converted these data to fit the Cartesian model by subtracting 1 to the polar values when two contacts of the forelimb with the treadmill belt occurred during one hindlimb step cycle (*i.e.* different stepping frequencies). This method renders an account of the intensity of the drift represented by the slope of the consecutive plots. (**C**) Hindlimbs coordination is expressed between 0 and 1 (*i.e.* theta) in a polar plot. The polar axis represents the delays from baseline (*i.e.* the innermost circle) to week 7 (*i.e.* the outermost) post-SCI. Circumference of the circles represent the normalized duration of right step cycle while the dots position on each circle represent the relative time position of the left foot contact averaged by group (see Alluin et al., 2011 for details). In addition, the size of each dot is proportional to the polar dispersion.

absence of treadmill training effect in the present study does not disclaim the beneficial effect of treadmill training after SCI but more likely represents the impact of continuous self-training of untrained SCI rats in their cage as previously suggested [26,27,49]. It is plausible that cage exercise in untrained and trained animals enhances their locomotor performance until a ceiling threshold is achieved beyond which any added treadmill training remains ineffective. In this context, it would be interesting in further experiment to challenge our combined strategy by increasing the severity of the spinal compression in order to lower the level of spontaneous recovery and reveal the potential benefits that might be concealed by the intrinsic locomotor capabilities. Further studies are required to elucidate the possibility that our combined therapy could improve functional recovery in a more severe compressive SCI with a lower degree of spontaneous locomotor recovery.

Other variables could also influence the outcomes of our training paradigm such as the duration and frequency of treadmill training and/or the optimal delay between SCI and the start of exercise training. An earlier study in spinal rats showed that the degree of locomotor recovery after SCI is correlated with the number of steps executed during each training session [53]. Therefore, it is plausible that the ten minutes duration of daily training in the present study might be insufficient to induce demonstrable activity-dependent functional improvement in clip compression SCI. Another variable is the impact of therapeutic time-window for initiating rehabilitation after SCI. In fact, studies by Smith and colleagues have shown the deleterious effect of swim training in acute phase of SCI on locomotor performance in rats with moderate contusive thoracic SCI [54]. The authors showed that starting training as early as 3 day after SCI could exert adverse effects on the recovery of locomotion by exacerbating the inflammatory response. Further studies are necessary to evaluate the impact of different variables in rehabilitation paradigms in SCI including time-window, frequency and duration of motor training.

Potential effects of combined ChABC and growth factors on fore-and hindlimbs coupling

Based on the absence of specific results induced by treadmill training, rats in the present study were consequently gathered into two experimental groups regardless of their training status: ChABC+GFs and vehicle treated groups. This was to focus on the effects of pharmacological treatments while increasing the statistical power of this new approach. Our kinematics analyses of ChABC+GFs and vehicle treated groups showed that injured rats generally regained plantar stepping with occasional weight bearing (not measured) and no evidence of forelimb-hindlimb coordination on treadmill (Fig. 7B). This recovery pattern corresponds to a BBB score of 9 to 10 which represents the baseline of our injury model as described previously [6,11]. However, although the anteroposterior coupling was globally disrupted in all animals of the present study, a subset of the ChABC+GFs treated group showed evidence of shorts bouts of coordinated frequency between forelimbs and hindlimbs (*i.e.* 3–5 consecutive step cycles) during their locomotor sequences 7 weeks after SCI (see few horizontal alignments of 3–5 consecutive black dots between 0–4, 5–8 and 15–20 forelimb step cycles in Fig. 7B). This transient period of coordination could be due to the perturbation of forelimb or hindlimb movements resulting in temporary forelimb-hindlimb synchronization. However, the fact that it was only evident in the ChABC+GFs group raises the potential benefits of the combined ChABC + GF treatment in establishing functional connections between upper and lower segments of the spinal cord.

It is noteworthy to mention that previous studies showing positive effects of ChABC on axonal regeneration and the potential functional connections used open field behavioural tasks to visually assess locomotion including coordination [11–13,19,22,44]. In the present study, we used precise measurement of coordination parameters using kinematics to assess fine locomotor improvements, which are normally unobservable or difficult to assess in open field evaluations. Given this, it is possible that moderate improvements in anteroposterior coupling may have occurred after ChABC treatment that had remained undetected in previous investigations. It is also possible that false positive anteroposterior coupling was observed on a short-term

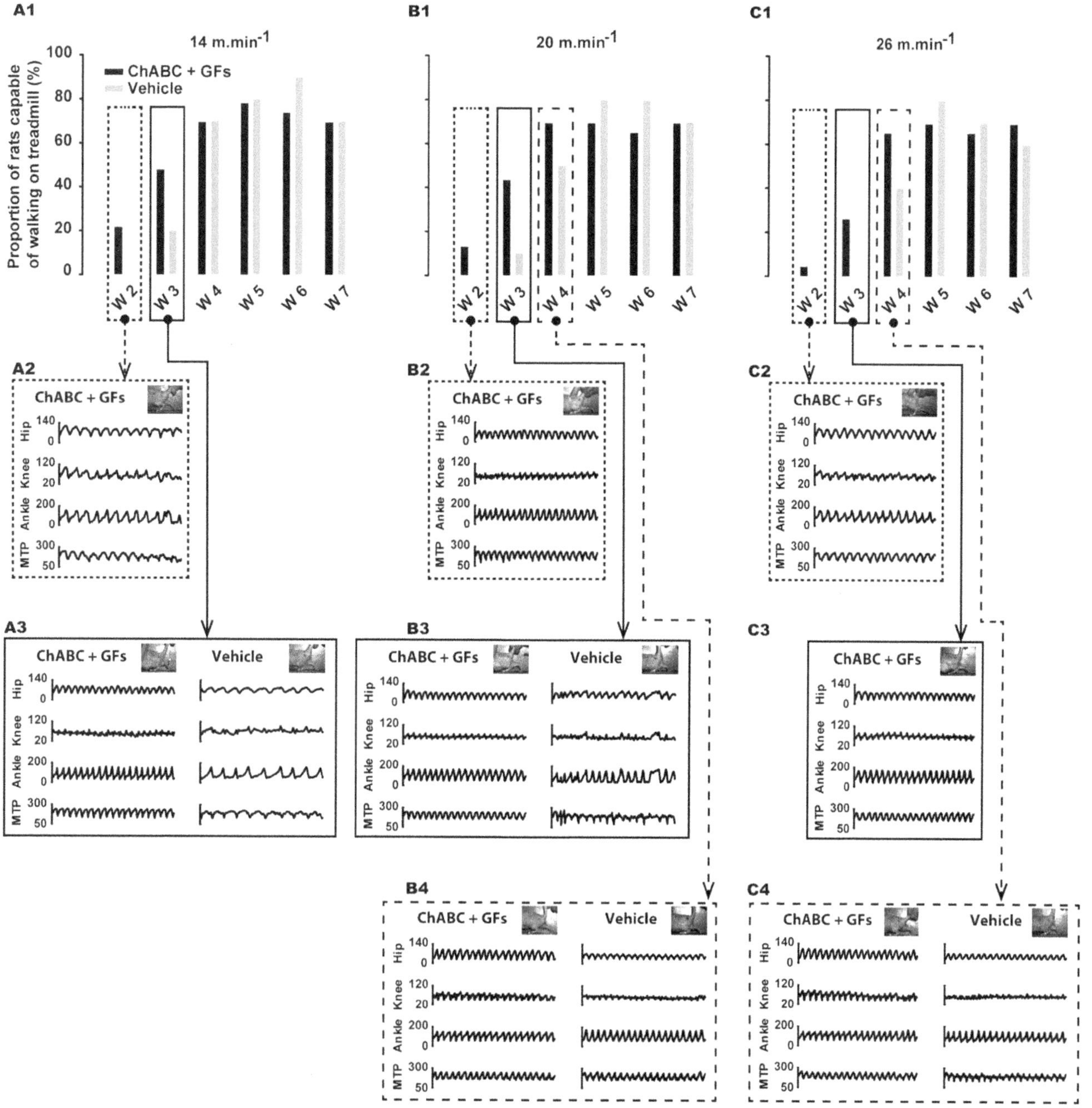

Figure 8. Frequency of rats that have recovered locomotion on treadmill at the three studied velocities and at the different time points throughout the recovery period. (**A1**, **B1** and **C1**), percent of rats capable of walking on treadmill at 14, 20 and 26 m.min^{-1} respectively, before and each week of the recovery period for ChABC+GFs and Vehicle groups. (**A2** and **A3**), raw angular excursions of hip, knee, ankle and MTP joints extracted from representative rats walking at 14 m.min^{-1} at week 2 and 3 respectively. (**B2**, **B3** and **B4**), raw angular excursions of hip, knee, ankle and MTP joints extracted from representative rats walking at 20 m.min^{-1} at week 2, 3 and 4 respectively. (**C2**, **C3** and **C4**), similar to B2, B3 and B4 for 26 m.min^{-1}. Data in A1, B1 and C1 are expressed in percentage of the group while the other panels below show angular data expressed in degrees.

scale. Nonetheless, in the present study, transient occurrences of anteroposterior coupling detected in ChABC+GFs treated group did not reach statistical significance. Future studies involving detailed analysis of interlimb coordination in a greater number of animals are essential to clarify the potential effect of ChABC+GFs treatment on forelimb-hindlimb coupling during locomotion in rat compressive SCI.

Some evidence of early locomotor recovery induced by the ChABC and GF treatments

Interestingly, our data on the percentage of rats capable of walking on treadmill at different time points after SCI, revealed not only a trend for an earlier recovery of locomotion in ChABC + GFs treated group, but also the improvement of stepping regularity and quality at early stages after SCI as demonstrated by comparison of raw angular excursions from representative rats

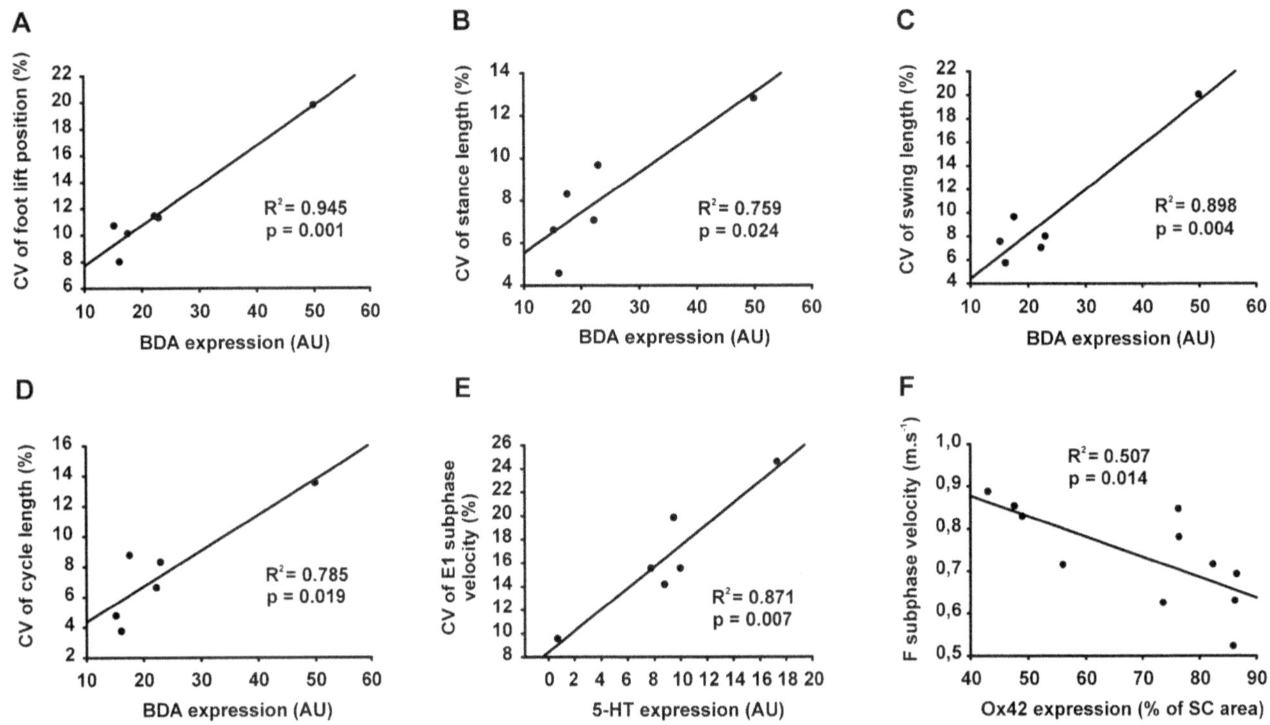

Figure 9. Relationships between behavior and neuroanatomical parameters. Given the absence of significant difference between groups for the behavioral features, available data from all rats were plotted together regardless of the groups. Given that the tissue preparation was different from one labelling protocol to the other, some animals were blindly selected in each group for each different procedure. In addition, among these selected animals not all have recovered the locomotion 7 weeks after SCI (as shown in Fig. 9 A1, B1 and C1). Taken together, this double restriction explains the limited number of plotted data in the present figure. (**A**) Global expression of BDA labeling from the spinal cord section studied was plotted against the coefficient of variation (CV) of the foot position at the onset of the swing phase. (**B**) Graph depicts overall BDA expression against the CV of stance phase length. (**C**) Overall BDA expression against the CV of swing phase length is shown. (**D**) Overall BDA expression against the CV of the step cycle length is depicted. (**E**) Graph shows overall 5-HT expression plotted against the CV of E1 subphase (*i.e.* 2nd part of the swing phase: extension of the hindlimb before foot contact) velocity. (**F**) Overall Ox42 expression is shown against averaged velocity of the F subphase (*i.e.* 1st part of the swing phase: initial flexion of the hindlimb following the foot lift). BDA and 5-HT quantifications are expressed in arbitrary unit (AU), CV is expressed in percentage of the mean and Ox42 labeling is expressed in percentage of the total spinal cord (SC) area. The coefficient of determination (R^2) and statistical significance (p) are given on each panel.

in both groups in Figure 8. Although these data did not reach statistical significance using our experimental design, the persistent trends at several consecutive time points and velocities suggest a possible effect of combined pharmacological treatment on the spinal cellular mechanisms early after the lesion. Immediately after SCI, influx of the inflammatory cells as well as the spinal shock occurs that targets the motoneurons below the lesion resulting in immediate loss of hindlimb movements and reflexes. This initial spinal shock is then followed by a gradual recovery of reflexes and, depending of the severity of lesion, regain of some motor functions. In the present study, we show a significant decrease in the presence of OX42 (CD11b) expressing macrophages/microglia in ChABC+GFs treated rats compared to vehicle counterparts (Fig. 3) suggesting the immunomodulatory effects of ChABC+GFs treatment on the injury induced-inflammatory response. Decrease in the inflammatory response in ChABC+GFs treated group may suggest a reduced period of spinal shock in these animals that could result in an earlier return of locomotor function observed in some of these animals. Here also, further investigations are needed to delineate the modulatory roles of these treatments on the recruitment of inflammatory cells as well as the impact of neuroinflammation inhibition on the time course of locomotor recovery after SCI.

Greater gait variability after SCI as a sign of greater supraspinal influence?

The correlation between the quantitative histological assessments and variability in the kinematic readouts is of interest. Such variability could be interpreted to mean that the step cycles are simply variable in nature or that the neuroplasticity induced by our treatment is aberrant and disrupting but it could also mean that the variability in the kinematic parameters reflect greater adaptability of these readouts. For instance, in a robotic locomotor performance in which the variability is dictated by the immediate environment only, such an automatic rhythmic behavior could be considered at the end of a spectrum where locomotion is principally defined by the operation of a spinal circuitry. However, it is considered that after partial SCI there are descending fibers re-innervating the spinal cord in an attempt to impose correcting inputs to the spinal cord. This might lead to a seemingly disorganized pattern but a pattern towards optimizing the motor performance despite the spinal lesion. We presume that the greater variability of the locomotor pattern may represent an attempt at a much more long-term functional recovery of the spinal cord. For instance, we can surmise that some degree of incoordination between the fore- and hindlimbs, as observed in the present study, might require adaptive corrections leading to a more apparent variability in the hindlimb step cycles. Our previous work in cats involved in a dual spinal lesion paradigm indicates that kinematic parameters of complete spinal cats are less variable than of hemisected cats suggesting that remnant descending pathways play a role in attempting to regulate the step cycle [55]. Similarly, in the present rat experiments, it could be postulated that as more supraspinal inputs reach the spinal cord through plastic mechanisms, the more variable step cycles may be represent as an attempt to continuously adapt the step cycles to the supraspinal inputs.

On the other hand, the recovery of hindlimb locomotion after partial spinal lesions depends also on intrinsic changes within the spinal cord itself. Indeed, several experiments in cats have shown that, after a thoracic hemisection, the spinal cord below the spinal lesion is durably changed since, after a further complete spinal section, the spinal cord can immediately express hindlimb locomotion whereas it usually takes 2–3 weeks of training to achieve such level of performance [56–59]. That such changes do occur in the spinal cord itself has consequences on the overall locomotor behavior of the animal since remnant inputs will encounter a more excitable spinal cord that has been changed by the previous lesion. In the present study, the large spinal lesion produced by the compression also leaves a great deal of autonomy to the spinal cord below the crush. It is therefore likely that such intrinsic spinal mechanisms also take place and those changes in intrinsic circuitry and neuroanatomical plasticity occurring below the lesion are part of the mechanisms leading to a seemingly faster optimal recovery of the hindlimb locomotor behavior [27].

Limitations and stringency of our behavioral assessment

Here, we assessed locomotor parameters on a treadmill but not as such changes in posture, in reflex transmission or in autonomic functions and it could be that some of the neuroanatomical changes seen reflect modifications of these parameters. Furthermore, changes in neuroanatomy and function may not be necessarily synergistic as seen here and in previous studies in which combined treatment of anti-Nogo-A antibody and training showed different beneficial effects but not synergistic [60]. Moreover, all parameters of improvement at a given time point may not reflect all the underlying processes that might be controlled by intrinsic neural mechanisms as well as environmental mechanisms such as provided by locomotor training. Thus, locomotor recovery after SCI can be defined from several points of views and with different degree of precision. Precise kinematic analyses such as employed here may be a double-edge sword. They provide an objective measurement of some specific parameters (step length for instance) but may fail to provide a complete global depiction of locomotion since not all kinematic parameters can be considered all the time at various speeds and epochs after SCI. Furthermore, the continuous scrolling of the belt during treadmill locomotion may provide afferent feedbacks from the hindlimbs, stimulating the locomotor system to generate locomotor movements and probably change the balance between spinal and supraspinal contributions to the control of locomotion decreasing the role of the supraspinal control while increasing that of the spinal circuitry.

Conclusions

Our findings demonstrate the beneficial effects of combined ChABC, growth factors and locomotor training on enhancing structural plasticity of the injured cord and despite an impressive spontaneous locomotor recovery observed in our model; we report modest neurobehavioral improvement in treated animals. However, the lack of significant kinematic evidence of sustained functional improvement beyond the spontaneous recovery, at least using our stringent video-based field-by-field analysis, suggests that additional approaches such as cell therapies and/or more appropriate locomotor training may be needed to optimize this therapeutic strategy.

Author Contributions

Conceived and designed the experiments: OA SKA MGF SR. Performed the experiments: OA SKA MKG HDM. Analyzed the data: OA SKA MKG HDM. Contributed to the writing of the manuscript: OA SKA SR MGF.

References

1. Sekhon LH, Fehlings MG (2001) Epidemiology, demographics, and pathophysiology of acute spinal cord injury. Spine 26: S2–12.
2. Tator CH (1998) Biology of Neurological Recovery and Functional Restoration after Spinal Cord Injury. Neurosurgery 42: 696–708.
3. van Hedel HJ, Dietz V (2010) Rehabilitation of locomotion after spinal cord injury. Restor Neurol Neurosci 28: 123–134.
4. Wilson JR, Grossman RG, Frankowski RF, Kiss A, Davis AM, et al. (2012) A clinical prediction model for long-term functional outcome after traumatic spinal cord injury based on acute clinical and imaging factors. J Neurotrauma 29: 2263–2271.
5. Fawcett JW, Curt A, Steeves JD, Coleman WP, Tuszynski MH, et al. (2007) Guidelines for the conduct of clinical trials for spinal cord injury as developed by the ICCP panel: spontaneous recovery after spinal cord injury and statistical power needed for therapeutic clinical trials. Spinal Cord 45: 190–205.
6. Karimi-Abdolrezaee S, Eftekharpour E, Wang J, Morshead C, Fehlings M (2006) Delayed Transplantation of Adult Neural Stem Cells Promotes Remyelination and functional recovery after Spinal Cord Injury. The Journal of Neuroscience, March 29, 26(13): 3377–3389.
7. Fouad K, Dietz V, Schwab ME (2001) Improving axonal growth and functional recovery after experimental spinal cord injury by neutralizing myelin associated inhibitors. Brain Res Brain Res Rev 36: 204–212.
8. Keirstead HS, Nistor G, Bernal G, Totoiu M, Cloutier F, et al. (2005) Human embryonic stem cell-derived oligodendrocyte progenitor cell transplants remyelinate and restore locomotion after spinal cord injury. J Neurosci 25: 4694–4705.
9. Lu P, Wang Y, Graham L, McHale K, Gao M, et al. (2012) Long-distance growth and connectivity of neural stem cells after severe spinal cord injury. Cell 150: 1264–1273.
10. Lu P, Blesch A, Graham L, Wang Y, Samara R, et al. (2012) Motor axonal regeneration after partial and complete spinal cord transection. J Neurosci 32: 8208–8218.
11. Karimi-Abdolrezaee S, Eftekharpour E, Wang J, Schut D, Fehlings MG (2010) Synergistic effects of transplanted adult neural stem/progenitor cells, chondroitinase, and growth factors promote functional repair and plasticity of the chronically injured spinal cord. J Neurosci 30: 1657–1676.
12. Bradbury EJ, Moon LD, Popat RJ, King VR, Bennett GS, et al. (2002) Chondroitinase ABC promotes functional recovery after spinal cord injury. Nature 416: 636–640.
13. Garcia-Alias G, Petrosyan HA, Schnell L, Horner PJ, Bowers WJ, et al. (2011) Chondroitinase ABC combined with neurotrophin NT-3 secretion and NR2D expression promotes axonal plasticity and functional recovery in rats with lateral hemisection of the spinal cord. J Neurosci 31: 17788–17799.
14. Fouad K, Schnell L, Bunge MB, Schwab ME, Liebscher T, et al. (2005) Combining Schwann cell bridges and olfactory-ensheathing glia grafts with chondroitinase promotes locomotor recovery after complete transection of the spinal cord. J Neurosci 25: 1169–1178.
15. Karimi-Abdolrezaee S, Schut D, Wang J, Fehlings MG (2012) Chondroitinase and growth factors enhance activation and oligodendrocyte differentiation of endogenous neural precursor cells after spinal cord injury. PLoS One 7: e37589.
16. Wang D, Ichiyama RM, Zhao R, Andrews MR, Fawcett JW (2011) Chondroitinase combined with rehabilitation promotes recovery of forelimb function in rats with chronic spinal cord injury. J Neurosci 31: 9332–9344.
17. Massey JM, Hubscher CH, Wagoner MR, Decker JA, Amps J, et al. (2006) Chondroitinase ABC digestion of the perineuronal net promotes functional collateral sprouting in the cuneate nucleus after cervical spinal cord injury. J Neurosci 26: 4406–4414.
18. Tom VJ, Kadakia R, Santi L, Houle JD (2009) Administration of chondroitinase ABC rostral or caudal to a spinal cord injury site promotes anatomical but not functional plasticity. J Neurotrauma 26: 2323–2333.
19. Lee H, McKeon RJ, Bellamkonda RV (2010) Sustained delivery of thermostabilized chABC enhances axonal sprouting and functional recovery after spinal cord injury. Proc Natl Acad Sci U S A 107: 3340–3345.

20. Garcia-Alias G, Barkhuysen S, Buckle M, Fawcett JW (2009) Chondroitinase ABC treatment opens a window of opportunity for task-specific rehabilitation. Nat Neurosci 12: 1145–1151.
21. Kanno H, Pressman Y, Moody A, Berg R, Muir EM, et al. (2014) Combination of engineered Schwann cell grafts to secrete neurotrophin and chondroitinase promotes axonal regeneration and locomotion after spinal cord injury. J Neurosci 34: 1838–1855.
22. Alilain WJ, Horn KP, Hu H, Dick TE, Silver J (2011) Functional regeneration of respiratory pathways after spinal cord injury. Nature 475: 196–200.
23. Carter LM, McMahon SB, Bradbury EJ (2011) Delayed treatment with chondroitinase ABC reverses chronic atrophy of rubrospinal neurons following spinal cord injury. Exp Neurol 228: 149–156.
24. Barritt AW, Davies M, Marchand F, Hartley R, Grist J, et al. (2006) Chondroitinase ABC promotes sprouting of intact and injured spinal systems after spinal cord injury. J Neurosci 26: 10856–10867.
25. Bukhari N, Torres L, Robinson JK, Tsirka SE (2011) Axonal regrowth after spinal cord injury via chondroitinase and the tissue plasminogen activator (tPA)/plasmin system. J Neurosci 31: 14931–14943.
26. Jakeman LB, Hoschouer EL, Basso DM (2011) Injured mice at the gym: review, results and considerations for combining chondroitinase and locomotor exercise to enhance recovery after spinal cord injury. Brain Res Bull 84: 317–326.
27. Alluin O, Karimi-Abdolrezaee S, Delivet-Mongrain H, Leblond H, Fehlings MG, et al. (2011) Kinematic study of locomotor recovery after spinal cord clip compression injury in rats. J Neurotrauma 28: 1963–1981.
28. Fouad K, Metz GA, Merkler D, Dietz V, Schwab ME (2000) Treadmill training in incomplete spinal cord injured rats. Behav Brain Res 115: 107–113.
29. Hutchinson KJ, Gomez-Pinilla F, Crowe MJ, Ying Z, Basso DM (2004) Three exercise paradigms differentially improve sensory recovery after spinal cord contusion in rats. Brain 127: 1403–1414.
30. Gauthier MK, Kosciuczyk K, Tapley L, Karimi-Abdolrezaee S (2013) Dysregulation of the neuregulin-1-ErbB network modulates endogenous oligodendrocyte differentiation and preservation after spinal cord injury. Eur J Neurosci.
31. Karimi-Abdolrezaee S, Eftekharpour E, Fehlings MG (2004) Temporal and spatial patterns of Kv1.1 and Kv1.2 protein and gene expression in spinal cord white matter after acute and chronic spinal cord injury in rats: implications for axonal pathophysiology after neurotrauma. Eur J Neurosci 19: 577–589.
32. Fehlings MG, Tator CH (1995) The relationships among the severity of spinal cord injury, residual neurological function, axon counts, and counts of retrogradely labeled neurons after experimental spinal cord injury. Exp Neurol 132: 220–228.
33. Eftekharpour E, Karimi-Abdolrezaee S, Wang J, Morshead C, Fehlings M (2007) Myelination of Congenitally Dysmyelinated Spinal Cord Axons by Adult Neural Precursor Cells Results in Formation of Nodes of Ranvier and Improved Axonal Conduction. The Journal of Neuroscience 27: 3416–3428.
34. Karimi-Abdolrezaee S, Schreyer DJ (2002) Retrograde repression of growth-associated protein-43 mRNA expression in rat cortical neurons. J Neurosci 22: 1816–1822.
35. Seif GI, Nomura H, Tator CH (2007) Retrograde axonal degeneration "dieback" in the corticospinal tract after transection injury of the rat spinal cord: a confocal microscopy study. J Neurotrauma 24: 1513–1528.
36. Ciranna L (2006) Serotonin as a Modulator of Glutamate- and GABA-Mediated Neurotransmission: Implications in Physiological Functions and in Pathology. Curr Neuropharmacol 4: 101–114.
37. Jordan LM, Liu J, Hedlund PB, Akay T, Pearson KG (2008) Descending command systems for the initiation of locomotion in mammals. Brain Res Rev 57: 183–191.
38. Schmidt BJ, Jordan LM (2000) The role of serotonin in reflex modulation and locomotor rhythm production in the mammalian spinal cord. Brain Res Bull 53: 689–710.
39. Husch A, Van Patten GN, Hong DN, Scaperotti MM, Cramer N, et al. (2012) Spinal cord injury induces serotonin supersensitivity without increasing intrinsic excitability of mouse V2a interneurons. J Neurosci 32: 13145–13154.
40. Gris P, Tighe A, Levin D, Sharma R, Brown A (2007) Transcriptional regulation of scar gene expression in primary astrocytes. Glia 55: 1145–1155.
41. Rolls A, Shechter R, London A, Segev Y, Jacob-Hirsch J, et al. (2008) Two faces of chondroitin sulfate proteoglycan in spinal cord repair: a role in microglia/macrophage activation. PLoS Med 5: e171.
42. Busch SA, Horn KP, Silver DJ, Silver J (2009) Overcoming macrophage-mediated axonal dieback following CNS injury. J Neurosci 29: 9967–9976.
43. Novotna I, Slovinska L, Vanicky I, Cizek M, Radonak J, et al. (2011) IT delivery of ChABC modulates NG2 and promotes GAP-43 axonal regrowth after spinal cord injury. Cell Mol Neurobiol 31: 1129–1139.
44. Starkey ML, Bartus K, Barritt AW, Bradbury EJ (2012) Chondroitinase ABC promotes compensatory sprouting of the intact corticospinal tract and recovery of forelimb function following unilateral pyramidotomy in adult mice. Eur J Neurosci 36: 3665–3678.
45. Fouad K, Pearse DD, Tetzlaff W, Vavrek R (2009) Transplantation and repair: combined cell implantation and chondroitinase delivery prevents deterioration of bladder function in rats with complete spinal cord injury. Spinal Cord 47: 727–732.
46. Mountney A, Zahner MR, Sturgill ER, Riley CJ, Aston JW, et al. (2013) Sialidase, chondroitinase ABC, and combination therapy after spinal cord contusion injury. J Neurotrauma 30: 181–190.
47. Yang YG, Jiang DM, Quan ZX, Ou YS (2009) Insulin with chondroitinase ABC treats the rat model of acute spinal cord injury. J Int Med Res 37: 1097–1107.
48. Caggiano AO, Zimber MP, Ganguly A, Blight AR, Gruskin EA (2005) Chondroitinase ABCI improves locomotion and bladder function following contusion injury of the rat spinal cord. J Neurotrauma 22: 226–239.
49. Heng C, de Leon RD (2009) Treadmill training enhances the recovery of normal stepping patterns in spinal cord contused rats. Exp Neurol 216: 139–147.
50. Ichiyama R, Potuzak M, Balak M, Kalderon N, Edgerton VR (2009) Enhanced motor function by training in spinal cord contused rats following radiation therapy. PLoS One 4: e6862.
51. Kuerzi J, Brown EH, Shum-Siu A, Siu A, Burke D, et al. (2010) Task-specificity vs. ceiling effect: step-training in shallow water after spinal cord injury. Exp Neurol 224: 178–187.
52. Caudle KL, Brown EH, Shum-Siu A, Burke DA, Magnuson TS, et al. (2011) Hindlimb immobilization in a wheelchair alters functional recovery following contusive spinal cord injury in the adult rat. Neurorehabil Neural Repair 25: 729–739.
53. Cha J, Heng C, Reinkensmeyer DJ, Roy RR, Edgerton VR, et al. (2007) Locomotor ability in spinal rats is dependent on the amount of activity imposed on the hindlimbs during treadmill training. J Neurotrauma 24: 1000–1012.
54. Smith RR, Brown EH, Shum-Siu A, Whelan A, Burke DA, et al. (2009) Swim training initiated acutely after spinal cord injury is ineffective and induces extravasation in and around the epicenter. J Neurotrauma 26: 1017–1027.
55. Barriere G, Frigon A, Leblond H, Provencher J, Rossignol S (2010) Dual spinal lesion paradigm in the cat: evolution of the kinematic locomotor pattern. J Neurophysiol 104: 1119–1133.
56. Barriere G, Leblond H, Provencher J, Rossignol S (2008) Prominent role of the spinal central pattern generator in the recovery of locomotion after partial spinal cord injuries. J Neurosci 28: 3976–3987.
57. Martinez M, Delivet-Mongrain H, Leblond H, Rossignol S (2012) Effect of locomotor training in completely spinalized cats previously submitted to a spinal hemisection. J Neurosci 32: 10961–10970.
58. Martinez M, Delivet-Mongrain H, Rossignol S (2013) Treadmill training promotes spinal changes leading to locomotor recovery after partial spinal cord injury in cats. J Neurophysiol 109: 2909–2922.
59. Rossignol SS, B.J.; Jordan,L.M (2014) Spinal plasticity underlying the recovery of locomotion after injury. In: Selzer MEC, S.; Cohen,L.G.; Kwakkel,G.; Miller,R.H., editor. Textbook of Neural Repair and Rehabilitation. Cambridge: Cambridge University Press.
60. Maier IC, Ichiyama RM, Courtine G, Schnell L, Lavrov I, et al. (2009) Differential effects of anti-Nogo-A antibody treatment and treadmill training in rats with incomplete spinal cord injury. Brain 132: 1426–1440.

Permissions

All chapters in this book were first published in PLOS ONE, by The Public Library of Science; hereby published with permission under the Creative Commons Attribution License or equivalent. Every chapter published in this book has been scrutinized by our experts. Their significance has been extensively debated. The topics covered herein carry significant findings which will fuel the growth of the discipline. They may even be implemented as practical applications or may be referred to as a beginning point for another development.

The contributors of this book come from diverse backgrounds, making this book a truly international effort. This book will bring forth new frontiers with its revolutionizing research information and detailed analysis of the nascent developments around the world.

We would like to thank all the contributing authors for lending their expertise to make the book truly unique. They have played a crucial role in the development of this book. Without their invaluable contributions this book wouldn't have been possible. They have made vital efforts to compile up to date information on the varied aspects of this subject to make this book a valuable addition to the collection of many professionals and students.

This book was conceptualized with the vision of imparting up-to-date information and advanced data in this field. To ensure the same, a matchless editorial board was set up. Every individual on the board went through rigorous rounds of assessment to prove their worth. After which they invested a large part of their time researching and compiling the most relevant data for our readers.

The editorial board has been involved in producing this book since its inception. They have spent rigorous hours researching and exploring the diverse topics which have resulted in the successful publishing of this book. They have passed on their knowledge of decades through this book. To expedite this challenging task, the publisher supported the team at every step. A small team of assistant editors was also appointed to further simplify the editing procedure and attain best results for the readers.

Apart from the editorial board, the designing team has also invested a significant amount of their time in understanding the subject and creating the most relevant covers. They scrutinized every image to scout for the most suitable representation of the subject and create an appropriate cover for the book.

The publishing team has been an ardent support to the editorial, designing and production team. Their endless efforts to recruit the best for this project, has resulted in the accomplishment of this book. They are a veteran in the field of academics and their pool of knowledge is as vast as their experience in printing. Their expertise and guidance has proved useful at every step. Their uncompromising quality standards have made this book an exceptional effort. Their encouragement from time to time has been an inspiration for everyone.

The publisher and the editorial board hope that this book will prove to be a valuable piece of knowledge for researchers, students, practitioners and scholars across the globe.

List of Contributors

Karla Menezes, Daiana Vieira Lopes, Aline Silva Cruz, João Ricardo Lacerda de Menezes, Tatiana Coelho-Sampaio and Maria Isabel Doria Rossi
Institute of Biomedical Sciences, Federal University of Rio de Janeiro, Rio de Janeiro, Rio de Janeiro, Brazil

Marcos Assis Nascimento and Juliana Pena Gonçalves
Institute of Biophysics Carlos Chagas Filho, Federal University of Rio de Janeiro, Rio de Janeiro, Rio de Janeiro, Brazil

Bianca Curzio and Martin Bonamino
National Institute of Cancer, Rio de Janeiro, Rio de Janeiro, Brazil

Radovan Borojevic
Excellion, Petrópolis, Rio de Janeiro, Brazil

Anne Jacobi and Anja Schmalz
Institute of Clinical Neuroimmunology, Ludwig-Maximilians University Munich, Munich, Germany

Florence M. Bareyre
Institute of Clinical Neuroimmunology, Ludwig-Maximilians University Munich, Munich, Germany
Munich Cluster for Systems Neurology (SyNergy), Munich, Germany

Yu Mi Park, Su Kyoung Seo and Jong Eun Lee
Department of Anatomy, Yonsei University College of Medicine, Seoul, Republic of Korea
BK 21 Project for Medical Science, Yonsei University College of Medicine, Seoul, Republic of Korea

Won Taek Lee, Kiran Kumar Bokara, Jae Hwan Kim and Kyung Ah Park
Department of Anatomy, Yonsei University College of Medicine, Seoul, Republic of Korea

Seung Hwa Park
Department of Anatomy, Konkuk University College of Medicine, Seoul, Republic of Korea

Midori A. Yenari
Department of Neurology, University of California San Francisco and Veterans Affairs Medical Center, San Francisco, California, United States of America

Yan Sun, Chong-Chong Xu, Lu Gao, Li-Xiang Ma, Rui-Xi Li and Yu-Wen Peng
Department of Anatomy, Histology and Embryology, Shanghai Medical College, Fudan University, Shanghai, China

Jin Li
Institutes of Biomedical Sciences, Fudan University, Shanghai, China

Xi-Yin Guan and Guo-Pei Zhu
Department of Radiation Oncology, Shanghai Cancer Hospital, Fudan University, Shanghai, China

Yingpeng Liu, Kathy Keefe, Xiaoqing Tang, Shen Lin and George M. Smith
Shriners Hospitals Pediatric Research Center, Temple University School of Medicine, Philadelphia, Pennsylvania, United States of America

Norman R. Saunders, Natassya M. Noor, Katarzyna M. Dziegielewska, Benjamin J. Wheaton and Mark D. Habgood
Department of Pharmacology & Therapeutics, The University of Melbourne, Victoria, Australia

Shane A. Liddelow
Department of Pharmacology & Therapeutics, The University of Melbourne, Victoria, Australia
Department of Neurobiology, Stanford University, Stanford, California,
United States of America

David L. Steer and A. Ian Smith
Department of Biochemistry and Molecular Biology, Monash University, Clayton, Victoria, Australia

C. Joakim Ek
Department of Neuroscience and Physiology, University of Gothenburg, Gothenburg, Sweden

Matthew J. Wakefield
Walter & Eliza Hall Institute of Medical Research, Victoria, Australia
Department of Genetics, The University of Melbourne, Victoria, Australia

Helen Lindsay
Walter & Eliza Hall Institute of Medical Research, Victoria, Australia
Institute of Molecular Life Sciences, University of Zurich, Zurich, Switzerland

Jessie Truettner and W. Dalton Dietrich
The Miami Project to Cure Paralysis, University of Miami, Miller School of Medicine, Miami, Florida, United States of America

Robert D. Miller
Center for Evolutionary & Theoretical Immunology, Department of Biology, University of New Mexico, Albuquerque, New Mexico, United States of America

D. Ryan Ormond, Craig Shannon, Julius Oppenheim, Kaushik Das, Raj Murali and Meena Jhanwar-Uniyal
Department of Neurosurgery, New York Medical College, Valhalla, New York, United States of America

Richard Zeman
Department of Cell Biology and Anatomy, New York Medical College, Valhalla, New York, United States of America

Steve Lacroix, Isabelle Pineau, Sébastien A. Lévesque and Catherine-Alexandra
Centre de recherche du Centre hospitalier universitaire (CHU) de Québec - CHUL et Département de médicine molé culaire, Faculté de médecine, Université Laval, Québec, Canada

Laura K. Hamilton, Alexandre Vaugeois, Stéfanny Beaudoin, Christian Breault-Dugas, Grégoire and Karl J. L. Fernandes
Department of Neurosciences, Faculty of Medicine, Centre de recherche du Centre hospitalier de ĺUniversité de Montréal (CRCHUM), and Groupe de recherche sur le système nerveux central (GRSNC), Université de Montréal, Quebec, Canada

Liping Ma and Harsh P. Khatri
W. M. Keck Center for Collaborative Neuroscience and Department of Cell Biology and Neuroscience, Rutgers University, Piscataway, New Jersey, United States of America

Yan-Qin Shen
Center for Neuroscience, Shantou University Medical College, Shantou, Guangdong Province, People's Republic of China
Department of Basic Medicine, Jiangnan University Medical School, Wuxi, Jiangsu Province, People's Republic of China

Melitta Schachner
W. M. Keck Center for Collaborative Neuroscience and Department of Cell Biology and Neuroscience, Rutgers University, Piscataway, New Jersey, United States of America
Center for Neuroscience, Shantou University Medical College, Shantou, Guangdong Province, People's Republic of China

Alessandro Graziano
Department of Physiology and Pharmacology, Drexel University College of Medicine, Philadelphia, Pennsylvania, United States of America

Guglielmo Foffani
School of Biomedical Engineering, Science and Health Systems, Drexel University, Philadelphia, Pennsylvania, United States of America
Hospital Nacional de Parapléjicos, Servicio de Salud de Castilla-La Mancha, Toledo, Spain

Eric B. Knudsen
School of Biomedical Engineering, Science and Health Systems, Drexel University, Philadelphia, Pennsylvania, United States of America

Jed Shumsky
Department of Neurobiology and Anatomy, Drexel University College of Medicine, Philadelphia, Pennsylvania, United States of America

Karen A. Moxon
School of Biomedical Engineering, Science and Health Systems, Drexel University, Philadelphia, Pennsylvania, United States of America
Department of Neurobiology and Anatomy, Drexel University College of Medicine, Philadelphia, Pennsylvania, United States of America

Anna Victoria Leonard and Emma Thornton
School of Medical Sciences, University of Adelaide, Adelaide, South Australia, Australia

Robert Vink
Division of Health Sciences, University of South Australia, Adelaide, South

Australia, Australia

Steffen Franz, Mareva Ciatipis, Beatrice Sandner, Armin Blesch and Norbert Weidner
Spinal Cord Injury Center, Heidelberg University Hospital, Heidelberg, Germany

Kathrin Pfeifer, Birthe Kierdorf and Ulrich Bogdahn
Department of Neurology, University of Regensburg, Regensburg, Germany

Beate Winner
3ZKF Junior Group III and BMBF Research Group Neuroscience, Interdisciplinary Center for Clinical Research, Nikolaus-Fiebiger Center for Molecular Medicine, Friedrich-Alexander University-Erlangen-Nürnberg, Erlangen, Germany

Myungsik Yoo, Muntasir Khaled, Kurt M. Gibbs and Jonghun Kim
W. M. Keck Center for Collaborative Neuroscience and Department of Cell Biology and Neuroscience, Rutgers University, Piscataway, New Jersey, United States of America

Björn Kowalewski and Thomas Dierks
Department of Chemistry, Biochemistry I, Bielefeld University, Universitätsstr Bielefeld, Germany

Melitta Schachner
W. M. Keck Center for Collaborative Neuroscience and Department of Cell Biology and Neuroscience, Rutgers University, Piscataway, New Jersey, United States of America
Center for Neuroscience, Shantou University Medical College, Shantou, Guandong Province, People's Republic of China

Sam Joshva Baskar Jesudasan, Kathryn G. Todd and Ian R. Winship
Centre for Neuroscience, University of Alberta, Edmonton, Alberta, Canada
Neurochemical Research Unit, Department of Psychiatry, University of Alberta, Edmonton, Alberta, Canada

Hae Young Shin, Min Jung Kwon and Dong Hoon Hwang
Department of Brain Science, Ajou University School of Medicine, Suwon, Republic of Korea
Neuroscience Graduate Program, Department of Biomedical Sciences, Ajou University School of Medicine, Suwon, Republic of Korea

Hyosil Kim and KiYoung Lee
Neuroscience Graduate Program, Department of Biomedical Sciences, Ajou University School of Medicine, Suwon, Republic of Korea
Department of Biomedical Informatics, Ajou University School of Medicine, Suwon, Republic of Korea

Byung Gon Kim
Department of Brain Science, Ajou University School of Medicine, Suwon, Republic of Korea
Neuroscience Graduate Program, Department of Biomedical Sciences, Ajou University School of Medicine, Suwon, Republic of Korea
Department of Neurology, Ajou University School of Medicine, Suwon, Republic of Korea

Yoshiomi Kobayashi, Go Itakura, Hiroki Iwai, Soraya Nishimura and Tsunehiko Konomi
Department of Orthopedic Surgery, School of Medicine, Keio University, Tokyo, Japan
Department of Physiology, School of Medicine, Keio University, Tokyo, Japan

Yohei Okada, Akimasa Yasuda, Satoshi Nori, Yoshiaki Toyama and Masaya Nakamura
Department of Orthopedic Surgery, School of Medicine, Keio University, Tokyo, Japan

Keigo Hikishima
Department of Physiology, School of Medicine, Keio University, Tokyo, Japan
Central Institute for Experimental Animals, Kanagawa, Japan

Kanehiro Fujiyoshi
Department of Orthopedic Surgery, National Hospital Organization Murayama Medical Center, Tokyo, Japan

Osahiko Tsuji
Department of Orthopedic Surgery, Saitama Social Insurance Hospital, Saitama, Japan

Shinya Yamanaka
Center for iPS Cell Research and Application (CiRA), Kyoto, Japan

Hideyuki Okano
Department of Physiology, School of Medicine, Keio University, Tokyo, Japan

Olivier Alluin, Hugo Delivet-Mongrain and Serge Rossignol
Multidisciplinary Team in Locomotor Rehabilitation of the Canadian Institutes of Health Research (CIHR) and Groupe de Recherche sur le Système Nerveux Central (GRSNC) of the Fonds de Recherche du Québec - Santé (FRQS), Department of Physiology, University of Montreal, Montreal, Quebec, Canada

Marie-Krystel Gauthier
The Department of Physiology and Pathophysiology and the Spinal Cord Research Center, University of Manitoba, Winnipeg, Manitoba, Canada

Michael G. Fehlings
Department of Surgery and Spinal Program, University of Toronto; Toronto Western Research Institute, University Health Network, Toronto, Ontario, Canada

Soheila Karimi-Abdolrezaee
The Department of Physiology and Pathophysiology and the Spinal Cord Research Center, University of Manitoba, Winnipeg, Manitoba, Canada
Regenerative Medicine Program and Manitoba Institute of Child Health, Winnipeg, Manitoba, Canada

Index